Advances in Ocular Imaging

Advances in Ocular Imaging

Editor: Bryce Strong

AMERICAN
MEDICAL PUBLISHERS
www.americanmedicalpublishers.com

AMERICAN
MEDICAL PUBLISHERS
www.americanmedicalpublishers.com

Cataloging-in-Publication Data

Advances in ocular imaging / edited by Bryce Strong.
p. cm.
Includes bibliographical references and index.
ISBN 978-1-63927-859-6
1. Eye--Imaging. 2. Eye--Diseases--Diagnosis. 3. Eye--Anatomy.
4. Optical data processing. 5. Ophthalmoscopy. 6. Ophthalmology.
I. Strong, Bryce.
RE79.I42 A38 2023
616.075 45--dc23

American Medical Publishers,
41 Flatbush Avenue,
1st Floor, New York,
NY 11217, USA

ISBN 978-1-63927-859-6 (Hardback)

Contents

Preface

This book aims to highlight the current researches and provides a platform to further the scope of innovations in this area. This book is a product of the combined efforts of many researchers and scientists, after going through thorough studies and analysis from different parts of the world. The objective of this book is to provide the readers with the latest information of the field.

Ocular imaging is a technology that allows quantitative examination of the posterior segment of the eye. This is a diagnostic tool that helps detect changes in the optic nerve head (ONH), the nerve fiber layer (NFL), and the macula. Such changes may be associated with glaucoma. Ocular imaging devices play a pivotal role in clinical glaucoma assessment due to their ability to obtain micron scale measurements. There are three major devices for ocular diagnostic imaging, namely, scanning laser polarimetry (SLP), confocal scanning laser ophthalmoscopy (CSLO), and optical coherence tomography (OCT). The real-time, non-invasive, and high-resolution images of the eye are provided by all three devices. The first technology, SLP, is used to determine the thickness of the nerve by assessing the birefringence of polarized light as it is reflected from the eye. The second technology, CSLO, is a confocal microscopy technique that has high transverse resolution. This book is compiled in such a manner, that it will provide in-depth knowledge about the theory and practice of ocular imaging. It is appropriate for students seeking detailed information in this area as well as for experts.

I would like to express my sincere thanks to the authors for their dedicated efforts in the completion of this book. I acknowledge the efforts of the publisher for providing constant support. Lastly, I would like to thank my family for their support in all academic endeavors.

Editor

1

Predictive Equation for Angle Opening Distance at 750 μm After Laser Peripheral Iridotomy in Primary Angle Closure Suspects

*Xinbo Gao†, Yuying Zhou†, Chengguo Zuo, Liming Chen, Jiawei Ren, Huishan Lin, Yunru Liao, Haijun Gong, Huanling Hu and Mingkai Lin**

State Key Laboratory of Ophthalmology, Zhongshan Ophthalmic Center, Sun Yat-sen University, Guangzhou, China

***Correspondence:**
Mingkai Lin
linmk@mail.sysu.edu.cn

†These authors have contributed equally to this work and share first authorship

Aim: The aim of this study was to investigate the changes in anterior segment parameters as assessed by ultrasound biomicroscopy (UBM) after laser peripheral iridotomy (LPI) and to propose a prediction equation for the width of the angle after LPI.

Design: This was a prospective study.

Participants: The participants included 100 subjects with primary angle closure suspect (PACS).

Methods: Anterior segment UBM parameters were measured, whereas AOD750 was chosen to indicate the width of the angle associated with gonioscopic angle closure, as found in a prior study.

Main Outcome Measures: Angle parameters, iris parameters, anterior chamber parameters and ciliary body parameters.

Results: All angle parameters increased after LPI, including the mean angle opening distance at 750 μm (AOD750), mean angle opening distance at 500 μm from the scleral spur (AOD500), mean angle opening distance at 750 μm from the scleral spur (AOD750), and mean angle recess area at 750 μm from the scleral spur (ARA750). Among iris parameters and ciliary body parameters, the iris thickness at 2,000 μm (IT2000), iris curvature (IC), and trabecular-ciliary process distance (ICPD) were reduced after LPI. The final equation consisted of four parameters: anterior chamber depth (ACD), iris thickness at 750 μm from the scleral spur (IT750), AOD750, and lens vault (LV). This equation explained 42.7% of the variability in the angle opening indicator AOD750 after LPI, whereas in the plateau iris configuration subgroup, the accuracy of the prediction equation reached the highest a maximum of 68.6%.

Conclusions: There was an increase in angle opening and iris flattening after LPI. An equation involving four angle parameters was constructed, this equation which could explained 42.7% of the variability in the angle opening indicator AOD750 after LPI whereas in the plateau iris configuration subgroup, the accuracy of the prediction equation reached a maximum of 68.6%.

Keywords: LPI, UBM and glaucoma, angle opening distance, primary angle closure suspects, predictive equation

INTRODUCTION

The incidence of angle-closure glaucoma is between 1.1% and 1.6% in China. By 2050, the total incidence of glaucoma in China may reach 3.48% (1). The prevalence of primary angle-closure suspect (PACS) is significantly higher than that of primary angle-closure (PAC) or primary angle-closure glaucoma (PACG) (2). Laser peripheral iridotomy (LPI) is an option for the treatment of PACS because it can establish a channel, relieve the pupil block component, and flatten the iris plane, thus increasing the width of the anterior chamber angle (3, 4). However, the effect of LPI on the induction of angle opening is not consistent, and the actual role of LPI is still controversial. Twenty percent of PACS patients still had iridotrabecular contact after LPI treatment (3). A previous study found that for every 0.1 mm decrease in the angle opening distance at 750 μm from the scleral spur (AOD750), the odds of developing gonioscopic angle closure increased by a factor of 3.27 (5). To predict the post-procedural effect of LPI, it is necessary to establish a prediction equation for the degree of angle opening after LPI based on the morphological structure of the eye.

As an objective and relatively reliable imaging method, ultrasound bomicroscopy (UBM) can reproducibly measure the parameters of the anterior chamber. Recent studies have explored the correlation between LPI-induced angle widening and baseline parameters (including angle parameters, anterior chamber parameters, iris parameters, and others) (6). The predictors of angle opening after LPI were identified as baseline central anterior chamber depth (cACD), AOD750, iris curvature (IC) and lens vault (LV) (7–9), and their proposed prediction accuracy for post-procedural angle opening distance based on pre-procedural baseline parameters ranged from 10 to 40%. However, the equation to predict the angle opening distance after LPI did not have high predictive value. In this study, we used UBM to establish the relationship between the angle opening distance after LPI and baseline parameters, and we proposed a predictive equation for the angle opening distance after LPI to predict the post-procedural effect of this technique.

MATERIALS AND METHODS

Design and Participants

All tests and treatments were carried out at the Zhongshan Ophthalmic Clinical Research Center, a tertiary hospital in Guangzhou, China. The experiment was approved by the Ethical Committee of Zhongshan Ophthalmic Center. The experiment was carried out according to the principles of the Declaration of Helsinki. From September 2019 to September 2020, patients diagnosed with PACS who underwent LPI were enrolled. All the participants provided written informed consent. The inclusion criteria were as follows: (1) PACS was diagnosed according to International Society for Geographical and Epidemiological Ophthalmology (ISGEO) definition, in which patients with narrow angles that $\geq$6h clock hours circumstances pigmented trabecular meshwork was not visible under non-indentation gonioscopy); (2) no peripheral anterior iris synechiae were found on gonioscopic examination; (3) intraocular pressure (IOP) $\leq$ 21 mmHg; and (4) no abnormalities were found on fundus examination. The exclusion criteria included serious general health problems, previous intraocular surgery, previous iridoplasty, and inability to undergo LPI due to the opacity of the media.

Pre-procedural and Post-procedural Evaluation

All patients underwent routine ophthalmic examinations, including the Humphrey visual field examination, IOP examination, slit-lamp examination, gonioscopy, and UBM examination. An experienced ophthalmologist performed gonioscopy in a dark room with a slit lamp. The Scheie method was used to classify the angle.

Two senior glaucoma experts, associate chief physician Zuo Chengguo and attending physician Gao Xinbo, divided PACS patients into pupillary block type, a plateau iris configuration, and a mixed mechanism type according to their UBM images before LPI. If the two glaucoma doctors disagreed on a patient's classification, a third senior glaucoma expert, chief physician Lin Mingkai, made the final judgement. We distinguished the mechanism of angle closure according to the following definitions (10):

1. Pupillary block angle type: iris bombe alone is present in at least two quadrants.
2. Plateau iris configuration: the iris profile is flat, and the iris root is shifted forward as a result of anterior positioning of the ciliary processes, making the iridocorneal angle narrow and the anterior chamber deep.
3. Mixed mechanism angle type: a combination of the pupillary block angle type and the plateau iris configuration.

One of the glaucoma specialists treated this cohort using a VISULAS® 532s diode laser (Carl Zeiss Meditec, Inc.) Two percent pilocarpine eye drops were used for pretreatment. LPI was performed at the thinnest part of the iris (at the 10–12 o'clock and 12–2 o'clock positions). The signs of full-thickness perforation were the forward movement of aqueous matter from the posterior chamber to the anterior chamber and the dispersion of pigment. The diameter of the perforation was approximately 200 μm. Immediately after surgery, all eyes were immediately treated with prednisolone and at least one drug to lower intraocular pressure. All patients were given 1% prednisolone six times on the day of LPI and six times a day for the next week. Two to three weeks after LPI, we obtained and evaluated UBM images. **Figure 1** illustrated the three types of angle-closure mechanisms before and after LPI.

Ultrasound Biomicroscopy Examination

A technician performed ultrasound biomicroscopy (SW-3200L, Suoer, Tianjin) before and after LPI. When the subjects gazed at the calibration object with the opposite eye, we obtained four-quadrant angle structure images and one central anterior chamber image. From 12 o'clock, the eyeballs of all patients were examined clockwise (the visual angle was kept at approximately 20 degrees, and the control was adjusted). After topical anesthesia, the probe was placed perpendicular to the ocular

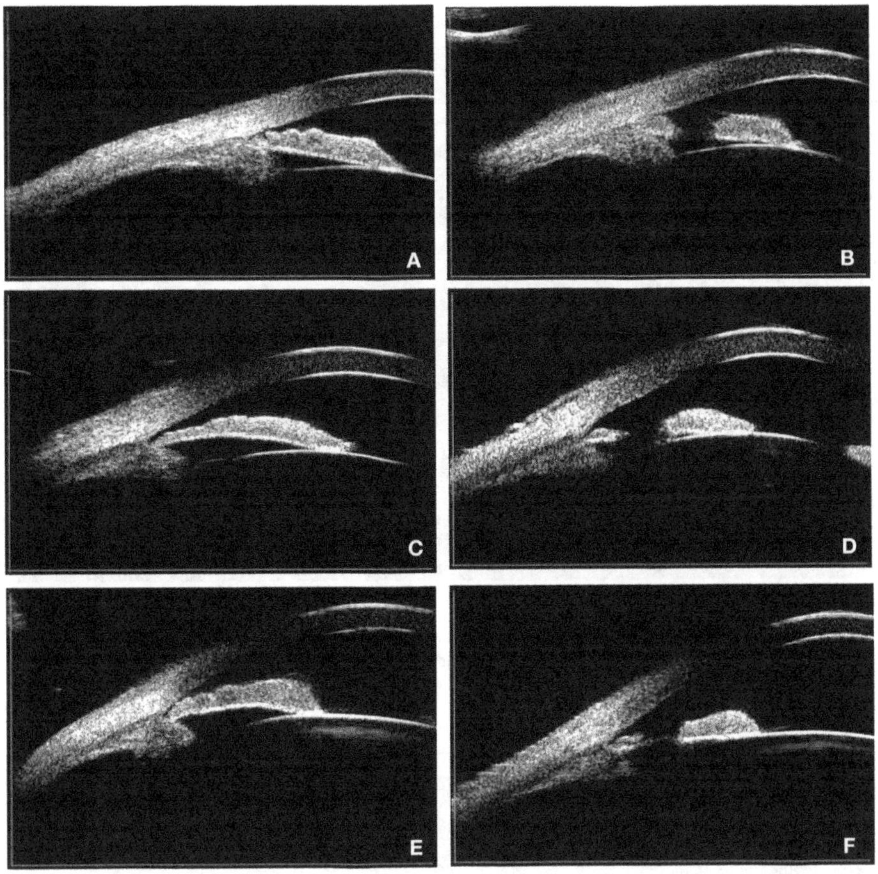

FIGURE 1 | Illustrated the three types of angle-closure mechanisms before and after LPI. **(A)** Typical plateau iris configuration before LPI, the peripheral iris is thick. **(B)** Typical plateau iris configuration after LPI, the peripheral iris is still thick. **(C)** Typical pupillary block type picture before LPI, iris bombe can be observed. **(D)** Typical pupillary block type picture after LPI, the iris is flattened. **(E)** Typical mixed mechanism type before LPI. **(F)** Typical mixed mechanism type after LPI, the iris is flattened slightly.

surface, and normal saline was used as the coupling agent. The gain was set between 60 and 80 dB to maximize the field of view of the imaging structure and minimize "noise". We attempted to ensure that the scleral spur, the angle, the ciliary body, and half the iris chord length were clearly visible.

Qualitative and Quantitative Analysis of Ultrasound Biomicroscopy

All UBM parameters namely, anterior chamber depth (ACD), anterior chamber width (ACW), LV, IC, trabecular-ciliary process distance at 750 μm (TCPD750), iris-ciliary process distance at 750 μm (ICPD750), ciliary body thickness (CBT0), angle recess area (ARA), iris thickness at 750 μm (IT750), and iris thickness (IT2000), were obtained using the UBM technique (SW-3200L, Suoer, Tianjin).

Figures 2, 3 illustrated their calculation method, the ACD was defined as the axial distance between the corneal endothelium and the anterior lens surface. The ACW was defined as the distance between the two scleral spurs (SS). The LV was defined as the perpendicular distance from the anterior pole of the lens to the horizontal line between the scleral spurs. The IC was defined as the vertical distance between the highest point of the back bulge of the iris and the line between the iris root and the edge of the pupil. TCPD750 was defined as a line extending from the corneal endothelium 750 μm anterior to the SS toward the ciliary processes. ICPD750 was defined as the posterior surface of the iris 750 μm anterior to the SS toward the ciliary processes. CBT0 was defined as ciliary body thickness at the point of the SS. Anterior opening distances of 250, 500, and 750 μm were measured on a line perpendicular to the plane of the trabecular surface 250, 500, and 750 μm, anterior to the scleral spur and extended to meet the surface of the iris. The ARA was the area bounded by the anterior surface of the iris surface, corneal endothelium, and the line perpendicular to the trabecular surface plane to the iris surface, starting from 750 μm before the scleral puncture. IT750 and IT2000 are defined as iris thickness at 750 and 2,000 μm, respectively, from the SS.

Statistical Analysis

SPSS software (IBM SPSS Statistics 23.0) was used for statistical analysis. Data with a normal distribution are reported as the means ± SDs. The paired t-test was used to compare

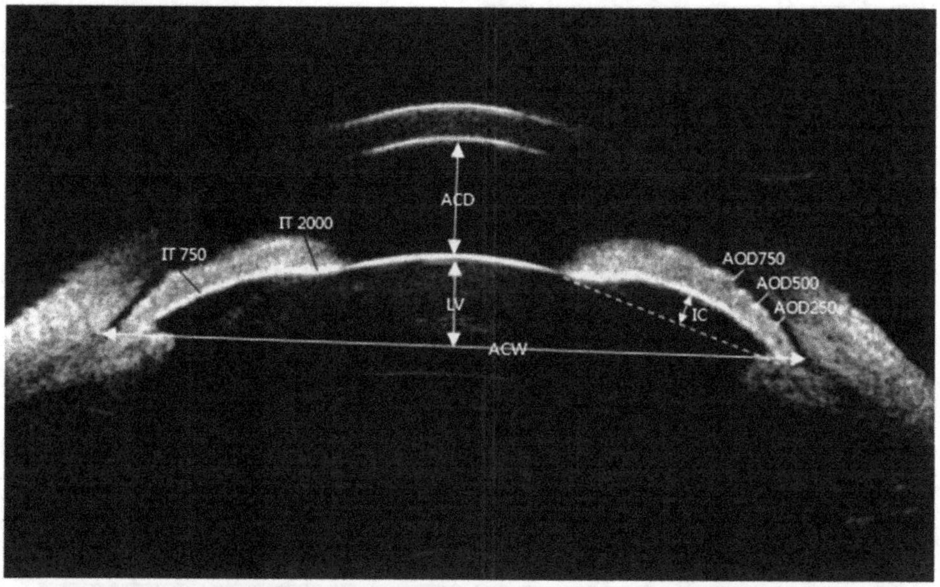

FIGURE 2 | Ultrasound biomicroscopic (UBM) images of ACD, LV, ACW, AOD250, AOD500, AOD750, IT750, IT2000, and IC. ACD, anterior chamber depth; LV, lens vault; ACW, anterior chamber width; AOD250, angle opening distance at 250 μm from the scleral spur; AOD500, angle opening distance at 500 μm from the scleral spur; AOD750, angle opening distance at 750 μm from the scleral spur.

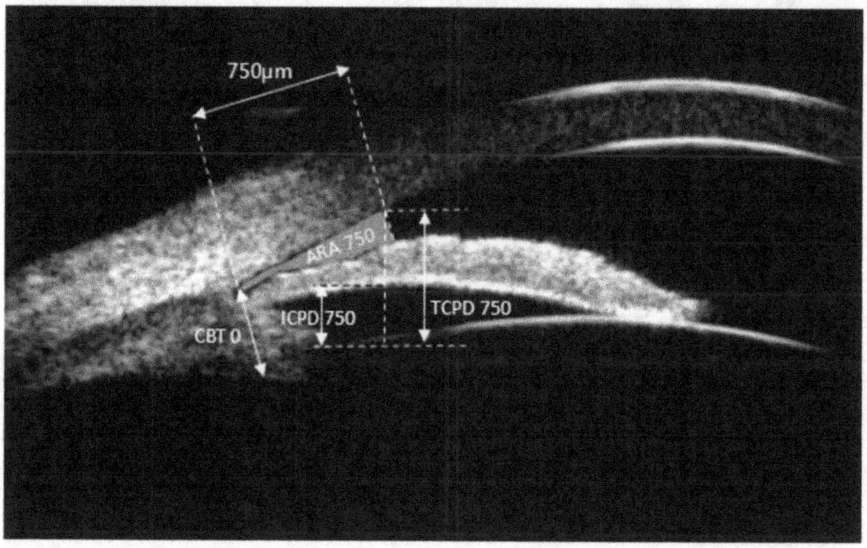

FIGURE 3 | Ultrasound biomicroscopic (UBM) images ARA750, ICPD750,TCPD750, CBT0. ARA750, angle recess area at 750 μm from the scleral spur; ICPD750, iris-ciliary process distance at 750 μm; TCPD750, trabecular-ciliary process distance at 750 μm; CBT0, ciliary body thickness at the point of the scleral spur.

the differences in UBM parameters before and after LPI. The AOD750 after LPI and baseline parameters AOD750, angle opening distance at 500 μm from the scleral spur (AOD500), AOD750, angle recess area at 750 μm from the scleral spur (ARA750), ACD, LV, IT750, IT2000, IC, CBT0, TCPD750, and ICPD750 were analyzed by univariable and multiple linear regression analysis. $P < 0.05$ was considered statistically significant.

RESULTS

Demographics and Baseline Clinical Characteristics of the Study Population

A total of 100 subjects were analyzed, including 38 with the pupillary block type (38.0%), 12 with the plateau iris configuration (12.0%), and 50 with the mixed mechanism type (50.0%) (**Table 1**). The mean age across all participants was 58.14

TABLE 1 | Demographics and Baseline demographic and clinical examination.

Varaible	Pupillary block (*N* = 38)	Plateau iris (*N* = 12)	Mixed mechanism (*N* = 50)	*P*-value
Age, yr, mean (SD)	59.82 (7.79)	57.42 (7.56)	57.04 (8.58)	>0.05
Female gender,%	81.6%	50.0%	74.0%	<0.001

TABLE 2 | Univariable and multivariable linear regression analysis for baseline predictors of AOD750 after laser peripheral iridotomy.

	Univariate			Multivariate		
Baseline parameters	**B(SE)**	**β**	***P*-value***	**B(SE)**	**β**	***P*-value***
Age	−1.639 (1.955)	−0.086	0.404			
Gender	22.000 (36.429)	0.062	0.547			
AOD250	0.272 (0.176)	0.158	0.126			
AOD500	0.709 (0.161)	0.415	<0.001			
AOD750	0.570 (0.112)	0.467	<0.001	0.381 (0.110)	0.312	0.001
IT750	'−0.698 (0.221)	−0.312	0.002	'−0.865 (0.183)	−0.386	<0.001
IT2000	'−0.168 (0.183)	−0.095	0.362			
TCPD750	0.285 (0.094)	0.300	0.003			
ICPD750	0.145 (0.075)	0.197	0.055			
ARA750	0.001 (0.000)	0.306	0.003			
IC	'−110.303 (182.231)	−0.063	0.546			
ACD	213.936 (57.993)	0.357	<0.001	180.882 (54.004)	0.302	0.001
ACW	2.551 (22.410)	0.012	0.910			
LV	108.065 (41.185)	0.263	0.010	83.119 (33.662)	0.202	0.015
CBTO	92.747 (94.634)	0.100	0.330			

**P* <0.05 indicate statistical significance.*
AOD250, angle opening distance at 250 μm from the scleral spur; AOD500, angle opening distance at 500 μm from the scleral spur; AOD750, angle opening distance at 750 μm from the scleral spur; IT750, iris thickness at 750 μm from the scleral spur; IT2000, iris thickness at 2000 μm from the scleral spur; TCPD750, trabecular-ciliary process distance at 750 μm from the scleral spur; ICPD750, iris-ciliary process distance at 750 μm from the scleral spur; ARA750, angle recess area at 750 μm from the scleral spur; IC, iris curvature; ACD, anterior chamber depth; ACW, anterior chamber width; LV, lens vault; CBTO, ciliary body thickness at the point of the scleral spur.

years (range, 33–74 years; standard deviation, 8.20 years), and the majority were females (74.0%).

Univariable and Multivariable Linear Regression Analysis for Baseline Predictors of AOD750 After Laser Peripheral Iridotomy

Linear regression analyses were performed to determine the baseline parameters that predict post-procedure angle widening, defined as AOD750 after LPI (**Table 2**). Greater baseline AOD500, AOD750, TCPD750, ARA750, ACD, and LV predicted higher odds of angle widening after LPI ($P < 0.05$ for all). Multiple linear regression ($R^2 = 0.427$, $P < 0.001$) showed that greater baseline IT750 ($P < 0.001$) was associated with a lower likelihood of angle widening, whereas greater baseline AOD750 ($P = 0.001$), ACD ($P = 0.001$) and LV ($P = 0.015$) predicted a higher likelihood of angle widening after LPI (P < 0.001).

The predictive equation was thus generated as follows:

$$\begin{aligned} \text{After} - \text{LPIAOD750} = {} & 177.340 + 180.882 * \text{ACD} - 0.865 \\ & * \text{IT750} + 0.381 * \text{AOD750} \\ & + 83.119 * \text{LV} \end{aligned}$$

Stepwise Multiple Linear Regression Analysis of AOD750 in the Different Angle Closure Groups

Table 3 presents the results of the stepwise multiple linear regression analyses for factors associated with AOD750 after LPI. The equation consisted of four parameters (ACD, IT750, AOD750, and LV) and explained 42.7% of the variability in AOD750. In the mixed mechanism group, AOD750 was the only significant variable ($P < 0.05$), explaining 11.4% of the variability in AOD750. In the Pupillary block, the equation consisted of two parameters (AOD750 and ICPD750) explaining 54.2% of the variability in AOD750. In the plateau iris configuration group, the equation consisted of two parameters (IT750 and AOD250), explaining 68.6% of the variability in AOD750.

Changes in Mean Anterior Segment Parameters Before and After Laser Peripheral Iridotomy

All angle parameters increased after LPI, including mean angle opening distance at 250 μm from the scleral spur (AOD250) (160.84 μm pre-procedurally vs 232.68 μm post-procedurally; $P < 0.001$) mean AOD500 (205.68 μm pre-procedurally vs. 311.94 μm post-procedurally; $P < 0.001$); mean AOD750 (297.98

TABLE 3 | Stepwise multiple linear regression analysis of AOD750 in the different angle-closure groups.

Variables in group	Variable	Regression coefficient(β)	Equation R squared
Total	IT750	−0.386	0.427
	AOD750	0.312	0.427
	LV	0.202	0.427
	ACD	0.302	0.427
Pupillary block	AOD750	0.771	0.542
	ICPD750	0.347	0.542
Mixed mechanism	AOD750	0.477	0.114
plateau iris configuration	IT750	−0.639	0.686
	AOD250	0.590	0.686

IT750, iris thickness at 750 μm from the scleral spur; AOD750, angle opening distance at 750 μm from the scleral spur; LV, lens vault; ACD, anterior chamber depth; ICPD750, iris-ciliary process distance 750; AOD250, angle opening distance at 250 μm from the scleral spur.

TABLE 4 | Changes in mean anterior segment parameters before and after laser peripheral iridotomy.

Parameter	Pre-LPI mean (SD)	Post-LPI mean (SD)	*P*-value*
Angle parameters			
AOD250 (μm)	160.84 (91.29)	232.68 (108.71)	<0.001
AOD500 (μm)	205.68 (91.81)	311.94 (120.73)	<0.001
AOD750 (μm)	297.98 (128.60)	460.33 (156.94)	<0.001
ARA750 (μm²)	125094.63 (54632.66)	176316.46 (62266.55)	<0.001
Anterior chamber parameters			
ACD (mm)	2.07 (0.26)	2.09 (0.26)	0.062
LV (mm)	0.44 (0.38)	0.47 (0.42)	0.079
ACW (mm)	11.24 (0.73)	11.46 (0.77)	0.004
Iris parameters			
IT750 (μm)	280.59 (70.05)	289.59 (70.30)	0.212
IT2000 (μm)	326.45 (88.45)	360.85 (99.10)	0.002
IC (mm)	0.28 (0.09)	0.01 (0.04)	<0.001
Ciliary body parameters			
CBT0 (mm)	0.99 (0.17)	1.00 (0.16)	0.830
TCPD750 (μm)	1031.57 (165.38)	1033.14 (153.22)	0.920
ICPD750 (μm)	586.32 (212.96)	459.61 (202.77)	<0.001

**P <0.05 represented statistical significance.*
AOD250, angle opening distance at 250 μm from the scleral spur; AOD500, angle opening distance at 500 μm from the scleral spur; AOD750, angle opening distance at 750 μm from the scleral spur; ARA750, angle recess area at 750 μm from the scleral spur; ACD, anterior chamber depth; LV, lens vault; ACW, anterior chamber width; IT750, iris thickness at 750 μm from the scleral spur; IT2000, iris thickness at 2,000 μm from the scleral spur; IC, iris curvature; CBT0, ciliary body thickness at point of the scleral spur; TCPD750, trabecular-ciliary process distance at 750 μm from the scleral spur; ICPD750, iris-ciliary process distance at 750 μm from the scleral spur.

μm pre-procedurally vs. 460.33 μm post-procedurally; $P < 0.001$); and mean ARA750 (125094.63 μm² pre-procedurally vs. 176316.46 μm² post-procedurally; $P < 0.001$). For all angle parameters, the ACW increased after LPI (11.24 mm pre-procedurally vs. 11.46 m post-procedurally; $P < 0.001$). Among iris parameters and ciliary body parameters, IT at 2,000 μm (326.45 μm pre-procedurally vs. 360.85 μm post-procedurally; P = 0.01), IC (0.28 mm pre-procedurally vs. 0.01 mm post-procedurally; $P < 0.001$), and ICPD (586.32 μm pre-procedurally vs. 459.61 μm post-procedurally; $P < 0.001$) were lower after LPI (**Table 4**).

DISCUSSION

In a recent study, He (11) noted that patients identified through community-based screening faced no immediate threat to their vision, and so widespread prophylactic laser peripheral iridotomy was not recommended. However, we speculated that patients identified through hospital-based screening might have different results. AOD750 was found to be associated with gonioscopic angle closure; therefore, we proposed a formula to predict the variability in AOD750 after LPI.

In previous studies, only one or two baseline predictive parameters were found for AOD or the percentage change in mean AOD after laser peripheral iridotomy. For example, the equation of How (7) explained 13% of the variability of the percentage change in mean AOD750; the equation of Zebardast (9) explained 34% of the variability of the change in AOD750 before and after the operation; and Atalay (12) found that in APAC patients, baseline iris thickness explained one-third of the variability of the change in AOD750. They found that post-procedural AOD750 was related to baseline parameters such as LV, IT750, IOP, PD, male sex, axial length, angle width, ACD and IC. These equations all explained less of the change in AOD750 than the one generated in this study, which fit the data well and explained 42.7% of the variability of AOD750 after LPI.

In contrast to previous studies based on anterior-segment - OCT, our study included ciliary body parameters such as TCPD and ICPD by using UBM. Linear regression analyses determined that greater baseline TCPD750 predicted higher odds of AOD750 after LPI ($P < 0.05$). Our study included four baseline parameters in the final equation, which enabled superior accuracy.

In the multivariable analysis equation, the larger the baseline ACD, LV, and AOD750 before the operation, the wider the angle was after LPI, which may be due to the larger anterior chamber depth and the narrower distance between the trabecular meshwork and the ciliary body at baseline, which allows the angle to become flatter after LPI, thus leading to greater angle opening.

In addition, among the subgroups with different angle-closure mechanisms, we found that the prediction equation for the plateau iris configuration subgroup was the most accurate, followed by the pupillary block subgroup and the mixed mechanism subgroup. LPI may have a limited ability to induce angle opening in patients with a plateau iris configuration. The AOD750 after LPI depended only on the size of AOD250 and IT750 at baseline. Recent studies have suggested that LPI alone has a limited therapeutic effect on patients with plateau iris configuration and may need to be combined with laser peripheral iridoplasty (LPIP), which is consistent with our findings (10, 13).

In this study, 100 patients with PACS were observed. It was found that the anterior chamber angle was widened, the ACD was deepened, the IC was decreased and the distance between the iris and the ciliary body was significantly shortened after LPI in a Guangzhou population with PACS, which is consistent with previous research results (14–17). The angle opening distance was related to the baseline ACD, IT750, AOD750, and LV before LPI. In the pupillary block subgroup, there was a significant correlation between the angle opening distance after LPI and the baseline IC, which is consistent with previous studies. Previous studies have suggested that greater baseline IC is associated with a higher likelihood of angle widening (8, 16).

The limitations of this study are as follows. Although AOD750 was used as the standard in this study, the magnitude of AOD750 does not directly define the quality of LPI. Second, two different senior doctors performed the gonioscopy, and, as in other studies, there must inevitably exist some inter-observer variability due to the subjective nature of gonioscopy. Third, our equation was based on univariable and multivariable linear regression equations. However, some baseline parameters may have no linear correlation with the AOD or percentage change in mean AOD after LPI. This may have caused us to miss some important baseline predictors. We will conduct further prospective studies to verify the reproducibility and accuracy of the proposed equation. Finally, non-standardized UBM gain parameters may affect the accuracy, reproducibility and further analysis of the results.

In conclusion, our study found that AOD750 was correlated with baseline ACD, IT750, AOD750 and LV, and we could predict the post-procedural AOD angle according to the structural parameters of the pre-procedural angle. Our findings could serve as a valuable reference to inform clinical work.

ETHICS STATEMENT

The studies involving human participants were reviewed and approved by Ethical Committee of Zhongshan Ophthalmic Center. Written informed consent for participation was not required for this study in accordance with the national legislation and the institutional requirements.

AUTHOR CONTRIBUTIONS

ML and XG: design and conduct of the study. LC and HH: collection of data. YZ and CZ: analysis of data. JR, HL, YL, and HG: preparation of the manuscript. All authors review and final approval of the manuscript.

REFERENCES

1. Song P, Wang J, Bucan K, Theodoratou E, Rudan I, Chan KY National and subnational prevalence and burden of glaucoma in China: A systematic analysis. *J Glob Health.* (2017) 7:020705. doi: 10.7189/jogh.07.020705
2. Qu W, Li Y, Song W, Zhou X, Kang Y, Yan L, et al. Prevalence and risk factors for angle-closure disease in a rural Northeast China population: a population-based survey in Bin County, Harbin. *Acta Ophthalmol.* (2011) 89:e515–20. doi: 10.1111/j.1755-3768.2011.02146.x
3. He M, Friedman DS, Ge J, Huang W, Jin C, Lee PS, et al. Laser peripheral iridotomy in primary angle-closure suspects: biometric and gonioscopic outcomes: the Liwan Eye Study. *Ophthalmology.* (2007) 114:494–500. doi: 10.1016/j.ophtha.2006.06.053
4. Radhakrishnan S, Chen PP, Junk AK, Nouri-Mahdavi K, Chen TC. Laser peripheral iridotomy in primary angle closure: a report by the American academy of ophthalmology. *Ophthalmology.* (2018) 125:1110–20. doi: 10.1016/j.ophtha.2018.01.015
5. Nongpiur ME, Aboobakar IF, Baskaran M, Narayanaswamy A, Sakata LM, Wu R, et al. Association of Baseline Anterior Segment Parameters With the Development of Incident Gonioscopic Angle Closure. *JAMA Ophthalmol.* (2017) 135:252–8. doi: 10.1001/jamaophthalmol.2016.5847
6. Do T, Nguyen Xuan H, Dao Lam H, Tran Tien D, Nguyen Thi Thuy G, Nguyen Do Ngoc H, et al. Ultrasound biomicroscopic diagnosis of angle-closure mechanisms in Vietnamese subjects with unilateral angle-closure glaucoma. *J Glaucoma.* (2018) 27:115–20. doi: 10.1097/IJG.0000000000000856
7. How AC, Baskaran M, Kumar RS, He M, Foster PJ, Lavanya R, et al. Changes in anterior segment morphology after laser peripheral iridotomy: an anterior segment optical coherence tomography study. *Ophthalmology.* (2012) 119:1383–7. doi: 10.1016/j.ophtha.2012.01.019
8. Huang G, Gonzalez E, Lee R, Osmonavic S, Leeungurasatien T, He M, et al. Anatomic predictors for anterior chamber angle opening after laser peripheral iridotomy in narrow angle eyes. *Curr Eye Res.* (2012) 37:575–82. doi: 10.3109/02713683.2012.655396
9. Zebardast N, Kavitha S, Krishnamurthy P, Friedman DS, Nongpiur ME, Aung T, et al. Changes in anterior segment morphology and predictors of angle widening after laser iridotomy in South Indian eyes. *Ophthalmology.* (2016) 123:2519–26. doi: 10.1016/j.ophtha.2016.08.020
10. Chen S, Lv J, Fan S, Zhang H, Xie L, Xu L, et al. Multi-mechanism Angle Closure Study group. Laser peripheral iridotomy versus laser peripheral iridotomy plus laser peripheral iridoplasty in the treatment of multi-mechanism angle closure: study protocol for a randomized controlled trial. *Trials.* (2017) 18:130. doi: 10.1186/s13063-017-1860-4
11. He M, Jiang Y, Huang S, Chang DS, Munoz B, Aung T, et al. Laser peripheral iridotomy for the prevention of angle closure: a single-center, randomized controlled trial. *Lancet.* (2019) 393:1609–18. doi: 10.1016/S0140-6736(18)32607-2
12. Atalay E, Nongpiur ME, Baskaran M, Sharma S, Perera SA, Aung T. biometric factors associated with acute primary angle closure: comparison of the affected and fellow eye. *Invest Ophthalmol Vis Sci.* (2016) 57:5320–5. doi: 10.1167/iovs.16-20006
13. Lee JR, Choi JY, Kim YD, Choi J. Laser peripheral iridotomy with iridoplasty in primary angle closure suspect: anterior chamber analysis by pentacam. *Korean J Ophthalmol.* (2011) 25:252–6. doi: 10.3341/kjo.2011.25.4.252
14. Ang BC, Nongpiur ME, Aung T, Mizoguchi T, Ozaki M. Changes in Japanese eyes after laser peripheral iridotomy: an anterior segment optical coherence tomography study. *Clin Exp Ophthalmol.* (2016) 44:159–65. doi: 10.1111/ceo.12673

15. Ang GS, Wells AP. Factors influencing laser peripheral iridotomy outcomes in white eyes: an anterior segment optical coherence tomography study. *J Glaucoma.* (2011) 20:577–83. doi: 10.1097/IJG.0b013e3181f7b26f
16. Lee KS, Sung KR, Shon K, Sun JH, Lee JR. Longitudinal changes in anterior segment parameters after laser peripheral iridotomy assessed by anterior segment optical coherence tomography. *Invest Ophthalmol Vis Sci.* (2013) 54:3166–70. doi: 10.1167/iovs.13-11630
17. Mansoori T, Balakrishna N. Anterior segment morphology after laser iridotomy in primary angle closure suspects. *Clin Exp Optom.* (2018) 101:333–8. doi: 10.1111/cxo.12631

2

Microvascular Structure Changes After Intravitreal Ranibizumab Injection in Retinal Vein Occlusion Patients with and without Macular Ischemia

Ziyi Zhu [1], Yongan Meng [1], Igor Kozak [2], Manyun Xie [1], Youling Liang [1], Bin Yan [1], Liang Zhou [1], Pingbo Ouyang [1], Xiaoxi Yao [3] and Jing Luo [1,4]*

[1] *Department of Ophthalmology, The Second Xiangya Hospital, Central South University, Changsha, China,* [2] *Hunan Clinical Research Center of Ophthalmic Disease, Changsha, China,* [3] *Moorfields Eye Hospital UAE, Abu Dhabi, United Arab Emirates,* [4] *Shenzhen College of International Education, Shenzhen, China*

***Correspondence:**
Jing Luo
luojing001@csu.edu.cn

Purpose: To investigate the changes in the macular microvascular structure after anti-vascular endothelial growth factor (anti-VEGF) treatment in retinal vein occlusion (RVO) patients with and without macular ischemia.

Methods: A total of 39 patients were divided into the macular ischemia group ($n = 22$) and the nonischemia group ($n = 17$) at baseline. All the patients received an intravitreal injection of ranibizumab with a 3+ pro re nata (PRN) regimen. The foveal avascular zone (FAZ) areas, macular vessel density (VD), and macular ischemic index (ISI) were evaluated at baseline and 3 and 6 months after treatment.

Results: After treatment, some patients in the macular ischemia group achieved obvious reperfusion in macular nonperfusion areas. The VD and macular ISI improved in RVO patients, but the changes in VD and macular ISI were different in the two groups. The improvement of best corrected visual acuity (BCVA) was positively correlated with the improvement of macular perfusion status. Macular perfusion remained stable in most patients in RVO and only one patient had macular ischemia aggravation.

Conclusion: The macular microvascular structures were stable in most RVO patients after anti-VEGF treatment. At the same time, some patients with macular ischemia presented reperfusion in macular nonperfusion areas, and still a few patients presented aggravated macular ischemia. Macular ISI is a good way to evaluate macular perfusion status in RVO compared to VD.

Keywords: anti-VEGF treatment, macular ischemia, OCTA, ischemic index, RVO, vessel density (VD)

INTRODUCTION

Retinal ischemia caused by retinal vein occlusion (RVO) has been of great concern in clinical studies and is present in ~66% of main branch RVO (BRVO) and ischemic central RVO (CRVO) cases (1, 2). Anti-vascular endothelial growth factor (VEGF) treatment, as a first-line treatment for RVO, has been proven to significantly improve macular edema. However, it has been controversial whether anti-VEGF treatment aggravates ischemia. Terui et al. (3) reported increased nonperfusion areas after anti-VEGF treatment in several cases. However, other studies have suggested that retinal ischemia develops gradually and irreversibly, irrespective of anti-VEGF treatment (4, 5). Campochiaro et al. (6) have shown that anti-VEGF treatment not only effectively improves macular edema but also prevents the progression of nonperfusion areas. In contrast, some researchers still believe that no reperfusion occurs after anti-VEGF treatment, which may be due to limited sample sizes and short observation periods; the number of patients was 9 and 14, and the observation time was only 3 months in those studies (7, 8). Moreover, no study has compared the different anti-VEGF treatments in RVO patients with and without macular ischemia.

Thus, we aimed to investigate the effects of ranibizumab with a 3+ pro re nata (PRN) regimen on macular perfusion status in RVO patients with and without macular ischemia. We wished to analyze the changes in macular perfusion and focus on whether the macular nonperfusion (MNP) area improved after anti-VEGF treatment, especially in RVO patients with macular ischemia. Optical coherence tomography angiography (OCTA) measurement values have been used as biomarkers in monitoring disease progression and treatment response in many clinical studies (9). Therefore, we quantified foveal avascular zone (FAZ) areas, capillary density, and macular ischemic index (ISI) in the macular region by using OCTA.

MATERIALS AND METHODS

Patients

This study followed the tenets of the Declaration of Helsinki. All the patients gave informed written consent before participating in this study. All the procedures were performed in accordance with the Ethical Standards of the Second Xiangya Hospital of Central South University Committee and the ethical review approval number was 2017-053. The study period was between September 2018 and December 2019 and all the patients were diagnosed with RVO. Only one eye of each patient was included in the study. All the eyes were injected with 0.3 mg of ranibizumab at monthly intervals for the first 3 months and given additional interval injections according to the PRN regimen. All the patients were evaluated for 6 months. Before the first intraocular injection, all the patients underwent fluorescein angiography (FA) and OCTA, which showed whether a patient had apparent ischemia and nonperfusion areas. The exclusion criteria were poor OCTA image quality before grouping patients, Q-score below 7, the opacity of refractive media, the presence of significant residual motion artifacts, and severely disrupted anatomical features of the macular area (such as severe cystoid macular edema) leading to the segmentation errors. Then, the patients were divided into two groups, namely, the macular ischemia group and the nonischemia group. The macular ischemia group was defined as the presence of retinal capillary loss or nonperfusion in the Early Treatment Diabetic Retinopathy Study (ETDRS) grid center subfield according to the CRYSTAL study (10). Additional exclusion criteria included patients with retinal arterial occlusion; retinal treatment or major ocular surgery within the prior 6 months; vision loss caused by any other retinal disease, including severe diabetic retinopathy and age-related macular degeneration (AMD); intraocular pressure $\geq$ 25 mm Hg; refractive error (myopia > 6 D or hyperopia > 3D); poor refractive media; and other systemic diseases that required hospitalization.

Ranibizumab (RBZ, Lucentis; Genentech Incorporation, South San Francisco, California, USA) is a monoclonal antibody against VEGF-A that effectively reduces VEGF concentrations by blocking VEGF binding to VEGF receptors (11). Some large multicenter clinical trials, including the Treatment of Macular Edema following Branch Retinal Vein Occlusion: Evaluation of Efficacy and Safety (BRAVO) and the Treatment of Macular Edema following Central Retinal Vein Occlusion: Evaluation of Efficacy and Safety (CRUISE) studies, have proven that ranibizumab effectively improved visual acuity (VA) and macular edema and affected retinal nonperfusion (12, 13).

Image Acquisition and Data Measurement

All the OCTA images were acquired by the AngioVue OCT System version 2018.0.0.14 (RTVue XR Avanti, Optovue Incorporation, Fremont, California, USA) by using the split-spectrum amplitude decorrelation angiography (SSADA) algorithm to detect blood flow and provided a new method for rapid imaging of detailed microvasculature at the distinct depths (14). The system reduced artifacts by motion correction technology (MCT) and three-dimensional (3D) projection artifact removal (PAR) to remove artifacts and PAR differentiated *in-situ* OCTA signals from the projection artifacts and removed the projection artifacts (14). AngioVue provided an automated software algorithm to generate the boundaries of the superficial capillary plexus (SCP) (from the internal limiting membrane (ILM) to 10 μm above the inner plexiform layer (IPL)) and deep capillary plexus (DCP) (from 10 μm above the IPL to 10 μm below the outer plexiform layer(OPL)). Additionally, the boundary of the FAZ area was from the ILM to 10 μm below the OPL, while the segmentation boundaries could also be adjusted and corrected by manual segmentation (15). Parameters of blood flow status in the macular region are derived from a 6 × 6 mm macular scan grid instead of a traditional 3 × 3 mm macular scan grid. This provides a new method to analyze the changes in macular ischemia after anti-VEGF treatment. The central foveal thickness (CFT), as an average value within a circular 1 mm diameter area centered in the fovea, was automatically measured by OCTA. The values of the FAZ area and vessel density (VD) were also automatically calculated by OCTA software when the segmentation boundaries were corrected. Tsui et al. (16) proposed the concept of ISI and provided us with a new way to evaluate the ischemic state in retinal vascular diseases by calculating areas of ischemia as a percentage of the total calculated visible retina in ultrawide-field angiography (UWFA) images. We similarly applied the macular ISI concept to analyze macular ischemia status by using OCTA. Macular ISI was calculated by areas of nonperfusion area as a percentage of the total calculated area. The calculation formula is as follows:

$$Macular\ ISI = \frac{Nonperfusion\ area}{Measurement\ area\ (6\ mm \times 6\ mm\ diameter\ circle\ area)} \times 100\% = \frac{Measurement\ area - Perfusion\ area - FAZ\ area}{Measurement\ area}$$

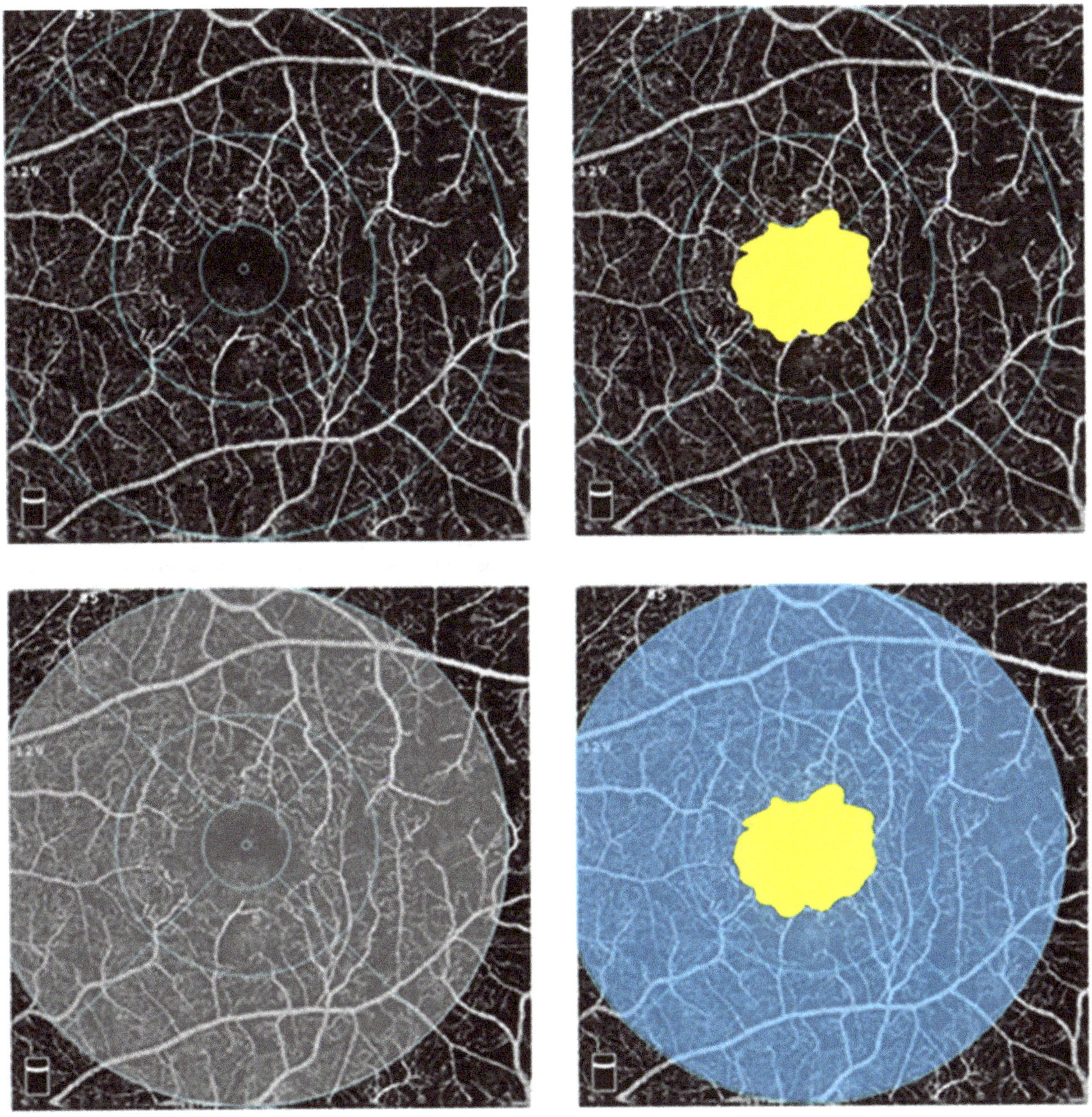

FIGURE 1 | Optical coherence tomography angiography (OCTA) images in superficial capillary plexus (6 × 6 mm). The foveal avascular zone (FAZ) area measurement is located in the yellow area, vessel density (VD) measurement is located in the gray area, and ischemic index (ISI) measurement is located in the blue area.

$$\times 100\% = \left(1 - \frac{Perfusion\ area + FAZ\ area}{Measurement\ area}\right)$$

$$\times 100\% = \left(1 - \frac{\frac{VD}{100\%} \times Measurement\ area + FAZ\ area}{Measurement\ area}\right) \times 100\%$$

$$Measurement\ area = 3\ mm \times 3\ mm \times \pi = 28.27\ mm2$$

$$Macular\ ISI = \left(1 - \frac{VD}{100\%} - \frac{FAZ\ area}{28.27}\right) \times 100\%$$

An example is shown in **Figure 1**. The FAZ area measurement is located in the yellow area, VD measurement is located in the gray area, and macular ISI measurement is located in the blue area. The macular ISI mainly excludes the influence of changes in the FAZ area and more intuitively represents the ischemic state in the macular region with a larger macular ISI indicating more severe ischemia and non-perfusion.

TABLE 1 | Characteristics of the macular ischemia group and the nonischemia group at baseline.

		Macular ischemia group (n = 22)	Nonischemia group (n = 17)	Total (n = 39)
Gender (male:female)		9:13	11:6	20:19
CRVO:BRVO		7:15	7:10	14:25
Age (years)		57.8 ± 7.6	56.4 ± 8.0	57.2 ± 7.7
BCVA (logMAR)		0.85 ± 0.42	0.54 ± 0.37	0.71 ± 0.42
CFT (μm)		324 ± 128	398 ± 152	357 ± 142
IOP (mmHg)		16.0 ± 2.2	16.9 ± 2.2	16.4 ± 2.2
FAZ area (mm^2)		0.463 ± 0.249	0.351 ± 0.130	0.414 ± 0.210
VD (%)	SCP	40.2 ± 4.6	48.0 ± 3.0	43.6 ± 5.5
	DCP	41.3 ± 4.4	45.4 ± 3.6	43.1 ± 4.5
ISI (%)	SCP	57.8 ± 4.5	50.6 ± 2.9	54.6 ± 5.3
	DCP	56.9 ± 4.6	53.3 ± 3.8	55.3 ± 4.6

BCVA, best corrected visual acuity; CFT, central foveal thickness; IOP, intraocular pressure; FAZ, foveal avascular zone; VD, vessel density; ISI, ischemic index; SCP, superficial capillary plexus.

TABLE 2 | Changes in the BCVA, CFT, FAZ area, VD, and macular ISI between the macular ischemia group and the nonischemia group.

	BCVA/logMAR	CFT/μm	FAZ area/mm^2	VD		ISI	
				Superficial-VD/%	Deep-VD/%	Superficial-ISI/%	Deep-ISI/%
Macular ischemia group							
Month 0	0.85 ± 0.42	324 ± 128	0.463 ± 0.249	40.2 ± 4.6	41.3 ± 4.4	57.8 ± 4.5	56.9 ± 4.6
Month 3	0.61 ± 0.35*	293 ± 98	0.447 ± 0.190	41.7 ± 4.8*	41.7 ± 4.1	56.1 ± 4.7*	56.3 ± 4.4
Month 6	0.60 ± 0.41	280 ± 77	0.465 ± 0.247	41.7 ± 5.2	41.3 ± 3.1	56.0 ± 4.9	57.0 ± 3.5
Nonischemia group							
Month 0	0.54 ± 0.37	398 ± 152	0.351 ± 0.130	48.0 ± 3.0	45.4 ± 3.6	50.6 ± 2.9	53.3 ± 3.8
Month 3	0.36 ± 0.30*	347 ± 106	0.346 ± 0.126	47.9 ± 4.2	44.3 ± 3.3	51.0 ± 4.4	54.4 ± 3.5
Month 6	0.29 ± 0.24	311 ± 95	0.336 ± 0.110	49.4 ± 4.6	47.4 ± 3.9*	49.4 ± 4.5	51.5 ± 4.0*

*$p < 0.05$.
BCVA, best corrected visual acuity; CFT, central foveal thickness; FAZ, foveal avascular zone; VD, vessel density; ISI, ischemic index.

Statistical Analysis

The main measurements, including best corrected visual acuity (BCVA), CFT, FAZ area, superficial and deep VD, and macular ISI in this study, were tested by the Kolmogorov–Smirnov test ($p > 0.05$ was set as statistically significant). At 0, 3, and 6 months, changes in FAZ area, blood flow, and macular ISI were evaluated by the paired sample t-test. Moreover, $p < 0.05$ indicated statistical significant. Statistical analysis was performed by using the Statistical Package for the Social Sciences (SPSS) version 25.0 (SPSS Incorporation, Chicago, Illinois, USA).

RESULTS

We enrolled 39 patients with RVO in two groups: the macular ischemia group ($n = 22$) and the nonischemia group ($n = 17$). The characteristics of the patients at baseline are shown in **Table 1**. The patients in the macular ischemia group showed ischemic changes, such as FAZ area expansion, MNP, decrease in blood flow density, and increase in macular ISI, especially in the superficial layer.

The changes in FAZ area, CFT, VD, and macular ISI are listed in **Table 2** and the changes in the macular perfusion status in the macular ischemia group are depicted in **Figure 2**. In the macular ischemia group, the logarithm of the minimum angle of resolution (logMAR) BCVA changed from 0.85 ± 0.42 to 0.61 ± 0.35 ($p < 0.001$) and then to 0.60 ± 0.41 ($p = 0.908$) and the FAZ area and CFT showed no significant changes. The superficial layer VD and macular ISI changed significantly at 3 months and remained stable until the endpoint. The superficial layer VD changed from 40.2 ± 4.6% to 41.7 ± 4.8% ($p = 0.009$) and then to 41.7 ± 5.2% ($p = 0.966$), whereas the superficial macular ISI changed from 57.8 ± 4.5% to 56.1 ± 4.7% ($p = 0.010$) and then to 56.0 ± 4.9% ($p = 0.902$) at the endpoint. Moreover, the VD and macular ISI remained stable during the study period in the deep layer. In the nonischemia group, the logMAR BCVA changed from 0.54 ± 0.37 to 0.36 ± 0.30 ($p = 0.008$) and then to 0.29 ± 0.24 ($p = 0.533$). The deep layer VD changed from 45.4 ± 3.6 to 44.3 ± 3.3% ($p = 0.135$) and then to 47.4 ± 3.9% ($p = 0.023$), whereas the deep macular ISI changed from 53.3 ± 3.8 to 54.4 ± 3.5% ($p = 0.150$) and then to 51.5 ± 4.0% ($p = 0.030$) at the endpoint.

At 6 months, from a total of 22 patients with macular ischemia at baseline, nine patients had increased superficial VD by more than 1%, seven patients had increased superficial VD by more

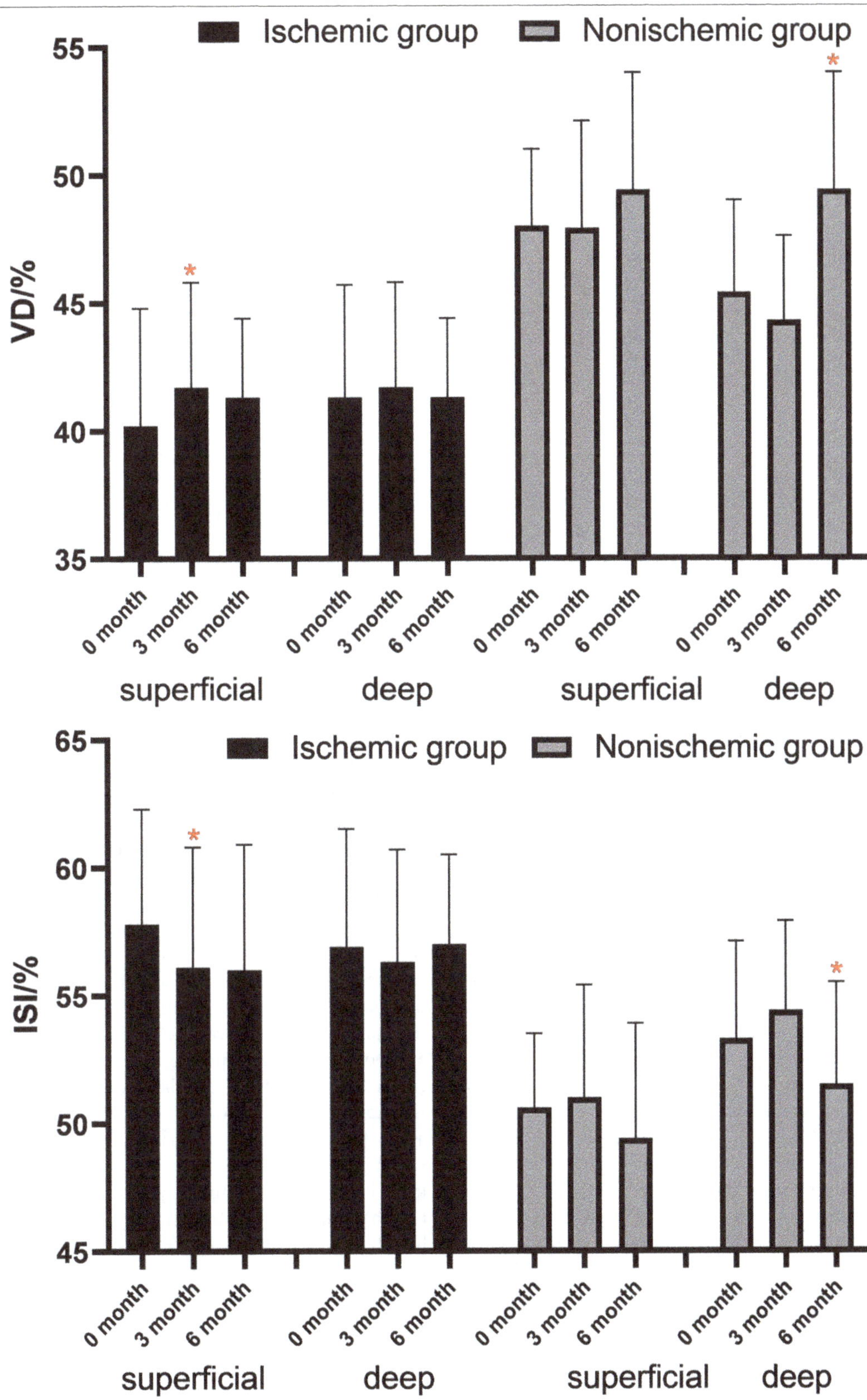

FIGURE 2 | Changes of VD and ISI in the macular ischemia group after antivascular endothelial growth factor (VEGF) treatment. $^{*}p < 0.05$.

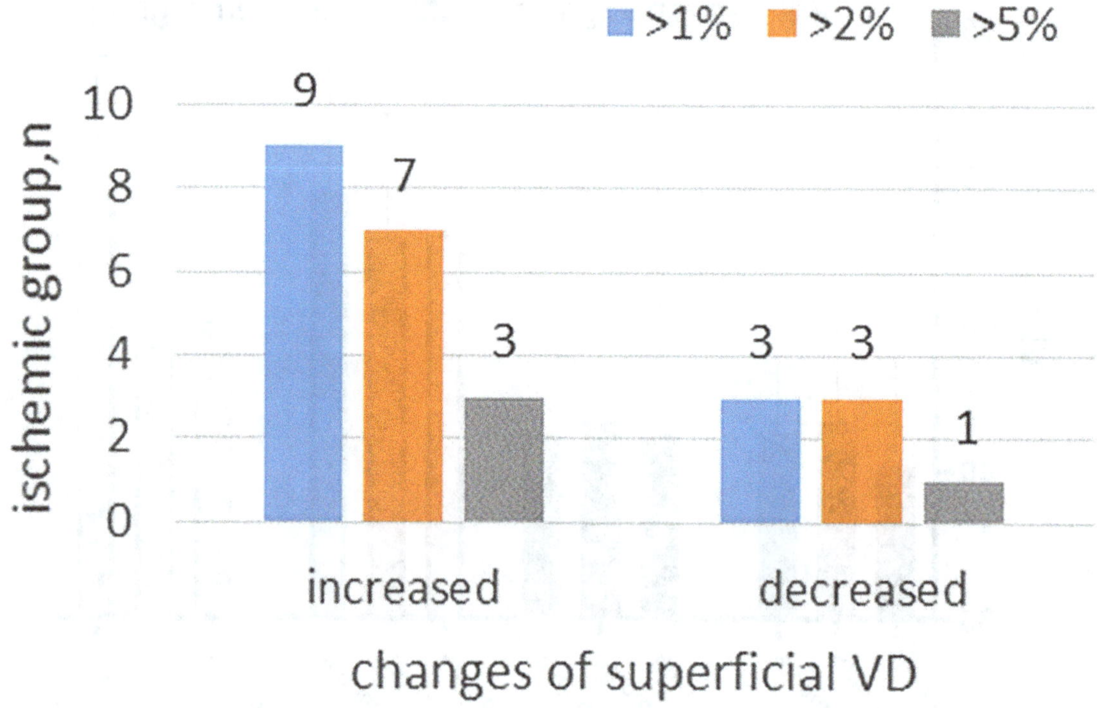

FIGURE 3 | The distribution of the number of patients with VD changes.

than 2%, and three patients had increased superficial VD by more than 5%. Only three patients had decreased superficial VD by more than 1%, three patients had decreased superficial VD by more than 2%, and two patients had decreased superficial VD by more than 5% (**Figure 3**). Three patients demonstrated reperfusion and only one patient had an enlarged MNP area. The VD and macular ISI remained stable during the study period in the nonischemia group.

Some patients with macular ischemia demonstrated reperfusion of previously nonperfused areas (**Figures 4**, **5**), and the red arrows indicate the growth of new capillaries and reperfusion in the MNP areas. There was still one patient with macular ischemia that was aggravated after receiving treatment (**Figure 6**) and the red arrows indicate that the nonperfusion area gradually increased and macular ischemia was aggravated.

Figure 7 shows the Pearson correlation analysis of the changes in BCVA and macular perfusion indexes in all the RVO patients. The changes in both the superficial and deep layer of VD were negatively correlated with the changes in the logMAR BCVA and the changes in both the superficial and deep layer macular ISI were positively correlated with the changes in the logMAR BCVA.

DISCUSSION

Retinal ischemia was the main sign of aggravation of RVO and approximately one-third of nonischemic CRVO converted to ischemic CRVO within 3 years (1, 2). Studies have also demonstrated that the capillary density and morphology have a significant association with the severity of RVO. Furthermore, the baseline BCVA in ischemic eyes was usually worse than that in nonischemic eyes. The extent of ischemia in the macular region was closely associated with the prognosis of BCVA, where patients with greater macular perfusion status were more likely to show a better improvement in macular edema and BCVA (17–19). Thus, it is valuable to evaluate macular perfusion status. At present, most studies use VD to evaluate macular perfusion status; however, the disadvantage is that the changes in VD can be influenced by changes in the FAZ area. Thus, we use macular ISI as an evaluation index. Tsui et al. (16) first proposed the concept of ISI to evaluate the ischemic state by calculating areas of ischemia as a percentage of the total calculated visible retina. We applied the macular ISI concept to analyze macular ischemia status. The concept of macular ISI provides us with a new way to evaluate the ischemic state in macular ischemia status and excludes the influence of changes in the FAZ area; thus, it could more intuitively represent the ischemic state in the macular region. Macular ISI was highly correlated with blood flow density in both the superficial and deep layers. However, when the area of the FAZ changes greatly, macular ISI evaluating the change in macular perfusion status is more accurate than VD.

In this study, we mainly adopted OCTA as the main evaluation method to observe the macular perfusion status. OCTA is highly consistent with FA in showing the vessels in the macular area and is not affected by the leakage of fluorescein. OCTA is noninvasive, repeatable, and easily operable, and it is subtler than FA in displaying macular area capillaries (14).

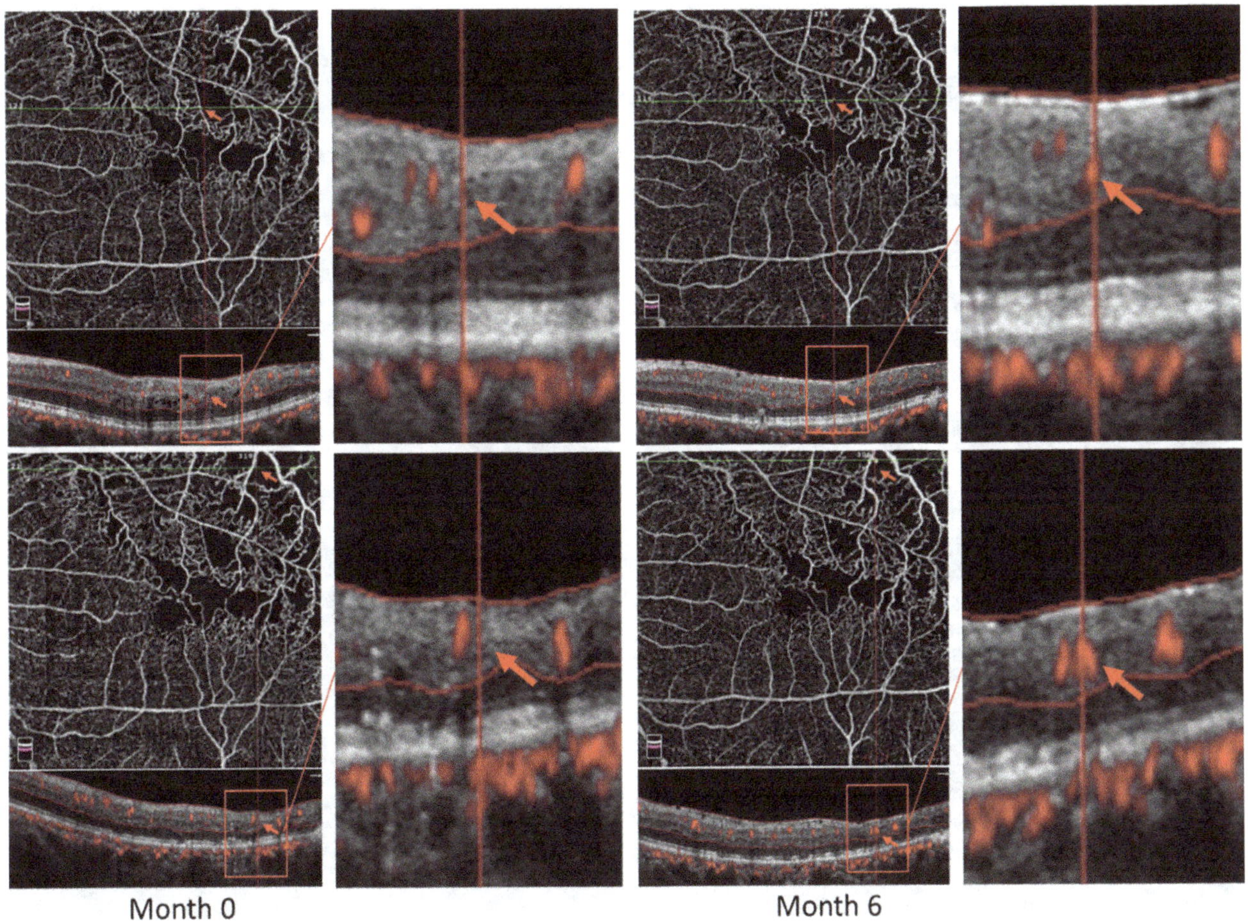

FIGURE 4 | Reperfusion occurred in the left eye of a 56-year-old male with macular ischemia after receiving anti-VEGF treatment. Red arrows indicate the growth of new capillaries and reperfusion in the macular nonperfusion areas.

OCTA has obvious advantages in quantifying VD, FAZ areas, and nonflow areas. Previous studies in RVO have also shown that OCTA detected nonperfusion areas and superficial and deep capillary abnormalities more often than FA and OCTA measurements values may serve as biomarkers for monitoring disease progression and treatment response (32).

In OCTA, total VD is divided into SCP and DCP. The status of superficial VD is associated with macular edema development, whereas VD in the deep plexus is important for the oxygen requirements of photoreceptors and the outer retina (20). Researchers suggest that microvascular changes, such as MNP areas of the RVO, are observed more obviously in the deep plexus than in the superficial plexus (21). Deep VD is related to choriocapillaris blood flow and is more susceptible to ischemia.

Overall, this study indicates that anti-VEGF treatment has a positive effect on macular ischemia and improves macular perfusion status in most cases. Our data suggested that the changes in VD and macular ISI were different in the macular ischemia group and the nonischemia group. In the RVO with macular ischemia, macular ischemia decreased significantly after anti-VEGF treatment, especially in the superficial retinal layer, and the VD and macular ISI in the deep plexus remained stable without exacerbation of ischemia. In the nonischemia group, VD and macular ISI still improved in the deep layer at 6 months. In addition, the improvement in BCVA was positively correlated with the improvement in macular perfusion status.

The improvement in VD and macular ISI was different between the macular ischemia group and the nonischemia group. Why is there such a difference between the two groups? Our data showed that the superficial VD in the macular ischemia group decreased more significantly than deep VD and the superficial macular ISI increased more significantly than deep macular ISI at baseline compared with the nonischemic group. The DCP, where the inner nuclear layer, is located maybe highly vulnerable to ischemia because the DCP supplies oxygen to the photoreceptor and upregulates VEGF more strongly than it does in the SCP (22, 23). Therefore, we suspect that in the macular ischemia group, anti-VEGF treatment can improve retinal hypoxia and give priority to oxygen supply to SCP. As SCP did not show severe ischemia and hypoxia, DCP improved in the nonischemia group. This speculation needs to be confirmed in future studies.

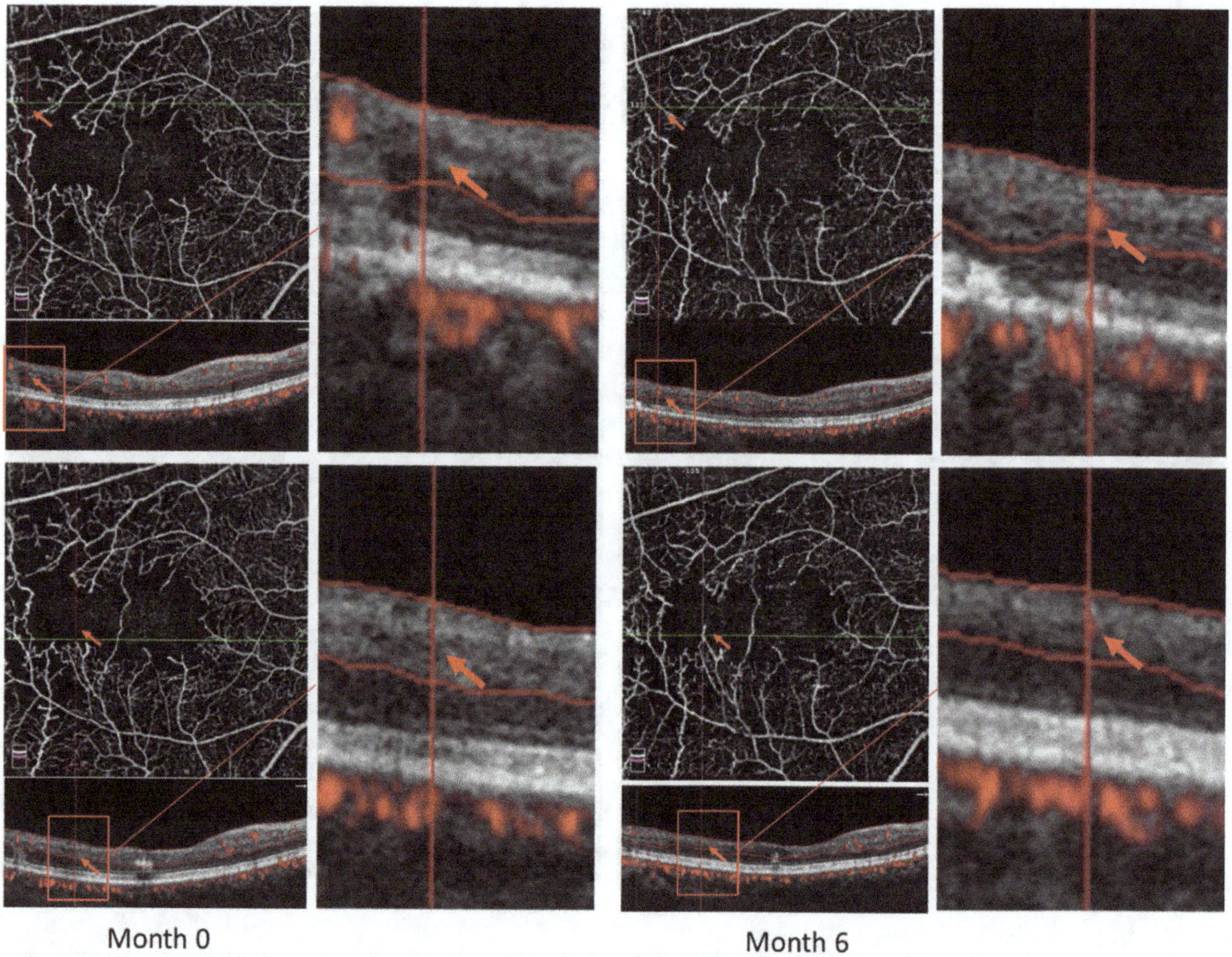

FIGURE 5 | Reperfusion occurred in the right eye of a 57-year-old female with macular ischemia after receiving anti-VEGF treatment. Red arrows indicate the growth of new capillaries and reperfusion in the macular nonperfusion areas.

Macular perfusion was not aggravated in most patients with RVO. In the macular ischemia group, the number of patients with increased superficial VD was more than the number of patients with decreased superficial VD in 6 months. Notably, some patients even demonstrated reperfusion after anti-VEGF treatment in the nonperfusion areas. Vascular reperfusion should be differentiated from neovascularization and collateral vessels. First, the shape of the reperfused vasculature is almost the same as that of the original vasculature, while neovascularization is usually dilated and tortuous. Second, OCTA also showed that there are no neovascularization or collateral vessels. The development of neovascularization usually appears in the superficial layer and has a tendency to break through the internal limiting membrane (ILM) and grows into the vitreous cavity, while the reperfused vasculature in this study was at a deep layer on OCTA instead of the superficial layer and did not break through the ILM. In addition, collateral vessels usually form in the acute phase in RVO (24). In this study, the reperfusion of RVO occurred more than 3 months after anti-VEGF treatment and OCTA confirmed that it was not collateral circulation.

The mechanism of these changes caused by anti-VEGF treatment is still unclear. Animal experiments have proven that the suppression of VEGF causes reperfusion of the closed vessels (25). Studies have demonstrated that anti-VEGF treatment could not only reduce autophagy and apoptosis rates and activate ischemia-damaged microglia to protect the retinal ganglion cells and bipolar cells, further normalize peripheral cells, stabilize the basement membrane, but also reopen closed retinal vessels, prevent the progression of vessel closure, and improve retinal ischemia (26, 27). Recently, Seo et al. (28) found that anti-VEGF treatment inhibited the upregulation of VEGF in both the superficial and deep capillary plexuses by decreasing the leukocyte aggregation and retinal hyperpermeability.

However, one case in this study was found that macular ischemia was aggravated after anti-VEGF treatment, which is consistent with some early studies. Takayuki et al. observed the deterioration of retinal perfusion status in BRVO, but

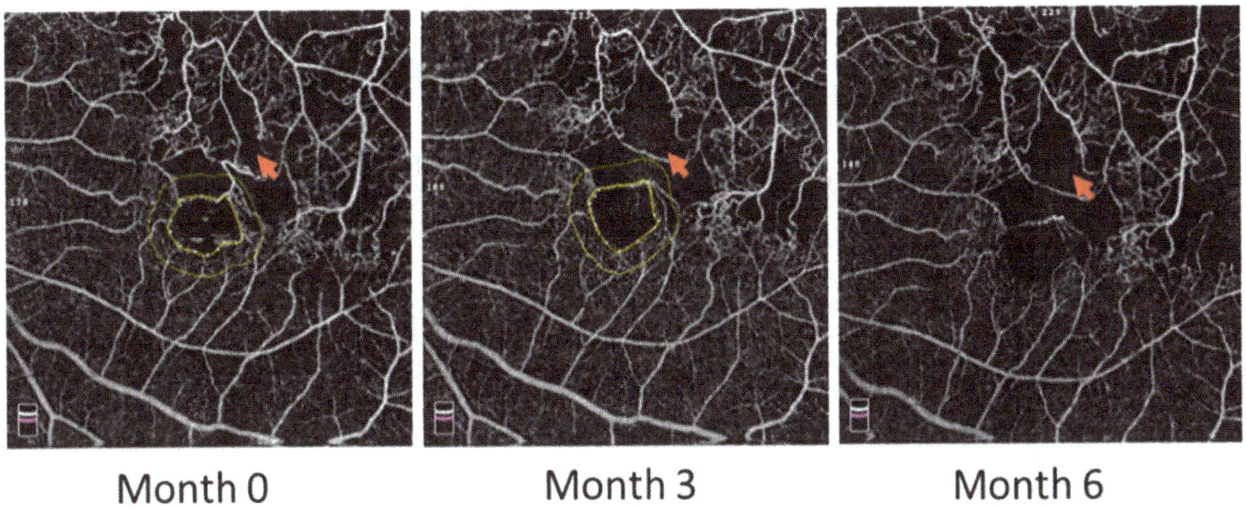

FIGURE 6 | Macular ischemia aggravated in the left eye of a 60-year-old male after receiving anti-VEGF treatment. Red arrows indicate the nonperfusion area gradually increased and macular ischemia aggravated.

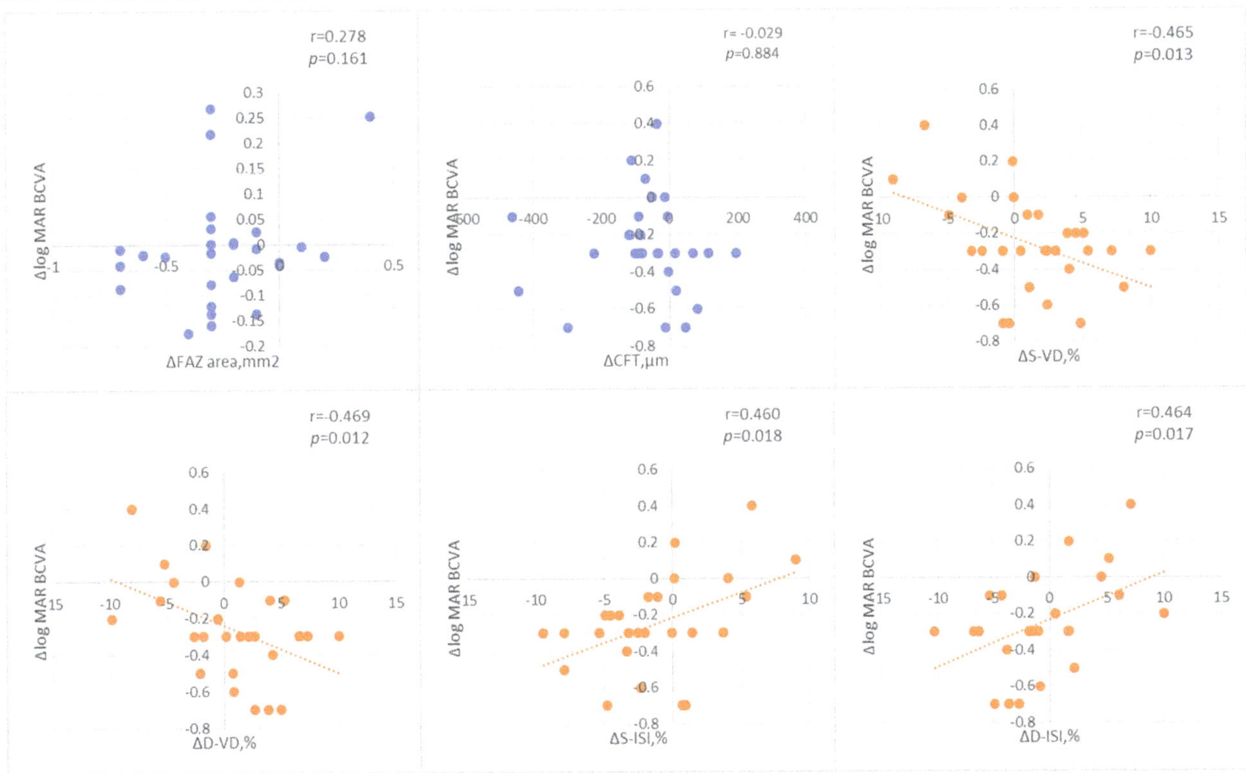

FIGURE 7 | The Pearson correlation analysis of the changes of best corrected visual acuity (BCVA) and macular perfusion indexes.

only a few (1.7%) patients presented a significant increase in nonperfusion areas (NPAs) greater than 1.0 in the disk area (3). However, a natural history of RVO showed that retinal ischemia would develop gradually and irreversibly (3). Retinal ischemia aggravated in RVO patients after anti-VEGF therapy, especially in patients with preexisting retinal ischemia. The Central Vein Occlusion Study (CVOS) indicates the conversion rate from nonischemic RVO to ischemic RVO which is 3.3% by 4 months (29). This study found that only one case (5.9%) had a significant extension of MNP in 6 months and probably reflected a conversion from nonischemia to ischemia in few patients with RVO. Due to the great hemodynamic abnormalities in some RVO patients and retinal capillary endothelial cells in a state of oxidative stress, macular ischemia might be enlarged before macular capillaries completely closed (30, 31).

This study has several limitations. First, we adopted OCTA as the main evaluation method to observe the blood flow of the macular region and to quantify macular ischemia, but fluid may induce segmentation artifacts. Fluorescein Fundus Angiography (FFA) is still considered a good method in retinal imaging, especially, in the observation of changes in the dynamic blood flow and retinal capillary leakage, but it is an invasive method requiring venipuncture and contrast infusion with poor repeatability. Second, the observation period and sample size are relatively short and small, respectively. A larger sample size and a longer observation period will benefit the determination of how anti-VEGF plays a role in improving macular ischemia and retinal ischemia.

In conclusion, macular ISI is a good way to evaluate the macular perfusion status in RVO. The changes in VD and macular ISI were different in the macular ischemia group and the nonischemia group. The macular microvascular structures were stable in most RVO patients after anti-VEGF treatment. At the same time, some patients with macular ischemia presented reperfusion in MNP areas, and still, a few patients presented aggravated macular ischemia. In addition, BCVA was positively correlated with macular perfusion status in RVO.

ETHICS STATEMENT

The studies involving human participants were reviewed and approved by Ethics Committee of the Second Xiangya Hospital of Central South University (Registration Number: 2010 K059). The patients/participants provided their written informed consent to participate in this study. Written informed consent was obtained from the individual(s) for the publication of any potentially identifiable images or data included in this article.

AUTHOR CONTRIBUTIONS

ZZ and JL were responsible for the conception and design of this research and wrote the draft. ZZ, YM, YL, BY, and PO acquired the data. ZZ, YM, and XY analyzed and interpreted the data. IK, MX, and LZ revised the manuscript critically. The manuscript benefited from the use of editorial service of American Journal Experts (AJE). All authors have read and approved the final manuscript.

REFERENCES

1. McIntosh RL, Rogers SL, Lim L, Cheung N, Wang JJ, Mitchell P, et al. Natural history of central retinal vein occlusion: an evidence-based systematic review. *Ophthalmology.* (2010) 117:1113–23.e15. doi: 10.1016/j.ophtha.2010.01.060
2. Rogers SL, McIntosh RL, Lim L, Mitchell P, Cheung N, Kowalski JW, et al. Natural history of branch retinal vein occlusion: an evidence-based systematic review. *Ophthalmology.* (2010) 117:10941101.e5. doi: 10.1016/j.ophtha.2010.01.058
3. Terui T, Kondo M, Sugita T, Ito Y, Kondo N, Ota I, et al. Changes in areas of capillary nonperfusion after intravitreal injection of bevacizumab in eyes with branch retinal vein occlusion. *Retina.* (2011) 31:1068–74. doi: 10.1097/IAE.0b013e31820c83c2
4. Li JK, Wei F, Jin XH, Dai YM, Cui HS, Li YM. Changes in vitreous VEGF, bFGF and fibrosis in proliferative diabetic retinopathy after intravitreal bevacizumab. *Int J Ophthalmol.* (2015) 8:1202–6. doi: 10.3980/j.issn.2222-3959.2015.06.22
5. Bonini-Filho M, Costa RA, Calucci D, Jorge R, Melo LA Jr, Scott IU. Intravitreal bevacizumab for diabetic macular edema associated with severe capillary loss: one-year results of a pilot study. *Am J Ophthalmol.* (2009) 147:1022–30, 1030.e1–5. doi: 10.1016/j.ajo.2009.01.009
6. Campochiaro PA, Wykoff CC, Shapiro H, Rubio RG, Ehrlich JS. Neutralization of vascular endothelial growth factor slows progression of retinal nonperfusion in patients with diabetic macular edema. *Ophthalmol.* (2014) 121:1783–9. doi: 10.1016/j.ophtha.2014.03.021
7. Couturier A, Rey PA, Erginay A, Lavia C, Bonnin S, Dupas B, et al. Widefield OCT-angiography and fluorescein angiography assessments of nonperfusion in diabetic retinopathy and edema treated with anti-vascular endothelial growth factor. *Ophthalmology.* (2019) 126:1685–94. doi: 10.1016/j.ophtha.2019.06.022
8. Bonnin S, Dupas B, Lavia C, Erginay A, Dhundass M, Couturier A, et al. Perfusion. *Retina.* (2019) 39:426–34. doi: 10.1097/IAE.0000000000002422
9. Koulisis N, Kim AY, Chu Z, Shahidzadeh A, Burkemper B, Olmos de Koo LC, et al. Quantitative microvascular analysis of retinal venous occlusions by spectral domain optical coherence tomography angiography. *PLoS ONE.* (2017) 12:e0176404. doi: 10.1371/journal.pone.0176404
10. Larsen M, Waldstein SM, Boscia F, Gerding H, Monés J, Tadayoni R, et al. CRYSTAL Study Group. Individualized ranibizumab regimen driven by stabilization criteria for central retinal vein occlusion: twelve-month results of the CRYSTAL study. *Ophthalmology.* (2016) 123:1101–11. doi: 10.1016/j.ophtha.2016.01.011
11. Presta LG, Chen H, O'Connor SJ, Chisholm V, Meng YG, Krummen L, et al. Humanization of an anti-vascular endothelial growth factor monoclonal antibody for the therapy of solid tumors and other disorders. *Cancer Res.* (1997) 57:4593–9.
12. Brown DM, Campochiaro PA, Bhisitkul RB, Ho AC, Gray S, Saroj N, et al. Sustained benefits from ranibizumab for macular edema following branch retinal vein occlusion: 12-month outcomes of a phase III study. *Ophthalmology.* (2011) 118:1594–602. doi: 10.1016/j.ophtha.2011.02.022
13. Campochiaro PA, Brown DM, Awh CC, Lee SY, Gray S, Saroj N, et al. Sustained benefits from ranibizumab for macular edema following central retinal vein occlusion: twelve-month outcomes of a phase III study. *Ophthalmology.* (2011) 118:2041–9. doi: 10.1016/j.ophtha.2011.02.038
14. Jia Y, Tan O, Tokayer J, Potsaid B, Wang Y, Liu JJ, et al. Split-spectrum amplitude-decorrelation angiography with optical coherence tomography. *Opt Express.* (2012) 20:4710–25. doi: 10.1364/OE.20.004710
15. Hwang TS, Zhang M, Bhavsar K, Zhang X, Campbell JP, Lin P, et al. Visualization of 3 distinct retinal plexuses by projection-resolved optical coherence tomography angiography in diabetic retinopathy. *JAMA Ophthalmol.* (2016) 134:1411–9. doi: 10.1001/jamaophthalmol.2016.4272

16. Tsui I, Williams BK Jr, Kok YO, Heilweil G, Schwartz SD. Reliability of ischemic index grading in common retinal vascular diseases. *Ophthalmic Surg Lasers Imaging Retina.* (2015) 46:618–25. doi: 10.3928/23258160-2015 0610-04
17. Samara WA, Shahlaee A, Sridhar J, Khan MA, Ho AC, Hsu J. Quantitative optical coherence tomography angiography features and visual function in eyes with branch retinal vein occlusion. *Am J Ophthalmol.* (2016) 166:76–83. doi: 10.1016/j.ajo.2016.03.033
18. Ghashut R, Muraoka Y, Ooto S, Iida Y, Miwa Y, Suzuma K, et al. An optical coherence tomography angiography study. *Retina.* (2018) 38:1571–80. doi: 10.1097/IAE.0000000000001749
19. Kadomoto S, Muraoka Y, Ooto S, Miwa Y, Iida Y, Suzuma K, et al. An optical coherence tomography angiography study. *Retina.* (2018) 38:272–82. doi: 10.1097/IAE.0000000000001541
20. Ota M, Tsujikawa A, Murakami T, Kita M, Miyamoto K, Sakamoto A, et al. Association between integrity of foveal photoreceptor layer and visual acuity in branch retinal vein occlusion. *Br J Ophthalmol.* (2007) 91:1644–9. doi: 10.1136/bjo.2007.118497
21. Tan PE, Yu PK, Balaratnasingam C, Cringle SJ, Morgan WH, McAllister IL, et al. Quantitative confocal imaging of the retinal microvasculature in the human retina. *Invest Ophthalmol Vis Sci.* (2012) 53:5728–36. doi: 10.1167/iovs.12-10017
22. Birol G, Wang S, Budzynski E, Wangsa-Wirawan ND, Linsenmeier RA. Oxygen distribution and consumption in the macaque retina. *Am J Physiol Heart Circ Physiol.* (2007) 293:H1696–704. doi: 10.1152/ajpheart.00221.2007
23. Wangsa-Wirawan ND, Linsenmeier RA. Retinal oxygen: fundamental and clinical aspects. *Arch Ophthalmol.* (2003) 121:547–57. doi: 10.1001/archopht.121.4.547
24. Suzuki N, Hirano Y, Tomiyasu T, Kurobe R, Yasuda Y, Esaki Y, et al. Collateral vessels on optical coherence tomography angiography in eyes with branch retinal vein occlusion. *Br J Ophthalmol.* (2019) 103:1373–9. doi: 10.1136/bjophthalmol-2018-313322
25. Liu Y, Shen J, Fortmann SD, Wang J, Vestweber D, Campochiaro PA. Reversible retinal vessel closure from VEGF-induced leukocyte plugging. *JCI Insight.* (2017) 2:e95530. doi: 10.1172/jci.insight.95530
26. Palmhof M, Lohmann S, Schulte D, Stute G, Wagner N, Dick HB, et al. Fewer functional deficits and reduced cell death after ranibizumab treatment in a retinal ischemia model. *Int J Mol Sci.* (2018) 19:1636. doi: 10.3390/ijms19061636
27. Inai T, Mancuso M, Hashizume H, Baffert F, Haskell A, Baluk P, et al. Inhibition of vascular endothelial growth factor (VEGF) signaling in cancer causes loss of endothelial fenestrations, regression of tumor vessels, and appearance of basement membrane ghosts. *Am J Pathol.* (2004) 165:35–52. doi: 10.1016/S0002-9440(10)63273-7
28. Seo EJ, Choi JA, Koh JY, Yoon YH. Aflibercept ameliorates retinal pericyte loss and restores perfusion in streptozotocin-induced diabetic mice. *BMJ Open Diabetes Res Care.* (2020) 8:e001278. doi: 10.1136/bmjdrc-2020-001278
29. The Central Vein Occlusion Study Group. Natural history and clinical management of central retinal vein occlusion. Erratum in: Arch Ophthalmol (1997) 115(10):1275. *Arch Ophthalmol.* (1997) 115:486–91. doi: 10.1001/archopht.1997.01100150488006
30. Pollack A, Leiba H, Oliver M. Progression of nonischemic central retinal vein occlusion. *Ophthalmologica.* (1997) 211:13–20. doi: 10.1159/000310861
31. Laatikainen L, Kohner EM. Fluorescein angiography and its prognostic significance in central retinal vein occlusion. *Br J Ophthalmol.* (1976) 60:411–8. doi: 10.1136/bjo.60.6.411
32. Tsai G, Banaee T, Conti FF, Singh RP. Optical coherence tomography angiography in eyes with retinal vein occlusion. *J Ophthalmic Vis Res.* (2018) 13:315–32. doi: 10.4103/jovr.jovr_264_17

3

Clinical and Ultrasound Biomicroscopic Characteristics of Congenital Fibrovascular Pupillary Membrane-Induced Secondary Glaucoma

Yingting Zhu[1†], Lei Fang[1†], Yimin Zhong[1], Julius Oatts[2], Ying Han[2], Shufen Lin[1], Liming Chen[1], Xiaodi Zhou[1], Yihua Su[1], Pingping Liu[1] and Xing Liu[1]*

[1] State Key Laboratory of Ophthalmology, Zhongshan Ophthalmic Center, Sun Yat-sen University, Guangzhou, China,
[2] Department of Ophthalmology, School of Medicine, University of California, San Francisco, San Francisco, CA, United States

***Correspondence:**
Xing Liu
drliuxing@163.com

† These authors have contributed equally to this work and share first authorship

Purpose: The purpose of this study was to describe and summarize the clinical features of congenital fibrovascular pupillary membrane-induced secondary glaucoma (CFPMSG).

Design: Cross-sectional case series.

Methods: Eyes of 32 patients with CFPMSG were enrolled. Demographic data, including gender, laterality, age at presentation, and age at onset of glaucoma were collected. Patients underwent comprehensive ophthalmic examinations and ultrasound biomicroscopy (UBM). CFPMSG eyes were classified into three groups based on UBM findings and intergroup analysis was performed using ANOVA.

Results: The average age at presentation was 2.4 ± 4.6 months (mean ± SD) and at glaucoma onset was 3.8 ± 4.5 months. Compared to normal fellow eyes, all affected eyes had increased intraocular pressure (IOP), axial length, corneal diameter, and central corneal thickness, and decreased anterior chamber depth (ACD) (all $P \leq 0.001$). Twenty-two affected eyes (68.8%) had evidence of glaucomatous optic neuropathy. Based on iris configuration on UBM, eyes were classified as 53% type I ("U" shape), 34% type II ("Y" shape), and 13% type III (no anterior chamber). IOP in types II (33.8 ± 5.9 mmHg) and III (35.2 ± 5.9 mmHg) was significantly higher than in type I eyes (26.5 ± 5.1 mmHg). The ACD was shallower in type II compared to type I ($P = 0.045$).

Conclusion: Congenital fibrovascular pupillary membrane-induced secondary glaucoma is characterized by ocular hypertension, corneal enlargement and edema, axial length elongation, and glaucomatous optic neuropathy. Glaucoma in this condition is secondary to pupillary block and angle-closure. UBM provides important information for the diagnosis and classification of CFPMSG. This novel classification system demonstrated varying levels of severity and may guide on management of this disease.

Keywords: congenital fibrovascular pupillary membrane, secondary glaucoma, ultrasound biomicroscopy, clinical characteristics, classification

INTRODUCTION

Congenital fibrovascular pupillary membrane (CFPM) refers to a condition where a congenital white membrane covers part or all of the pupil and may be accompanied by anterior chamber angle dysplasia (1). It is most commonly unilateral. It was originally believed to be the result of abnormal migration and differentiation of anterior chamber neural crest cells, but a recent histopathological study suggests that it is a variant of persistent fetal vasculature (2, 3). If the membrane blocks the pupil completely, iris bombé and anterior chamber angle closure may occur. Additionally, children with CFPM may demonstrate progressive occlusion of the pupil leading to deprivational amblyopia or/and increased intraocular pressure (IOP) leading to optic nerve damage and irreversible vision loss (4).

Most cases of CFPM are sporadic. The first reported cases in 1986 were called congenital pupil-iris-lens membrane with goniodysgenesis (1). Subsequent cases have been described (2–7), though without detailed imaging of the anterior chamber. More recently, another group described the clinical characteristics of 13 cases of CFPM, though reported unsatisfactory surgical results with a high recurrence rate and poor surgical success (8). This emphasizes the importance of better understanding and classifying this condition to improve visual outcomes.

While the slit-lamp examination is useful in visualizing pupillary membranes, ultrasound biomicroscopy (UBM), a widely used anterior segment modality using ultrahigh-frequency sound, can provide a more detailed and complete view of the anterior segment pathology. To our knowledge, this is the first study to use UBM to image and classify CFPM. This novel classification system may provide better insight into the pathophysiology of congenital fibrovascular pupillary membrane-induced secondary glaucoma (CFPMSG).

METHODS

Patients

This was a retrospective cross-sectional study of all children with CFPMSG seen at the Zhongshan Ophthalmic Center, Sun Yat-sen University, between 2013 and 2020. This study was approved by the Zhongshan Ophthalmic Center Institution Review and Ethics Board (2020KYPJ121). All parents of the patients provided informed consent following the Declaration of Helsinki. Inclusion criteria were (1) age <16 years, (2) unilateral presentation, (3) presence of a fibrovascular membrane attached to the iris stroma adjacent to the pupil, and (4) initial IOP >21 mmHg. Exclusion criteria included patients with bilateral disease or other types of glaucoma. Demographic data were collected, including gender, age at referral to our clinic, age at presentation, age at onset of glaucoma, eye laterality, and parental chief complaint.

Ophthalmic Examination

Examinations under anesthesia were performed using chloral hydrate 10% and topical anesthesia. All patients underwent hand-held slit-lamp biomicroscopy (Keeler, Bucks, England) and slit-lamp photography (BX900; Haag-Streit AG, Koniz, Switzerland). Corneal opacity was classified as mild (iris details clearly visible), moderate (iris details partially visible), or severe (no iris details visible) (9). Horizontal corneal diameter (HCD) was defined as the white-to-white distance from 3 to 9 o'clock, measured using a caliper. IOP was measured using a Tono-pen Avia (Reichert, Depew, New York, USA). A- and B-scan ultrasonography were performed to measure the axial length (AL) and evaluate the posterior segment of the eye (Quantel Medical, CF, France; Nidek US-1800, Japan). The cross-section image of the optic nerve head was evaluated. It was considered glaucomatous cupping when we observed a depression anterior to the optic nerve, which is limited to the papilla (10). All ultrasound examinations were carried out by a single experienced examiner (PPL).

Ultrasound Biomicroscopy

UBM was performed under anesthesia with 50 MHz resolution and the patient was in the supine position (model SW-3200L; Tianjin Suowei Electronic Technology Co, Ltd., Tianjin, China). Saline was used as the coupling agent, and the probe was always perpendicular to the ocular surface. UBM images of the anterior segment were obtained under standard room illumination with axial and radial scans at the 3, 6, 9, and 12 o'clock positions. We selected high-quality images from each o'clock's position and one image of the central anterior chamber to measure anterior chamber parameters and estimation of pupil position. Central corneal thickness (CCT) was measured on UBM in the center of the cornea from the inner surface of the corneal endothelium to the outer epithelial surface. Anterior chamber depth (ACD) was measured as the axial distance from the corneal endothelium to the anterior lens surface. If the anterior lens surface was not visible due to the membrane, the most posterior point of the iris synechiae in front of the lens was used as the reference point. Iris configuration was recorded and classified. All UBM examinations were carried out by a single experienced examiner (LMC).

Statistical Analysis

Descriptive statistics were reported as means and SD, medians and ranges, or numbers and percentages as appropriate. The normality of the continuous variable distribution was examined using the Kolmogorov–Smirnov test. For comparison between affected and unaffected eyes, Student's paired t-test or Kruskal–Wallis H-test was used according to whether variables conformed to a normal distribution. The ANOVA or Pearson's chi-squared test and Fisher's exact test were used for comparison between UBM-defined CFPMSG subtypes. Bonferroni correction was used for multiple comparisons, statistical significance was defined as $P < 0.05$. All statistical analysis was performed using SPSS software, version 22.0 (SPSS, Inc., Chicago, IL, USA).

TABLE 1 | Demographic data of patients with congenital fibrous pupillary membrane-induced secondary glaucoma.

Variables	
Gender, n (%)	
Male	17 (53.1%)
Laterality, n (%)	
Right	18 (56.3%)
Age at first presentation, months	
Median (range)	0 (0–24)
Age at onset of glaucoma, months	
Median (range)	3.0 (0–24)
Age at referral, months	
Median (range)	4.3 (1–24)
Chief complaint, n (%)	
Enlarged or cloudy cornea	15 (46.9%)
White pupil	11 (34.4%)
Epiphora and photophobia	3 (9.4%)
Ocular redness and pain	2 (6.3%)
Vomiting	1 (3.1%)

TABLE 2 | Comparison between affected and fellow eyes in subjects with congenital fibrous pupillary membrane-induced secondary glaucoma at the time of referral.

Variables	Affected eye	Fellow eye	*P*-value*
IOP, mmHg			
Mean (SD)	30.1(6.6)	14.6(3.0)	**<0.001**
Range	17.3–43.4	8.5–20.6	
HCD, mm			
Mean (SD)	12.3 (0.9)	10.8(0.4)	**<0.001**
Range	10.5–14.0	10–11.5	
AL, mm			
Mean (SD)	22.7(1.8)	19.3(1.5)	**<0.001**
Range	19.5–26.6	16.6–21.8	
CCT, μm			
Mean (SD)	629.3(110.7)	528.3(34.9)	**<0.001**
Range	450.0–920.0	460.0–580.0	
ACD, mm			
Mean (SD)	1.50(0.99)	2.19(0.33)	**0.001**
Range	0–3.92	1.62–2.70	
Corneal opacity, n (%)			
Mild	23 (71.9%)	–	
Moderate	9 (28.1%)	–	
Severe	0(0%)		
Corectopia, n (%)			
None	4 (12.5%)	–	
Superior	3 (9.4%)	–	
Nasal	11 (34.4%)	–	
Temporal	14 (43.8%)	–	

ACD, anterior chamber depth; AL, axial length; CCT, central corneal thickness; HCD, horizontal corneal diameter; IOP, intraocular pressure; mmHg, millimeters of mercury. Independent samples t-tests were used for continuous variables.
**Comparison between fellow eye and affected eye.*
P-values with statistical significance (<0.05) are highlighted in bold.

RESULTS

Demographics

In total, 32 eyes of 32 patients with CFPMSG were included in this study, and demographic data are summarized in **Table 1**. Seventeen patients were noted to have an abnormality by their parents (such as white pupil) at birth, and four (24%) presented with symptoms associated with glaucoma (cloudy cornea, corneal enlargement, epiphora, photophobia, ocular redness, eye pain, and vomiting) within 1 month of age. The remaining 15 patients had no symptoms at birth, and 12 of them (80%) were first noticed and presented with glaucomatous symptoms at a median age of 3 months. All patients but one were born at full term. Two of the children were twins with unaffected twin siblings. Systemic conditions included G6PD deficiency (2) and congenital heart disease (1). No other abnormalities, including facial, dental, or umbilical malformations, were reported. There was no family history of pupillary abnormalities or glaucoma. All of the subjects were negative in serological tests for rubella.

Ophthalmic Examination

A comparison of clinical data between affected and unaffected eyes is shown in **Table 2**. IOP, AL, HCD, and CCT were all significantly higher in affected eyes compared to normal fellow eyes (P < 0.001). Mean ACD was 1.50 ± 0.99 mm in affected eyes compared to 2.19 ± 0.33 mm in unaffected eyes (P = 0.001). All patients presented with IOP > 21 mmHg. Seven patients presented with HCD <12 mm with a median age at the time of referral of 9 months (range 1–24 months), which is significantly older than the rest of patients with the median age at the referral of whom of 4 months (range 1–10 months) (P = 0.033). Moreover, based on the AL-to-age data of Sampaolesi and Caruso (11), we found that four of seven patients (57.1%) with HCD <12 mm had initial AL within normal range, while four of 25 patients (16%) with HCD ≥ 12 mm did. All patients had a white membrane covering the pupil and iris bombé with peripheral anterior synechiae. Most patients (87.5%) had pupil displacement. B-scan ultrasound showed optic nerve cupping in 22 eyes (68.8%).

Ultrasound Biomicroscopy Classification

Based on the iris configuration and ACD, we classified CFPMSG into three types (**Figure 1**, **Table 3**).

Type I ("U" shape) was found in 17 eyes (53%). It was characterized as 360-degree iridolenticular adhesions with resultant iris bombé and peripheral iridocorneal contact. A thick and hyperreflective structure blocked the pupil, pupillary margin, pupillary membrane, and was completely adherent to the anterior

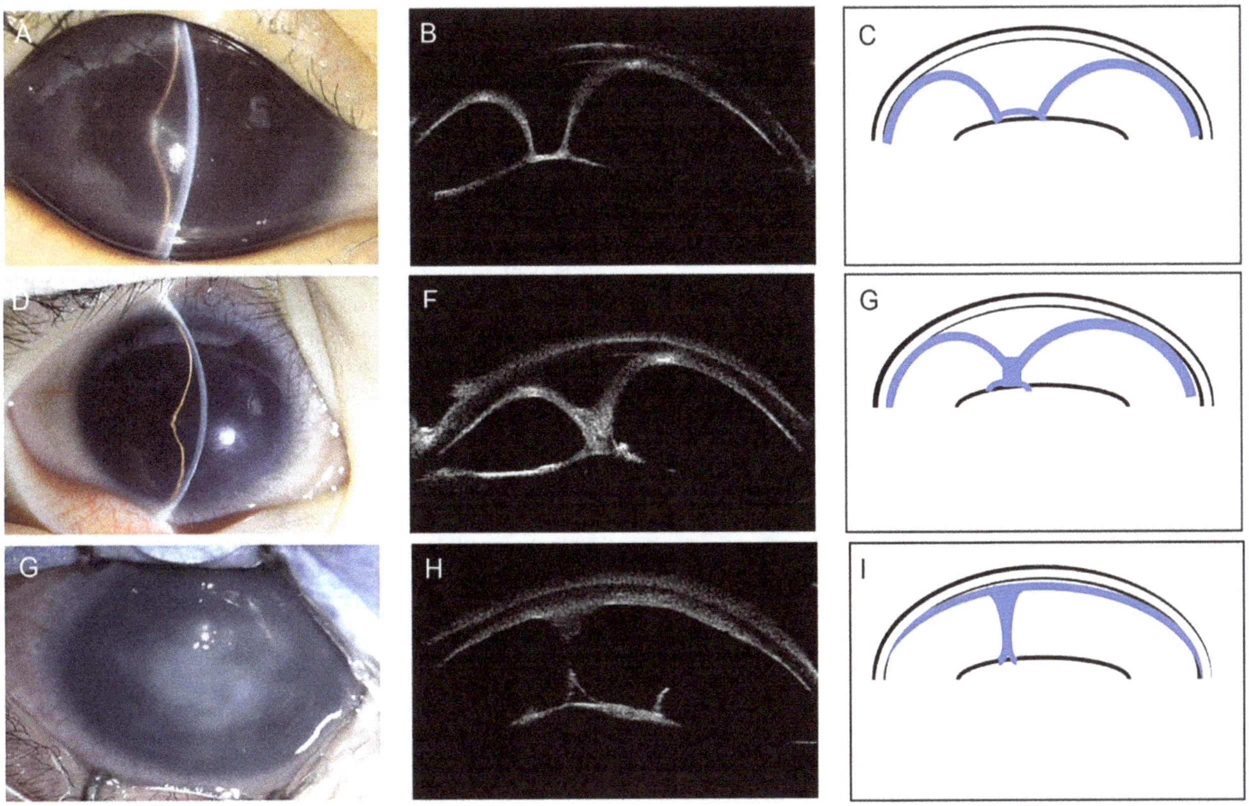

FIGURE 1 | Anterior segment photography, corresponding ultrasound biomicroscopy (UBM) images, and schematic illustrations demonstrating the three different types of congenital fibrovascular pupillary membrane-induced secondary glaucoma (CFPMSG). **(A–C)** Type I CFPMSG: "U"-shape configuration of iris, with complete pupillary obstruction with a fibrovascular membrane and iris bombé with peripheral anterior synechiae, but some central anterior chamber depth. **(D–F)** Type II CFPMSG: "Y"-shape configuration of iris with more severe iris bombé and peripheral anterior synechiae and central iris adhesion to the fibrotic membrane. **(G–I)** Type III CFPMSG: absent anterior chamber depth detectable, manifested as complete iris-cornea contact.

surface of the lens. In this group, the median age at referral was 4 months with moderate IOP elevation.

Type II ("Y" shape) was found in 11 eyes (34%). It was characterized by more severe iris bombé with fibrotic adhesions not only between the iris and lens but also between the elevated portions of the iris blocking the pupil. The thick hyperreflective membrane in this type is larger with iris-iris adhesion. The median age at referral was 4.7 months. The IOP detected at the referral of type II eyes was significantly higher than type I eyes ($P = 0.002$) and ACD was shallower than type I ($P = 0.045$).

Type III [absent anterior chamber (AC)] was found in four eyes (13%). It was characterized by the complete absence of the anterior chamber due to total iridocorneal opposition. Some strands of the iris can be seen connected to the membrane on the anterior surface of the lens. The median age at referral was 7.0 months. Mean IOP was significantly higher than that of type I eyes ($P = 0.008$), but not type II eyes ($P = 0.654$). ACD was shallower than type I ($P < 0.001$) and type II ($P = 0.006$).

We also compared other clinical characteristics, including AL, HCD, and CCT between types and found no significant difference ($P = 0.350$, 0.614, and 0.648, respectively). There were more eyes with glaucomatous optic neuropathy in type III, though this did not achieve statistical significance ($P = 0.353$).

Case Report

One patient presented with an interesting clinical course worth highlighting given progression to secondary glaucoma within 3 weeks (**Figure 2**). Her mother noted a cloudy pupil in the left eye at birth. On the first examination at 3 months of age, the IOP was 11 mmHg in the right eye and 12 mmHg in the left eye. The slit-lamp examination showed a slightly larger pupil on the left associated with a white vascular band partially adherent to the inferior border of the pupil. Mild segmental iris bombé was found, but the central and peripheral ACD was still detectable with ACD of 3.5 corneal thickness. Dilated fundus examination was not possible due to the pupillary membrane, but the B-scan showed no optic nerve damage. Three weeks later, the examination was notable for increased IOP in the left eye (11.5 mmHg right eye and 23.8 mmHg left eye) and severe corneal edema. The central AC depth was 1.47 mm with peripheral iridocorneal touch. UBM demonstrated complete pupillary obstruction by the membrane adherent to the anterior lens capsule leading to iris bombé and peripheral anterior synechiae, consistent with type I CFPMSG. B-scan ultrasound demonstrated optic nerve cupping on the left and there was AL asymmetry (19.82 mm right eye and 21.49 mm left eye).

TABLE 3 | Comparison between different configurations of congenital fibrous pupillary membrane-induced secondary glaucoma.

Variables	Type I, "U" shape ($n = 17$)	Type II, "Y" shape ($n = 11$)	Type III, absent AC ($n = 4$)	*P*-values
Age at first presentation, months				
Median (range)	0 (0–24.0)	0 (0–7.0)	1.3 (0–5.0)	0.685
Age at glaucoma onset, months				
Median (range)	2.0 (0–24.0)	3.0 (0–7.0)	3.5 (1.5–7.0)	0.972
Age at referral, months				
Median (range)	4.0 (1.0–24.0)	4.7 (2.5–9.0)	7.0 (2.0–8.0)	0.966
IOP, mmHg				
Mean (SD)	26.5(5.1)	33.8(5.9)	35.2(5.9)	**0.002[a]**/ 0.654[b]/ **0.008[c]**
HCD, mm				
Mean (SD)	12.3(1.0)	12.1(0.8)	12.6(0.8)	0.63
AL, mm				
Mean (SD)	22.3(1.8)	23.3(1.8)	23.1(1.5)	0.35
CCT, μm				
Mean (SD)	628.1(79.9)	611.8(140.1)	700.0(144.2)	0.648
ACD, mm				
Mean (SD)	1.97(0.92)	1.34(0.62)	0	**0.045[a]/ 0.006[b]/ <0.001[c]**
Optic nerve cupping, n (%)	11(64.7%)	7(63.6%)	4(100%)	0.353

ACD, anterior chamber depth; AL, axial length; CCT, central corneal thickness; HCD, horizontal corneal diameter; IOP, intraocular pressure; mmHg, millimeters of mercury. ANOVA was used for continuous variables. The Pearson's chi-squared test and the Fisher's exact test were used for the categoric variables.

[a]Comparison between type II and type I.

[b]Comparison between type III and type II.

[c]Comparison between type III and type I.

P-values with statistical significance (<0.05) are highlighted in bold.

DISCUSSION

In this study, we summarize the clinical characteristics and propose a novel classification system of CFPMSG base on UBM images of 32 subjects: the largest series of this rare condition published to date. Overall, the clinical presentation (early-onset ocular hypertension, corneal enlargement and edema, AL elongation, and optic nerve cupping) was consistent with total pupillary blockage in the setting of the fibrotic membrane. UBM images confirmed obstruction of aqueous flow from the posterior chamber to the anterior chamber resulting in iris bombé and angle-closure glaucoma.

Secondary glaucoma is seen in CFPM often presents at an early age (12), and in our cohort, onset was between birth and 2 years of age with a median of 3 months. This early onset is consistent with prior reports of this condition, emphasizing the importance of early referral to a specialist. This early onset also supports prior suppositions that the pathophysiology likely occurs during embryogenesis. Unlike a similar condition, persistent pupillary membrane, which is thought to be a static condition, we found evidence of post-natal progression with CFPM. The normal anterior chamber angle continues to develop post-natally, which may explain the post-natal changes we observed in CFPM, such as the patient with no signs of glaucoma at 3 months of age who progressed to have iris bombe 1 month later. Enlargement and thickening of pupil-iris membrane led to pupil block and iris bombé, peripheral anterior synechia, and vision-threatening acute angle-closure glaucoma. Our study elucidated that the age at onset of glaucoma was around 1 month later than the age at presentation. In one of our cases (**Figure 2**), we also found the sudden elevation of IOP due to the seclusion of the pupil by the fibrovascular membrane. For this reason, close follow-up on patients with fibrotic pupillary membranes is recommended to monitor for the development of secondary glaucoma.

Given the rarity of this condition and a small number of reported cases, the incidence of secondary glaucoma is unknown. Due to our inclusion criteria, all of our CFPM cases had glaucoma. Of the cases of this condition previously published (**Table 4**), seven patients had glaucoma (4, 12–15). Given this and the secondary corneal edema associated with glaucoma, UBM is

TABLE 4 | Summary of previous cases reports of the congenital fibrovascular pupillary membrane.

No.	Author	Year	Cases	Secondary glaucoma	Age at glaucoma onset	IOP at glaucoma onset (mmHg)
1	T. Avitabile et al.	2000	1	1	14 months	25
2	Richard M. Robb	2001	7	1	4.5 months	32
3	Gerhard W. Cibis	2004	9	3	7 days	45
					14 days	40
					2 months	40
4	Alexander Demidenko et al.	2009	1	1	3 days	45
5	Michiko Kandori et al.	2010	1	1	6 months	60

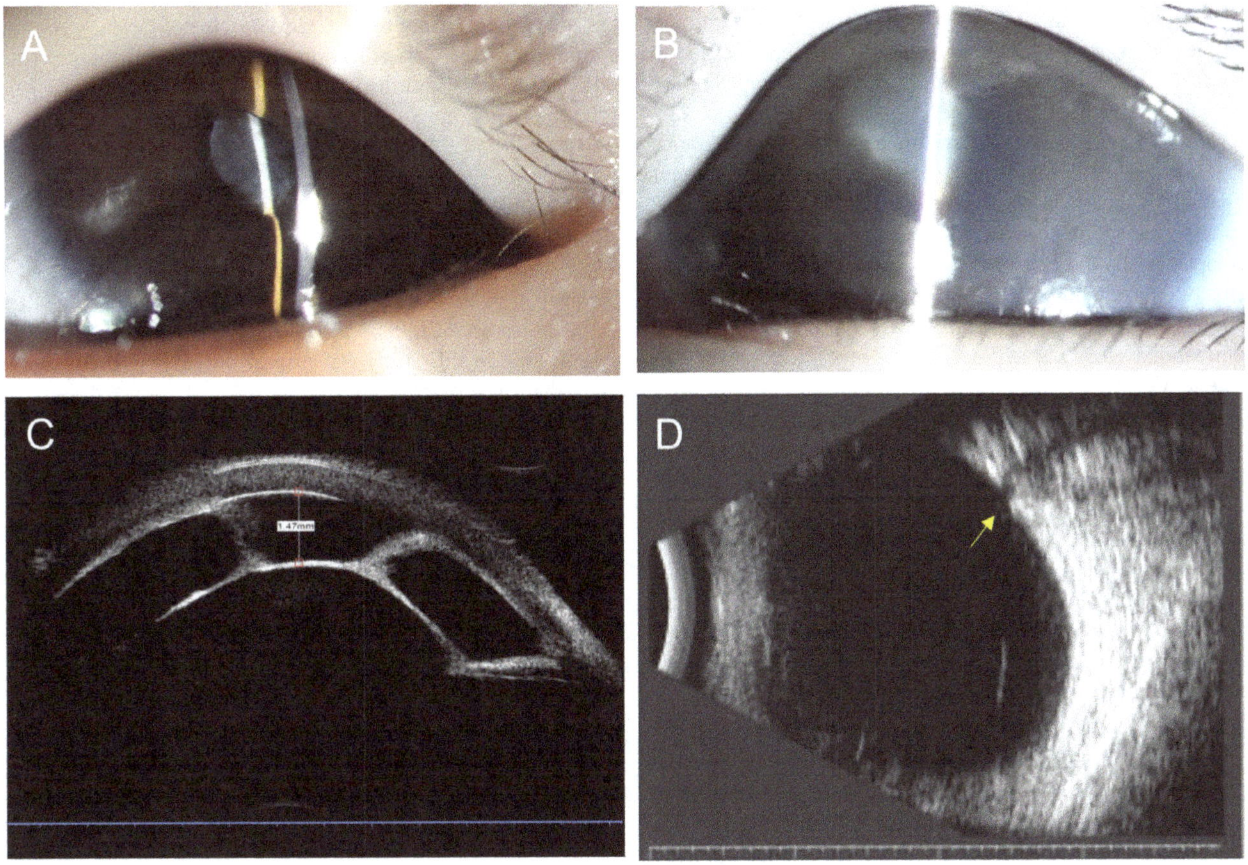

FIGURE 2 | Anterior segment photography, ultrasound biomicroscopy (UBM), and B-scan ultrasonography of a 4-month-old child with congenital fibrous pupillary membrane-induced secondary glaucoma. **(A)** Anterior segment photograph at 3 months of age showing a clear cornea and normal central and peripheral anterior chamber depth. The pupil is covered by a white vascularized membrane with a few areas of posterior synechiae. **(B)** Anterior segment photograph at 4 months of age showing moderate corneal edema, iris bombé with the very shallow peripheral anterior chamber, and posterior synechiae covering 360 degrees of the pupil. **(C)** UBM demonstrates a fibrous membrane adherent to the anterior lens capsule covering the entire pupil leading to iris bombé and peripheral anterior synechiae. Central anterior depth measured 1.47 mm. **(D)** B-scan ultrasound image demonstrates significant cupping of the optic nerve as the yellow arrow shown.

a useful adjunct in the identification and classification of anterior chamber involvement. As the UBM exam showed, there was no marked inflammatory activity. Therefore, we excluded the diagnosis of uveitis. UBM can be used to closely document and monitor abnormal attachments between the membrane and the iris, changes in ACD, membrane contracture, and malposition of the lens and ciliary processes (13).

With UBM, we created a classification system based on the three phenotypes identified in our cohort. The majority of patients were in type I ("U" shape). The second most common was in type II ("Y" shape). The rarest and most severe type was type III (absent AC). Children with different UBM types of CFPMSG demonstrated different clinical characteristics. IOP was significantly higher in both types II and III patients than in type I patients and the ACD became shallower from type I to III, due to more severe manifestation of pupil block and iris bombé. In our cases, patients with type III were referred at a later age and presented with the most severe situation of secondary glaucoma. This partially demonstrated the severity increased with the duration of onset.

We found thickening of CCT in all three types of eyes, which may suggest the possibility of cornea decompensation even in a mild form of CFPMSG and close follow-up on corneal condition is important. Progression of CFPMSG from type I to III may occur with a more convex shape of iris and further shallowing of central anterior chamber subsequently leading to elevated IOP and optic nerve cupping. We also found the onset of secondary glaucoma at a younger age will be vulnerable to cornea enlargement and AL elongation. Therefore, it is necessary to have an early and close UBM follow-up for patients with CFPMSG to detect AC changes and disease progression.

Various treatment approaches for CFPM have been described. For patients without signs of secondary glaucoma, observation with or without adjuvant amblyopia treatment may be suitable for patients with normal IOP, deep anterior chamber, and sufficient pupillary opening. In cases with progressive growth and adhesion of the pupillary membrane which leads to microcoria and coretopia, timely membrane removal and separation, iridectomy, and anterior chamber reformation are required for preventing poor visual outcome (4, 16, 17). In eyes with secondary glaucoma, surgical excision of the membrane is the recommended treatment. For patients with iris bombé and extensive posterior synechiae, peripheral iridectomy, synechiolysis, goniosynechialysis, and pupilloplasty should all be considered dependent on the extent of the membrane (1, 4, 12). Since early detection facilitated early treatment, early surgical treatment is also recommended for preventing progressive and pathologic changes of CFPMSG.

There were several limitations to this study. First, given the rarity of this condition, only 32 cases are included, and another study is warranted to validate and confirm the clinical significance of the proposed classification system. Second, most of the enrolled subjects were younger than 1 year old, limiting visual acuity outcomes. Finally, the ages at which parents first noted symptoms were subjective and susceptible to recall bias and mild inaccuracy.

In conclusion, we describe the largest group of children with CFPMSG and presented a novel classification system based on UBM findings. Secondary glaucoma in this condition is due to pupillary block and angle-closure and requires surgical intervention. Unlike other congenital pupillary abnormalities, CFPMSG may be a progressive condition. UBM classification provides new insight into the diagnosis and monitoring of CFPMSG and may play a role in treatment planning.

ETHICS STATEMENT

The studies involving human participants were reviewed and approved by Zhongshan Ophthalmic Center Institution Review and Ethics Board (2020KYPJ121). Written informed consent to participate in this study was provided by the participants' legal guardian/next of kin.

AUTHOR CONTRIBUTIONS

XL contributed to study decisions and clinical supervision. YTZ and LF were responsible for records review, data analysis, and manuscript writing. YMZ, JO, and YH contributed to data analysis and manuscript revision. SL, LC, XZ, YS, and PL contribute to ophthalmic examination and data record. All authors contributed to the article and approved the submitted version.

REFERENCES

1. Cibis GW, Waeltermann JM, Hurst E, Tripathi RC, Richardson W. Congenital pupillary-iris-lens membrane with goniodysgenesis. *Ophthalmology.* (1986) 93:847–52. doi: 10.1016/S0161-6420(86)33659-5
2. Cibis GW TR, Tripathi BJ. Surgical removal of congenital pupillary-Iris-lens membrane. *Ophthalmic Surg Lasers.* (1994) 259:580–3. doi: 10.3928/1542-8877-19940901-06
3. Lambert SR, Buckley EG, Lenhart PD, Zhang Q, Grossniklaus HE. Congenital fibrovascular pupillary membranes: clinical and histopathologic findings. *Ophthalmology.* (2012) 119:634–41. doi: 10.1016/j.ophtha.2011.08.043
4. Cibis GW, Walton DS. Congenital pupillary-iris-lens membrane with goniodysgenesis. *J AAPOS.* (2004) 8:378–83. doi: 10.1016/j.jaapos.2004.04.010
5. Lambert SR AL, Taylor D. Congenital idiopathic microcoria. *Am J Ophthalmol.* (1988) 1065:590–4. doi: 10.1016/0002-9394(88)90592-2
6. Chu ER, Taranath DA. Another case of congenital pupillary-iris-lens membrane with goniodysgenesis. *J Pediatr Ophthalmol Strabismus.* (2010) 47:e1–3. doi: 10.3928/01913913-20100510-01
7. Deshpande N SS, Krishnadas SR. Pupillary-iris-lens membrane with goniodysgenesis: a case report. *Indian J Ophthalmol.* (2006) 544:275–6. doi: 10.4103/0301-4738.27957
8. Liang TW, Zhang CY, Bai DY, Peng CX, Bai XQ, Wu Q, et al. Clinical characteristics and treatment of congenital fibrovascular pupillary membranes. *Zhonghua Yan Ke Za Zhi.* (2018) 54:849–54. doi: 10.3760/cma.j.issn.0412-4081.2018.11.010
9. Temkar S, Gupta S, Sihota R, Sharma R, Angmo D, Pujari A, et al. Illuminated microcatheter circumferential trabeculotomy versus combined trabeculotomy-trabeculectomy for primary congenital glaucoma: a randomized controlled trial. *Am J Ophthalmol.* (2015) 159:490–7.e2. doi: 10.1016/j.ajo.2014.12.001
10. Tongu MTS, Borges MJH, Giovedi MRA, Cohen R, Almeida GV. Reliability of echographic examination for the study of optic nerve cupping. *Arquivos Brasileiros de Oftalmologia.* (1999) 62:265–8. doi: 10.5935/0004-2749.19990010
11. Roberto Sampaolesi RC. Ocular echometry in the diagnosis of congenital glaucoma. *Arch ophthalmol.* (1982) 100:574–7. doi: 10.1001/archopht.1982.01030030576003
12. RM R. Fibrous congenital iris membranes with pupillary distortion. *Trans Am Ophthalmol Soc.* (2001) 99:45–51.
13. Avitabile T, Castiglione E, Marano E, Reibaldi M. Congenital pupillary-iris-lens membrane with goniodysgenesis: clinical history and ultrabiomicroscopic findings. *J Pediatr Ophthalmol Strabismus.* (2002) 394:248–50. doi: 10.3928/0191-3913-20020701-17
14. Demidenko A, Jakobiec FA, Hanna E, Walton DS. Congenital pupillary-iris-lens membrane with goniodysgenesis: histopathologic findings in an enucleated eye. *J Pediatr Ophthalmol Strabismus.* (2010) 47:178–82. doi: 10.3928/01913913-20100505-09
15. Kandori M, Saishin Y, Kusaka S, Shimojyo H, Otori Y, Tano Y. Pupilloplasty for congenital pupillary-iris-lens membrane with 25-gauge vitreous cutter. *Acta Ophthalmol.* (2010) 88:e289–90. doi: 10.1111/j.1755-3768.2009.01698.x
16. Wang Q, Zhou F, Chen W, Chen J, Ouyang Z, Lin Z, et al. A safe treatment for congenital fibrovascular pupillary membrane. *Eur J Ophthalmol.* (2020) 305:1143–8. doi: 10.1177/1120672119859666
17. Demidenko A JF, Hanna E, Walton DS. Congenital pupillary-iris-lens membrane with goniodysgenesis: a rare cause of glaucoma and vision loss. *Int Ophthalmol Clin.* (2009) 491:83–8. doi: 10.1097/IIO.0b013e318192442b

4

Vascular Abnormalities in Peripapillary and Macular Regions of Behcet's Uveitis Patients Evaluated by Optical Coherence Tomography Angiography

Chun Yan[1†], *Fan Li*[1†], *Min Hou*[2†], *Xiaoyuan Ye*[1], *Lishi Su*[1], *Yixin Hu*[1], *Jiawen Luo*[1] and *Wei Chi*[1*]

[1] State Key Laboratory of Ophthalmology, Zhongshan Ophthalmic Center, Sun Yat-sen University, Guangzhou, China,
[2] Department of Ophthalmology, Luoyang Central Hospital, Zhengzhou University, Luoyang, China

***Correspondence:**
Wei Chi
chiwei@mail.sysu.edu.cn

†These authors have contributed equally to this work

Purpose: To investigate the involvement of peripapillary zone vascular abnormalities in Behcet's uveitis (BU) and associated visual dysfunction. We evaluated the retinal and choroidal microvascular features in both macular and peripapillary areas of BU patients to identify vascular abnormalities contributing to reduced best-corrected visual acuity (BCVA) using optical coherence tomography angiography (OCTA).

Methods: A prospective, observational study was conducted in 24 eyes of 13 patients with BU and 24 eyes of 15 healthy participants as controls. They received a standard eye examination and were recorded by OCTA measurements of macular and peripapillary areas. The vascular densities of superficial capillary plexus (SCP) and deep capillary plexus (DCP), choroidal flow area, radial peripapillary capillary network (RPCN) density, foveal avascular zone (FAZ) area and perimeter, full retinal thickness (FRT), and peripapillary retinal nerve fiber layer thickness (pRNFLT) were measured.Correlations among microvascular, structural, and functional changes were assessed.

Results: Our findings uncovered that the vascular density was significantly reduced in the peripapillary zone of BU eyes compared to healthy eyes, especially in the inferior subfield of the RPCN. The vascular densities of SCP and DCP quadrants within the macular zone had no significant difference between BU and control groups except for DCP density of the nasal parafoveal quadrant. Both FAZ area and perimeter were greater but without statistical significance in the BU group. Compared to healthy eyes, the choriocapillaris flow area was smaller while the FRT and pRNFLT were greater in the BU group. Notably, there was a significant correlation between the reduction in RPCN vascular density and decreased BCVA in BU patients.

Conclusion: Based on OCTA, vascular changes associated with BU are more prominent in the peripapillary zone than those in the macular zone. The vascular density of the RPCN could serve as a sensitive indicator to monitoring BU pathogenic progression and treatment response using a non-invasively method of OCTA.

Keywords: Behcet's disease, retinal microstructure, optical coherence tomography angiography (OCTA), Behcet's uveitis, vasculitis

INTRODUCTION

Behcet's disease (BD) is a multisystem immune-mediated disorder manifested by recurrent uveitis (Behcet's uveitis, BU), oral or genital ulcers, and skin lesions (1–3). BD has a worldwide distribution (4), and over two-thirds of BD cases present with bilateral recurrent uveitis and stubborn retinal microvasculitis (5–7). BU is one of the most stubborn and refractory uveitis entity in the worldwide, leading to severe vision loss.

Fluorescein angiography (FA) can detect both the leaky and the occlusive nature of retinal vasculitis in BU (6). However, the invasiveness (8) and time consuming restrict the application of FA in long-term follow-ups of BU patients. Moreover, FA cannot visualize multiple layers of the retinal vasculature separately or resolve radial peripapillary and deep capillary networks clearly (9). In comparison, OCTA is a non-invasive and transformative imaging technique that can quantify the retinal and disc microcirculation rapidly and accurately down to the capillary level (10). Furthermore, OCTA can reveal the retinal vascular structure layer by layer, which provides micromesh information about structural damage (11). Combined with structural optical coherence tomography (12), OCTA enables a more comprehensive understanding of vascular abnormalities in some eye diseases, including diabetic retinopathy (13), glaucoma (14, 15), age-related macular degeneration (16), retinal vein obstruction (17, 18), and Vogt-Koyanagi-Harada disease (19).

Previous OCTA studies have revealed macular vascular abnormalities in BU patients, including perifoveal capillary disorders (20, 21), reduced vascular density (22). However, no reports have been made on performing peripapillary analyses of patients with BU using OCTA, so the associations between OCTA-based peripapillary zone abnormalities and visual dysfunction remain unclear. We aim to comprehensively analyze vascular and structural changes in the macular and peripapillary zones of BU patients using OCTA and to examine the associations with best-corrected visual acuity (BCVA) deficits.

In the present study, we disclosed a significant decrease in vascular density within the peripapillary region of BU patients compared to healthy subjects. Further, BCVA was positively correlated with vascular density in the peripapillary region, suggesting that the density of radial peripapillary capillaries may be a novel indicator for disease progression and prognosis among BU patients.

MATERIALS AND METHODS

Study Design and Ethical Approval

This cross-sectional comparative study was approved by the Ethics Committee of Zhongshan Ophthalmic Center (Guangzhou, China 2019KYPJ127) and conducted in compliance with the principles of the Declaration of Helsinki. Informed consent was obtained from each participant prior to enrollment.

Study Subjects

Inclusion criteria were patients fulfilling the diagnostic criteria for BU developed by the International Study Group for Behcet's Disease (ISGBD) (23)and presenting with posterior uveitis or panuveitis characterized by retinal vasculitis and manifestations of optic nerve and/or macular inflammation. Investigational work-ups (e.g., serological testing for syphilis, chest x-ray, tuberculin skin test, and anterior chamber tap for viral polymerase chain reaction) were performed in selected cases to rule out conditions mimicking BU. Patients with other retinal and/or optic nerve diseases or who underwent intraocular surgery other than for uncomplicated cataract were excluded. Age- and sex-matched healthy individuals were recruited as a control group. Poor quality OCTA images resulting from media opacities, eye movements, or incorrect auto-segmentation were also excluded from further analysis.

All patients received detailed ophthalmic examinations, including the assessment of BCVA, slit-lamp biomicroscopy, intraocular pressure assessment, and dilated fundus examination. Color fundus photography and FA were also performed, followed by OCTA scan (Optovue Inc., Fremont, CA, USA).

Layer and Sector Segmentation in OCTA

En-face OCTA slabs of the superficial capillary plexus (SCP), deep capillary plexus (DCP), choriocapillaris, and retinal layers within the macular zone, and the radial peripapillary capillary network (RPCN) within the peripapillary zone were automatically segmented by the built-in software AngioVue (Software Version 2017.1, RTVue XR Avanti, AngioVue). The software automatically divided the peripapillary and macular (parafovea and perifovea) regions into four sectors (temporal, superior, nasal, and inferior) for quadrant analysis and two hemispheres (superior-hemi and inferior-hemi) defined by a horizontal line drawn through the disc or foveal center. The diagrams of layer and sector segmentation within macular and peripapillary regions are displayed in **Figures 1, 2**.

Macular Parameter Measurements

A 6.0 × 6.0-mm macular cube OCTA scan centered on the fovea was acquired to obtain the following parameters: (1) vascular densities of SCP and DCP (defined as % areas occupied) in separate sectors of the macular region; (2) vascular flow area in the choriocapillaris, calculated within a 1-mm radius circle centered on the fovea; (3) foveal avascular zone (FAZ) parameters, including FAZ area and perimeter, quantified in the retina slab extending from the inner limiting membrane (ILM) to the outer plexiform layer (OPL); (4) full retinal thickness (FRT), which was set to incorporate the slab from the ILM to the retinal pigment epithelium (RPE) and was generated from different subfields of the macular region.

Peripapillary Parameter Measurements

Each studied eye underwent a 4.5 × 4.5-mm cube OCTA scan centered on the optic disc. The parameters measured in the peripapillary zone included (1) radial peripapillary capillary network (RPCN) vascular densities (exclusive of large vessels) and (2) peripapillary retinal nerve fiber layer thickness (pRNFLT)

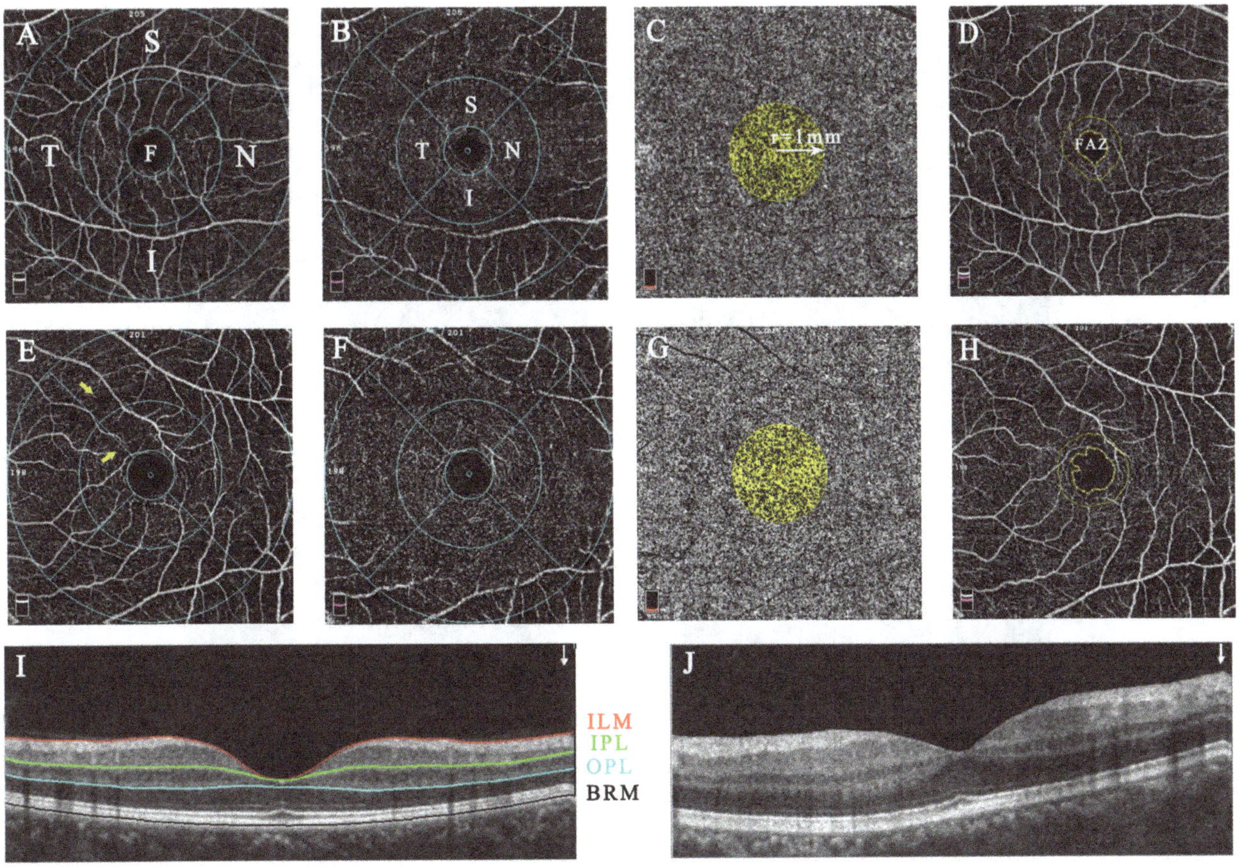

FIGURE 1 | The representative macular image diagram of layer and sector segmentation and vascular parameter measurements in healthy **(A–D,I)** and Behcet's uveitis subjects **(E–H,J).** The images were acquired within a 6.0 × 6.0-mm macular cube scan centered on the fovea in 4 default en-face slabs: the SCP (ILM to IPL; **A,E**), the DCP (IPL to OPL; **B,F**), the CC (BRM to BRM+30 μm; **C,G**), and the retina slab (ILM to OPL; **D,H**). B-scan image shows the place of segmentation **(I,J).** The SCP and DCP layers were overlaid by the ETDRS grid comprised of 3 concentric rings of 1, 3, and 6-mm diameter; The fovea, parafovea, and perifovea were defined as the inner circle, medial annulus, and outer annulus, respectively. The vascular density was automatically measured in different subfields of SCP and DCP **(A,B,E,F).** The CC flow area was calculated within a 1-mm radius circle centered at the fovea **(C,G)**. The FAZ area and perimeter were quantified basing on the retina slab, and automated FAZ boundary detection was performed by the AngioVue software **(D,H)**. Capillary arcade disruptions with rarefaction of vessels (yellow arrow) were present in the temporal and superior sectors of the BU patient. F, fovea; S, superior; T, temporal; I, inferior; N, nasal; SCP, superficial capillary plexus; ILM, inner limiting membrane; IPL, inner plexiform layer; OPL, outer plexiform layer; CC, choriocapillaris; BRM, Bruch's membrane; DCP, deep capillary plexus; ETDRS, the Early Treatment Diabetic Retinopathy Study; FAZ, foveal avascular zone.

calculated from the ILM to the nerve fiber layer (NFL) across different peripapillary sectors.

Statistical Analyses

Statistical analyses were performed using SPSS version 24 (SPSS Inc., Chicago, IL). All quantitative data are presented as mean ± standard deviation (SD). Conformity to the normal distribution was tested using the Shapiro–Wilk procedure. Independent samples *t*-test was used to compare normally distributed data and Mann-Whitney U test to compare non-normally distributed data. Pearson χ^2 test was used to compare categorical variables. Pearson's correlation analyses were performed among log MAR BCVA, peripapillary parameters, and macular parameters. A *P* value < 0.05 (two-tailed) was considered statistically significant for all tests.

RESULTS

Demographic Summary

Thirteen BU patients and 15 healthy participants were enrolled in this study at the Zhongshan Ophthalmic Center, Sun Yat-Sen University, China, between July 2019 and October 2019. Demographic data and clinical details are summarized in **Table 1**. There were no significant differences in mean age or sex ratio between groups. In the BU group, two eyes were excluded from analysis due to poor-quality images. Among included patients (mean age 32.9 ± 15.2 years, range 14–56 years), ocular involvement was bilateral in 12 cases (92.3%) and unilateral in one (7.7%). The log MAR BCVA ranged from 0 to 1.70 and the mean was 0.87 ± 0.62.

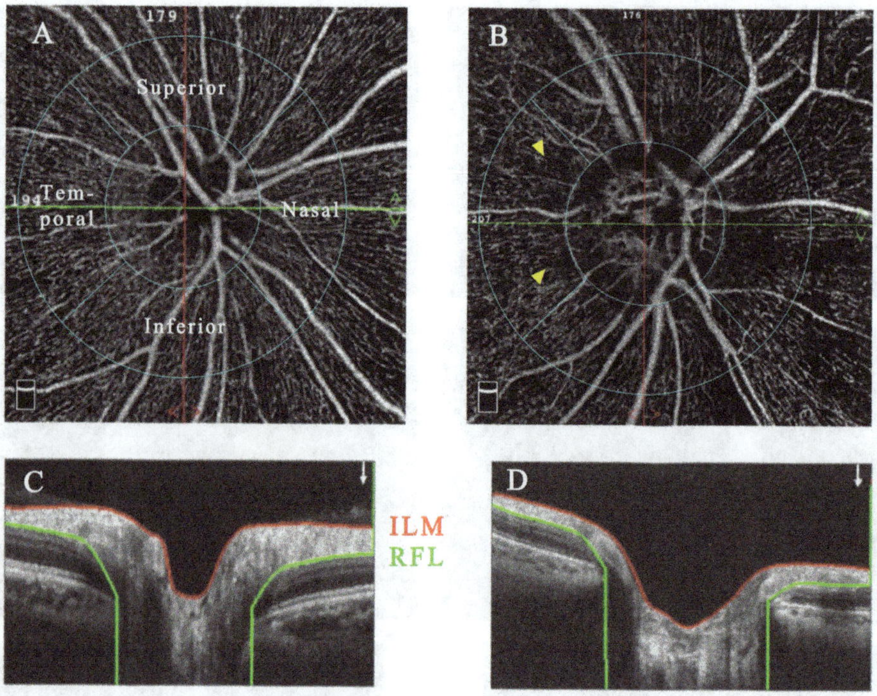

FIGURE 2 | The representative RPCN OCTA images with accompanying B-scan images of healthy **(A,C)** and Behcet's uveitis eyes **(B,D)**. RPCN images were acquired between the ILM and NFL within a 4.5 × 4.5-mm cube scan centered on the optic disc. The peripapillary region was an annular area with 1-mm-width, and the inner concentric ring was defined by the disc boundary. Grayish areas of capillary non-perfusion/hypoperfusion were observed in OCTA images of a Behcet's uveitis patient (yellow arrowhead). OCTA, optical coherence tomography angiography; RPCN, radial peripapillary capillary network; NFL, nerve fiber layer.

TABLE 1 | Characteristics of BU Patients and Normal Controls.

Characteristics	BU	Normal	*P value*
Subjects (eyes)	13 (24)	15 (24)	
Gender, male (ratio)	7 (53.8%)	5 (33.3%)	0.149
Age, years (range)	32.9 ± 15.2 (14–56)	38.5 ± 12.4 (19–58)	0.257
Laterality			
Unilateral (ratio)	12 (92.3%)	NA	
Bilateral (ratio)	1 (7.7%)	NA	
log MAR BCVA	0.87 ± 0.62	NA	

BU, Behcet's uveitis; log MAR, logarithm of the minimum angle resolution; BCVA, best-corrected visual acuity.

Macular Microcirculation Parameters

The microcirculation analyses of the macular region for BU and healthy eyes are summarized in **Table 2**. The flow area in the choriocapillaris was dramatically lower in BU eyes than controls ($P = 0.009$). The vascular densities of both SCP and DCP within the macular region did not differ significantly between BU and healthy eyes, except in the nasal parafoveal quadrant of the DCP ($P = 0.048$, **Supplementary Table 1**), whereas qualitative vascular abnormalities were presented in the SCP of BU patients (**Figure 1**). Both FAZ area and perimeter were identifiably greater in the BU group, but without significance compared to healthy controls.

TABLE 2 | Comparison of FAZ Parameters, Flow Area and Vascular Densities between BU and Normal Eyes.

Variables	BU	Normal	*P value*
Flow area-Choriocapillaris (mm^2, at 1 mm radius)	1.91 ± 0.24	2.37 ± 0.13	0.007**
FAZ area (mm^2)	0.99 ± 2.07	0.38 ± 0.25	0.629
FAZ perimeter (mm)	3.52 ± 4.04	2.19 ± 0.30	0.959
Vascular density-SCP (%)			
Whole image	45.81 ± 5.12	45.07 ± 4.07	0.618
Fovea	23.26 ± 15.58	17.81 ± 6.57	0.133
Parafovea	42.41 ± 6.02	44.34 ± 5.77	0.301
Perifovea	47.75 ± 6.55	46.04 ± 4.15	0.326
Vascular density-DCP (%)			
Whole image	44.41 ± 7.41	44.16 ± 7.48	0.912
Fovea	33.26 ± 16.45	31.79 ± 10.46	0.741
Parafovea	45.89 ± 8.97	50.79 ± 7.72	0.070
Perifovea	46.38 ± 7.79	44.93 ± 8.12	0.563

*FAZ, foveal avascular zone; BU, Behcet's uveitis; SCP, superficial capillary plexus; DCP, deep capillary plexus. All data are presented as Mean ± SD. **p < 0.01.*

RPCN Vessel Parameters

The RPCN vessel parameters measured from BU and healthy eyes are summarized in **Table 3**. The RPCN vascular densities were significantly lower in BU eyes compared to healthy eyes

TABLE 3 | Comparison of Vascular Density in the RPCN between BU and Normal Eyes.

Variables	BU	Normal	*P value*
Peripapillary	48.54 ± 3.66	51.66 ± 5.06	0.005**
Superior hemi	48.84 ± 4.49	51.97 ± 5.57	0.004**
Inferior hemi	48.15 ± 3.54	51.35 ± 4.92	0.031*
Inferior	47.70 ± 5.19	54.12 ± 5.80	0.000**
Superior	47.87 ± 6.05	53.12 ± 5.77	0.002**
Temporal	53.70 ± 5.04	52.13 ± 8.69	0.947
Nasal	44.91 ± 4.20	48.45 ± 4.03	0.004**

*RPCN, radial peripapillary capillary network; BU, Behcet's uveitis. All data are presented as Mean ± SD. *p < 0.05. **p < 0.01.*

TABLE 4 | Comparison of FRT and pRNFLT Measurements Evaluated between BU and Normal Eyes.

Variables	BU	Normal	*P value*
FRT (μm)			
Whole image	338.25 ± 56.90	290.17 ± 18.46	0.001**
Superior-hemi	338.33 ± 58.55	293.67 ± 16.78	0.001**
Inferior-hemi	337.83 ± 56.98	286.78 ± 20.17	0.000**
Fovea	334.83 ± 155.48	236.17 ± 28.37	0.005**
Parafovea	377.04 ± 87.33	322.50 ± 14.50	0.006**
Perifovea	338.67 ± 54.64	290.39 ± 20.30	0.000**
pRNFLT (μm)			
Peripapillary	154.48 ± 62.73	116.63 ± 12.37	0.009**
Superior-hemi	152.09 ± 56.19	117.71 ± 12.68	0.010*
Inferior-hemi	151.65 ± 70.71	115.42 ± 13.40	0.024*
Inferior	189.00 ± 86.73	144.17 ± 19.48	0.034*
Superior	183.26 ± 76.36	139.75 ± 17.34	0.013*
Temporal	123.09 ± 42.97	82.48 ± 15.84	0.000**
Nasal	139.00 ± 88.78	103.67 ± 19.98	0.075

*FRT, full retinal thickness; pRNFLT, peripapillary retinal nerve fiber layer thickness; BU, Behcet's uveitis. All data are presented as Mean ± SD. *p < 0.05. **p < 0.01.*

in all sectors ($P < 0.05$) except for the temporal quadrant ($P = 0.947$). Qualitative vascular abnormalities were also observed in the peripapillary region of BU eyes (**Figure 2**).

FRT and pRNFLT Parameters

The OCTA findings of FRT and pRNFLT parameters in BU and healthy eyes are summarized in **Table 4**. The FRT values in the different sectors within the macular region were significantly greater in BU patients than healthy subjects ($P < 0.05$), the more subtly separated analysis of FRT listed in **Supplementary Table 2**. Similar tendencies were also detected in the pRNFLT, with significantly higher values in all sectors of BU patients compared to controls ($P < 0.05$) with the exception of the nasal quadrant ($P = 0.075$).

Correlations Among Parameters

We first analyzed the correlation between OCTA-based parameters and log MAR BCVA in BU eyes. While there were no correlations between log MAR BCVA and macular parameters (including FAZ area, FAZ perimeter, FRT, choriocapillaris flow area, SCP density, and DCP density), RPCN vascular density was negatively correlated with log MAR BCVA ($r = -0.692$, $p = 0.013$). The pRNFLT showed no significant correlation with BCVA. Pearson correlation coefficients and corresponding P values are listed in **Table 5, Supplementary Table 3.**

The results of correlation analysis between peripapillary and parafoveal vascular densities in BU patients are summarized in **Table 6**, which reveals a positive association of vascular density between the temporal quadrant of the RPCN and the nasal quadrant of both the parafoveal DCP ($r = 0.490$, $p = 0.018$) and SCP ($r = 0.309$, $p = 0.023$). Across the entire region, however, there were no significant correlations between parafoveal vascular densities (including the vascular density of the SCP and DCP) and peripapillary vascular density. No attractive correlation was located in vascular densities of fovea and perifovea compared to that of peripapillary region (**Supplementary Table 4**).

Additionally, thicker pRNFLT was correlated with increased FRT in the fovea and parafovea ($r = 0.534$, $P = 0.009$; $r = 0.454$, $P = 0.029$, respectively). In healthy eyes only, there was a positive correlation between RPCN vascular density and pRNFLT ($r = 0.521$, $p = 0.009$). The correlations associated with pRNFLT are summarized in **Table 7**.

DISCUSSION

BU is a potentially blinding disorder characterized by relapsing-remitting panuveitis with retinal vasculitis involving macular and peripapillary vessels. Not only does it cause extensive vascular leakage or arterial occlusion, but it also triggers severe vitreous opacity (24). As prolonged immunomodulatory therapy in a long-time follow-up is essential for the management of BU (25), the non-invasive OCTA is more suitable for observing microvascular changes compared with invasive FA.

The RPCN cannot be visualized by FA. Alternatively, Engelke and colleagues demonstrated that retinal microvascular changes in the peripapillary region can be evaluated successfully using OCTA (26). Previous studies have identified decreased peripapillary vascular density in glaucoma (14, 27) and non-arteritic anterior ischemic optic neuropathy (28) using OCTA. Therefore, we examined the involvement of peripapillary vasculature in BU using OCTA and found reduced RPCN vascular density in multiple sectors compared to controls, highlighting the potential of OCTA for monitoring disease status among BU patients.

Several studies have conducted quantitative and qualitative assessments of macular zone using OCTA. Vascular abnormalities, including macular capillary hypoperfusion, disorganization, and rarefaction were revealed by qualitative assessment in BU patients (20, 21). Consistent with these reports, macular vascular disorders were also presented in our study cohort (**Figure 1**). Previous quantitative analyses of the macular vasculature revealed significant reductions in both SCP and DCP densities among BU patients (22, 29). However, the analysis

TABLE 5 | The Results of Pearson Correlation Analyses between log MAR BCVA and Vascular Densities in BU Group.

Variables	Peripapillary	Fovea		Parafovea		Perifovea	
	RPCN-VD	SCP-VD	DCP-VD	SCP-VD	DCP-VD	SCP-VD	SCP-VD
log MAR BCVA	−0.692 (0.013)*	0.082 (0.789)	−0.258 (0.394)	0.119 (0.698)	−0.286 (0.344)	0.311 (0.301)	−0.253 (0.405)

*BU, Behcet's uveitis; log MAR, logarithm of the minimum angle resolution; RPCN, radial peripapillary capillary network; BCVA, best-corrected visual acuity; SCP, superficial capillary plexus; DCP, deep capillary plexus; VD, vascular density. All data are presented as Pearson correlation coefficients and their corresponding P values. *p < 0.05.*

TABLE 6 | The Results of Pearson Correlation Analyses between RPCN and Parafoveal Vascular Densities in BU Group.

Variables		Parafovea		Nasal quadrant of parafovea	
		SCP-VD	DCP-VD	SCP-VD	DCP-VD
RPCN-VD	Peripapillary	0.180 (0.935)	0.251 (0.249)		
	Peri-temporal			0.309 (0.023)*	0.490 (0.018)*

*BU, Behcet's uveitis; RPCN, radial peripapillary capillary network; SCP, superficial capillary plexus; DCP, deep capillary plexus; VD, vascular density; Peri-temporal, temporal quadrant of peripapillary. All data are presented as Pearson correlation coefficients and their corresponding P values. *p < 0.05.*

TABLE 7 | The Results of Pearson Correlation Analyses between RNFLT and Macular FRT/ RPCN Vascular Density in BU and Normal Eyes.

Variables		FRT-Macular			RPCN-VD-PP
		Fovea	Parafovea	Perifovea	
RNFLT-PP	BU	0.534 (0.009)**	0.454 (0.029)*	0.148 (0.500)	0.252 (0.246)
	Normal	−0.260 (0.297)	0.311 (0.209)	0.063 (0.804)	0.521 (0.009)**

*BU, Behcet's uveitis; RNFLT, retinal nerve fiber layer thickness; PP, peripapillary; FRT, full retinal thickness; RPCN, radial peripapillary capillary network; VD, vascular density. All data are presented as Pearson correlation coefficients and their corresponding P values. *p < 0.05. **p < 0.01.*

was limited in the parafovea and absent in the perifovea. We found no significant differences in macular vascular densities within parafoveal and perifoveal subfields between groups. Thus, the macular vessel involvement in our BU group was insufficient to be statistically differentiated by OCTA, possibly because our study included patients with retinal edema, which can interfere with vascular quantitative assessment. Significant correlations were found between vascular density in the RPCN temporal sector and vascular densities in the nasal parafoveal DCP and SCP, which could result from the specific nasal position of anatomic feature that the optical nerve head is located in the nasal position of in the macula. In addition, we found a significantly reduced choriocapillaris flow area lower in BU patients compared to healthy controls.

The reasonable unifying explanation for the differences in vascular involvement among regions, is that the extent of damage is associated with the vascular structure and susceptibility to ischemia (even though vasculature damages in BU eyes occur across retinal layers). The RPCN may be more prone to ischemic damage because of the correspondingly dense in unmyelinated nerve fibers with high metabolic demands (9). Besides, the RPCN radiates out of the ONH and branches directly from the central retinal artery and the peripapillary area also contains principal intraretinal vessels compared with macular area (9, 30). Hence, the RPCN vascular density could be more vulnerable to flow changes in larger vessels. Further clinical and histopathological examinations are warranted to clarify the regional evolution of vascular deficits during disease progression and associated functional changes.

When sufficient capillary non-perfusion occurs surrounding the fovea in BU patients, the enlargement and irregularity of foveal avascular zone (FAZ) could be detected by OCTA. A wider FAZ suggests more severe vascular dysfunction, our research demonstrated larger FAZ area and perimeter in BU group compared to controls, although the difference did not reach statistical significance. Likewise, a previous study also demonstrated no significant FAZ changes in BU eyes (31) but significant FAZ differences have been detected (32, 33). The discrepancy in different studies suggests further validation by expanding sample size and that FAZ measurements may not be sufficiently sensitive metrics for determining retinal involvement in BU.

Among anatomic parameters measured, FRT and the pRNFLT were notably greater in BU patients than controls, probably due to retinal edema. We conducted correlation analyses to further clarify the relationship between RNFL thickness and vascular density in the peripapillary region. We found a correlation between RPCN vascular density and pRNFLT in healthy subjects, consistent with previous work (34), but not in BU patients, which may be due to retinal edema and segmentation artifacts.

The main limitation of our study is the relatively small sample size, so these findings require validation, preferably in multi-center studies. A second limitation is the cross-sectional study design, which precluded the assessment of vascular changes during different disease phases. A longitudinal study may reveal the evolution of vascular abnormalities and associations with BCVA deficits.

Nonetheless, our study reveals novel vascular changes in the peripapillary region of the BU retina using OCTA and associations with visual dysfunction. Patients exhibited marked reductions in vascular densities within the peripapillary region, and decreased flow density in the peripapillary zone was mightily associated with poorer BCVA. Taken together, our study indicates that OCTA is a valuable modality for monitoring the microvascular changes associated with BU, and that RPCN vascular density could serve as a sensitive indicator of disease progression and therapeutic response among BU patients.

ETHICS STATEMENT

The studies involving human participants were reviewed and approved by the Ethics Committee of Zhongshan Ophthalmic Center (Guangzhou, China 2019KYPJ127). The patients/participants provided their written informed consent to participate in this study.

AUTHOR CONTRIBUTIONS

WC, CY, FL, and MH contributed to conception and design of the study. MH, FL, and JL organized the database. CY and XY performed the statistical analysis. CY, FL, and MH wrote the first draft of the manuscript. XY, LS, YH, and WC wrote sections of the manuscript. All authors contributed to manuscript revision, read, and approved the submitted version.

ACKNOWLEDGMENTS

We would like to acknowledge the assistance of Guandi Chen at Zhongshan Ophthalmic Center for her contribution to assisting in examining the patients and providing images.

REFERENCES

1. He Y, Wang C, Su G, Deng B, Ye Z, Huang Y, et al. Decreased expression of A20 is associated with ocular Behcet's Disease (BD) but not with Vogt-Koyanagi-Harada (VKH) disease. *Br J Ophthalmol.* (2018) 102:1167–72. doi: 10.1136/bjophthalmol-2017-311707
2. Tong B, Liu X, Xiao J, Su G. Immunopathogenesis of Behcet's Disease. *Front Immunol.* (2019) 10:665. doi: 10.3389/fimmu.2019.00665
3. Muruganandam M, Rolle NA, Sibbitt WL, Cook GB, Emil NS, Fangtham M, et al. Characteristics of Behcet's disease in the American Southwest. *Semin Arthritis Rheum.* (2019) 49:296–302. doi: 10.1016/j.semarthrit.2019.03.003
4. Leonardo NM, McNeil J. Behcet's disease: is there geographical variation? a review far from the silk road. *Int J Rheumatol.* (2015) 2015:945262. doi: 10.1155/2015/945262
5. Cunningham ET, Tugal-Tutkun I, Khairallah M, Okada AA, Bodaghi B, Zierhut M. Behçet Uveitis. *Ocul Immunol Inflamm.* (2017) 25:2–6. doi: 10.1080/09273948.2017.1279840
6. Tugal-Tutkun I, Ozdal PC, Oray M, Onal S. Review for diagnostics of the year: multimodal imaging in Behçet Uveitis. *Ocul Immunol Inflamm.* (2017) 25:7–19. doi: 10.1080/09273948.2016.1205100
7. Pei M, Zhao C, Gao F, Qu Y, Liang A, Xiao J, et al. Analysis of parafoveal microvascular abnormalities in Behcet's Uveitis using projection-resolved optical coherence tomographic angiography. *Ocul Immunol Inflamm.* (2019) 29:1–6. doi: 10.1080/09273948.2020.1807201
8. Liu W, Li H, Shah RS, Shu X, Linsenmeier RA, Fawzi AA, et al. Simultaneous optical coherence tomography angiography and fluorescein angiography in rodents with normal retina and laser-induced choroidal neovascularization. *Opt Lett.* (2015) 40:5782–5. doi: 10.1364/OL.40.005782
9. Spaide RF, Fujimoto JG, Waheed NK, Sadda SR, Staurenghi G. Optical coherence tomography angiography. *Prog Retin Eye Res.* (2018) 64:1–55. doi: 10.1016/j.preteyeres.2017.11.003
10. Zhang S, Wu C, Liu L, Jia Y, Zhang Y, Zhang Y, et al. Optical coherence tomography angiography of the peripapillary retina in primary angle-closure glaucoma. *Am J Ophthalmol.* (2017) 182:194–200. doi: 10.1016/j.ajo.2017.07.024
11. Çömez A, Beyoglu A, Karaküçük Y. Quantitative analysis of retinal microcirculation in optical coherence tomography angiography in cases with Behçet's disease without ocular involvement. *Int Ophthalmol.* (2019) 39:2213–21. doi: 10.1007/s10792-018-1059-z
12. Toshev AP, Schuster AK, Ul Hassan SN, Pfeiffer N, Hoffmann EM. Optical coherence tomography angiography of optic disc in eyes with primary open-angle glaucoma and normal-tension glaucoma. *J Glaucoma.* (2019) 28:243–51. doi: 10.1097/IJG.0000000000001184
13. Carnevali A, Sacconi R, Corbelli E, Tomasso L, Querques L, Zerbini G, et al. Optical coherence tomography angiography analysis of retinal vascular plexuses and choriocapillaris in patients with type 1 diabetes without diabetic retinopathy. *Acta Diabetol.* (2017) 54:695–702. doi: 10.1007/s00592-017-0996-8
14. Liu L, Jia Y, Takusagawa HL, Pechauer AD, Edmunds B, Lombardi L, et al. Optical coherence tomography angiography of the peripapillary retina in glaucoma. *JAMA Ophthalmol.* (2015) 133:1045–52. doi: 10.1001/jamaophthalmol.2015.2225
15. Manalastas PIC, Zangwill LM, Daga FB, Christopher MA, Saunders LJ, Shoji T, et al. The association between macula and onh optical coherence tomography angiography (OCT-A) vessel densities in glaucoma, glaucoma suspect, and healthy eyes. *J Glaucoma.* (2018) 27:227–32. doi: 10.1097/IJG.0000000000000862

16. Lee SC, Tran S, Amin A, Morse LS, Moshiri A, Park SS, et al. Retinal vessel density in exudative and nonexudative age-related macular degeneration on optical coherence tomography angiography. *Am J Ophthalmol.* (2020) 212:7–16. doi: 10.1016/j.ajo.2019.11.031
17. Deng Y, Cai X, Zhang S, Su L, Chen H, Lin Y, et al. Quantitative analysis of retinal microvascular changes after conbercept therapy in branch retinal vein occlusion using optical coherence tomography angiography. *Ophthalmologica.* (2019) 242:69–80. doi: 10.1159/000499608
18. Deng Y, Zhong QW, Zhang AQ, Cai XJ, Lu MZ, Zhang SC, et al. Microvascular changes after conbercept therapy in central retinal vein occlusion analyzed by optical coherence tomography angiography. *Int J Ophthalmol.* (2019) 12:802–8. doi: 10.18240/ijo.2019.05.16
19. Luo K, Cai H, Hu Y, Jin C, Gan X, Deng Y, et al. Distinguishing microvasculature features of vogt-koyanagi-harada in patients in acute and convalescent phases using optical coherence tomography angiography. *Ocul Immunol Inflamm.* (2020) 29:1–7. doi: 10.1080/09273948.2019.1695856
20. Khairallah M, Abroug N, Khochtali S, Mahmoud A, Jelliti B, Coscas G, et al. Optical coherence tomography angiography in patients with Behçet Uveitis. *Retina.* (2017) 37:1678–91. doi: 10.1097/IAE.0000000000001418
21. Accorinti M, Gilardi M, De Geronimo D, Iannetti L, Giannini D, Parravano M. Optical coherence tomography angiography findings in active and inactive ocular Behçet disease. *Ocul Immunol Inflamm.* (2020) 28:589–600. doi: 10.1080/09273948.2019.1612452
22. Koca S, Onan D, Kalayci D, Alli N. Comparison of optical coherence tomography angiography findings in patients with Behçet's disease and healthy controls. *Ocul Immunol Inflamm.* (2020) 28:806–13. doi: 10.1080/09273948.2019.1635167
23. Criteria for diagnosis of Behçet's disease. International study group for Behçet's disease. *Lancet.* (1990) 335:1078–80. doi: 10.1016/0140-6736(90)92643-V
24. Takeuchi M, Hokama H, Tsukahara R, Kezuka T, Goto H, Sakai J, et al. Risk and prognostic factors of poor visual outcome in Behcet's disease with ocular involvement. *Graefes Arch Clin Exp Ophthalmol.* (2005) 243:1147–52. doi: 10.1007/s00417-005-0005-8
25. Eser Ozturk H, Oray M, Tugal-Tutkun I. Tocilizumab for the treatment of Behçet Uveitis that failed interferon alpha and anti-tumor necrosis factor-alpha therapy. *Ocul Immunol Inflamm.* (2018) 26:1005–14. doi: 10.1080/09273948.2017.1355471
26. Engelke H, Shajari M, Riedel J, Mohr N, Priglinger SG, Mackert MJ, et al. Angiography in optic disc drusen: comparison with structural and functional parameters. *Br J Ophthalmol.* (2020) 104:1109–13. doi: 10.1136/bjophthalmol-2019-314096
27. Liu L, Edmunds B, Takusagawa HL, Tehrani S, Lombardi LH, Morrison JC, et al. Projection-resolved optical coherence tomography angiography of the peripapillary retina in glaucoma. *Am J Ophthalmol.* (2019) 207:99–109. doi: 10.1016/j.ajo.2019.05.024
28. Wright Mayes E, Cole ED, Dang S, Novais EA, Vuong L, Mendoza-Santiesteban C, et al. Optical coherence tomography angiography in nonarteritic anterior ischemic optic neuropathy. *J Neuroophthalmol.* (2017) 37:358–64. doi: 10.1097/WNO.0000000000000493
29. Cheng D, Shen M, Zhuang X, Lin D, Dai M, Chen S, et al. Inner retinal microvasculature damage correlates with outer retinal disruption during remission in Behçet's posterior Uveitis by optical coherence tomography angiography. *Invest Ophthalmol Vis Sci.* (2018) 59:1295–304. doi: 10.1167/iovs.17-23113
30. Pournaras CJ, Riva CE. Retinal blood flow evaluation. *Ophthalmologica.* (2013) 229:61–74. doi: 10.1159/000338186
31. Eser-Ozturk H, Ismayilova L, Yucel OE, Sullu Y. Quantitative measurements with optical coherence tomography angiography in Behçet Uveitis. *Eur J Ophthalmol.* (2020) 31:1047–55. doi: 10.1177/11206721209 20214
32. Goker YS, Yilmaz S, Kiziltoprak H, Tekin K, Demir G. Quantitative analysis of optical coherence tomography angiography features in patients with nonocular Behcet's disease. *Curr Eye Res.* (2019) 44:212–8. doi: 10.1080/02713683.2018.1530361
33. Türkcü FM, Sahin A, Karaalp Ü, Çinar Y, Sahin M, Özkurt ZG, et al. Automated quantification of foveal avascular zone and vascular density in Behçet's disease. *Ir J Med Sci.* (2020) 189:349–54. doi: 10.1007/s11845-019-02051-2
34. She X, Guo J, Liu X, Zhu H, Li T, Zhou M, et al. Reliability of vessel density measurements in the peripapillary retina and correlation with retinal nerve fiber layer thickness in healthy subjects using optical coherence tomography angiography. *Ophthalmologica.* (2018) 240:183–90. doi: 10.1159/000485957

5

Ultrasound Biomicroscopy Might Predict the Outcome of Phacoemulsification-Visco Dissection in Medically Controlled Primary Angle-Closure Glaucoma Eye with Extensive Peripheral Anterior Synechia

Haijun Gong [1,2†], Xu Dong [1,3†], Bingru Zheng [1], Xinbo Gao [1], Liming Chen [1], Simin Zhang [1], Chengguo Zuo [1] and Mingkai Lin [1*]*

[1] State Key Laboratory of Ophthalmology, Guangdong Provincial Key Laboratory of Ophthalmology and Visual Science, Zhongshan Ophthalmic Center, Sun Yat-sen University, Guangzhou, China, [2] Guangdong Provincial Key Laboratory of Malignant Tumor Epigenetics and Gene Regulation, Department of Ophthalmology, Sun Yat-sen Memorial Hospital, Sun Yat-sen University, Guangzhou, China, [3] The Fourth People's Hospital of Shenyang, Shenyang, China

***Correspondence:**
Mingkai Lin
linmk@mail.sysu.edu.cn
Chengguo Zuo
chengguozuo@163.com

† These authors have contributed equally to this work

Objective: The treatment procedures of primary angle-closure glaucoma (PACG) with extensive peripheral anterior synechia (PAS) is a subject of debate. This study is to investigate the clinical features of phacoemulsification (Phaco)-visco dissection in medically controlled PACG patients with PAS > 180° and evaluate the predictability of Ultrasound Biomicroscopy (UBM) parameters on postoperative intraocular pressure (IOP).

Methods: 48 eyes (48 patients) with acute angle-closure glaucoma (AACG) and 30 eyes (30 patients) with chronic angle-closure glaucoma (CACG) were prospectively included. All patients underwent phaco-viscogoniolysis and foldable lens implantation and were followed for 1 year after surgery. We analyzed preoperative and postoperative IOP, the numbers of anti-glaucoma medicine, the visual field value, the extent of PAS, and UBM parameters alterations, and evaluated the correlation between preoperative UBM parameters and one-year postoperative IOP.

Results: IOP reduced significantly from 16.24 ± 4.33 to 14.49 ± 3.69 mmHg in AACG group and from 16.16 ± 3.69 mmHg to 14.31 ± 4.12 mmHg in CACG group, and PAS decreased significantly from 270 ± 60.33 to 171 ± 56.44° in AACG group and from 285 ± 70.46 to 168 ± 61.32° in CACG group, and the number of anti-glaucoma drugs decreased significantly in both groups. Several UBM parameters, including anterior chamber depth, trabecular iris angle, and peripheral iris thickness 500 increased while iris convex reduced considerably in the two groups, and angle opening distance 500 and trabecular-meshwork ciliary process angle increased significantly only in AACG group. One-year postoperative IOP correlated with preoperative angle opening distance 500 and trabecular iris angle negatively and iris convex positively.

Conclusion: Phaco-visco dissection can effectively reduce IOP, the numbers of glaucomatous medications, and PAS in medically controlled PACG patients with extensive PAS. UBM parameters might be valuable for analyzing postoperative anterior segment structure and predicting postoperative IOP of Phaco-visco dissection in PACG patients with extensive PAS.

Keywords: primary angle-closure glaucoma, ultrasound biomicroscopy, phacoemulsification, visco dissection, predictability

INTRODUCTION

Primary angle-closure glaucoma (PACG) is a leading cause of blindness in East Asia (1). East Asians have the well-known anatomic configurations, including a shallower anterior chamber depth (ACD), shorter axis length (AL), thicker lens, and smaller radius of the cornea than Westerners, thereby causing a higher prevalence of PACG (2). The classical clinical classification of PACG includes acute angle-closure glaucoma (AACG) and chronic angle-closure glaucoma (CACG), in which the anterior chamber angle can be permanently closed by peripheral anterior synechia (PAS). Previous studies reported that PACG patients with extensive PAS >180 degrees should be the candidates for filtering surgery because of their inefficient trabecular meshwork cellular capability and insufficient medical therapeutic effect (3). Although sole-filtering surgery or combined glaucoma and cataract surgery can cause a remarkable intraocular pressure (IOP) decrease, unfortunately, these procedures also bring about a high risk of short- and long-term complications, such as filtering bleb scarring and shallow anterior chamber (4).

Phacoemulsification-goniosynechialysis (PEGS) has been reported to have a lowering effect on IOP and reduce the use of antiglaucoma drugs in patients with medically uncontrolled (primary angle closure) PAC (5), AACG (6), medically controlled CACG (7), and primary open angle glaucoma (POAG) (8). Evidence suggested cataract extraction by phacoemulsification (Phaco) can result in an IOP decrease due to its effects including, but not limited to, ultrasound on the trabecular meshwork cellular, mechanical washout on the trabecular meshwork, and uveal tract outflow (9). Additionally, tearing off PAS from the anterior chamber angle wall by PEGS is an effective procedure to reestablish outflow structure and increase drainage of aqueous humor (10). Our clinical work used an alternative safe and minor procedure—combined Phaco and visco dissection in some medical controlled PACG patients with PAS and observed a relatively long-term controlled IOP. It indicated medically controlled PACG eye with PAS >180° might have remaining aqueous outflow function and can also be the candidates for combined Phaco and visco dissection. However, there is limited information related to the clinical outcome and the preoperative predictors in these patients. Ultrasound biomicroscopy (UBM) is a non-invasive imaging technique and widely be used to assess the morphology changes of glaucoma and measure the anterior segment structure. Interestingly, numerous studies have shown UBM parameters changes and have diagnostic capabilities following cataract surgery in patients with glaucoma (11–13). Therefore, evaluating the quantitative changes of preoperative and postoperative characters and understanding the link between UBM parameters and clinical features in PACG with extensive PAS might help ophthalmologists manage this disease.

In this study, we analyzed the effect of combined Phaco-visco dissection on IOP, numbers of antiglaucoma drops, and PAS degrees in PACG patients with PAS >180° and IOP controlled before surgery. Meanwhile, we used UBM to detect the morphologic changes of anterior segment parameters and hopefully explored their prediction roles in postoperative IOP.

METHODS

Participants

This prospective case series evaluated patients between January 2018 and December 2019 at the Zhongshan Ophthalmic Center, Sun Yat-sen University. This study was approved by the medical ethics committee of Zhongshan Ophthalmic Center and was performed following the Declaration of Helsinki's tenets.

This study evaluated 78 eyes of 78 patients, including 48 AACG patients and 30 CACG patients. The AACG patients had an elevated IOP history (acute, subacute, and intermediate attacks) and symptoms remission before inclusion. The time between controlling and attack of AACG ranged from 1 month to 2 months. At the time of surgery, no change in glaucoma medication administration and visual field parameters and target IOP < 21 mmHg in the last 1 month was considered a medically controlled condition in AACG and CACG group. In both groups, each patient had preoperative gonioscopy showing PAS >180° and had a typical visual field and optical nerve defects, coexisting cataract, and the best corrected visual acuity (BCVA) <0.5 (decimal). In two eyes of each participant, we selected the eye with more severe PAS. The exclusion criteria were having a history of intraocular surgery, laser iridotomy, extra non-glaucoma laser conditions, ocular trauma, intraocular inflammation, ischemic disease, and secondary glaucoma histories such as vascular glaucoma, pseudoexfoliation, pigmentary glaucoma, glaucomatocyclitic syndrome, lens, and corticosteroid-induced glaucoma.

Examination and Surgical Procedure

Baseline parameters were evaluated 1 week before surgery, and the follow-up examinations were 1 day, 1 week, 1 month, and then every 3 months till 1 year. Baseline demographics, the number of medications before and after the operation, visual acuity testing, IOP, MD (mean deviation) value of the visual field, slit-lamp examination, and ophthalmoscopy results were recorded. Angle structure was evaluated with a Zeiss four-mirror gonio lens. The PAS degree was evaluated by senior glaucoma subspecialists and confirmed by the same surgeon to keep the examination consistency. The visual field was measured by automated program 24-2 threshold perimetry (Humphrey 750i, Zeiss, Germany). UBM examinations were performed 1 week before surgery and 1 month, 6 months, and 1 year after surgery. Anterior parameters including ACD, angle-opening distance 500 (AOD500), scleral ciliary process angle (SCPA), trabecular-meshwork ciliary process angle (TCPA), trabecular ciliary process distance (TCPD), trabecular iris angle (TIA), peripheral iris thickness 500 (IT500), ciliary body thickness (CBT), and iris convex (IC) were obtained using the UBM technique (SW-3200L, Suoer, China). **Figures 1**, **2** illustrated their calculation method: ACD was the length from the front lens surface to the corneal endothelium; AOD500 was defined as the distance between the point of the posterior corneal surface at 500 mm from the scleral spur and the anterior iris surface; TCPD has defined the perpendicular distance between a point spreading out from scleral spur to the corneal endothelium at 500 mm and the ciliary processes; CBT was detected at 1 mm posterior from the scleral spur; TIA was the angle passing through a point on the corneal endothelium at 500 mm from the scleral spur and the point on the iris vertically opposite, and it represents the open degrees of anterior angle; SCPA was the angle between the tangent line

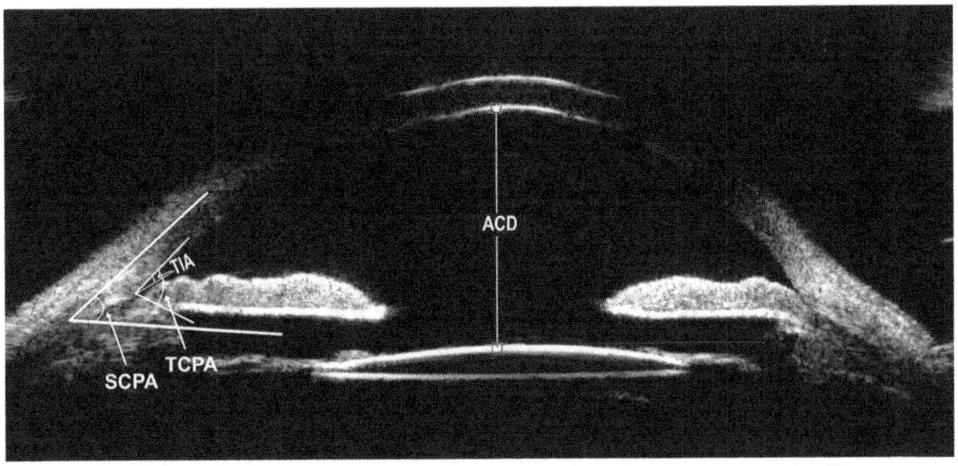

FIGURE 1 | Ultrasound biomicroscopic (UBM) image of ACD, TIA, TCPA, SCPA. ACD, anterior chamber depth. TIA, trabecular iris angle. TCPA, trabecular-meshwork ciliary process angle. SCPA, scleral ciliary process angle.

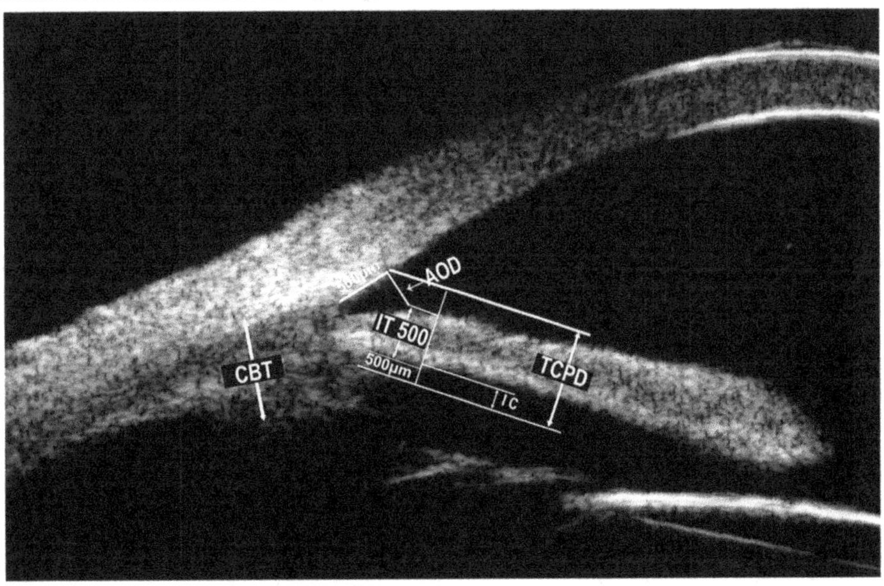

FIGURE 2 | Ultrasound biomicroscopic (UBM) image of AOD500, TCPD, IT500, CBT, IC. AOD500, angle opening distance 500. TCPD, trabecular ciliary process distance. IT500, peripheral iris thickness 500. CBT, ciliary body thickness. IC, iris convex.

TABLE 1 | Patients characteristics.

	AACG ($n = 48$)	CACG ($n = 30$)	P
Age (years)	68.07 ± 3.97	66.87 ± 2.38	0.139
Sex (M: F)	19:29	12:18	0.971
Laterality (OD: OS)	26:22	13:17	0.352
Preoperative BCVA (decimal)	0.37 ± 0.13	0.43 ± 0.12	0.071
Preoperative MD (dB)	−17.59 ± 10.16	−15.23 ± 12.20	0.231
Range	−29.62 to −2.36	−28.43 to −1.19	

BCVA, best corrected visual acuity; MD, mean deviation.

TABLE 2 | The changes of preoperative and 1-year postoperative clinical parameters.

	Preoperative value	Postoperative value	P
IOP (mmHg)			
AACG	16.24 ± 4.33	14.49 ± 3.69	0.012*
CACG	16.16 ± 3.69	14.31 ± 4.12	0.009*
P	0.519	0.104	
NO. Eye drop (n)			
AACG	1.74 ± 1.46	1.12 ± 0.94	0.007*
CACG	2.23 ± 1.54	1.20 ± 0.76	0.001*
P	0.274	0.035*	
Degree of PAS (degrees)			
AACG	270 ± 60.33	171 ± 56.44	<0.001*
CACG	285 ± 70.46	168 ± 61.32	<0.001*
P	0.402	0.595	
MD (dB)			
AACG	−17.59 ± 10.16	−16.34 ± 11.03	0.381
CACG	−15.23 ± 12.20	−14.15 ± 11.65	0.912
P	0.354	0.547	

**Means $p < 0.05$. IOP, intraocular pressure; PAS, peripheral anterior synechia; MD, mean deviation.*

to the scleral surface and the axis of the ciliary processes, and it represents the ciliary body location; TCPA was defined as the angle between the line on corneal endothelium at 500 mm from the scleral spur and the front surface of ciliary processes; IT500 was detected from the iris point 500 mm and represented iris thickness and location; IC was measured as the perpendicular length between iris apex and the lowest point of pupillary margin to the iris rear surface's highest point.

All surgeries were performed by one surgeon who used the same procedure. It was performed by topical anesthesia, 3-mm corneal incision, continuous circular capsulorhexis using a 27-gauge bent needle, and standard phacoemulsification. A single-piece acrylic IOL (SA60AT, Alcon, US) was inserted into the posterior chamber through the corneal incision. According to preoperative records, viscoelastic material was used to strip the most peripheral iris from angle adhesion positions bluntly after lens implantation. Then we used an irrigation-aspiration system to remove the remaining viscoelastic material from the anterior chamber. After surgery, all patients were treated with topical corticosteroids, antibiotics, and antiglaucoma medications. Topical antibiotics and steroids were trapped within 6 weeks. All patients were followed 1 day, 1 week, 2 weeks, 1 month, and then every 3 months till 1 year after surgery. To evaluate the long-term IOP and PAS reduction, we only compare the preoperative and 1-year postoperative parameters.

Statistics Methods

SPSS version 21.0 for Social Sciences (IBM SPSS Inc., NY, US) was used for statistical analysis. All numerical data were expressed as mean ± SD, and the Student t-test was performed to compare all parameter variations from baseline. Gender and laterality differences were assessed by Chi-square test. Pearson correlation was used to study the correlation between 1-year postoperative IOP and preoperative UBM characteristics. A p-value < 0.05 was considered statistically significant.

RESULTS

Table 1 provides the baseline characteristics of all 78 participants. The mean age of subjects was 68.07 ± 3.97 years in the AACG group and 66.87 ± 2.38 years in the CACG group. There were no statistically significant differences in all demographic features and preoperative visual acuity and MD value between the AACG and CACG groups.

Table 2 shows the clinical features of preoperative and 1-year postoperative stages, including IOP, numbers of lowering IOP eye drops and, the extent of PAS and MD value in the two groups. IOP decreased significantly in the two groups, from 16.24 ± 4.33 to 14.2 ± 3.6 mmHg in the AACG group and from 16.16 ± 3.69 to 14.31 ± 4.12 mmHg in the CACG group. The PAS degree also reduced remarkably in both groups, from 270 ± 60.33 to 171 ± 56.44° in the AACG group and from 285 ± 70.46 to 168 ± 61.32° in the CACG group. Meanwhile, both groups had a meaningful decrease in numbers of antiglaucoma drugs, from 1.74 ± 1.46 to 1.12 ± 0.94 in the AACG group and from 2.23 ± 1.54 to 1.20 ± 0.76 in the CACG group. There was also a significant difference in the numbers of postoperative antiglaucoma drugs between the AACG and the CACG group. However, the MD value did not differ significantly in both groups.

Table 3 provides the changes of UMB parameters. Each value in the four positions (12, 3, 6, and 9 o'clock) was measured, and their mean value was selected for analysis. The increase in ACD, TIA, and IT500 and decrease in IC were statistically significant in both groups, whereas AOD500 and TCPA just increased significantly within the AACG group only following the surgery. In the meanwhile, compared with the CACG group, the AACG group had a lower postoperative value in AOD500, TIA, and IC.

Table 4 shows the correlation between 1-year postoperative IOP and preoperative UBM parameters in two groups. Postoperative IOP was negatively correlated with preoperative AOD ($R = -0.383, p = 0.043$) and TIA ($R = -0.383, p = 0.043$), and related to preoperative IC positively ($R = 0.557, p = 0.003$). There was also a significant correlation between preoperative IOP and 1-year postoperative in both CACG group ($R = 0.475, p = 0.015$) and AACG group ($R = 0.442, p = 0.023$).

TABLE 3 | The changes of preoperative and 1-year postoperative UBM parameters.

UBM parameters	Preoperative value	Postoperative value	*P*
ACD (mm)			
AACG	1.77 ± 0.31	3.33 ± 0.55	<0.001*
CACG	1.78 ± 0.23	3.21 ± 0.58	<0.001*
P	0.345	0.523	
AOD500 (mm)			
AACG	0.012 ± 0.022	0.075 ± 0.059	<0.001*
CACG	0.0785 ± 0.0616	0.1882 ± 0.6977	0.610
P	0.112	0.002*	
TIA (degrees)			
AACG	1.168 ± 2.266	7.684 ± 6.226	<0.001*
CACG	1.6390 ± 1.5588	8.0773 ± 6.4486	0.001*
P	0.124	0.016*	
TCPD (mm)			
AACG	0.4639 ± 0.1167	0.5235 ± 0.1152	0.120
CACG	0.4616 ± 0.1182	0.5348 ± 0.1096	0.121
P	0.234	0.315	
SPCA (degrees)			
AACG	37.7347 ± 4.721	39.7911 ± 2.8719	0.128
CACG	38.5801 ± 4.3325	39.2944 ± 2.7639	0.668
P	0.345	0.521	
TCPA (degrees)			
AACG	46.6730 ± 9.8928	56.7547 ± 10.6560	0.004*
CACG	49.2000 ± 11.2269	56.6045 ± 10.5147	0.097
P	0.081	0.124	
IT500(mm)			
AACG	0.3635 ± 0.0615	0.4404 ± 0.0652	<0.001*
CACG	0.3516 ± 0.0709	0.4357 ± 0.0936	0.018*
P	0.106	0.539	
CBT (mm)			
AACG	0.6878 ± 0.1313	0.7193 ± 0.1241	0.452
CACG	0.6922 ± 0.1641	0.7087 ± 0.1627	0.802
P	0.775	0.732	
IC (mm)			
AACG	0.2304 ± 0.1034	0.0969 ± 0.0819	<0.001*
CACG	0.6953 ± 0.1732	0.1838 ± 0.3945	<0.001*
P	0.007*	0.003*	

**Means $p < 0.05$. ACD, anterior chamber depth; AOD500, angle opening distance 500; TIA, trabecular iris angle; TCPD, trabecular ciliary process distance; SCPA, scleral ciliary process angle; TCPA, trabecular-meshwork ciliary process angle; IT500, peripheral iris thickness 500; CBT, ciliary body thickness; IC, iris convex.*

TABLE 4 | Correlation coefficients between preoperative UBM parameters and 1-year postoperative IOP in two groups.

Variables	AACG		CACG	
	R	*P*	R	*P*
ACD	0.205	0.187	−0.071	0.440
AOD500	−0.383	0.043*	0.450	0.155
TIA	−0.383	0.043*	−0.450	0.155
TCPD	−0.320	0.078	0.000	0.500
SPCA	0.141	0.272	0.143	0.380
TCPA	−0.294	0.098	−0.179	0.351
IT500	0.333	0.070	−0.036	0.470
CBT	0.058	0.402	0.214	0.322
IC	0.577	0.033*	0.179	0.351

**Means $p < 0.05$. ACD, anterior chamber depth; AOD500, angle opening distance 500; TIA, trabecular iris angle; TCPD, trabecular ciliary process distance; SCPA, scleral ciliary process angle; TCPA, trabecular-meshwork ciliary process angle; IT500, peripheral iris thickness 500; CBT, ciliary body thickness; IC, iris convex.*

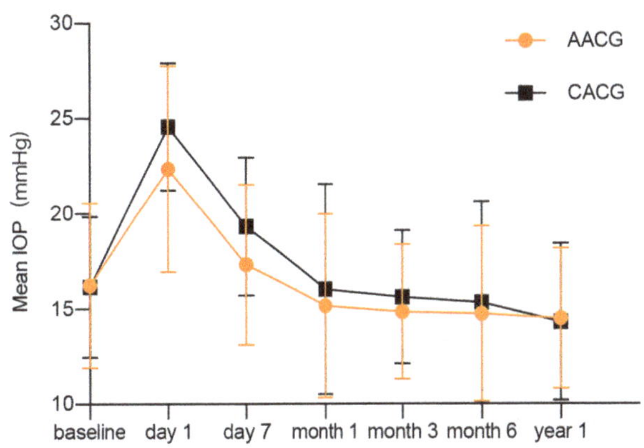

FIGURE 3 | The changes of intraocular pressure after surgery in acute angle-closure glaucoma and chronic angle-closure glaucoma patients.

For the 1-year follow-up period, none of the patients in both groups has an IOP spikes history (**Figure 3**). Assessment of intraoperative complications showed that two patients in the AACG group and three patients in the CACG group experienced intraoperative anterior chamber hemorrhage, but it didn't affect the final vision and IOP. None of the participants in both groups experienced severe complications within 1 year after surgery. Postoperative re-PAS occurred in six cases (12.5%) in the AACG group and seven cases (23.3%) in the CACG group, and the major sites were identical to the preoperative site but didn't require further intervention.

DISCUSSION

In this study, we first found IOP, degree of PAS, and anti-glaucoma medication decreased significantly in both AACG and CACG groups after Phaco-visco dissection surgery. According to PAS degrees, regarding numbers of antiglaucoma medication, and the condition of visual acuity and cataract severity, the surgical approach of PACG with PAS may be a subject of debate. Surgical treatment approaches in those patients include phacoemulsification, trabeculectomy, Phaco-trabeculectomy, goniosynechialysis, and Phaco-goniosynechialysis (14). A meta-analysis of angle-closure glaucoma reported that IOP in the PEGS group decreased significantly more than in Phaco alone group, and there was no statistical difference between PEGS group and Phaco-trabeculectomy/ trabeculectomy group (15).

This is in accordance with our study that Phaco-visco dissection has a satisfactory IOP decrease and a possible improvement of trabecular meshwork function in both groups. Therefore, using this lower-risk and simpler procedure rather than filtering surgery to restore the normal anterior chamber anatomic structure and clear the aqueous outflow from any obstruction will be appealing for those medically controlled patients with extensive PAS.

UBM is the most useful method of imagining anterior segment configurations and their clinic implications and evaluating the result of PACG treatment (16). Previous UBM studies showed these eyes have shorter TCPD and anteriorly positioned ciliary process (17). Sang Woo Park reported that the ACD, AOD500, TIA, TCPD, and SCPA increased significantly after the glaucoma triple procedure (18). The ciliary process position can directly influence TCPD. Nonaka reported, after Phaco surgery, ACD, AOD500, and TCPD increased due to widening of the angle, removal of the pupillary block, and reduction in the anterior position of the ciliary processes (19). Our study found similar results that ACD, TIA, and IT500 increased in both groups and AOD500 and TCPA just increased significantly in the AACG group following the surgery. The TCPD was also increased but had no statistical significance in both groups. We also found postoperative IOP was negatively associated with preoperative AOD and TIA and positively related to preoperative IC. It means higher preoperative AOD and TIA may easily lead to lower postoperative IOP, whereas thicker IC might cause higher postoperative IOP. We suppose it is because high AOD and TIA may induce a low incidence of anterior chamber angle-closure, but IC may represent a high pupillary block risk. These parameters may also hopefully be the predictors for the postoperative IOP accordingly when making the surgery decision.

This prospective study has several limitations. Small-scale and all participants from the same race in China is the principal limitation. To further verify our results and obtain stronger evidence of Phaco-visco dissection effects on those patients, large-scale randomized controlled trials are necessary for the prospective study. In addition, the clinical and UBM data for multiple time points should be included and assessed in the future study to provide more detailed information, such as long-term re-PAS rate and IOP level, thereby assisting clinicians regarding PACG patients' postoperative treatment and management.

In conclusion, we have shown that combined Phaco and visco dissection has an advantage in lowering IOP, decreasing numbers of antiglaucoma drops, and ameliorating anterior chamber angle structure and function in PACG patients with extensive PAS degree. UBM parameters may be possible predictors for the effect of Phaco and visco dissection on postoperative IOP.

ETHICS STATEMENT

The studies involving human participants were reviewed and approved by the medical ethics committee of Zhongshan Ophthalmic Center. The patients/participants provided their written informed consent to participate in this study.

AUTHOR CONTRIBUTIONS

ML, XD, and HG designed this study. BZ and XG collected and measured data. LC and SZ analyzed data. CZ and HG wrote this article and revised the manuscript. All authors discussed the results and commented on the manuscript.

REFERENCES

1. Wright C, Tawfik MA, Waisbourd M, Katz LJ. Primary angle-closure glaucoma: an update. *Acta Ophthalmol.* (2016) 94:217–25. doi: 10.1111/aos.12784
2. Chan EW, Li X, Tham Y-C, Liao J, Wong TY, Aung T, et al. Glaucoma in Asia: regional prevalence variations and future projections. *Br J Ophthalmol.* (2016) 100:78–85. doi: 10.1136/bjophthalmol-2014-306102
3. Razeghinejad MR, Myers JS. Contemporary approach to the diagnosis and management of primary angle-closure disease. *Surv Ophthalmol.* (2018) 63:754–68. doi: 10.1016/j.survophthal.2018.05.001
4. Olayanju JA, Hassan MB, Hodge DO, Khanna CL. Trabeculectomy-Related Complications in Olmsted County, Minnesota, 1985 Through 2010 *JAMA Ophthalmol.* (2015) 133:574–80. doi: 10.1001/jamaophthalmol.2015.57
5. Kameda T, Inoue T, Inatani M, Tanihara H, Japanese Phaco-Goniosynechialysis Multicenter Study Group. Long-term efficacy of goniosynechialysis combined with phacoemulsification for primary angle closure. *Graefes Arch Clin Exp Ophthalmol.* (2013) 251:825–30. doi: 10.1007/s00417-012-2091-8
6. Teekhasaenee C, Ritch R. Combined phacoemulsification and goniosynechialysis for uncontrolled chronic angle-closure glaucoma after acute angle-closure glaucoma. *Ophthalmology.* (1999) 106:669–74; discussion 674–75. doi: 10.1016/S0161-6420(99)90149-5
7. Lee C-K, Rho SS, Sung GJ, Kim NR, Yang JY, Lee NE, et al. Effect of goniosynechialysis during phacoemulsification on IOP in patients with medically well-controlled chronic angle-closure glaucoma. *J Glaucoma.* (2015) 24:405–9. doi: 10.1097/IJG.0000000000000043
8. Majstruk L, Leray B, Bouillot A, Michée S, Sultan G, Baudouin C, et al. Long term effect of phacoemulsification on intraocular pressure in patients with medically controlled primary open-angle glaucoma. *BMC Ophthalmol.* (2019) 19:149. doi: 10.1186/s12886-019-1157-3
9. Slabaugh MA, Chen PP. The effect of cataract extraction on intraocular pressure. *Curr Opin Ophthalmol.* (2014) 25:122–6. doi: 10.1097/ICU.0000000000000033
10. Rodrigues IA, Alaghband P, Beltran Agullo L, Galvis E, Jones S, Husain R, et al. Aqueous outflow facility after phacoemulsification with or without goniosynechialysis in primary angle closure: a randomised controlled study. *Br J Ophthalmol.* (2017) 101:879–85. doi: 10.1136/bjophthalmol-2016-309556

11. Kronberg BP, Rhee DJ. Anterior segment imaging and the intraocular pressure lowering effect of cataract surgery for open and narrow angle glaucoma. *Semin Ophthalmol.* (2012) 27:149–54. doi: 10.3109/08820538.2012.708810
12. Avetisov SE, Ambartsumian AR, Avetisov KS. [Diagnostic capabilities of ultrasound biomicroscopy in phaco surgery]. *Vestn Oftalmol.* (2013) 129:32–41.
13. Dada T, Mohan S, Bali SJ, Bhartiya S, Sobti A, Panda A. ultrasound biomicroscopic assessment of angle parameters in patients with primary angle closure glaucoma undergoing phacoemulsification. *Eur J Ophthalmol.* (2011) 21:559–65. doi: 10.5301/EJO.2011.6287
14. Zhang H, Tang G, Liu J. Effects of phacoemulsification combined with goniosynechialysis on primary angle-closure glaucoma. *J Glaucoma.* (2016) 25:e499–503. doi: 10.1097/IJG.0000000000000297
15. Liu Y, Li W, Jiu X, Lei X, Liu L, Yan C, et al. Systematic Review and Meta-Analysis of Comparing Phacoemulsification Combined with goniosynechialysis to other mainstream procedures in treating patients with angle-closure glaucoma. *Medicine.* (2019) 98:e17654. doi: 10.1097/MD.0000000000017654
16. Ünsal E, Eltutar K, Muftuoglu IK. Morphologic changes in the anterior segment using ultrasound biomicroscopy after cataract surgery and intraocular lens implantation. *Eur J Ophthalmol.* (2017) 27:31–8. doi: 10.5301/ejo.5000812
17. Cho HJ, Woo JM, Yang KJ. Ultrasound biomicroscopic dimensions of the anterior chamber in angle-closure glaucoma patients. *Korean J Ophthalmol.* (2002) 16:20–5. doi: 10.3341/kjo.2002.16.1.20
18. Park SW, Heo H, Yang KJ. Comparison of ultrasound biomicroscopic changes after glaucoma triple procedure and trabeculectomy in eyes with primary angle closure glaucoma. *J Glaucoma.* (2009) 18:311–5. doi: 10.1097/IJG.0b013e318184568e
19. Nonaka A, Kondo T, Kikuchi M, Yamashiro K, Fujihara M, Iwawaki T, et al. Angle widening and alteration of ciliary process configuration after cataract surgery for primary angle closure. *Ophthalmology.* (2006) 113:437–41. doi: 10.1016/j.ophtha.2005.11.018

6

Longitudinal Changes in Peripapillary Retinal Nerve Fiber Layer and Macular Ganglion Cell Inner Plexiform Layer in Progressive Myopia and Glaucoma Among Adolescents

*Hui Xiao, Yimin Zhong, Yunlan Ling, Xiaoyu Xu and Xing Liu**

State Key Laboratory of Ophthalmology, Zhongshan Ophthalmic Center, Sun Yat-sen University, Guangdong Provincial Key Laboratory of Ophthalmology and Visual Science, Guangdong Provincial Clinical Research Center for Ocular Diseases, Guangzhou, China

Correspondence:
Xing Liu
drliuxing@163.com

Purpose: This study aimed to investigate the differences in longitudinal changes in the peripapillary retinal nerve fiber layer (pRNFL) and macular ganglion cell plus inner plexiform layer (GCIPL) caused by progressive myopia and glaucoma among adolescents.

Design: This was a retrospective observational study.

Methods: A total of forty-seven and 25 eyes of 47 and 25 adolescents with myopia progression (MP) and glaucoma progression (GP), respectively, who were followed up at the Zhongshan Ophthalmic Center for at least 3 years, were included in the study. The pRNFL and GCIPL that measured at the initial and last visits were analyzed.

Results: The median follow-up period was 5 years for both two groups. During follow-up, the whole, superior, and inferior pRNFL decreased in both the MP and GP groups, ($p < 0.001$). Nasal pRNFL decreased in the MP group ($p < 0.001$) but had no significant difference in the GP group ($p = 0.19$). Temporal pRNFL was increased in the MP group ($p < 0.001$) but decreased in the GP group ($p < 0.001$). The average and sectoral GCIPL decreased in both groups ($p < 0.001$). The annual change rate of temporal pRNFL and pRNFL at 10-, 8-, 9-, and 7-clock-hour sectors and the inferotemporal GCIPL has better diagnostic value to differentiate glaucoma from myopia (the area under the receiver operating characteristic curve, AUC > 0.85).

Conclusion: Glaucoma and MP could cause loss of the pRNFL and GCIPL in adolescents; however, the loss patterns were different between the two groups. The temporal quadrant and 7-, 8-, 9-, and 10-clock-hour sector pRNFL and the inferotemporal GCIPL can help distinguish pRNFL and GCIPL loss caused by glaucoma or MP.

Keywords: adolescent, glaucoma, myopia, retinal nerve fiber layer, ganglion cell plus inner plexiform layer

INTRODUCTION

Glaucoma is the leading cause of irreversible blindness (1) and is characterized by the degeneration of the retinal ganglion cells (RGCs), with progressive loss of the retinal nerve fiber layer (RNFL) and the corresponding visual field (2). The previous studies (3, 4) have shown that the loss of the peripapillary retinal nerve fiber layer (pRNFL) and RGCs was more sensitive than the visual field test in detecting early glaucoma and the progression of glaucoma and was therefore a sensitive indicator for detecting glaucoma in the general population. However, the studies (5–7) have shown that myopia could also lead to the loss of pRNFL and RGCs, which makes it difficult to determine whether the loss of pRNFL is due to myopia or early glaucoma (8). As glaucoma is a chronic progressive neuropathy, longitudinal observation of the loss of pRNFL and RGCs in suspected cases is necessary to differentiate glaucoma from myopia. However, when it comes to adolescents, the problem becomes more confused. As myopia typically manifests and progresses in childhood and adolescence (9), the possible impact of myopia development and its effect on the RNFL and RGCs in adolescent myopia cannot be ignored. Previous cross-sectional studies (10, 11) reported a significant correlation between pRNFL and the spherical equivalent (SE) in Chinese and Caucasian students. One study (12) using long-wavelength swept-source optical coherence tomography (OCT) also found that the macular inner plexiform layer (IPL) plus ganglion cell layer (GCL) in children with myopia exhibited a small but statistically significant decrease over the course of 18 months. Thus, identifying the difference in the loss pattern of the pRNFL and RGCs caused by glaucomatous or myopic progression in adolescents is critical for the early detection of juvenile glaucoma. To date, most studies (6, 13) that have compared the pRNFL and RGCs between myopia and glaucoma were cross-sectional investigations on adults, which limits the insights that can be drawn from the data regarding the time course of pRNFL and RGCs changes associated with the progressive myopia and glaucoma during adolescence.

Therefore, this study retrospectively analyzed the long-term follow-up data of pRNFL and the ganglion cell plus inner plexiform layer (GCIPL) in patients with adolescent myopia and juvenile glaucoma at the Zhongshan Ophthalmic Center from September 2013 to December 2020. We compared the difference in loss patterns of the pRNFL and macular GCIPL between progressive myopia and glaucoma among adolescents to provide useful information that could differentiate glaucomatous progression from myopic progression.

MATERIALS AND METHODS

Study Participants

This retrospective observational study was approved by the Ethics Review Committee of the Zhongshan Ophthalmic Center and adhered to the tenets of the Declaration of Helsinki for research involving human subjects. Informed consent was obtained from the guardians of all participants involved in the study.

We retrospectively reviewed the medical records of patients with myopia and glaucoma in adolescents at the Zhongshan Ophthalmic Center, Sun Yat-sen University, between September 2013 and December 2020. The enrolled participants have been followed up for at least 3 years, with the complete routine ocular examination records and adequate quality pRNFL and macular GCIPL measurements at the initial and last visits.

The routine ocular examination records included comprehensive ophthalmological examination, cycloplegic refraction, best-corrected visual acuity (BCVA), intraocular pressure (IOP) measurement using a Goldmann applanation tonometer, and disk photography (Kowa non-myd a-D III; Kowa Optimed Inc., Aichi, Japan). The RNFL and GCIPL were obtained using OCT.

The inclusion criteria for progressive myopia in adolescents were as follows: (1) age <18 years at initial visit; (2) progression of myopia (SE) more than 1 D during the follow-up; (3) BCVA ≥20/25, with IOP <21 mmHg at each visit; (4) no glaucomatous optic neuropathy (GON) confirmed and agreed upon by two glaucoma specialists based on disk photography during the follow-up; and (5) no family history of glaucoma or intraocular surgery.

The inclusion criteria for progressed glaucoma in adolescents were as follows: (1) age <18 years at initial visit; (2) IOP >22 mmHg for at least two times measurements by Goldmann applanation tonometer, without treatment; (3) open angle; and (4) glaucoma progression (GP) confirmed by progression of the optic nerve defects during the follow-up. The GON progression was determined through the evaluation of the entire series of stereoscopic optic disk and red-free RNFL photographs by two glaucoma specialists (HX and XL) independently. The most recent photograph of each patient was compared with the baseline photograph. GP was defined as an increase in the extent of neuroretinal rim thinning, enhancement of disk excavation, and/or any widening, deepening, or new RNFL defects. The graders classified each glaucomatous eye as either stable or progressive. Cases were excluded if the opinions of the two observers differed.

The exclusion criteria were as follows: (1) blurred disk photography that cannot be evaluated; (2) poor OCT quality, defined by signal strength <6 or poor alignment on the individual OCT scans; (3) other retinal, uveal, neurological, or systemic diseases that could affect retinal results; and (4) prior ocular trauma and intraocular surgery history, except for glaucoma surgery. If data from both eyes were eligible for analysis, only one randomly selected eye from each patient was included in this study.

Peripapillary Retinal Nerve Fiber Layer and Macular Ganglion Cell Plus Inner Plexiform Layer Measurements

Measurements of the pRNFL and GCIPL were taken during the follow-up using Cirrus HD-OCT 5000 (Carl Zeiss Meditec, Inc., Dublin, CA, United States; version 10.0) and were subsequently analyzed. An optic disk cube 200 × 200 protocol centered at the optic disk center and a macular cube 512 × 128 scan protocol centered at the fovea were performed for all eyes. Participants were tested using the same device during the follow-up examinations.

The cup/disk area ratio (C/D) was automatically generated by the optic nerve head (ONH) algorithm used in Cirrus OCT software from the optic disk cube 200 × 200 protocol. The pRNFL software automatically extracted a peripapillary circle (3.46 mm in diameter) from the cube data set to measure pRNFL thickness. The average, four quadrants, and 12-clock-hour RNFL thickness were analyzed in this study. All of the clock positions for the left eye were converted to the right eye clock position and were recorded (i.e., the pRNFL of 1 o'clock for the left eye was recorded as 11 o'clock and 11 o'clock for the left was recorded as 1 o'clock).

The ganglion cell analysis algorithm was used to process the data obtained with the macular cube 512 × 128 scan protocol to calculate the macular GCIPL thickness within a 14.13-mm^2 elliptical annular area centered at the fovea. The algorithm identified the distance between the outer boundary of the RNFL and the IPL as the thickness of the GCIPL. The average and six sectoral (superior, superonasal, inferonasal, inferior, inferotemporal, and supertemporal) GCIPL thickness measurements were analyzed.

Statistical Analysis

Statistical analyses were performed using SPSS (version 20.0; SPSS Inc., Chicago, IL, United States). The Kolmogorov–Smirnov test was performed to test for normality. An independent *t*-test or Mann–Whitney *U* test (for non-parametric data) was used to compare the baseline data between the myopia and glaucoma groups. Baseline and follow-up pRNFL and GCIPL data were compared in each group using the pairwise *t*-test. The annual change rate was calculated as [(last visit–initial visit)/follow-up duration (years)]. General linear regression model was used to describe the association between the group and the annual change rate of the whole and regional RNFL/GCIPL, and the coeffect of initial age, initial refractive error, and annual refractive error change rate were also considered in the model. The area under the receiver operating characteristic curve (AUC) was used to evaluate the diagnostic value of the annual change rate of the mean and sectoral pRNFL and GCIPL between myopia and glaucoma groups. The significance level was set to 0.05 for a two-sided alternative hypothesis test.

RESULTS

A total of forty-seven eyes of 47 subjects in the adolescent myopia progression (MP) group and 25 eyes of 25 subjects in the GP group were included. The basic demographics of the two groups are listed in **Table 1**.

At the initial visit, the whole average and superior pRNFL were thinner in the glaucoma group ($p < 0.05$), whereas no statistically significant difference was found in the inferior, temporal, and nasal pRNFL between the two groups (**Figure 1A**), whereas the average and sectoral GCIPL in the glaucoma group were thinner than myopia group ($p < 0.05$) (**Figure 1B**).

TABLE 1 | Basic demographics of progressive myopia and progressive glaucoma eyes in adolescents.

	Myopia	Glaucoma	P
Number	47	25	–
Sex (Female, %)	41.55%	40.00%	–
Laterality (Right, %)	57.45%	60.00%	–
Age at initial visit (years, mean ± SD)	10.97 ± 2.30	12.76 ± 3.92	0.05*
SE at initial visit (D, mean ± SD)	−1.89 ± 0.92	−2.48 ± 1.74	0.12*
BCVA at initial visit (logMAR, mean ± SD)	−0.05 ± 0.07	−0.03 ± 0.07	0.64*
IOP at initial visit (mmHg, mean ± SD)	15.93 ± 1.83	23.77 ± 2.87	<0.001*
Follow-up period (years, median, IQR)	5 (4~6)	5 (3~6)	0.80†
Age at last visit (years, mean ± SD)	14.92 ± 2.70	17.00 ± 3.74	0.02*
SE at last visit (D, mean ± SD)	−4.60 ± 1.61	−4.64 ± 2.80	0.95*
BCVA at last visit (logMAR, mean ± SD)	−0.05 ± 0.07	0.01 ± 0.07	0.24*
IOP at last visit (mmHg, mean ± SD)	15.89 ± 1.78	18.38 ± 3.85	0.11*

logMAR, logarithm of the minimum angle of resolution; SE, spherical equivalent; BCVA, best-corrected visual acuity; IOP, intraocular pressure; SD, standard deviation, IQR, interquartile range.
**Independent t-test.*
†Mann–Whitney U test.

The pRNFL and GCIPL of the initial and last visits in the myopia and GP groups are shown in **Figures 2, 3** and **Table 2**. In both the myopia and glaucoma groups, the average thickness of the whole, superior, and inferior pRNFL decreased during follow-up ($p < 0.05$). Nasal pRNFL decreased in the myopia group ($p < 0.05$) during the follow-up period, but no statistically significant difference was observed in the glaucoma group ($p = 0.19$) between the initial and last visits. The temporal pRNFL was increased in the MP group ($p < 0.05$), but decreased in the GP group during follow-up ($p < 0.05$). In the MP group, the pRNFL thickness at the 10, 9, 8, and 7 o'clock sections increased during the follow-up, whereas the pRNFL thickness at the 12, 1, 2, 5, and 6 o'clock sections decreased. By contrast, no statistically significant differences were found in the pRNFL thickness at the 3, 4, and 11 o'clock sections during follow-up ($p = 0.08$, 0.08, and 0.57). In the GP group, the pRNFL thickness decreased at most of the clock-hour sections during follow-up, except at the 4 and 3 o'clock sections. The average and sectoral GCIPL became thinner during follow-up in both myopia and glaucoma groups ($p < 0.05$).

When the coeffect of initial age, initial refractive error, and annual refractive error change rate were considered, the annual change rates of most pRNFL parameters still showed significantly different between the myopia and glaucoma groups, except the nasal pRNFL and pRNFL at 1–5 and 11 o'clock. In terms of GCIPL, the annual change rates of average, superotemporal, inferotemporal, and inferior GCIPL had significant difference between the two groups (**Table 3**).

The AUCs of the annual change rate of pRNFL and GCIPL are shown in **Table 4**. The AUCs of the annual change rate

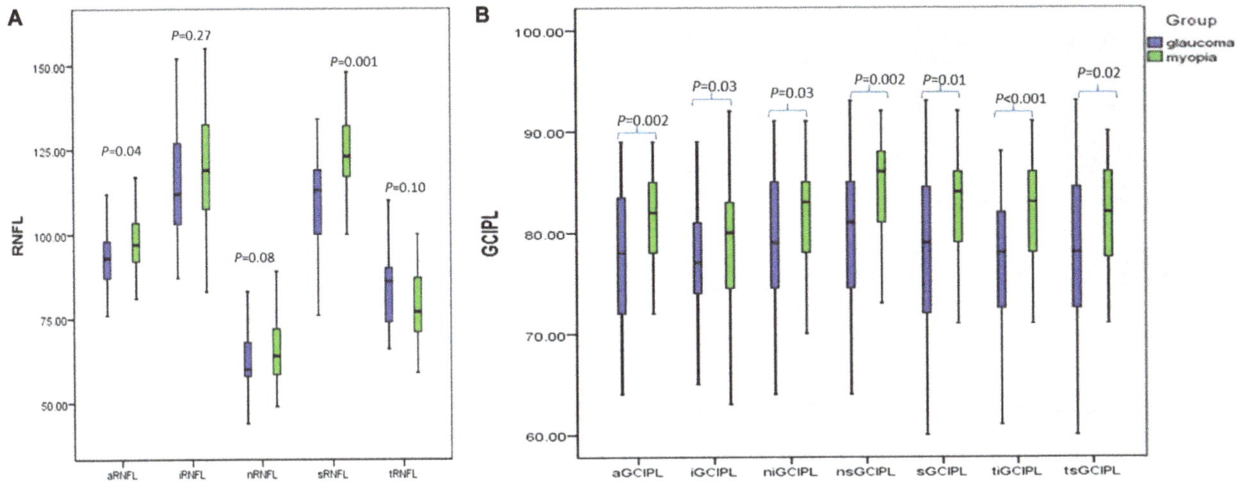

FIGURE 1 | Comparison of the pRNFL and the macular GCIPL between the glaucoma and myopia groups at initial visit. **(A)** Comparison of the pRNFL between the glaucoma and myopia groups at initial visit. **(B)** Comparison of the macular GCIPL between the glaucoma and myopia groups at initial visit. aRNFL, average retinal nerve fiber layer; iRNFL, inferior retinal nerve fiber layer; nRNFL, nasal retinal nerve fiber layer; sRNFL, superior retinal nerve fiber layer; tRNFL, temporal retinal nerve fiber layer; aGCIPL, average ganglion cell plus inner plexiform layer complex; iGCIPL, inferior ganglion cell and inner plexiform layer complex; niGCIPL: inferonasal ganglion cell plus inner plexiform layer complex; nsGCIPL, superonasal ganglion cell plus inner plexiform layer complex; sGCIPL, superior ganglion cell plus inner plexiform layer complex; tiGCIPL, inferotemporal ganglion cell plus inner plexiform layer complex; tsGCIPL, supertemporal ganglion cell plus inner plexiform layer complex.

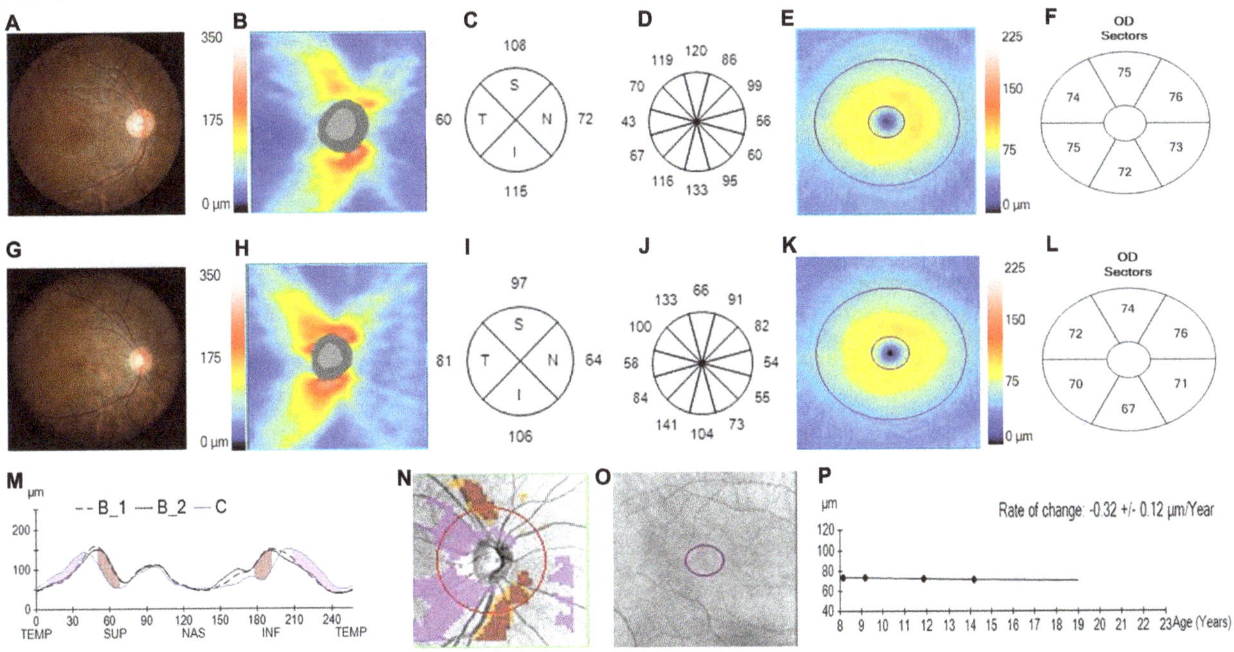

FIGURE 2 | Changes in the pRNFL and macular GCIPL in an adolescent with progressed myopia. **(A)** The fundus photograph of an adolescent myopia taken at initial visit in 2013. **(B)** The pRNFL thickness map taken at the initial visit. **(C)** The quadrantal pRNFL thickness at the initial visit. **(D)** The clock-hour pRNFL thickness at the initial visit. **(E)** The GCIPL thickness map taken at the initial visit. **(F)** The sectoral GCIPL thickness at the initial visit. **(G)** The fundus photograph of adolescent myopia taken at the last visit in 2018. **(H)** The pRNFL thickness map taken at the last visit. **(I)** The quadrantal pRNFL thickness at the last visit. **(J)** The clock-hour pRNFL thickness at the last visit. **(K)** The GCIPL thickness map taken at the last visit. **(L)** The sectoral GCIPL thickness at the last visit. **(M)** The pRNFL thickness profiles showing that the pRNFL thickness was possibly increased in the temporal quadrant (purple region), but was likely decreased in the superior and inferior quadrants (brown region) during the follow-up (B1, baseline 1; B2, baseline 2; C, current line). **(N)** The change possibility map of pRNFL thickness showing that the pRNFL thickness was possibly increased in the temporal quadrant (purple region), but was likely decreased in the superior and inferior quadrants (brown region) during the follow-up. **(O)** The change possibility map of GCIPL thickness showing neither possible increase nor possible loss in the entire GCIPL measured region during the follow-up. **(P)** The change trend line of GCIPL thickness profiles showing that the change rate of GCIPL was about -0.32 ± 0.12 µm/year.

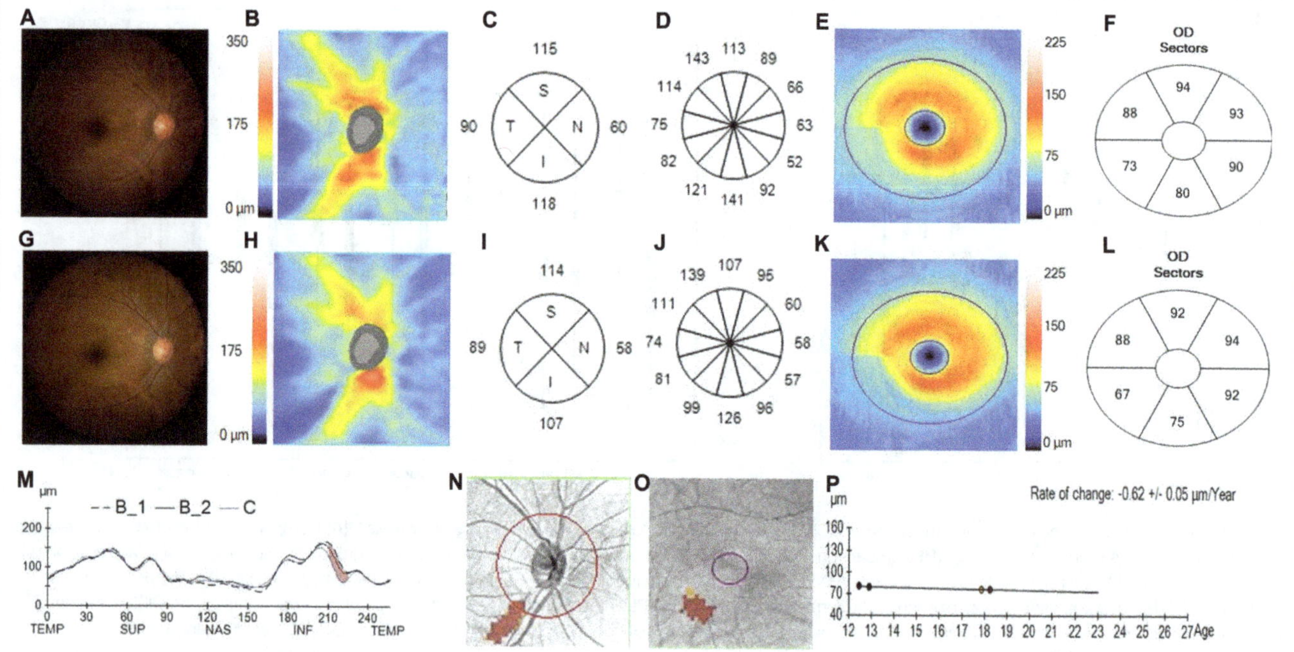

FIGURE 3 | Changes in the pRNFL and macular GCIPL in a progressed juvenile glaucoma. **(A)** The fundus photograph of a juvenile glaucoma case taken at the initial visit in 2014, with the white arrow showing a wedge defect of the RNFL corresponding to the narrowed inferior rim. **(B)** The pRNFL thickness map taken at the initial visit. **(C)** The quadrantal RNFL thickness at the initial visit. **(D)** The clock-hour RNFL thickness at the initial visit. **(E)** The GCIPL thickness map taken at the initial visit. **(F)** The sectoral GCIPL at the initial visit. **(G)** The fundus photograph of a juvenile glaucoma case taken at the last visit in 2019, with a considerable serious defect of the RNFL and narrower rim displayed on the photograph. **(H)** The RNFL thickness map taken at the last visit. **(I)** The quadrantal RNFL thickness at the last visit. **(J)** The clock-hour RNFL thickness at the last visit. **(K)** The GCIPL thickness map taken at the last visit. **(L)** The sectoral GCIPL at the last visit. **(M)** The pRNFL thickness profiles showing that the RNFL thickness was likely decreased in the inferotemporal region (brown region) during the follow-up (B1, baseline 1; B2, baseline 2; C, current line). **(N)** The change possibility map of RNFL thickness showing that the RNFL thickness was likely decreased in the inferotemporal region (brown region) during the follow-up. **(O)** The change possibility map of GCIPL thickness showing that GCIPL was likely decreased in the inferotemporal region (brown region) during the follow-up. **(P)** The change trend line of GCIPL thickness profiles showing that the change rate of GCIPL was about -0.62 ± 0.05 µm/year.

of pRNFL at the 10, 8, 9, and 7 o'clock sections, and also the temporal pRNFL and inferotemporal GCIPL, were above 0.85, which suggested that these parameters might be useful in differentiating whether the loss of pRNFL and GCIPL was caused by GP or MP (**Table 4**).

DISCUSSION

In this study, we retrospectively reviewed the longitudinal changes in the pRNFL and GCIPL among patients with adolescent myopia and juvenile glaucoma and compared the changes caused by progressed myopia and progressed glaucoma. Both progressed myopia and glaucoma could lead to a decrease in the average, superior, and inferior pRNFL. Temporal pRNFL showed an increase in the progressed myopia group, but decrease in the progressed glaucoma group. The GCIPL became thinner during follow-up in both the progressed myopia and glaucoma groups, and only the annual change rate of the inferotemporal and superotemporal GCIPL had a statistically significant difference between the two groups. The AUC analysis revealed that among the pRNFL and GCIPL parameters, the annual change rate of temporal pRNFL, inferotemporal GCIPL, and pRNFL at the 7, 8, 9, and 10 o'clock sectors had better diagnostic ability to differentiate progressed glaucoma from progressed myopia.

The previous cross-sectional studies (14–16) have confirmed that the distribution of pRNFL in eyes with myopia, especially in eyes with high myopia, is different from that in non-myopic eyes. Eyes with myopia displayed thicker temporal pRNFL and thinner superior, inferior, and nasal pRNFL (15, 16). Recently, Lee et al. (17) reported a decrease of the pRNFL on adult high myopia with time in a 2-year longitudinal study. However, the longitudinal databases of pRNFL in adolescents are still limited. This study revealed that with the progression of myopia in adolescents, the whole pRNFL decreased and shifted to the temporal quadrant gradually, which leads to an increase in temporal pRNFL and a reduction in the superior, inferior, and nasal pRNFL. There might be several factors which account for the result. First, the reduction in the whole pRNFL thickness may be due to the globe elongation that leads to mechanical stretching and thinning of the retina resulting from the progression of myopia over time (18). The previous studies have proved that the increase of myopia refraction is positively correlated with the increase of axial length (19, 20). In this study, though axial length data were lacked, the increase of myopia refraction might indirectly reflect the increase of axial length. Second, peripapillary atrophy, optic disk tilting, and rotation are very common in myopic eyes in Chinese

TABLE 2 | Comparison of the pRNFL and GCIPL between the initial and last visits.

	Myopia (mean ± SD) μ m			Glaucoma (mean ± SD) μ m		
	Initial visit	Last visit	*P*	Initial visit	Last visit	*P*
N (eye)	47	47		25	25	
Average RNFL	97.53 ± 8.60	94.78 ± 8.70	<0.001*	93.00 ± 9.12	81.12 ± 12.28	<0.001*
Superior RNFL	123.81 ± 12.26	115.31 ± 12.62	<0.001*	110.20 ± 14.50	95.24 ± 19.19	<0.001*
Temporal RNFL	79.38 ± 12.74	92.80 ± 14.59	<0.001*	85.20 ± 14.58	74.75 ± 10.19	0.01*
Inferior RNFL	119.64 ± 16.72	112.67 ± 14.73	<0.001*	115.00 ± 17.51	93.52 ± 20.21	<0.001*
Nasal RNFL	65.64 ± 8.99	61.34 ± 8.78	<0.001*	61.56 ± 10.49	60.68 ± 11.70	0.19
RNFL12′	121.21 ± 20.43	109.75 ± 20.84	<0.001*	107.80 ± 18.23	93.16 ± 22.45	<0.001*
RNFL11′	140.06 ± 20.02	141.58 ± 17.88	0.57	128.96 ± 24.69	111.00 ± 29.77	<0.001*
RNFL10′	92.28 ± 16.71	106.96 ± 20.71	<0.001*	97.24 ± 27.95	83.56 ± 18.94	0.01*
RNFL9′	61.54 ± 10.20	70.13 ± 10.19	<0.001*	64.44 ± 13.83	60.20 ± 12.66	0.10
RNFL8′	84.40 ± 17.75	100.31 ± 18.80	<0.001*	91.24 ± 12.16	80.36 ± 14.39	0.001*
RNFL7′	149.22 ± 23.61	154.55 ± 19.03	0.01*	144.48 ± 12.50	111.88 ± 24.68	<0.001*
RNFL6′	121.38 ± 28.07	106.78 ± 25.40	<0.001*	112.12 ± 25.83	92.88 ± 30.76	<0.001*
RNFL5′	88.82 ± 17.13	78.78 ± 14.30	<0.001*	85.20 ± 24.42	77.04 ± 25.42	0.03*
RNFL4′	57.74 ± 11.11	56.65 ± 11.11	0.08	55.80 ± 10.90	55.72 ± 10.46	0.98
RNFL3′	60.32 ± 10.94	57.62 ± 11.71	0.08	56.76 ± 10.40	57.52 ± 10.98	0.74
RNFL2′	75.74 ± 11.59	70.16 ± 12.58	<0.001*	74.08 ± 15.98	69.04 ± 17.22	0.06
RNFL1′	109.70 ± 18.22	95.82 ± 17.87	<0.001*	95.24 ± 17.16	81.16 ± 18.48	<0.001*
Average GCIPL	81.75 ± 4.94	78.84 ± 4.65	<0.001*	77.96 ± 7.20	71.33 ± 8.35	<0.001*
Superior GCIPL	82.85 ± 5.24	80.13 ± 4.86	<0.001*	79.96 ± 9.35	73.08 ± 11.96	0.002*
Superotemporal GCIPL	81.36 ± 5.08	79.78 ± 4.71	0.002*	77.91 ± 7.46	71.95 ± 9.91	<0.001*
Inferotemporal GCIPL	81.53 ± 5.72	78.89 ± 4.98	<0.001*	77.13 ± 7.58	65.96 ± 6.92	<0.001*
Inferior GCIPL	78.84 ± 6.33	74.67 ± 5.94	<0.001*	77.08 ± 6.54	67.83 ± 7.76	<0.001*
Inferonasal GCIPL	81.64 ± 5.44	76.63 ± 11.06	<0.001*	79.13 ± 7.32	73.79 ± 10.49	0.001*
Superonasal GCIPL	84.53 ± 5.05	81.31 ± 4.83	<0.001*	79.57 ± 8.22	73.83 ± 10.96	<0.001*

RNFL, retinal nerve fiber layer; GCIPL, ganglion cell plus inner plexiform layer.
**p < 0.05 for a two-sided alternative hypothesis test.*

population (21). As the progression of myopia, the occurrence of peripapillary atrophy, optic disk tilting, and rotation may lead to the redistribution of pRNFL (22) and a more temporally positioned superior or inferior peak locations (23). Third, the larger retinal vessels play a significant role in peripapillary RNFL thickness, since they comprise 13% of the total RNFL thickness (24). The previous study has reported that myopia status played effect on the superior and inferior vessel positions (25). The peaks of peripapillary RNFL profiles may change with superior and inferior vascular structures in myopia eyes (26).

A study conducted by Kanamori et al. (27) revealed that the RNFL thickness at the 7 o'clock position had the widest areas under the ROC curves for all parameters for early glaucomatous eyes (0.873). Lloyd et al. (28) found that the inferotemporal quadrant was the most common location for GP in ocular hypertension and early glaucoma. Kim et al. (29) reported that the progression of glaucoma had significantly higher rates on inferotemporal and supertemporal RNFL thicknesses. This study revealed in the glaucoma group, the greatest reduction in pRNFL was located at 7 o'clock sections These results confirm that the inferotemporal pRNFL is most vulnerable to glaucomatous damage. Moreover, despite the increase in refractive error in the glaucoma group being comparable to that in the myopia group in this study, the temporal pRNFL still became thinner in the glaucoma group. The greatest reduction region was more temporal in the glaucoma group than in the myopia group. The AUC analysis also showed that the annual pRNFL change rate at the 10, 8, 9, and 7 o'clock sections and also the temporal RNFL was above 0.90. The result may indicate that when considering the influence of myopia on the pRNFL, the change in temporal pRNFL may provide valuable information in addition to inferotemporal pRNFL in detecting glaucoma from myopia eyes.

A longitudinal study conducted by Lee et al. (30) reported that highly myopic eyes had thinner GCIPL and a significantly greater reduction in GCIPL over 3 years. Studies (31, 32) demonstrated that GCIPL thicknesses were significantly thinner with decreasing SE and also significantly thinner with increasing axial length. Miller et al. (13) found patient with high myopia experience thinning of non-temporal parameters ganglion cell-inner plexiform layer. Our study displayed similar results that both myopia and GP could lead to a decrease in the average and sectoral GCIPL, but the annual change rate of inferotemporal GCIPL in the GP group was much greater than that in the MP group. It has been proposed by Mill et al. that myopia-induced thinning of GCIPL is ubiquitous and most-pronounced with higher degrees of myopia, but that temporal GCIPL is least susceptible. A study (33) investigated the glaucoma detection

TABLE 3 | Annual change rate of RNFL and GCIPL between Glaucoma and Myopia groups.

Annual change rate	Myopia group (Mean ± SD) *N* = 47	Glaucoma group (Mean ± SD) *N* = 25	β coefficient (95% CI)	*p*
RNFL (μ m/year)				
Average RNFL	−0.55 ± 0.72	−3.55 ± 4.17	−3.30 (−4.61 ~ −2.00)	<0.001*
Superior RNFL	−1.81 ± 1.95	−3.78 ± 5.01	−2.24 (−4.17 ~ −0.68)	0.007*
Temporal RNFL	3.33 ± 2.27	−2.99 ± 3.76	−6.10 (−7.55 ~ −4.65)	<0.001*
Inferior RNFL	−1.73 ± 1.97	−6.50 ± 7.04	−5.39 (−7.72 ~ −3.05)	<0.001*
Nasal RNFL	−0.81 ± 1.75	−0.51 ± 3.54	0.01 (−1.22 ~ 1.23)	0.99
RNFL12′	−2.36 ± 3.64	−4.11 ± 4.59	−2.54 (−4.58~ −0.50)	0.02*
RNFL11′	0.59 ± 3.03	−2.46 ± 11.90	−3.02 (−0.6.50 ~ 0.45)	0.09
RNFL10′	3.75 ± 3.14	−3.12 ± 4.17	−6.43 (−8.15~ −4.71)	<0.001*
RNFL9′	2.16 ± 1.69	−1.16 ± 2.47	−3.13 (−4.11~ −2.15)	<0.001*
RNFL8′	3.82 ± 3.30	−3.71 ± 4.89	−7.08 (−9.16 ~ −5.00)	<0.001*
RNFL7′	1.07 ± 3.69	−10.15 ± 10.00	−10.74 (−14.25 ~ −7.23)	<0.001*
RNFL6′	−3.65 ± 3.87	−5.94 ± 6.08	−3.27 (−5.68 ~ 0.86)	0.01*
RNFL5′	−2.21 ± 2.61	−2.22 ± 5.31	−0.58 (−2.54 ~ 1.39)	0.56
RNFL4′	−1.44 ± 2.07	−0.66 ± 2.45	0.42 (−0.74 ~ 1.57)	0.47
RNFL3′	−1.62 ± 2.87	−0.38 ± 3.77	0.84 (−0.84 ~ 2.52)	0.32
RNFL2′	−1.00 ± 2.39	−1.55 ± 4.16	−0.73 (−2.37 ~ 0.92)	0.38
RNFL1′	−3.02 ± 3.37	−3.55 ± 3.69	−1.06 (−2.89 ~ 0.77)	0.25
GCIPL (μ m/year)				
Average GCIPL	−0.69 ± 0.73	−1.68 ± 1.64	−1.07 (−1.67~ − 0.48)	0.001*
Superior GCIPL	−0.63 ± 1.05	−1.48 ± 2.60	−0.87 (−1.80 ~ 0.06)	0.07
Superotemporal GCIPL	−0.37 ± 0.69	−1.36 ± 1.51	−0.87 (−1.42 ~ 0.32)	0.002*
Inferotemporal GCIPL	−0.67 ± 0.66	−2.93 ± 2.89	−2.40 (−3.34 ~ −1.45)	<0.001*
Inferior GCIPL	−0.98 ± 0.83	−2.40 ± 2.69	−1.70 (−2.60 ~ −0.81)	<0.001*
Inferonasal GCIPL	−1.47 ± 4.05	−1.18 ± 1.90	−0.40 (−1.40 ~ 2.21)	0.66
Superonasal GCIPL	−0.67 ± 0.82	−1.14 ± 1.21	−0.58 (−1.09 ~ −0.07)	0.05

RNFL, retinal nerve fiber layer; GCIPL, ganglion cell plus inner plexiform layer.
**p < 0.05 for a two-sided alternative hypothesis test.*

ability of the macular GCIPL in myopic preperimetric glaucoma (PPG) and found that the best parameter for discrimination of myopic PPG from myopic healthy eyes was inferotemporal macular GCIPL thickness. Our study's result was consistent with these results. The inferotemporal GCIPL corresponds to the inferotemporal and inferior pRNFL structures, which has been proven to be the region most vulnerable to glaucomatous damage. The reduction of inferotemporal GCIPL provided further evidence of the impairment of inferotemporal and inferior pRNFL. The AUC analysis reveals that the annual change rate of inferotemporal GCIPL had the greatest AUC among all sectoral GCIPL parameters in differentiating glaucoma from myopia confirmed inferotemporal GCIPL provide additional information beyond the temporal pRNFL in detecting GP.

There are some limitations in our study. Given that axial length measurement was not routinely performed for the patients involved in the study, we used SE. Despite associations that have been shown between SE and axial length (19, 20), and the pRNFL was also reported to be thinner with negative SE and longer AL (34), Guo et al. (35) reported significant axial elongation with minimal refraction changes among Chinese preschoolers, the effect of axial length change on pRNFL and GCIPL in adolescents still needs further study. Another limitation is that we did not collect data from a large sample size, which would have increased the power, and possibly strengthened the findings of our study. Despite this weakness, this study reported the preliminary results of the longitudinal changes in pRNFL and GCIPL between progressive myopia and glaucoma among adolescents and revealed that even though both GP and MP

TABLE 4 | The area under ROC curve (AUC) of the annual change rate of the pRNFL and the macular GCIPL to discriminate GP from MP.

Variable	Area under ROC curve	Variable	Area under ROC curve
Average RNFL	0.79 (0.66~0.92)	RNFL12′	0.58 (0.44~0.73)
Superior RNFL	0.64 (0.48~0.79)	RNFL11′	0.76 (0.64~0.89)
Temporal RNFL	0.81 (0.72~0.91)	RNFL10′	0.96 (0.92~1.00)*
Inferior RNFL	0.99 (0.90~1.00)*	RNFL9′	0.91 (0.83~0.98)*
Nasal RNFL	0.45 (0.29~0.60)	RNFL8′	0.94 (0.89~0.99)*
Average GCIPL	0.66 (0.52~0.80)	RNFL7′	0.95 (0.90~0.99)*
Superior GCIPL	0.58 (0.43~0.73)	RNFL6′	0.61 (0.48~0.74)
Superotemporal GCIPL	0.69 (0.54~0.83)	RNFL5′	0.45 (0.30~0.61)
Inferotemporal GCIPL	0.89 (0.81~0.96)*	RNFL4′	0.62 (0.49~0.76)
Inferior GCIPL	0.64 (0.49~0.78)	RNFL3′	0.62 (0.478~0.75)
Inferonasal GCIPL	0.51 (0.35~0.66)	RNFL2′	0.52 (0.378~0.66)
Superonasal GCIPL	0.65 (0.50~0.80)	RNFL1′	0.54 (0.39~0.68)

**The area under the receiver operating characteristic curve (AUC) above 0.85.*
RNFL, retinal nerve fiber layer; GCIPL, ganglion cell plus inner plexiform layer.

could cause reduction of the whole pRNFL and GCIPL in adolescents, the loss patterns of pRNFL and GCIPL were different between the two groups. The temporal (7, 8, 9, and 10 o'clock sectors) pRNFL plus the inferotemporal GCIPL can help to distinguish the loss of pRNFL and GCIPL caused by glaucoma or MP.

ETHICS STATEMENT

The studies involving human participants were reviewed and approved by the Ethics Review Committee of the Zhongshan Ophthalmic Center. Written informed consent to participate in this study was provided by the participants' legal guardian/next of kin.

AUTHOR CONTRIBUTIONS

HX: designing the study, analyzing the data, and writing the manuscript. YZ: collecting the data and editing the important part of the manuscript. YL and XX: collecting and analyzing the data. XL: designing the study and editing the important part of the manuscript. All authors met the ICMJE authorship criteria.

REFERENCES

1. Tham YC, Li X, Wong TY, Quigley HA, Aung T, Cheng CY. Global prevalence of glaucoma and projections of glaucoma burden through 2040: a systematic review and meta-analysis. *Ophthalmology.* (2014) 121:2081–90. doi: 10.1016/j.ophtha.2014.05.013
2. Casson RJ, Chidlow G, Wood JP, Crowston JG, Goldberg I. Definition of glaucoma: clinical and experimental concepts. *Clin Experiment Ophthalmol.* (2012) 40:341–9. doi: 10.1111/j.1442-9071.2012.02773.x
3. Quigley HA, Katz J, Derick RJ, Gilbderd D, Sommer A. An evaluation of optic disc and nerve fiber layer examinations in monitoring progression of early glaucoma damage. *Ophthalmology.* (1992) 99:19–28. doi: 10.1016/s0161-6420(92)32018-4
4. Daneshvar R, Yarmohammadi A, Alizadeh R, Henny S, Law SK, Caprioli J, et al. Prediction of glaucoma progression with structural parameters: comparison of optical coherence tomography and clinical disc parameters. *Am J Ophthalmol.* (2019) 208:19–29. doi: 10.1016/j.ajo.2019.06.020
5. Singh D, Mishra SK, Agarwal E, Sharma R, Bhartiya S, Dada T. Assessment of retinal nerve fiber layer changes by cirrus high-definition optical coherencetomography in myopia. *J Curr Glaucoma Pract.* (2017) 11:52–7. doi: 10.5005/jp-journals-10028-1223
6. Aref AA, Sayyad FE, Mwanza JC, Feuer WJ, Budenz DL. Diagnostic specificities of retinal nerve fiber layer, optic nerve head, and macular ganglion cell-inner plexiform layer measurements in myopic eyes. *J Glaucoma.* (2014) 23:487–93. doi: 10.1097/IJG.0b013e31827b155b
7. Sezgin Akcay BI, Gunay BO, Kardes E, Unlu C, Ergin A. Evaluation of the ganglion cell and retinal nerve fiber layer in low, moderate, and high myopia: a study by RTVue spectral domain optical coherence tomography. *Semin Ophthalmol.* (2017) 32:682–8. doi: 10.3109/08820538.2016.1170157
8. Choi YJ, Jeoung JW, Park KH, Kim DM. Glaucoma detection ability of ganglion cell-inner plexiform layer thickness by spectral-domain optical coherence tomography in high myopia. *Invest Ophthalmol Vis Sci.* (2013) 54:2296–304. doi: 10.1167/iovs.12-10530
9. Holden BA, Fricke TR, Wilson DA, Jong M, Naidoo KS, Sankaridurg P, et al. Global prevalence of myopia and high myopia and temporal trends from 2000 through 2050. *Ophthalmology.* (2016) 123:1036–42. doi: 10.1016/j.ophtha.2016.01.006
10. Chen L, Huang J, Zou H, Xue W, Ma Y, He X, et al. Retinal nerve fiber layer hickness in normal Chinese students aged 6 to 17 years. *Invest Ophthalmol Vis Sci.* (2013) 54:7990–7. doi: 10.1167/iovs.12-11252
11. Barrio-Barrio J, Noval S, Galdós M, Ruiz-Canela M, Bonet E, Capote M, et al. Multicenter Spanish study of spectral-domain optical coherence tomography in normal children. *Acta Ophthalmol.* (2013) 91:e56–63. doi: 10.1111/j.1755-3768.2012.02562.x
12. Read SA, Alonso-Caneiro D, Vincent SJ. Longitudinal changes in macular retinal layer thickness in pediatric populations: myopic vs non-myopic eyes. *PLoS One.* (2017) 12:e0180462. doi: 10.1371/journal.pone.0180462
13. Miller GD, Abu-Qamar O, Salim S. Evaluation of retinal nerve fiber layer, ganglion cell-inner plexiform layer, and optic nerve head in glaucoma suspects with varying myopia. *J Glaucoma.* (2021) 30:e213–21. doi: 10.1097/IJG.0000000000001834
14. Rauscher FM, Sekhon N, Feuer WJ, Budenz DL. Myopia affects retinal nerve fiber layer measurements as determined by optical coherence tomography. *J Glaucoma.* (2009) 18:501–5. doi: 10.1097/IJG.0b013e318193c2be
15. Kang SH, Hong SW, Im SK, Lee SH, Ahn MD. Effect of myopia on the thickness of the retinal nerve fiber layer measured by Cirrus HD optical coherence tomography. *Invest Ophthalmol Vis Sci.* (2010) 5:4075–83. doi: 10.1167/iovs.09-4737
16. Leung CKS, Yu M, Weinreb RN, Mak HK, Lai G, Ye C, et al. Retinal nerve fiber layer imaging with spectral-domain optical coherence tomography: interpreting the RNFL maps in healthy myopic eyes. *Invest Ophthalmol Vis Sci.* (2012) 53:7194–200. doi: 10.1167/iovs.12-9726
17. Lee MW, Kim JM, Shin YI, Jo YJ, Kim JY. Longitudinal changes in peripapillary retinal nerve fiber layer thickness in high myopia: a prospective, observational study. *Ophthalmology.* (2019) 126:522–8. doi: 10.1016/j.ophtha.2018.07.007
18. Jonas JB, Weber P, Nagaoka N, Ohno-Matsui K. Temporal vascular ARCADE width and angle in high axial myopia. *Retina.* (2018) 38:1839–47. doi: 10.1097/IAE.0000000000001786
19. Fan Q, Wang H, Jiang Z. Axial length and its relationship to refractive error in Chinese university students. *Cont Lens Anterior Eye.* (2021) 101470. doi: 10.1016/j.clae.2021.101470 [Epub ahead of print].
20. Jong M, Sankaridurg P, Naduvilath TJ, Li W, He M. The relationship between progression in axial length/corneal radius of curvature ratio and spherical equivalent refractive error in myopia. *Optom Vis Sci.* (2018) 95:921–9. doi: 10.1097/OPX.0000000000001281
21. Li Z, Guo X, Xiao O, Lee PY, Liu R, Wang D, et al. Optic disc features in highly myopic eyes: the ZOC-BHVI high myopia cohort study. *Optom Vis Sci.* (2018) 95:318–22. doi: 10.1097/OPX.0000000000001200
22. Hwang YH, Yoo C, Kim YY. Characteristics of peripapillary retinal nerve fiber layer thickness in eyes with myopic optic disc tilt and rotation. *J Glaucoma.* (2012) 21:394–400. doi: 10.1016/j.ophtha.2014.09.031
23. Hwang YH, Yoo C, Kim YY. Myopic optic disc tilt and the characteristics of peripapillary retinal nervefiber layer thicknessmeasured by spectral-domain optical coherence tomography. *J Glaucoma.* (2012) 21:260–5. doi: 10.1097/IJG.0b013e31820719e1
24. Hood DC, Fortune B, Arthur SN, Xing D, Salant JA, Ritch R, et al. Blood vessel contributions to retinal nerve fiber layer thickness profiles measured with optical coherence tomography. *J Glaucoma.* (2008) 17:519–28. doi: 10.1097/IJG.0b013e3181629a02
25. Wang M, Jin Q, Wang H, Baniasadi N, Elze T. Quantifying positional variation of retinal blood vessels in glaucoma. *PLoS One.* (2018) 13:e0193555. doi: 10.1371/journal.pone.0193555
26. Du J, Du Y, Xue Y, Wang H, Li Y. Factors associated with changes in peripapillary retinal nerve fibre layer thickness in healthy myopic eyes. *J Ophthalmol.* (2021) 2021:3462004. doi: 10.1155/2021/3462004

27. Kanamori A, Nakamura M, Escano MF, Seya R, Maeda H, Negi A. Evaluation of the glaucomatous damage on retinal nerve fiber layer thickness measured by optical coherence tomography. *Am J Ophthalmol.* (2003) 135:513–20. doi: 10.1016/s0002-9394(02)02003-2
28. Lloyd MJ, Mansberger SL, Fortune BA, Nguyen H, Torres R, Demirel S, et al. Features of optic disc progression in patients with ocular hypertension and early glaucoma. *J Glaucoma.* (2013) 22:343–8. doi: 10.1097/IJG.0b013e31824c9251
29. Kim HJ, Jeoung JW, Yoo BW, Kim HC, Park KH. Patterns of glaucoma progression in retinal nerve fiber and macular ganglion cell-inner plexiform layer in spectral-domain optical coherence tomography. *Jpn J Ophthalmol.* (2017) 61:324–33. doi: 10.1007/s10384-017-0511-3
30. Lee MW, Nam KY, Park HJ, Lim HB, Kim JY. Longitudinal changes in the ganglion cell-inner plexiform layer thickness in high myopia: a prospective observational study. *Br Ophthalmol.* (2020) 104:604–9. doi: 10.1136/bjophthalmol-2019-314537
31. Seo S, Lee CE, Jeong JH, Park KH, Kim DM, Jeoung JW. Ganglion cell-inner plexiform layer and retinal nerve fiber layer thickness according to myopia and optic disc area: a quantitative and three-dimensional analysis. *BMC Ophthalmol.* (2017) 17:22. doi: 10.1186/s12886-017-0419-1
32. Goh JP, Koh V, Chan YH, Ngo C. Macular ganglion cell and retinal nerve fiber layer thickness in children with refractive errors-an optical coherence tomography study. *J Glaucoma.* (2017) 26:619–25. doi: 10.1097/IJG.0000000000000683
33. Seol BR, Jeoung JW, Park KH. Glaucoma detection ability of macular ganglion cell-inner plexiform layer thickness in myopic preperimetric glaucoma. *Invest Ophthalmol Vis Sci.* (2015) 56:8306–13. doi: 10.1167/iovs.15-18141
34. Kang MT, Li SM, Li H, Liu LR, Wang Y, Yang Z, et al. Peripapillary retinal nerve fiber layer thickness and its association with refractive error in Chinese children: the Anyang childhood eye study. *Clin Exp Ophthalmol.* (2016) 44:701–9. doi: 10.1167/iovs.13-11958
35. Guo X, Fu M, Ding X, Morgan IG, Zeng Y, He M. Significant axial elongation with minimal change in refraction in 3- to 6-year-old Chinese preschoolers: the Shenzhen kindergarten eye study. *Ophthalmology.* (2017) 124:1826–38. doi: 10.1016/j.ophtha.2017.05.030

7

Optical Coherence Tomography Angiography Compared with Optical Coherence Tomography for Detection of Early Glaucoma With High Myopia

Pei-Yao Chang [1,2,3,4*], *Jiun-Yi Wang* [3,5], *Jia-Kang Wang* [1,2,4,6], *Tzu-Lun Huang* [1,4] *and Yung-Ray Hsu* [1,2,4]

[1] *Department of Ophthalmology, Far Eastern Memorial Hospital, New Taipei City, Taiwan,* [2] *Department of Medicine, National Taiwan University Hospital, Taipei, Taiwan,* [3] *Department of Healthcare Administration, Asia University, Taichung, Taiwan,* [4] *Department of Electrical Engineering, Yuan Ze University, Taoyuan City, Taiwan,* [5] *Department of Medical Research, China Medical University Hospital, China Medical University, Taichung, Taiwan,* [6] *Department of Healthcare Administration and Department of Nursing, Oriental Institute of Technology, New Taipei City, Taiwan*

Correspondence:
Pei-Yao Chang
peiyao@seed.net.tw

Purpose: To investigate the diagnostic abilities of the perfusion density (PD) and structural thickness parameters in the peripapillary and macular regions measured by optical coherence tomography angiography (OCTA) and optical coherence tomography (OCT) and to test if their diagnostic abilities of early glaucoma are different between highly myopic (HM) and non-highly myopic (NHM) patients.

Methods: A total of 75 glaucoma patients and 65 controls were included in the analyses. The glaucoma detection abilities of macular PD and peripapillary PD, along with macular ganglion cell-inner plexiform layer (mGCIPL) thickness and peripapillary retinal nerve fiber layer (pRNFL) thicknesses were compared between the HM and NHM group. Diagnostic ability was assessed by area under the receiver operating characteristics (AUC) curves, adjusted by age, axial length, and signal strength.

Results: The diagnostic ability of macular PD and mGCIPL thickness had no significant difference in both HM and NHM groups. However, the diagnostic ability of peripapillary PD except in the temporal section was significantly lower in the HM group than in the NHM group (all $p < 0.05$). The diagnostic ability of the superior, nasal, and average pRNFL thickness was also significantly lower in the HM group than in the NHM group (all $p < 0.05$).

Conclusion: This study demonstrated that although peripapillary PD and macular PD were both significantly reduced in patients with highly myopia, the diagnostic ability of peripapillary PD in HM patients was significantly lower than that in NHM patients, while macular PD was not. Macular OCTA along with OCT imaging should be included in the imaging algorithm in early glaucoma diagnosis in highly myopic patients.

Keywords: optic nerve head vessel density, retinal vessel density, retinal nerve fiber layer thickness, open angle glaucoma, high myopia

INTRODUCTION

Myopia is highly prevalent in Asia and high myopia has been considered an independent risk factor for glaucoma (1). Optic disc of highly myopic patients manifests structural change that mimics glaucoma. Early glaucoma diagnosis is crucial but challenging in myopic patients even for glaucoma specialists because the optic disc of myopic, especially highly myopic patients is usually accompanied by tilting/torsional, shallow cup, and peripapillary atrophy (2). Several studies have reported that myopic eyes have a thinner retinal nerve fiber layer (RNFL) and the pattern of peripapillary retinal nerve fiber layer (pRNFL) defect in high myopic glaucoma is different (3–5). The papillomacular bundle in highly myopic (HM) patients is more susceptible (4, 5) and the macular ganglion cell complex or ganglion cell-inner plexiform layer (GCIPL) thickness was reported to have comparable or even better glaucoma detection ability than pRNFL thickness in HM (6, 7). However, even with the pRNFL and macular GCIPL thickness measurement by spectral-domain optical coherence tomography (SD-OCT), it is still more difficult to detect an early glaucomatous change in highly myopic eyes than in emmetropic eyes (8, 9).

Vessel density parameters measured by OCT angiography (OCTA) in the peripapillary and macular regions in the glaucomatous eyes were significantly lower than those in the healthy eyes (10–13). Peripapillary/macular vessel density changes have been reported to be useful for differentiating between glaucoma and healthy eyes, especially in HM patients because vessel density measurement is less affected by the low reflectance of the RNFL or optic disc deformation (14, 15). That is, if the vessel density changes are more prominent than other structural changes at the early stage of glaucoma in HM, it would be helpful for this challenging early glaucoma diagnosis. Thus, we focused on the vessel density parameters in HM patients with early glaucoma to investigate the diagnostic abilities of the vessel density parameters in the peripapillary and macular regions and to test if their diagnostic abilities are different between HM and non-highly myopic (NHM) patients. We further compared their diagnostic abilities of structural OCT parameters, such as pRNFL and macular GCIPL thickness, with vessel density parameters to investigate their performance in early glaucoma diagnosis.

METHODS

Study Design and Procedure

This retrospective cross-sectional study collected medical records of patients who visited the glaucoma clinic in a medical center in northern Taiwan between January and June 2018. The inclusion criteria for all groups were age more than 20 years, best-corrected visual acuity ≥20/30, and open-angle confirmed by gonioscopy. Glaucomatous eyes were defined as glaucomatous damage to the optic disc as accompanied by two corresponding and reliable abnormal visual field (VF) examinations, regardless of the intraocular pressure (IOP). Subjects with evidence of retinal pathology, diabetes, hypertension, or non-glaucomatous optic nerve diseases were excluded, as well as eyes that had undergone previous laser therapy or ocular surgery, or the presence of any media opacities that prevented high-quality OCT scans. If both eyes of a patient were eligible, one eye was selected at random.

The study was performed in accordance with the tenets of the Declaration of Helsinki and was approved by the Institutional Review Board at Far Eastern Memorial Hospital (No. 107135-E). Informed consent was waived as personal identities in the retrospective data were recoded and delinked.

Measures

All of the subjects underwent a complete ophthalmic examination, which included measurement of visual acuity, IOP measurement through noncontact tonometry (CT-80, Topcon, Japan), refractive error measurement through autorefraction (Auto Refractometer AR-610; Nidek Co, Ltd., Tokyo, Japan), slit-lamp examination; gonioscopy; dilated fundus examination with simultaneous stereophotography of the optic disc, and red-free RNFL photography. VF testing was performed using a Humphrey Field Analyzer (SITA full threshold programs 30-2; Carl Zeiss Meditec, Inc., Dublin, CA, USA).

The refraction data were converted to spherical equivalents (SE), and the subjects were divided into two groups: an HM group (spherical equivalent <-6.00 diopters [D] and >-13.00 D) and an NHM group (spherical equivalent ≥ −6.00 D and < +0.5 D).

Glaucomatous optic disc changes were defined on stereoscopic color disc photography as a large cupping (>0.7 vertical cup/disc ratio), cup/disc asymmetry between the glaucomatous and normal eyes >0.2, neuroretinal rim thinning, notching, or excavation. Eyes with glaucomatous VF defects were defined as those with a glaucoma hemifield test result outside normal limits or a pattern standard deviation outside 95% of normal limits. Additionally, a cluster of three points with probabilities of 5% on the pattern deviation map in at least one hemifield, such as at least one point with a probability of 1%, or a cluster of two points with a probability of 1% was needed. A VF was defined as reliable when fixation losses were <20%, and each of the false-positive and false-negative rates was <15%. Normal eyes were defined as IOP <21 mm Hg, an absence of glaucomatous optic disc appearance as determined by two masked observers, and no perimetric defects.

Peripapillary (Optic Disc Cube 200 × 200 protocol) and macular (Macular Cube 512 × 128 protocol) scans (collectively referred to as ganglion cell analysis) were acquired using the Cirrus 5000 HD-OCT (Carl Zeiss Meditec, Inc.). Software released by the manufacturer was used to calculate pRNFL and mGCIPL thicknesses, as previously described (16). The pRNFL thickness was measured in a circle of 3.46 mm in diameter and the circumpapillary average, superior, inferior, temporal, and nasal quadrant thicknesses were analyzed. Regarding the macular GCIPL thickness, average and sectoral (superonasal, superior, superotemporal, inferotemporal, inferior, and inferonasal) were analyzed.

Optical coherence tomography angiography imaging of the radial peripapillary and macular capillaries was performed using the AngioPlex™ (Cirrus; Zeiss, Dublin, USA; software Version 11). Angiographic images were generated through OCT-based microangiography (OMAG) and the procedure for

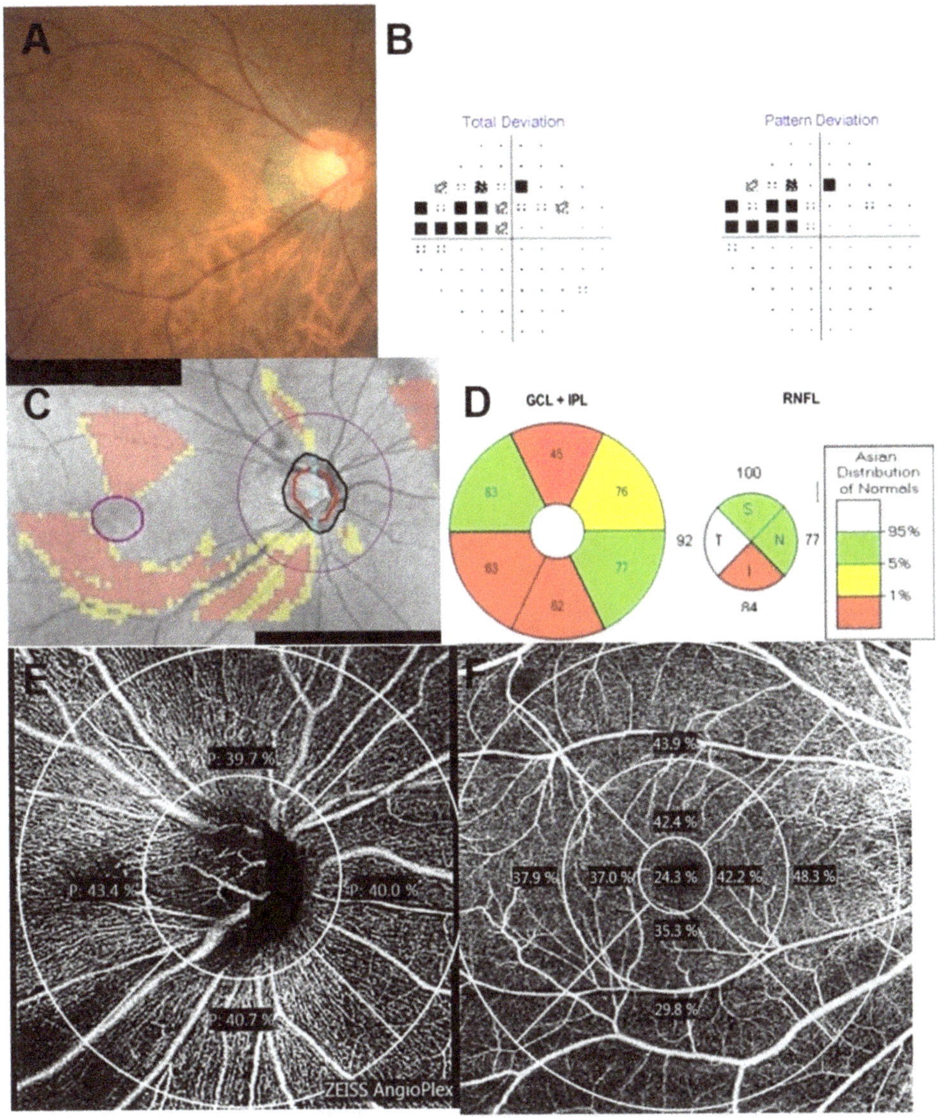

FIGURE 1 | Inferior disc excavation with inferior nerve fiber layer wedge defect of the right eye of a 42-year-old man with POAG **(A)**. Visual field (VF) results revealed defects at the corresponding superonasal site **(B)**. Combined retinal nerve fiber layer (RNFL) and GCIPL deviation maps indicated structural glaucomatous damage **(C)**. OCT scan showed the GCIPL thickness (μm) provided by the ganglion cell analysis report [**(D)**, left] and RNFL thickness (μm) (**(D)**, right) in each sector. OCT angiography image (Cirrus HD-OCT, version 11) of a 4.5 mm × 4.5 mm scan **(E)** exhibited radial peripapillary superficial perfusion (%) and a 6 mm × 6 mm scan **(F)** exhibited the superficial vessels at the macula. The grids represented the sectors across which the perfusion density (%) was calculated. The area between the inner two circles in the 6 mm × 6 mm scan represented the inner sectors, and the area between the outer two circles represented the outer sectors. GCIPL, ganglion cell-inner plexiform layer; OCT, optical coherence tomography; I, inferior; IN, inferonasal; IT, inferotemporal; N, nasal; S, superior; SN, superonasal; ST, superotemporal; T, temporal.

OCTA imaging using the Cirrus HD-OCT has been detailed previously (17). The optic nerve scan was imaged using a 4.5 mm^2 × 4.5 mm^2 scan and the macula scan using a 6 mm^2 × 6 mm^2 scan pattern. Angiometric software of the Cirrus HD-OCT automatically calculates perfusion density (defined as the total area of perfused vasculature per unit area in the region of interest) from the superficial retinal layer slab and radial outer region peripapillary capillaries. This software calculates the macular perfusion density parameters across four inner and four outer sectors of the Early Treatment Diabetic Retinopathy Study (ETDRS) grid over the macula. Inner and outer ring measurements were analyzed by sectoral locations (inferior, superior, nasal, and temporal). The software also calculates the radial peripapillary perfusion density across the four sectors (inferior, superior, nasal, and temporal) (**Figure 1**).

Image quality was assessed for all OCTA and OCT scans. Poor quality images, which were defined as those with a signal strength

TABLE 1 | Baseline characteristics of the control and glaucoma groups.

	Highly myopic, $n = 70$			Non-highly myopic, $n = 70$				
	Control, $n = 27$	Glaucoma, $n = 43$	P	Control, $n = 38$	Glaucoma, $n = 32$	P	$P^{\dagger}$	$P^{\ddagger}$
Age (y)	39.63 ± 7.63	42.63 ± 10.72	0.210	45.18 ± 8.56	54.94 ± 8.65	<0.001	0.009	<0.001
Sex (Male:Female)	11:16	28:15	0.046	21:17	24:8	0.086	0.248	0.359
SE (D)	−8.87 ± 2.00	−9.12 ± 2.30	0.642	−1.87 ± 2.05	−2.70 ± 2.01	0.091	<0.001	<0.001
Visual field index (%)	99.25 ± 0.99	94.30 ± 4.68	<0.001	99.30 ± 0.95	93.25 ± 4.98	<0.001	0.839	0.352
Mean deviation (dB)	−0.50 ± 1.42	−2.73 ± 2.22	<0.001	−0.12 ± 1.07	−2.98 ± 2.12	<0.001	0.262	0.621
Optic Disc area (mm^2)	1.84 ± 0.48	1.92 ± 0.56	0.526	2.19 ± 0.42	2.00 ± 0.56	0.109	0.002	0.539
Rim Area (mm)	1.23 ± 0.30	0.88 ± 0.24	<0.001	1.63 ± 2.44	0.82 ± 0.20	0.065	0.405	0.245
Average C/D ratio (%)	0.54 ± 0.12	0.70 ± 0.13	<0.001	0.62 ± 0.15	0.75 ± 0.07	<0.001	0.032	0.024
IOP at the scanning visit (mm Hg)	17.44 ± 4.02	15.72 ± 3.15	0.049	18.46 ± 4.61	14.69 ± 2.50	<0.001	0.358	0.130

†*Value for comparison between normal and glaucomatous eyes in the non-highly myopic group.*
‡*Value for comparison between highly and non-highly myopic groups.*

of <7, poor centration, or motion artifacts and segmentation errors, were excluded from the analysis.

Statistical Analysis

Data were analyzed using IBM SPSS version 22.0 (Armonk, NY: IBM Corp.). Descriptive statistics like the number for categorical data and the mean ± standard deviation for continuous data were used to demonstrate characteristics of the study participants and distributions of the biomarkers. A two-sample t-test was conducted to compare the variable distributions between controls and glaucoma cases in the HM group and in the NHM group, as well as between controls or between glaucoma cases in the two groups. Multivariable logistic regression models which included one major biomarker and adjusted for sex, age, and SE and signal strength were first conducted to estimate the likelihood of being glaucoma for the myopia group and the non-myopia group. Then the area under the receiver operating characteristic curves (AUCs) was calculated and compared between the two groups. The comparison between AUCs was based on the method demonstrated in Gonen (18). The significance level was set at 0.05 for all analyses.

RESULTS

In total, 181 individuals (81 normal and 100 primary open angle glaucoma patients) underwent OCTA measurements. Among them, 10 eyes (5.5%) with motion artifacts in OMAG scans, 20 eyes (11.05%) with a signal strength of <7, 4 eyes (2.2%) with poor structural scans of optic nerve head OCT images owing to decentration and 7 eyes (3.9%) with media opacity, such as vitreous floaters, were excluded. Finally, 140 eyes, comprising 65 healthy subjects and 75 glaucoma patients, were included in the analysis. All participants in the glaucoma group were treated with at least one type of ocular antihypertensive medication at the time of OCTA imaging. The demographic and ophthalmic characteristics of the four groups are summarized in **Table 1**. The mean age among NHM glaucoma patients was significantly higher than that in NHM control subjects, but the age was not significantly different in the HM group. The mean VF defect had no significant difference between the NHM glaucoma group (mean [SD], 2.98 [2.12]) and the HM glaucoma group (mean [SD], 2.73 [2.22]).

The macular perfusion density, comparing the normal and glaucomatous eyes in both the HM and NHM groups, was significantly different (all $p < 0.05$), except for the inner nasal ($p = 0.103$) in the HM group and inner nasal, inner temporal, and inner superior section in the NHM group. The optic disc perfusion, comparing the normal and glaucomatous eyes in both the HM and the NHM groups, was significantly different (all $p < 0.05$), except for the nasal ($p = 0.103$) in the HM group (**Table 2**). There was no significant difference in all sections of the macular perfusion density and the optic disc perfusion between the glaucoma patients in the HM group and those in the NHM group. The signal strength of the macular perfusion density, macular GCIPL thickness, pRNFL thickness, except for the optic disc perfusion was significantly higher in normal controls than in the glaucoma patients. The mGCIPL thickness in every section, except the temporal section in the HM group, was significantly thicker in controls than in the glaucomatous patients, whether in the NHM group or in the HM group. The pRNFL thickness in every section was significantly thinner in glaucomatous eyes than in controls, both in highly and non-highly myopic eyes (all $p < 0.05$, **Table 2**). The AUCs of structural and vascular parameters are shown in **Table 3**. The diagnostic ability of macular perfusion density and mGCIPL thickness had no significant difference between the HM and the NHM group. However, the diagnostic ability of optic disc flux index in every section and perfusion density except in the temporal section was significantly lower in the HM group than in the NHM group. The diagnostic ability of the superior, nasal, and average pRNFL thickness was also significantly lower in the HM group than in the NHM group. However, when comparing the AUCs of OCT and OCTA measurement, the diagnostic performance had no significant difference between outer region mean perfusion density/flux index and average pRNFL thickness and between outer mean macular perfusion density and average mGCIPL thickness (**Table 4**).

TABLE 2 | Vessel perfusion density parameters measured by optical coherence tomography angiography (OCTA) and structural parameters measured by optical coherence tomography (OCT).

	Highly myopic $n = 70$			Non-highly myopic $n = 70$				
	Control $n = 27$	Glaucoma $n = 43$	P	Control $n = 38$	Glaucoma $n = 32$	P	$P^{\dagger}$	$P^{\ddagger}$
Macula perfusion density								
Signal strength	8.7 ± 1.33	7.7 ± 1.26	0.002	8.84 ± 1.29	8.09 ± 1.2	0.015	0.674	0.175
Outer superior	0.45 ± 0.04	0.39 ± 0.07	<0.001	0.44 ± 0.04	0.38 ± 0.06	<0.001	0.781	0.856
Outer inferior	0.44 ± 0.05	0.33 ± 0.07	<0.001	0.44 ± 0.04	0.34 ± 0.08	<0.001	0.992	0.474
Outer temporal	0.39 ± 0.07	0.31 ± 0.09	0.001	0.39 ± 0.06	0.33 ± 0.07	<0.001	0.698	0.570
Outer nasal	0.49 ± 0.03	0.45 ± 0.07	0.001	0.48 ± 0.03	0.45 ± 0.05	0.006	0.210	0.884
Inner superior	0.43 ± 0.04	0.38 ± 0.1	0.006	0.41 ± 0.06	0.38 ± 0.07	0.138	0.141	0.855
Inner inferior	0.41 ± 0.06	0.35 ± 0.09	0.001	0.41 ± 0.05	0.38 ± 0.07	0.041	0.691	0.215
Inner temporal	0.4 ± 0.04	0.34 ± 0.1	0.002	0.4 ± 0.06	0.37 ± 0.07	0.123	0.894	0.157
Inner nasal	0.41 ± 0.05	0.38 ± 0.09	0.103	0.41 ± 0.05	0.4 ± 0.06	0.256	0.782	0.410
Inner mean	0.41 ± 0.04	0.37 ± 0.08	0.003	0.41 ± 0.05	0.38 ± 0.06	0.077	0.611	0.368
Outer mean	0.44 ± 0.04	0.37 ± 0.06	<0.001	0.44 ± 0.03	0.37 ± 0.05	<0.001	0.615	0.760
Full mean	0.43 ± 0.04	0.36 ± 0.06	<0.001	0.42 ± 0.04	0.37 ± 0.05	<0.001	0.608	0.661
Optic disc perfusion density								
Signal strength	8.48 ± 1.24	8.05 ± 1.36	0.213	8.74 ± 1.14	8.28 ± 1.09	0.102	0.423	0.428
Superior	0.43 ± 0.03	0.41 ± 0.03	0.007	0.43 ± 0.03	0.4 ± 0.03	<0.001	0.722	0.303
Inferior	0.43 ± 0.02	0.4 ± 0.04	<0.001	0.44 ± 0.02	0.4 ± 0.03	<0.001	0.073	1.000
Temporal	0.48 ± 0.02	0.46 ± 0.03	<0.001	0.48 ± 0.02	0.46 ± 0.03	0.013	0.320	0.702
Nasal	0.42 ± 0.02	0.42 ± 0.03	0.979	0.44 ± 0.02	0.42 ± 0.02	0.001	0.023	0.469
Outer region mean	0.44 ± 0.02	0.42 ± 0.02	<0.001	0.45 ± 0.02	0.42 ± 0.02	<0.001	0.168	0.616
Macular ganglion cell-inner plexiform layer thickness (mGCIPL) (μm)								
Signal strength	8.85 ± 0.99	8.02 ± 1.04	0.001	8.92 ± 0.88	8.31 ± 1.03	0.01	0.768	0.234
Superior	80.81 ± 5.07	70.67 ± 10	<0.001	84.39 ± 5.59	70.78 ± 10.58	<0.001	0.010	0.965
Inferior	75.56 ± 4.69	63.91 ± 8.42	<0.001	81.53 ± 5.32	64.09 ± 10.62	<0.001	<0.001	0.933
Superotemporal	80.15 ± 4.8	70.91 ± 9.07	<0.001	82.26 ± 5.3	67.03 ± 10.61	<0.001	0.104	0.093
Inferotemporal	78.89 ± 4.82	63.47 ± 7.42	<0.001	83.11 ± 5.11	62.59 ± 10.9	<0.001	0.001	0.698
Superonasal	80.96 ± 4.54	73.35 ± 11.74	<0.001	86.24 ± 5.95	76.94 ± 10.64	<0.001	<0.001	0.177
Inferonasal	79.26 ± 5.22	71.02 ± 9.5	<0.001	84.61 ± 5.37	71.66 ± 10.34	<0.001	<0.001	0.784
Average	79 ± 4.79	68.88 ± 6.83	<0.001	83.71 ± 5	68.75 ± 8.92	<0.001	<0.001	0.942
Peripapillary retinal nerve fiber layer thickness (pRNFL) (μm)								
Signal strength	7.96 ± 0.94	7.44 ± 1.03	0.003	8.47 ± 0.86	7.75 ± 0.84	0.001	0.027	0.171
Superior	108.33 ±13.29	95.3 ± 19.22	<0.001	127.57 ± 13.81	87.59 ± 17.79	<0.001	<0.001	0.080
Inferior	112 ± 11.24	82.91 ± 14.82	0.001	128.54 ± 14.06	82.41 ± 19.33	<0.001	<0.001	0.899
Temporal	84.74 ± 21.36	69.47 ± 14.42	0.496	72.84 ± 12.8	60.97 ± 14.01	<0.001	0.014	0.013
Nasal	65.52 ± 7.77	67.16 ± 10.83	<0.001	71.26 ± 10.86	64.94 ± 7.44	0.007	0.022	0.321
Average	93.52 ± 5.21	78.74 ± 10.26	0.003	100.53 ± 8.66	73.91 ± 10.14	<0.001	<0.001	0.046

†P-Value for comparison between control eyes in the highly and the nonhighly myopic groups.
‡P-Value for comparison between glaucomatous eyes in the highly and the nonhighly myopic groups.

DISCUSSION

Retinal vessel density as measured by OCTA was reduced in HM subjects (19, 20). In the meanwhile, pRNFL profile abnormalities also became more prominent with axial elongation in those with high myopia (4, 5, 8). It has been suggested that the peripapillary vessel density changes are useful for diagnosing highly myopic glaucoma (14). In this study, we compared the diagnostic ability of early glaucoma between HM and NHM eyes using OCT and OCTA. We found not only the diagnostic ability of pRNFL thickness, but also the diagnostic ability of peripapillary PD was significantly lower in differentiating highly myopic early glaucoma.

Shin et al. (15) reported that the peripapillary vessel density had a better global and regional correlation with VF mean sensitivity (VFMS) than pRNFL thickness in glaucoma patients with high myopia. They concluded that the peripapillary vessel density may be less affected by myopic changes compared with

TABLE 3 | Area under the receiver operation characteristic curves (AUC) values in highly and non-highly myopic eyes among normal and glaucomatous eyes.

	Highly myopic AUC (95%CI)	Non-highly myopic AUC(95%CI)	*P*
Optic disc perfusion density			
Superior	0.725(0.595–0.854)	0.891(0.814–0.967)	0.031
Inferior	0.808(0.704–0.913)	0.938(0.885–0.992)	0.030
Temporal	0.780(0.658–0.903)	0.865(0.775–0.955)	0.275
Nasal	0.646(0.511–0.781)	0.886(0.804–0.968)	0.003
Outer region mean	0.793(0.680–0.906)	0.941(0.890–0.993)	0.019
Macula perfusion density			
Outer superior	0.825(0.726–0.925)	0.886(0.802–0.969)	0.360
Outer inferior	0.917(0.841–0.993)	0.929(0.864–0.994)	0.813
Outer temporal	0.766(0.651–0.881)	0.863(0.774–0.952)	0.188
Outer nasal	0.791(0.679–0.903)	0.847(0.753–0.942)	0.447
Inner superior	0.721(0.597–0.845)	0.846(0.749–0.942)	0.119
Inner inferior	0.745(0.625–0.865)	0.850(0.755–0.945)	0.178
Inner temporal	0.734(0.615–0.853)	0.842(0.745–0.940)	0.167
Inner nasal	0.727(0.598–0.856)	0.843(0.747–0.940)	0.157
Inner mean	0.724(0.601–0.846)	0.844(0.747–0.941)	0.131
Outer mean	0.913(0.843–0.983)	0.913(0.849–0.977)	0.997
Full mean	0.845(0.750–0.940)	0.878(0.797–0.959)	0.605
Peripapillary retinal nerve fiber layer thickness (pRNFL) (μm)			
Superior	0.767(0.656–0.879)	0.979(0.953–1.000)	<0.001
Inferior	0.946(0.899–0.994)	0.983(0.962–1.000)	0.165
Temporal	0.798(0.687–0.908)	0.908(0.839–0.977)	0.096
Nasal	0.663(0.537–0.789)	0.884(0.807–0.961)	0.003
Average	0.915(0.849–0.980)	0.993(0.982–1.000)	0.021
Macular ganglion cell-inner plexiform layer thickness (mGCIPL) (μm)			
Superior	0.856(0.769–0.943)	0.949(0.899–0.999)	0.069
Inferior	0.927(0.861–0.992)	0.952(0.902–1.000)	0.544
Superotemporal	0.868(0.779–0.957)	0.953(0.902–1.000)	0.105
Inferotemporal	0.981(0.951–1.000)	0.959(0.902–1.000)	0.502
Superonasal	0.780(0.674–0.887)	0.883(0.802–0.964)	0.131
Inferonasal	0.826(0.730–0.922)	0.920(0.857–0.984)	0.107
Average	0.921(0.854–0.987)	0.965(0.927–1.000)	0.254

TABLE 4 | Comparisons of AUCs of the vessel perfusion density parameters and structural thickness.

	P-value	
	Highly myopic	**Non-highly myopic**
Optic outer region mean perfusion density vs Average pRNFL thickness	0.068	0.058
Outer inferior macular perfusion density vs Inferotemporal mGCIPL thickness	0.126	0.504
Outer mean macular perfusion density vs Average mGCIPL thickness	0.875	0.168

the pRNFL thickness. Our findings were consistent with their study that we found there was no significant difference in the optic disc perfusion between NHM and HM controls, while the pRNFL thickness in the HM controls was significantly lower than that in the NHM controls. Superficial microvascular network in highly myopic eyes may be stretched rather than lost (19), while glaucomatous vascular damage was found as a dropout of the microvasculature (21). However, Lee et al. (22) later reported that the vessel density was not superior to the pRNFL thickness in the correlation with VFMS when images with segmentation error with improper OCT results were excluded, which implies that as long as a correct and clear OCT image was taken, OCTA did not provide better topographic correlation with VFMS in highly myopic glaucoma patients. Moreover, in Shin's (15) and Lee's (22) study, they included moderate glaucoma (VF defect: 7.5 dB in Shin's study and 9.2 dB in Lee's study), while we included only patients with early glaucoma with VF mean defect <3 MD. To the best of our knowledge, no prior study has compared the diagnostic performance between OCT and OCTA in early glaucoma of highly myopic and non-highly myopic eyes. It is vital that the OCTA diagnostic performance is likely to depend on the severity of glaucoma. Studies have demonstrated that peripapillary vessel density parameters, while comparing with pRNFL thickness, had similar glaucoma diagnostic ability in NHM patients and suggested that the vessel density parameters showed limited clinical value in the early stage (10, 11, 13), which was consistent with our findings in NHM patients. In this study, we further demonstrated that in HM patients, OCTA did not provide better diagnostic ability than conventional structural OCT measurement, whether using the optic nerve head perfusion density or flux index parameter.

The distribution pattern of the pRNFL thickness in HM patients was changed with the superotemporal and inferotemporal RNFL bundles converging temporally. We found the superior, inferior, and nasal quadrants of pRNFL thickness were significantly thinner, while the temporal pRNFL thickness was significantly thicker in HM controls comparing to NHM controls. These findings are in agreement with those from previous studies (4, 8, 23). Akiyasu et al. (8) evaluated patients with similar severity of glaucoma (VF defect: 2.73 dB) as our study population and reported that the abilities of the SD-OCT to detect high myopic early glaucoma were higher if the control group was set with highly myopia comparing to non-highly myopia as the internal normal database in OCT instruments. Their conclusion, along with other studies, suggested OCT instruments should change the internal normal database to increase the glaucoma diagnostic ability in high myopic patients. In this study, we found even the normal controls were set with highly myopia, the glaucoma diagnostic ability was significantly lower in the HM group than in the NHM group whether using average pRNFL or superior thickness. Magnification effect due to longer axial length and difficulty in definition of disc margin due to peripapillary atrophy could not be completely eliminated even using high myopic patients as normal controls.

Ganglion cell complex and macular vessel density measurement showed similar efficiency to detect early glaucoma in NHM patients (12). In our study, the glaucoma diagnostic ability of macular PD and macular GCIPL had no significant difference between HM and NHM eyes. This might be because thinning of the macular inner retinal layer was more supposed to be due to glaucomatous retinal ganglion cell loss, rather than axial length elongation in high myopia (6). Lee et al. (14) had similar findings as ours that the glaucoma diagnostic ability of macular PD and macular GCIPL had no significant difference between HM and NHM patients; however, they further reported that the inferior vessel density ratio had better diagnostic performance comparing to the conventional parameters like inferior RNFL thickness or inferotemporal GCIPL thickness in HM than in NHM patients, which was different from our results. We found inferior macular vessel density and inferotemporal GCIPL thickness had no significant difference in early glaucoma diagnosis whether in HM or NHM patients. There are two points that need to be stressed. First, the highly myopic glaucoma patients in their study were much severer than those in our study in that their VF mean defect was 11.8 MD. Second, we analyzed the macular perfusion density directly provided by the commercial software instead of the vessel density ratio (i.e. outer macular vessel density/inner macular vessel density); hence, our results would be directly applicable to the clinical settings. Third, the sector definitions of radial peripapillary capillaries used in the present study were the ones automatically demarcated by the commercial software of OMAG measurements. However, the ETDRS grid used in Lee's study to define macular and peripapillary sector for perfusion density analysis was primarily developed for the diabetic retinopathy macular evaluation rather than glaucoma evaluation.

Potentially confounding factors (such as IOP, age, and refractive status) may affect vessel density measured by OCTA (9, 24, 25). Higher signal strength was related to higher RNFL thickness (26) and higher macular perfusion density (9) in healthy subjects. Image quality plays an important role in terms of the precision of a measurement. Even within a range of high-quality images, lower signal strength was found to be responsible for the apparent perfusion loss (27). Therefore, we adjusted the signal strength, age, and axial length in the AUC analysis to increase the diagnostic precision in our study.

Several issues need to be considered when interpreting the results of our current study. First, the definition of glaucoma in our study was based on the VF defect, although it did great help in diagnosing early glaucoma with high myopia, our findings might not directly apply to patients with very early preperimetric glaucoma who were not included in our study. Moreover, the results might not be the same in moderate to severe glaucoma. Second, we included only images with signal strength that exceeded the manufacturer's recommended standard. Peripapillary atrophy is common in high myopic eyes, mostly on the temporal side. We excluded peripapillary atrophy in the superior and inferior quadrant extending across from the 3.4-mm-diameter scan circle centered on the optic nerve head by Cirrus HD-OCT in this study. Therefore, the results of this study might only be applicable to eyes with high-quality OCT and OCTA images.

Our study had some limitations. First, because of its retrospective design, we did not investigate the blood pressure of the subjects or their anti-hypertensive medications and we did not measure axial length in advance. Second, the sector definitions of OCT and OCTA measurements used in the present study were the ones automatically demarcated by the software and we did not use other software to redefine the region of interest. It might not be fair to compare it directly since the scan area of vessel density and structural thickness was different; however, our study results provided clinicians the information of those parameters directly provided by commercial software of the Cirrus OCT and OCTA machines which we could easily get in clinical practice.

In conclusion, this study demonstrated that although peripapillary PD and macular PD were significantly reduced in early glaucoma with highly myopia, the diagnostic ability of peripapillary PD in HM patients was significantly lower than that in NHM patients, while macular PD was not. Macular OCTA along with OCT imaging should be included in the imaging algorithm in early glaucoma diagnosis in highly myopic patients.

ETHICS STATEMENT

The studies involving human participants were reviewed and approved by No.21, Sec. 2, Nanya S. Rd. Banciao Dist. Written informed consent for participation was not required for this study in accordance with the national legislation and the institutional requirements.

AUTHOR CONTRIBUTIONS

P-YC and J-YW contributed to conceptualization, investigation, writing, reviewing, and editing. J-YW contributed to methodology, validation, and formal analysis. Y-RH contributed to software, validation, and investigation. T-LH contributed to investigation and visualization. P-YC contributed to resources, data curation, writing original draft preparation, visualization, and funding acquisition. J-KW contributed to supervision, investigation, and project administration. All authors have read and agreed to the published version of the manuscript.

REFERENCES

1. Lam DS, Leung KS, Mohamed S, Chan WM, Palanivelu MS, Cheung CY, et al. Regional variations in the relationship between macular thickness measurements and myopia. *Invest Ophthalmol Vis Sci.* (2007) 48:376–82. doi: 10.1167/iovs.06-0426
2. Jonas JB, Dichtl A. Optic disc morphology in myopic primary open-angle glaucoma. *Graefes Arch Clin Exp Ophthalmol.* (1997) 235:627–33. doi: 10.1007/BF00946938
3. Teng MC, Poon YC, Hung KC, Chang HW, Lai IC, Tsai JC, et al. Diagnostic capability of peripapillary retinal nerve fiber layer parameters in time-domain versus spectral-domain optical coherence tomography for assessing glaucoma in high myopia. *Int J Ophthalmol.* (2017) 10:1106–12. doi: 10.18240/ijo.2017.07.14
4. Kimura Y, Hangai M, Morooka S, Takayama K, Nakano N, Nukada M, et al. Retinal nerve fiber layer defects in highly myopic eyes with early glaucoma. *Invest Ophthalmol Vis Sci.* (2012) 53:6472–8. doi: 10.1167/iovs.12-10319
5. Akashi A, Kanamori A, Nakamura M, Fujihara M, Yamada Y, Negi A. The ability of macular parameters and circumpapillary retinal nerve fiber layer by three SD-OCT instruments to diagnose highly myopic glaucoma. *Invest Ophthalmol Vis Sci.* (2013) 54:6025–32. doi: 10.1167/iovs.13-12630
6. Zhang Y, Wen W, Sun X. Comparison of several parameters in two optical coherence tomography systems for detecting glaucomatous defects in high myopia. *Invest Ophthalmol Vis Sci.* (2016) 57:4910–5. doi: 10.1167/iovs.16-19104
7. Nakano N, Hangai M, Noma H, Nukada M, Mori S, Morooka S, et al. Macular imaging in highly myopic eyes with and without glaucoma. *Am J Ophthalmol.* (2013) 156:511-23.e6. doi: 10.1016/j.ajo.2013.04.028
8. Akashi A, Kanamori A, Ueda K, Inoue Y, Yamada Y, Nakamura M. The ability of SD-OCT to differentiate early glaucoma with high myopia from highly myopic controls and nonhighly myopic controls. *Invest Ophthalmol Vis Sci.* (2015) 56:6573–80. doi: 10.1167/iovs.15-17635
9. Rao HL, Pradhan ZS, Weinreb RN, Reddy HB, Riyazuddin M, Sachdeva S, et al. Determinants of peripapillary and macular vessel densities measured by optical coherence tomography angiography in normal eyes. *J Glaucoma.* (2017) 26:491–7. doi: 10.1097/IJG.0000000000000655
10. Yarmohammadi A, Zangwill LM, Diniz-Filho A, Suh MH, Manalastas PI, Fatehee N, et al. Optical coherence tomography angiography vessel density in healthy, glaucoma suspect, and glaucoma eyes. *Invest Ophthalmol Vis Sci.* (2016) 57: 451–9. doi: 10.1167/iovs.15-18944
11. Rao HL, Kadambi SV, Weinreb RN, Puttaiah NK, Pradhan ZS, Rao DAS, et al. Diagnostic ability of peripapillary vessel density measurements of optical coherence tomography angiography in primary open-angle and angle-closure glaucoma. *Br J Ophthalmol.* (2017) 101:1066–70. doi: 10.1136/bjophthalmol-2016-309377
12. Hou H, Moghimi S, Zangwill LM, Shoji T, Ghahari E, Penteado RC, et al. Macula vessel density and thickness in early primary open-angle glaucoma. *Am J Ophthalmol.* (2019) 199:120–32. doi: 10.1016/j.ajo.2018.11.012
13. Chung JK, Hwang YH, Wi JM, Kim M, Jung JJ. Glaucoma diagnostic ability of the optical coherence tomography angiography vessel density parameters. *Curr Eye Res.* (2017) 42:1458–67. doi: 10.1080/02713683.2017.1337157
14. Lee K, Maeng KJ, Kim JY, Yang H, Choi W, Lee SY, et al. Diagnostic ability of vessel density measured by spectral-domain optical coherence tomography angiography for glaucoma in patients with high myopia. *Sci Rep.* (2020) 10:3027. doi: 10.1038/s41598-020-60051-0
15. Shin JW, Kwon J, Lee J, Kook MS. Relationship between vessel density and visual field sensitivity in glaucomatous eyes with high myopia. *Br J Ophthalmol.* (2018) 103:1827–33. doi: 10.1136/bjophthalmol-2018-313019
16. Kotowski J, Folio LS, Wollstein G, Ishikawa H, Ling Y, Bilonick RA, et al. Glaucoma discrimination of segmented cirrus spectral domain optical coherence tomography (SD-OCT) macular scans. *Br J Ophthalmol.* (2012) 96:1420–5. doi: 10.1136/bjophthalmol-2011-301021
17. Rosenfeld PJ, Durbin MK, Roisman L, Zheng F, Miller A, Robbins G, et al. ZEISS Angioplex spectral domain optical coherence tomography angiography: technical aspects. *Dev Ophthalmol.* (2016) 56:18–29. doi: 10.1159/000442773
18. M G. Comparison and covariate adjustment of ROC curves. In: Gonen M. *Anayzing Receiver Operating Characteristics Curves with SAS.* SAS Publishing (2007).
19. Li M, Yang Y, Jiang H, Gregori G, Roisman L, Zheng F, et al. Retinal microvascular network and microcirculation assessments in high myopia. *Am J Ophthalmol.* (2017) 174:56–67. doi: 10.1016/j.ajo.2016.10.018
20. Suwan Y, Fard MA, Geyman LS, Tantraworasin A, Chui TY, Rosen RB, et al. Association of myopia with peripapillary perfused capillary density in patients with glaucoma: an optical coherence tomography angiography study. *JAMA Ophthalmol.* (2018) 136:507–13. doi: 10.1001/jamaophthalmol.2018.0776
21. Akagi T, Iida Y, Nakanishi H, Terada N, Morooka S, Yamada H, et al. Microvascular density in glaucomatous eyes with hemifield visual field defects: an optical coherence tomography angiography study. *Am J Ophthalmol.* (2016) 168:237–49. doi: 10.1016/j.ajo.2016.06.009
22. Lee SH, Lee EJ, Kim TW. Comparison of vascular-function and structure-function correlations in glaucomatous eyes with high myopia. *Br J Ophthalmol.* (2020) 104:807–12. doi: 10.1136/bjophthalmol-2019-314430
23. Kang SH, Hong SW, Im SK, Lee SH, Ahn MD. Effect of myopia on the thickness of the retinal nerve fiber layer measured by Cirrus HD optical coherence tomography. *Invest Ophthalmol Vis Sci.* (2010) 51:4075–83. doi: 10.1167/iovs.09-4737
24. Wang X, Kong X, Jiang C, Li M, Yu J, Sun X. Is the peripapillary retinal perfusion related to myopia in healthy eyes? A prospective comparative study. *BMJ Open.* (2016) 6:e010791. doi: 10.1136/bmjopen-2015-010791
25. Rao HL, Pradhan ZS, Weinreb RN, Riyazuddin M, Dasari S, Venugopal JP, et al. A comparison of the diagnostic ability of vessel density and structural measurements of optical coherence tomography in primary open angle glaucoma. *PLoS ONE.* (2017) 12:e0173930. doi: 10.1371/journal.pone.0173930
26. Zhang X, Iverson SM, Tan O, Huang D. Effect of signal intensity on measurement of ganglion cell complex and retinal nerve fiber layer scans in fourier-domain optical coherence tomography. *Transl Vis Sci Technol.* (2015) 4:7. doi: 10.1167/tvst.4.5.7
27. Hirasawa K, Smith CA, West ME, Sharpe GP, Shuba LM, Rafuse PE, et al. Discrepancy in loss of macular perfusion density and ganglion cell layer thickness in early glaucoma. *Am J Ophthalmol.* (2021) 221:39–47. doi: 10.1016/j.ajo.2020.08.031

8

Changes of Peripapillary Retinal Nerve Fiber Layer in Childhood Glaucoma

Yuwen Wen, Yingting Zhu* and Yehong Zhuo*

State Key Laboratory of Ophthalmology, Zhongshan Ophthalmic Center, Sun Yat-sen University, Guangzhou, China

***Correspondence:**
Yingting Zhu
zhuyingting@gzzoc.com
Yehong Zhuo
zhuoyh@mail.sysu.edu.cn

Objectives: Retinal nerve fiber layer (RNFL) thickness has been detected by numerous studies about alterations and abnormalities in childhood glaucoma, but these studies have yielded inconsistent results about the RNFL thinning region. The investigation of characteristics of RNFL in pediatric patients would contribute to the deep understanding of the neuropathic mechanisms of childhood glaucoma. Thus, the degree of thinning in different quadrants deserves further discussion and exploration.

Method: A systematic literature search was conducted using the Cochrane Central Register of Controlled Trials, Medline, Embase, and PubMed databases to identify clinical studies published from inception to April 1, 2021.

Results: Ten studies were included in this review with a total of 311 children with glaucoma and 444 in nonglaucomatous controls. The results revealed that average peripapillary RNFL (pRNFL) thickness was attenuated in pediatric patients with glaucoma [weighted mean difference (WMD) = −20.75; 95% CI −27.49 to −14.01; $p < 0.00001$]. Additionally, pRNFL thickness in eight quadrants (superior, inferior, temporal, nasal, superotemporal, inferotemporal, superonasal, and inferonasal) had different levels of reduction in the pediatric group of glaucoma.

Conclusion: This study indicates that eight regions of RNFL thickness show various degrees of thinning in childhood glaucoma. However, caution is required in the interpretation of results due to marked heterogeneity. Future studies, especially larger samples and multicenter, need to confirm our results.

Keywords: childhood glaucoma, retinal nerve fiber layer (RNFL) thickness, glaucoma optic nerve damage, spectral-domain optical coherence tomography (SD-OCT), meta-analysis

INTRODUCTION

Glaucoma is a multifactorial, progressive optic neuropathy with unclear pathogenesis characterized by visual field deficits and cupping of the optic nerve (1–3). As a major cause of irreversible blindness, more than 70 million people worldwide are affected and approximately 10% of the patients with glaucoma are bilaterally blind (4, 5). Childhood glaucoma is a varied group of disorders occurring in children and adolescents younger than 16 years that requires careful attention to prevent vision loss throughout life. It is estimated that 5% of blindness in children worldwide is caused by childhood glaucoma (6). Primary congenital glaucoma (PCG) is the most common type of childhood glaucoma accounting for 32–47% (7, 8) and 70–80% of cases are bilateral (9, 10). Most of the patients with childhood glaucoma present within 6 months of birth with ~ 80% appearing before 1 year of age (11). Childhood glaucoma and its management not only have a marked impact on functional vision of children, but also reduced the quality of life of the patients, relatives, and caregivers (12–14). Hence, early diagnosis is crucial for children affected with glaucoma to receive timely and appropriate treatment.

The clinical visual field is regarded as the essential part of following-up and identifying neurological damage and progressive change in glaucoma. However, visual field testing in children is limited. Different from the adult patients, children have shortened duration for maintaining attention and learning curve, which requires correctly explaining the visual field findings (15, 16). The measurement of intraocular pressure (IOP) is another essential part of the diagnosis and follow-up of glaucoma. However, this detection of young children often has large fluctuation due to poor cooperation.

The pathological changes in glaucoma include cupping of the optic disk, thinning of the retinal nerve fiber layer (RNFL), and loss of the retinal ganglion cells (3, 17, 18). Recently, detection of glaucomatous structural changes has relied on the assessment of morphological changes within fundus photography or direct ophthalmoscopes such as cup-to-disk ratio (CDR) and bilateral asymmetry. A well-known phenomenon in pediatric glaucoma is that cupping of the optic disk can be reversible after remarkable IOP reduction, especially before 1 year of age (19–21). However, cupping reversal in childhood glaucoma may not be a good indicator to assess the improvement of optic nerve head health. Continued RNFL thinning was observed in some cases with IOP reduction and cupping reversal after treatment of glaucoma (22). Preoperative RNFL thickness is a key prognostic indicator of RNFL thinning progress even after surgery and visual prognosis. A precise evaluation of the RNFL is crucial for diagnosing and monitoring pediatric glaucoma.

With the appearance of spectral-domain optical coherence tomography (SD-OCT), it is possible to monitor the automatic segmentation of the individual retinal layers. It has been widely used in the diagnosis and follow-up of glaucoma in recent years. Being a simple, non-invasive, and safe imaging test, it has been intensely applied to measure and observe the change in the peripapillary retinal nerve fiber layer (pRNFL) (23). SD-OCT has dramatically improved image resolution and reliably detects glaucoma disease and progression in adults (24). Considering the difficulty of testing children, the most recent SD-OCT is designed to handheld OCT or overhead mounted OCT to make infants and young children benefit from this technology.

Recently, several studies using SD-OCT were performed to compare pRNFL thickness in children with glaucoma and healthy children and to convey conflicting results. Some researchers have reported the thinning of average pRNFL thickness in all sectors between pediatric glaucoma and controls (25–30). However, other studies have found that children with glaucoma and normal participants have comparable pRNFL thickness in some regions such as the temporal, nasal, and inferior nasal quadrants (31–34). Thus, the possible association of each sector between pRNFL thickness and childhood glaucoma remains unclear, which justifies the need for more studies on this issue. In this meta-analysis, we aimed to carry out a comprehensive overview of the characteristics of thinning RNFL in childhood glaucoma offered by SD-OCT applications. Furthermore, by analyzing the average eight quadrants of pRNFL thickness changes in pediatric glaucoma compared with the normal participants, we can investigate whether pRNFL thickness measurements are affected in childhood glaucoma and whether they could provide a diagnostic tool in assessing pediatric patients as in adults. Finally, this study also summarized similarities and differences of RNFL thickness between children and adults and the role of SD-OCT in childhood glaucoma.

MATERIALS AND METHODS

This review was conducted and reported according to the guidelines presented by the PRISMA statements and the Meta-Analyses and Systematic Reviews of Observational Studies statement (35, 36).

Literature Search

We searched Cochrane Central Register of Controlled Trials, Medline, Embase, and PubMed from database inception to April 1, 2021, with keywords: "childhood glaucoma," "pediatric glaucoma," "juvenile glaucoma," "retinal nerve fiber layer," "RNFL," "spectral-domain optical coherence tomography," and "SD-OCT." Manual searching of reference lists from all relevant retrieved articles was conducted to identify additional eligible studies. Eligible papers were screened by two authors independently and the duplicated and irrelevant studies were removed. After screening the abstracts, the remaining articles were checked by full-text review.

Inclusion and Exclusion Criteria

We enrolled the studies if all the inclusion criteria and no exclusion criteria were met as follows. The relative search and selection were shown as a flowchart (**Figure 1**).

In our meta-analysis, the inclusion criteria were (1) original articles reporting independent studies; (2) images with satisfactory quality that measured RNFL thickness by using SD-OCT; (3) satisfactory SD-OCT scan quality recorded in the article; (4) clinical trial, prospective or retrospective cross-sectional study, or case-control study; (5) comparison of pediatric patients with glaucoma and healthy controls or physiologic cupping controls; and (6) sample size ≥10 in each group. Moreover, studies were excluded if they met the following criteria: (1) the study groups were adult patients (aged 16 years or older); (2) RNFL thickness was not measured by SD-OCT; (3) reviews, letters, case reports, and studies with important data unavailable; and (4) studies without the healthy control group.

Data Extraction

The following information contained in all the eligible publications was retrieved independently by two authors:

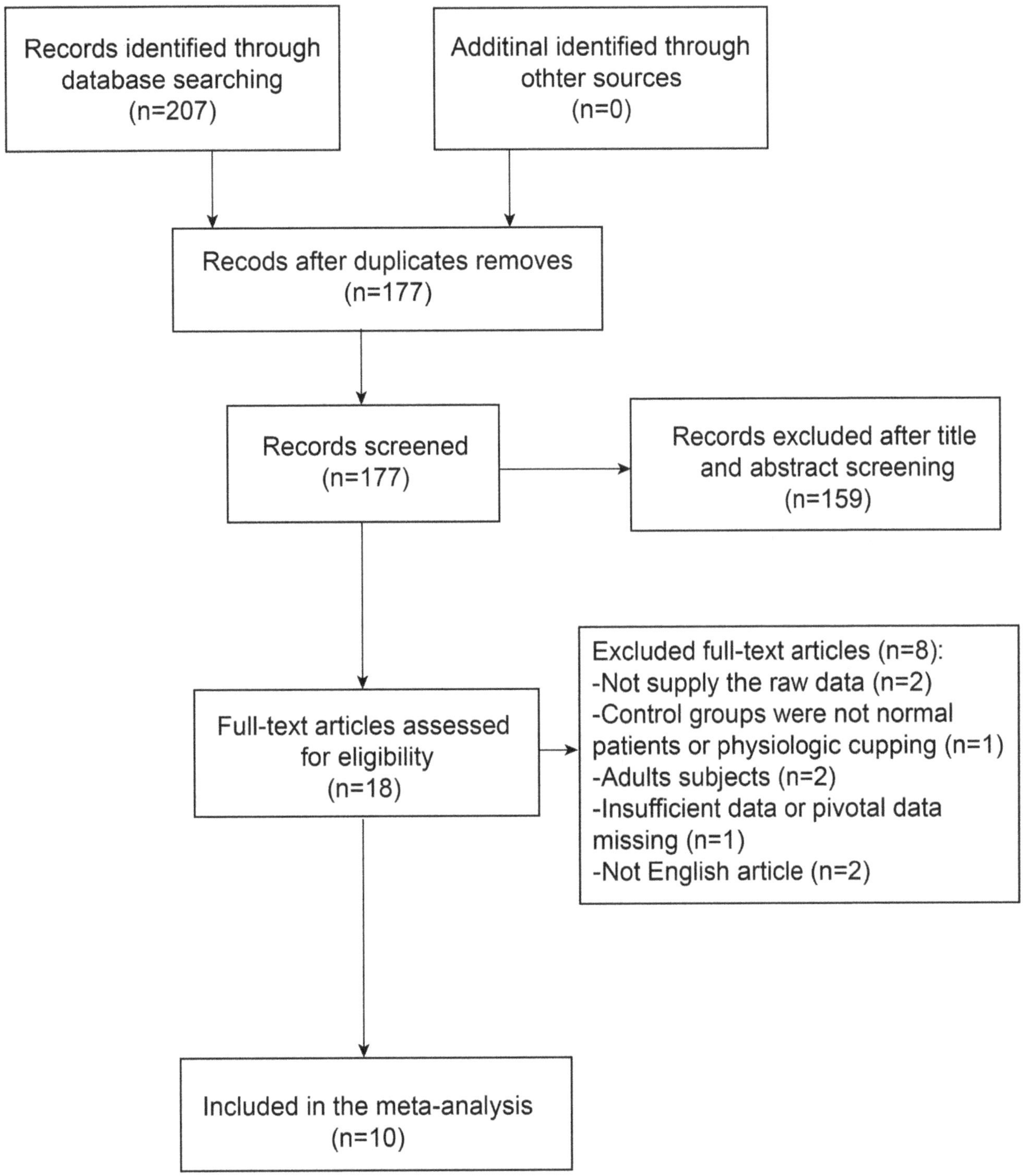

FIGURE 1 | Flowchart of study selection.

first author, country, year of publication, study type, SD-OCT manufacturer, glaucoma type, mean age, gender, CDR, number of participations, IOP, and average eight quadrants of pRNFL thickness. Discrepancies in data extraction were solved by discussion or by consulting the third author. Projecting a circle of 3.5 mm in diameter on the retina and divided into eight sectors totaling 360°. The pRNFL thickness parameters evaluated in these studies were average thickness (360° measurement), superior quadrant thickness (46°-135° including 45° superonasal sector and 45° superotemporal sector), inferior quadrant thickness (226–315° including 45° inferonasal sector and 45° inferotemporal sector), nasal quadrant thickness (136–225°), and temporal quadrant thickness (316–45°).

Quality Assessment

The Newcastle–Ottawa Scale (NOS) was used to assess the methodological quality of all the included studies. The NOS is a star system to judge quality based on three elements of a study: selection, comparability, and outcome or exposure. The maximum NOS score is nine and the study with a NOS score of ≥6 was considered to be of relatively high quality. Quality was assessed independently by the two reviewers and disagreements were resolved *via* discussion.

Statistical Analysis

We used Review Manager version 5.3 to perform the meta-analyses. The data of RNFL thickness were entered as a continuous variable. Means and standard deviations (SDs) were used to calculate the weighted mean differences (WMDs) for continuous outcomes. A $p < 0.05$ ($p < 0.05$) was regarded as the criterion for statistical significance. Substantial heterogeneity was defined as I2 values of more than 50%. We adopted a fixed effects model for analysis if there was no heterogeneity across studies ($p > 0.1$, I2 < 50%). Otherwise, a random effects model was used (DerSimonian and Kacker). The potential publication bias was evaluated by funnel plot and Egger's statistics.

RESULTS

Selection of Studies

The literature screening strategy was summarized and presented by a flowchart (**Figure 1**). In total, 207 pieces of literature were initially identified via the original search and 30 pieces were excluded due to duplication. In addition, 18 publications were left for further evaluation after screening titles and abstracts. Out of these reports, eight pieces could not provide useful or available data for meta-analysis. Thus, we excluded these publications that did not meet the inclusion criteria. Finally, a total of 10 studies, consisting of 311 patients with glaucoma and 444 controls, were included in the meta-analysis.

Characteristics and Quality Assessment of the Studies

During the enrollment period, a total of 755 participants (311 in the glaucoma group and 444 in the control group) were included in our meta-analysis. Six studies were performed in the USA and the other four studies were performed in the UK, Spain, India, and Germany. The characteristics and qualities of these studies are shown in **Table 1**.

Meta-Analysis of Childhood Glaucoma Group Compared With a Healthy Control Group

Analysis of average pRNFL thickness between the group of children with glaucoma and children without glaucoma in eight studies showed significant heterogeneity (I2 = 89%). Hence, the random effects model was used for data analysis. The meta-analysis showed that the average pRNFL thickness in the pediatric glaucoma group was decreased significantly than the non-glaucomatous group (WMD = −20.75; 95% CI −27.49–−14.01; $p < 0.00001$, **Figure 2**).

In addition, we also examined the difference in pRNFL thickness between patients with glaucoma and healthy controls in each quadrant and there was significant difference in pRNFL thickness between those two groups in the superior (WMD = −30.80; 95% CI −47.00 to −14.59; $p < 0.00001$), inferior (WMD = −31.81; 95% CI −46.04 to −17.58; $p < 0.00001$), nasal (WMD = −11.61; 95% CI −17.21 to −6.02; $p < 0.00001$), temporal (WMD = −10.07; 95% CI −14.84 to −5.30; $p < 0.00001$), superotemporal (WMD = −34.71; 95% CI −47.52 to −21.90; $p = 0.03$), inferotemporal (WMD = −22.44; 95% CI −43.26 to −1.61; $p = 0.002$), inferonasal (WMD = −26.45; 95% CI −38.59 to −14.30; $p = 0.03$), and superonasal quadrant (WMD = −24.99; 95% CI −37.04 to −12.93; $p = 0.04$) between the glaucoma group and healthy control (**Figure 3**).

Publication Bias

Due to the few eligible studies in our meta-analysis, funnel plots were easily seen as asymmetrical and we could not claim or deny bias for certain. Therefore, the funnel plot and Egger's statistics were not interpretable (data are not shown).

DISCUSSION

To the best of our knowledge, this review and meta-analysis are the first systematic synthesizing currently available observational studies to investigate the pRNFL thickness in childhood glaucoma. In this comprehensive meta-analysis, we investigated the specific regions of reduced pRNFL thickness in childhood glaucoma. As expected, the average pRNFL thickness was significantly thinner in the pediatric patients with glaucoma than in the healthy controls. There were also significant differences in pRNFL thickness between the groups in the superior, inferior, nasal, temporal, superotemporal, inferotemporal, superonasal, and inferonasal quadrants. We additionally observed the tendency of pRNFL thinning among the different regions in pediatric glaucoma of which the nasal and temporal quadrants demonstrated a small reduction in pRNFL thickness. The present meta-analysis showed that childhood glaucoma is strongly associated with changes in pRNFL thickness in the peripapillary region.

In our view, one of the important sources of high heterogeneity may have been the different inclusion criteria and adjusted factors across the studies. First, there were differences in types of childhood glaucoma and only the two pieces of literature mentioned the severity of glaucoma. Second, the exclusion criteria of individual studies differed greatly. For example, one study excluded patients with juvenile open-angle glaucoma (JOAG) that was considered an inherently progressive disease, while others included them or did not state whether JOAG was included. Additionally, the age range of childhood glaucoma was large, which may be a confounding variable in heterogeneity analysis. Third, although the pooled results of our study showed a significant decrease in superior, inferior, and

TABLE 1 | Characteristics of included studies.

Reference	Country	Study type	SD-OCT brand	Glaucoma	No. of participants		Gender (Male)		Age (Y), mean ± SD		CDR, mean ± SD		IOP (mm Hg)		Quality scaling (NOS)
					Case	Control	Case	Control	Case	Control	Case	Control	Case	Control	
Lever et al. (34)	Germany	3	Heidelberg spectralis	PCG, JOAG, other types	19	53	NA	NA	11.2 ± 3.5	12.2 ± 3.5	0.8	0.6	18.7 ± 7.2	14.5 ± 2.7	7
Michelle et al. (31)	USA	1	Heidelberg spectralis	G/SG	39	57	22	28	5.9 ± 5.9	2.3 ± 1.5	NA	NA	23 ± 8	14 ± 3	7
Perucho-González et al. (32)	USA	2	Heidelberg spectralis	PCG	59	87	NA	NA	9.61 ± 3.23	8.47 ± 2.99	NA	NA	19.11 ± 4.23	13.95 ± 1.98	6
Pilat et al. (33)	UK	2	Envisu 2,300	PCG	20	20	10	11	4.64 ± 2.79	4.73 ± 2.81	0.668 ± 0.173	0.398 ± 0.178	17.68 ± 6.52	NA	8
Xu et al. (30)	USA	3	Heidelberg spectralis	PCG	20	15	11	6	9.7 ± 3.3	11.2 ± 3.3	0.4 ± 0.2	0.7 ± 0.1	15.4 ± 3.6	16.5 ± 3.6	8
Morales-Fernandez et al. (27)	Spain	2	Heidelberg spectralis	PCG	40	60	24	24	11.20 ± 3.94	10.90 ± 2.46	0.52 ± 0.29	0.24 ± 0.14	NA	NA	7
Silverstein et al. (28)	USA	NA	Heidelberg spectralis	PCG/ JOAG	37	43	20	22	9.9 ± 3.3 (PCG) 13.1 ± 2.0 (JOAG)	11.1 ± 3.1 (PC) 12.3 ± 3.2 (N)	0.52 ± 0.29 (PCG) 0.83 ± 0.2 (JOAG)	0.7 ± 0.11 (PCG) 0.21 ± 0.12	NA	NA	6
Ghasia et al. (26)	USA	1	Optovue RTVue	G/SG	12	13	6	6	11.5 ± 3.5	10 ± 2.5	0.4 ± 0.2	0.1 ± 0.1	NA	NA	8
Srinivasan et al. (29)	India	4	Heidelberg spectralis	PCG	37	41	20	22	10.1 ± 3.6	13.6 ± 3.2	NA	NA	30.2 ± 5.9	NA	8
Ghasia et al. (25)	USA	1	Heidelberg spectralis	MG/M-to-SG	28	55	15	30	12 ± 1.08 (MG) 13 ± 1.6 (M-to-SG)	11 ± 0.75 (PC) 12 ± 3 (N)	0.43 ± 0.04 (MG) 0.72 ± 0.04 (M-to-SG)	0.67 ± 0.02 (PC) 0.15 ± 0.03 (N)	NA	NA	7

1, Prospective cross-sectional study; 2, Observational cross-sectional study; 3, Retrospective observational case series; 4, Case–control study. OCT, optical coherence tomography; G, glaucoma; SG, suspect glaucoma; PCG, primary congenital glaucoma; JOAG, juvenile open-angle glaucoma; MG, mild glaucoma; M-to-SG, moderate-to-severe glaucoma; PC, physiologic cupping; N, normal; NA, not available; CDR, cup-to-disc ratio; IOP, intraocular pressure.

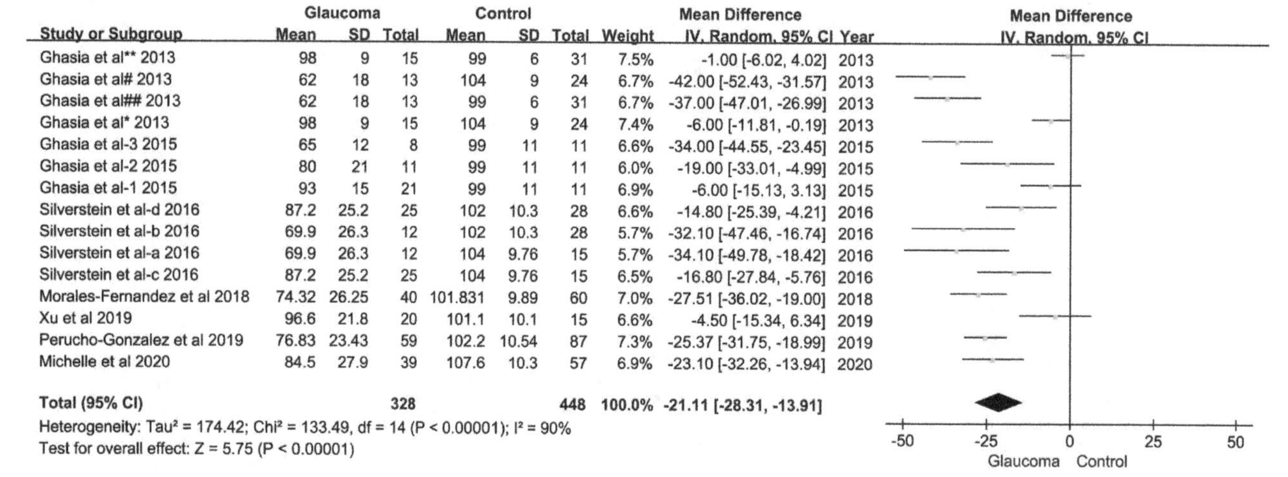

FIGURE 2 | Forest plots of weighted mean difference (WMD) in the glaucoma group and healthy control group for average peripapillary retinal nerve fiber layer (RNFL) thickness. Horizontal lines are 95% CIs.

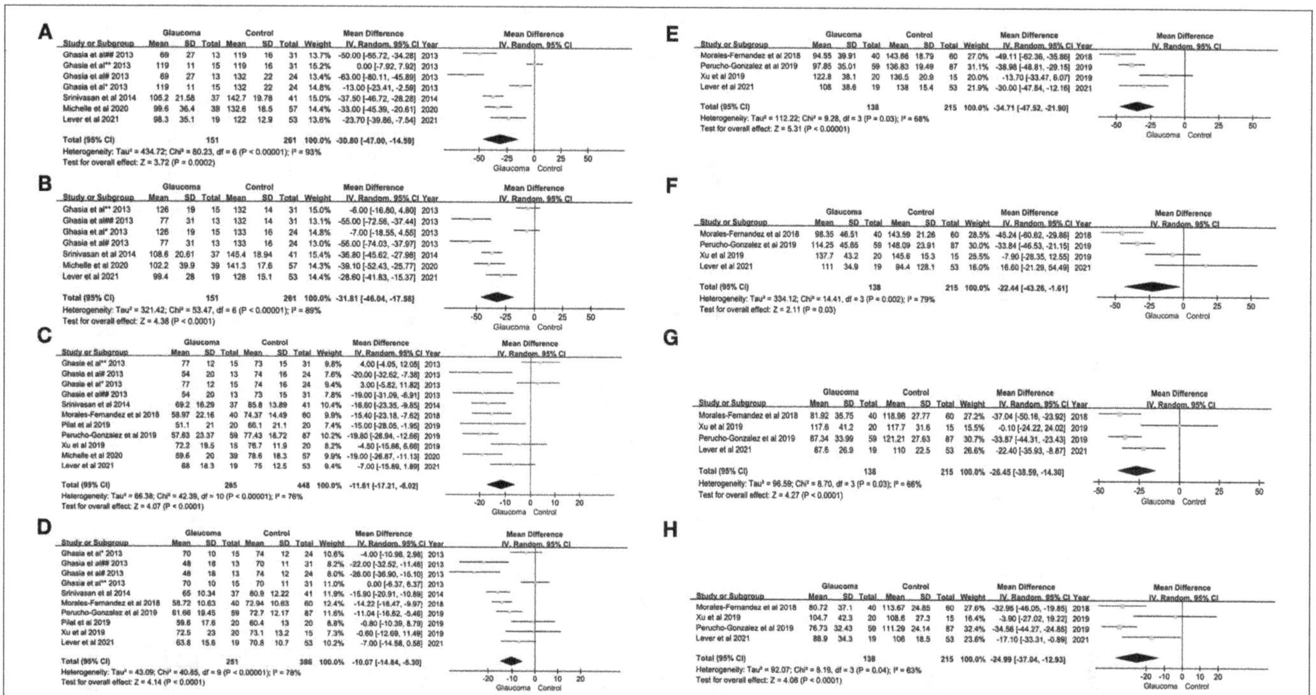

FIGURE 3 | Forest plots of weighted mean difference (WMD) in the glaucoma group and healthy control group for peripapillary RNFL thickness in eight quadrants. Horizontal lines are 95% CIs. **(A)** Superior; **(B)** Inferior; **(C)** Nasal; **(D)** Temporal; **(E)** Superotemporal; **(F)** Inferotemporal; **(G)** Superonasal; and **(H)** Inferonasal. #, Moderate-to-severe glaucoma vs. normal; ##, Moderate-to-severe glaucoma vs. physiologic cupping; *, Mild glaucoma vs. normal; **, Mild glaucoma vs. physiologic cupping; 1, glaucoma suspect/preperimetric glaucoma vs. normal; 2, mild glaucoma vs. normal; 3, moderate/severe glaucoma vs. normal; a, JOAG vs. normal; b, JOAG vs. physiologic cupping; c, PCG vs. normal; d, PCG vs. physiologic cupping. RNFL, retinal nerve fiber layer; JOAG, juvenile open-angle glaucoma; PCG, primary congenital glaucoma.

superotemporal quadrants, we could not speculate which regions had the most significant reduction in children with glaucoma due to a large 95% CI, which is probably related to the severity of glaucoma.

It is reported that the pRNFL thickness in the superior and inferior quadrants is thicker and the temporal and nasal quadrants are relatively thinner in healthy adults (37–39). Turk et al. (40) evaluated 107 healthy Turkish children aged 6–16 years using SD-OCT and found that the average pRNFL thickness was 106.45 ± 9.41 μm, inferotemporal pRNFL (the thickest sector) thickness was 144.64 ± 17.16 μm, and nasal pRNFL (the thinnest sector) thickness was 71.54 ± 10.03 μm. Zhu et al. (41) examined

2,105 12-year-old healthy students using SD-OCT and reported that the average pRNFL thickness was 103.08 ± 1.2 μm and the pRNFL thickness was thicker with shorter axial length and higher hyperopia. Rotruck et al. (42) reported that the mean global pRNFL thickness of healthy children aged 0–5 years old was 107.6 ± 10.3 μm and it was not dependent on age. In general, the thickest region of pRNFL in healthy children is the inferior quadrant, which is thicker than in adults and not dependent on age but showed a negative relationship with axial length (41–44). The pRNFL thickness may attenuate subsequently because of physiologic growth in axial length during the growth and development of children. However, this corresponding change of normal eyes in pRNFL thickness is considerably less than the variability compared with pathological progression and should not be clinically significant (30, 45). Moreover, children with large CDRs were considered as the potential hazard of a glaucomatous process. However, the study (46) revealed that the degree of optic nerve cupping does not correlate with the RNFL thickness. Normal eyes and physiologic cupping showed equivalence in the several measurement parameters between all macular layers and pRNFL (28). Hence, the data can be analyzed by incorporating both normal controls and physiologic cupping simultaneously.

More attention should be given when the pRNFL thickness thinning exceeds approximately 8 μm because it is a likely sign of the probable clinical change (30). Compared to the other optic disc parameters, pRNFL thickness has a higher diagnostic accuracy of glaucoma, especially in the superior and inferior regions (27, 47). Studies have shown that RNFL thinning commonly begins with the inferior and superior sectors and then affects nasal and temporal regions in adult patients and the temporal RNFL quadrant is most conserved in glaucoma (48, 49). This phenomenon may be explained by the preservation of central vision in patients with glaucoma, which is mainly fed by the temporal RNFL fibers (50–52). The changes of pRNFL thickness are meaningful in these children with less severe glaucomatous optic nerve damage, where the damage of visual function may be difficult to measure. Thus, the superior and inferior pRNFL might be optimal to reflect glaucomatous changes, which is consistent with the results of our meta-analysis. In the adult patients with pseudoexfoliation glaucoma, one of the subtypes of open-angle glaucoma, the temporal RNFL thickness is not significantly different from the healthy controls. Our results, however, showed otherwise. In our meta-analysis, the temporal pRNFL thickness was thinning but the superonasal sectors were not different from normal eyes (48). This indicates that childhood glaucoma has its characteristics of RNFL thinning. Furthermore, a larger lamina cribrosa curvature index (LCCI) was perceived as the first indication of prognosis for faster progressive RNFL thinning. Primary congenital glaucoma (PCG) had significantly deeper cups than adults with primary open angle glaucoma emphasizing the importance of measuring cup depth besides concerning CDR (53, 54). Therefore, additional research is needed to demonstrate these differences with the development and preservation of visual function in childhood glaucoma and glaucoma in adults. Our focus should be especially on cup depth and morphology of lamina cribrosa testing RNFL thinning by SD-OCT in pediatric patients. Some of the included studies elucidated the stage of glaucoma (25, 26) and others were not (27–33), which may influence our meta-analysis of RNFL thickness. These could explain the high degree of statistical heterogeneity between the studies in the meta-analysis.

Spectral domain optical coherence tomography is a valuable tool in diagnosing and monitoring visual loss, especially for pediatric glaucoma. It provides an objective and quantitative scan with three-dimensional images, increased speed of image acquisition, and improved axial resolution for early diagnosis and monitoring of disease progression. This device has proved to be useful in the management of pediatric glaucoma as it provides objective RNFL thickness measurements in children (45). The advantages of SD-OCT compared to OCT devices in the past are short exposure durations and automatic eye-tracking systems. SD-OCT has higher sensitivity and specificity compared to the past OCT devices in detecting RNFL thickness. Its overall diagnostic precision of detecting and measuring localized RNFL defects in patients with glaucoma was also relatively higher than conventional fundus photographs (55, 56). Consequently, SD-OCT has potential clinical value in evaluating progression and follow-up for pediatric glaucoma as an effective means.

However, it was challenging to obtain high-quality images for children with glaucoma in the past due to poor cooperation, the opacity of refractive media, and unsuitable examination equipment. Poor-quality images often make it difficult for ophthalmologists to judge the progression of the disease. Delaying in diagnosis and treatment can increase the risk of irreversible optic nerve damage and even blindness. With the technical improvement and development of new instruments, the emergence of handheld OCT and overhead-mounted OCT solved this problem perfectly. The high-quality image can be acquired and analyzed by handheld and overhead-mounted OCT in very young patients. Updated SD-OCT has presented benefits for improved clinical management and study of the pathophysiology associated with childhood glaucoma (31, 33).

To some extent, there were several limitations to this study that need to be considered. First, the number of included studies as well as the included pediatric patients with glaucoma in each study was relatively small. In addition, childhood glaucoma is rare and there are some limitations to acquire good-quality imaging such as nystagmus or poor media opacity. Second, the severity of glaucoma was verified to be related to the mean pRNFL global thickness in children older than 6 years (40, 44), but we were unable to analyze the association between pRNFL thickness and the severity of pediatric glaucoma due to lack of sufficient studies providing data on the severity of glaucoma. Third, included studies of this meta-analysis were applied in four different SD-OCT devices (8 Heidelberg, 1 Envisu, and 1 Optovue). A primary concern was the measurement differences between manufacturers, which were statistically significant in the past and the clinical implication of this difference is less clear (57). However, this study believed that there were no statistically significant differences between devices for any particular area imaged and no major differences were noted for any of the parameters across OCT devices (58). Fourth, as a non-negligible factor, axial length affects RNFL measurement in the direction of thinner RNFL because of physiological growth or pathological factors such as high myopia (59). Therefore, future studies should obtain a random distribution of myopic and non-myopic participants in both normal and glaucomatous subgroups. Fifth, although, we had demonstrated specific regions of thinning pRNFL in pediatric glaucoma, the lack of studies about early-stage changes and progression in childhood glaucoma is a current limitation.

CONCLUSION

In summary, our meta-analysis indicates that patients with childhood glaucoma have significantly reduced average eight quadrants RNFL thickness compared with healthy controls. We also observed a non-uniformity in the thinning of the pRNFL in different quadrants. Therefore, we suggest that the segmentation of peripapillary RNFL thickness as measured by SD-OCT can provide valuable information for the diagnosis and follow-up of childhood glaucoma. Moreover, a standardized and reproducible measurement technique of RNFL thickness needs to be introduced and utilized in children. In future research, further studies with multicenter and larger sample sizes, prospective and longitudinal studies are required to confirm the present results of this meta-analysis.

AUTHOR CONTRIBUTIONS

YW was responsible for designing the review protocol, writing the protocol and report, conducting the search, screening potentially eligible studies, extracting and analyzing data, interpreting results, updating reference lists, and creating figures and tables. YiZ was responsible for designing the review protocol and screening potentially eligible studies and contributed to writing the report, extracting and analyzing data, and interpreting results. YeZ contributed to the design of the review protocol, arbitrating potentially eligible studies, extracting and analyzing data, and interpreting results provided feedback on the report. All authors listed have made a substantial, direct and intellectual contribution to the work, and approved it for publication.

REFERENCES

1. Flaxman SR, Bourne R, Resnikoff S, Ackland P, Braithwaite T, Cicinelli MV, et al. Global causes of blindness and distance vision impairment 1990-2020: a systematic review and meta-analysis. *Lancet Glob Health.* (2017) 5:e1221–34. doi: 10.1016/S2214-109X(17)30393-5
2. Bourne R, Flaxman SR, Braithwaite T, Cicinelli MV, Das A, Jonas JB, et al. Magnitude, temporal trends, and projections of the global prevalence of blindness and distance and near vision impairment: a systematic review and meta-analysis. *Lancet Glob Health.* (2017) 5:e888–97. doi: 10.1016/S2214-109X(17)30293-0
3. Jonas JB, Aung T, Bourne RR, Bron AM, Ritch R, Panda-Jonas S. Glaucoma. *Lancet.* (2017) 390:2183–93. doi: 10.1016/S0140-6736(17)31469-1
4. Weinreb RN, Aung T, Medeiros FA. The pathophysiology and treatment of glaucoma: a review. *JAMA.* (2014) 311:1901–11. doi: 10.1001/jama.2014.3192
5. Quigley HA, Broman AT. The number of people with glaucoma worldwide in 2010 and 2020. *Br J Ophthalmol.* (2006) 90:262–7. doi: 10.1136/bjo.2005.081224
6. Gilbert C, Rahi J, West K. Visual impairment and blindness in children. In: Johnson GJ, Minassian DC, Weale RA, West SK, editors. *The Epidemiology of Eye Disease.* 3rd ed. London: Imperial College Press (2012). p. 267–368.
7. Hoguet A, Grajewski A, Hodapp E, Chang TC. A retrospective survey of childhood glaucoma prevalence according to childhood glaucoma research network classification. *Indian J Ophthalmol.* (2016) 64:118–23. doi: 10.4103/0301-4738.179716
8. Ben-Zion I, Tomkins O, Moore DB, Helveston EM. Surgical results in the management of advanced primary congenital glaucoma in a rural pediatric population. *Ophthalmology.* (2011) 118:231–5. doi: 10.1016/j.ophtha.2010.02.027
9. François J. Congenital glaucoma and its inheritance. *Ophthalmologica.* (1980) 181:61–73. doi: 10.1159/000309028
10. Franks W, Taylor D. Congenital glaucoma–a preventable cause of blindness. *Arch Dis Child.* (1989) 64:649–50. doi: 10.1136/adc.64.5.649
11. Papadopoulos M, Cable N, Rahi J, Khaw PT. The British infantile and childhood glaucoma (BIG) eye study. *Invest Ophthalmol Vis Sci.* (2007) 48:4100–6. doi: 10.1167/iovs.06-1350
12. Dahlmann-Noor A, Tailor V, Bunce C, Abou-Rayyah Y, Adams G, Brookes J, et al. Quality of life and functional vision in children with glaucoma. *Ophthalmology.* (2017) 124:1048–55. doi: 10.1016/j.ophtha.2017.02.024
13. Gothwal VK, Bharani S, Mandal AK. Impact of surgery on the quality of life of caregivers of children with congenital glaucoma. *Ophthalmology.* (2016) 123:1161–2. doi: 10.1016/j.ophtha.2015.11.013
14. Zhu Y, Gao J, Li X, Yang Q, Lian Y, Xiao H, et al. Burden, positive aspects, and predictive variables of caregiving: a study of caregivers of patients with pediatric glaucoma. *J Ophthalmol.* (2019) 2019:6980208. doi: 10.1155/2019/6980208
15. Blumenthal EZ, Haddad A, Horani A, Anteby I. The reliability of frequency-doubling perimetry in young children. *Ophthalmology.* (2004) 111:435–9. doi: 10.1016/j.ophtha.2003.06.018
16. Safran AB, Laffi GL, Bullinger A, Viviani P, de Weisse C, Désangles D, et al. Feasibility of automated visual field examination in children between 5 and 8 years of age. *Br J Ophthalmol.* (1996) 80:515–8. doi: 10.1136/bjo.80.6.515
17. Burgoyne CF, Morrison JC. The anatomy and pathophysiology of the optic nerve head in glaucoma. *J Glaucoma.* (2001) 10(Suppl 1):S16–8. doi: 10.1097/00061198-200110001-00007

18. Quigley HA, Nickells RW, Kerrigan LA, Pease ME, Thibault DJ, Zack DJ. Retinal ganglion cell death in experimental glaucoma and after axotomy occurs by apoptosis. *Invest Ophthalmol Vis Sci.* (1995) 36:774–86.
19. Harju M, Saari J, Kurvinen L, Vesti E. Reversal of optic disc cupping in glaucoma. *Br J Ophthalmol.* (2008) 92:901–5. doi: 10.1136/bjo.2007.135350
20. Lesk MR, Spaeth GL, Azuara-Blanco A, Araujo SV, Katz LJ, Terebuh AK, et al. Reversal of optic disc cupping after glaucoma surgery analyzed with a scanning laser tomograph. *Ophthalmology.* (1999) 106:1013–8. doi: 10.1016/S0161-6420(99)00526-6
21. Azuara-Blanco A, Spaeth GL. Methods to objectify reversibility of glaucomatous cupping. *Curr Opin Ophthalmol.* (1997) 8:50–4. doi: 10.1097/00055735-199704000-00009
22. Ely AL, El-Dairi MA, Freedman SF. Cupping reversal in pediatric glaucoma–evaluation of the retinal nerve fiber layer and visual field. *Am J Ophthalmol.* (2014) 158:905–15. doi: 10.1016/j.ajo.2014.07.030
23. Budenz DL, Anderson DR, Varma R, Schuman J, Cantor L, Savell J, et al. Determinants of normal retinal nerve fiber layer thickness measured by stratus OCT. *Ophthalmology.* (2007) 114:1046–52. doi: 10.1016/j.ophtha.2006.08.046
24. Puzyeyeva O, Lam WC, Flanagan JG, Brent MH, Devenyi RG, Mandelcorn MS, et al. High-resolution optical coherence tomography retinal imaging: a case series illustrating potential and limitations. *J Ophthalmol.* (2011) 2011:764183. doi: 10.1155/2011/764183
25. Ghasia FF, Freedman SF, Rajani A, Holgado S, Asrani S, El-Dairi M. Optical coherence tomography in paediatric glaucoma: time domain versus spectral domain. *Br J Ophthalmol.* (2013) 97:837–42. doi: 10.1136/bjophthalmol-2012-302648
26. Ghasia FF, El-Dairi M, Freedman SF, Rajani A, Asrani S. Reproducibility of spectral-domain optical coherence tomography measurements in adult and pediatric glaucoma. *J Glaucoma.* (2015) 24:55–63. doi: 10.1097/IJG.0b013e31829521db
27. Morales-Fernandez L, Jimenez-Santos M. Martinez-de-la-Casa JM, Sanchez-Jean R, Nieves M, Saenz-Frances F, et al. Diagnostic capacity of SD-OCT segmented ganglion cell complex versus retinal nerve fiber layer analysis for congenital glaucoma. *Eye.* (2018) 32:1338–44. doi: 10.1038/s41433-018-0077-4
28. Silverstein E, Freedman S, Zéhil G, Jiramongkolchai K, El-Dairi M. The macula in pediatric glaucoma: quantifying the inner and outer layers via optical coherence tomography automatic segmentation. *J AAPOS.* (2016) 20:332–6. doi: 10.1016/j.jaapos.2016.05.013
29. Srinivasan S, Addepalli UK, Rao HL, Garudadri CS, Mandal AK. Spectral domain optical coherence tomography in children operated for primary congenital glaucoma. *Brit J Ophthalmol.* (2014) 98:162–5. doi: 10.1136/bjophthalmol-2012-302486
30. Xu L, Freedman SF, Silverstein E, Muir K, El-Dairi M. Longitudinal reproducibility of spectral domain optical coherence tomography in children with physiologic cupping and stable glaucoma. *J AAPOS.* (2019) 23:261–2. doi: 10.1016/j.jaapos.2019.05.012
31. Go MS, Barman NR, Kelly MP, House RJ, Rotruck JC, El-Dairi MA, et al. Overhead mounted optical coherence tomography in childhood glaucoma evaluation. *J Glaucoma.* (2020) 29:742–9. doi: 10.1097/IJG.0000000000001567
32. Perucho-González L, de La Casa JMM, Sáenz-Francés F, Morales-Fernandez L, Méndez-Hernández CD, Sánchez-Jean R, et al. Retinal nerve fiber layer thickness in children with primary congenital glaucoma measured by spectral domain optical coherence tomography. *J AAPOS.* (2019) 23:91–4. doi: 10.1016/j.jaapos.2017.03.023
33. Pilat AV, Shah S, Sheth V, Purohit R, Proudlock FA, Abbott J, et al. Detection and characterisation of optic nerve and retinal changes in primary congenital glaucoma using hand-held optical coherence tomography. *BMJ Open Ophthalmol.* (2019) 4:e194. doi: 10.1136/bmjophth-2018-000194
34. Lever M, Halfwassen C, Unterlauft JD, Bechrakis NE, Manthey A, Böhm M. The Paediatric glaucoma diagnostic ability of optical coherence tomography: a comparison of macular segmentation and peripapillary retinal nerve fibre layer thickness. *Biology.* (2021) 10:260. doi: 10.3390/biology10040260
35. Moher D, Liberati A, Tetzlaff J, Altman DG. Preferred reporting items for systematic reviews and meta-analyses: the PRISMA statement. *PLoS Med.* (2009) 6:e1000097. doi: 10.1371/journal.pmed.1000097
36. Stroup DF, Berlin JA, Morton SC, Olkin I, Williamson GD, Rennie D, et al. Meta-analysis of observational studies in epidemiology: a proposal for reporting. Meta-analysis of observational studies in epidemiology (MOOSE) group. *JAMA.* (2000) 283:2008–12. doi: 10.1001/jama.283.15.2008
37. Bowd C, Weinreb RN, Williams JM, Zangwill LM. The retinal nerve fiber layer thickness in ocular hypertensive, normal, and glaucomatous eyes with optical coherence tomography. *Arch Ophthalmol.* (2000) 118:22–6. doi: 10.1001/archopht.118.1.22
38. Schuman JS, Hee MR, Puliafito CA, Wong C, Pedut-Kloizman T, Lin CP, et al. Quantification of nerve fiber layer thickness in normal and glaucomatous eyes using optical coherence tomography. *Arch Ophthalmol.* (1995) 113:586–96. doi: 10.1001/archopht.1995.01100050054031
39. Varma R, Bazzaz S, Lai M. Optical tomography-measured retinal nerve fiber layer thickness in normal latinos. *Invest Ophthalmol Vis Sci.* (2003) 44:3369–73. doi: 10.1167/iovs.02-0975
40. Turk A, Ceylan OM, Arici C, Keskin S, Erdurman C, Durukan AH, et al. Evaluation of the nerve fiber layer and macula in the eyes of healthy children using spectral-domain optical coherence tomography. *Am J Ophthalmol.* (2012) 153:552–9. doi: 10.1016/j.ajo.2011.08.026
41. Zhu BD, Li SM, Li H, Liu LR, Wang Y, Yang Z, et al. Retinal nerve fiber layer thickness in a population of 12-year-old children in central China measured by iVue-100 spectral-domain optical coherence tomography: the Anyang childhood eye study. *Invest Ophthalmol Vis Sci.* (2013) 54:8104–11. doi: 10.1167/iovs.13-11958
42. Rotruck JC, House RJ, Freedman SF, Kelly MP, Enyedi LB, Prakalapakorn SG, et al. Optical coherence tomography normative peripapillary retinal nerve fiber layer and macular data in children 0-5 years of age. *Am J Ophthalmol.* (2019) 208:323–30. doi: 10.1016/j.ajo.2019.06.025
43. Larsson E, Molnar A, Holmström G. Repeatability, reproducibility and interocular difference in the assessments of optic nerve OCT in children– a Swedish population-based study. *BMC Ophthalmol.* (2018) 18:270. doi: 10.1186/s12886-018-0940-x
44. Yanni SE, Wang J, Cheng CS, Locke KI, Wen Y, Birch DG, et al. Normative reference ranges for the retinal nerve fiber layer, macula, and retinal layer thicknesses in children. *Am J Ophthalmol.* (2013) 155:354–60. doi: 10.1016/j.ajo.2012.08.010
45. El-Dairi MA, Asrani SG, Enyedi LB, Freedman SF. Optical coherence tomography in the eyes of normal children. *Arch Ophthalmol.* (2009) 127:50–8. doi: 10.1001/archophthalmol.2008.553
46. Mocan MC, Machen L, Jang I, Cao D. the relationship between optic nerve cup-to-disc ratio and retinal nerve fiber layer thickness in suspected pediatric glaucoma. *J Pediat Ophth Strab.* (2020) 57:90–6. doi: 10.3928/01913913-20200117-02
47. González-García AO, Vizzeri G, Bowd C, Medeiros FA, Zangwill LM, Weinreb RN. Reproducibility of RTVue retinal nerve fiber layer thickness and optic disc measurements and agreement with Stratus optical coherence tomography measurements. *Am J Ophthalmol.* (2009) 147:1067–74. doi: 10.1016/j.ajo.2008.12.032
48. Baniasadi N, Paschalis EI, Haghzadeh M, Ojha P, Elze T, Mahd M, et al. Patterns of retinal nerve fiber layer loss in different subtypes of open angle glaucoma using spectral domain optical coherence tomography. *J Glaucoma.* (2016) 25:865–72. doi: 10.1097/IJG.0000000000000534
49. Hua Z, Fang Q, Sha X, Yang R, Hong Z. Role of retinal nerve fiber layer thickness and optic disk measurement by oct on early diagnosis of glaucoma. *Eye Sci.* (2015) 30:7–12. doi: 10.3969/j.issn.1000-4432.2015.01.002
50. Maurice C, Friedman Y, Cohen MJ, Kaliner E, Mimouni M, Kogan M, et al. Histologic RNFL thickness in glaucomatous versus normal human eyes. *J Glaucoma.* (2016) 25:447–51. doi: 10.1097/IJG.0000000000000286
51. Wu H, de Boer JF, Chen TC. Diagnostic capability of spectral-domain optical coherence tomography for glaucoma. *Am J Ophthalmol.* (2012) 153:815–26. doi: 10.1016/j.ajo.2011.09.032
52. Lee VW, Mok KH. Retinal nerve fiber layer measurement by nerve fiber analyzer in normal subjects and patients with glaucoma. *Ophthalmology.* (1999) 106:1006–8. doi: 10.1016/S0161-6420(99)00524-2
53. Lee EJ, Kim TW, Kim JA, Kim GN, Kim JM, Girard M, et al. Elucidation of the strongest factors influencing rapid retinal nerve fiber layer thinning in glaucoma. *Invest Ophthalmol Vis Sci.* (2019) 60:3343–51. doi: 10.1167/iovs.18-26519

54. Lee EJ, Kim TW, Kim H, Lee SH, Girard M, Mari JM. Comparison between lamina cribrosa depth and curvature as a predictor of progressive retinal nerve fiber layer thinning in primary open-angle glaucoma. *Ophthalmol Glaucoma.* (2018) 1:44–51. doi: 10.1016/j.ogla.2018.05.007
55. Wu XS, Xu L, Jonas JB, Zhang L, Yang H, Chen CX. Agreement between spectral domain optical coherence tomography and retinal nerve fiber layer photography in chinese. *J Glaucoma.* (2012) 21:228–33. doi: 10.1097/IJG.0b013e3182070cc6
56. Sung KR, Kim DY, Park SB, Kook MS. Comparison of retinal nerve fiber layer thickness measured by Cirrus HD and Stratus optical coherence tomography. *Ophthalmology.* (2009) 116:1264–70. doi: 10.1016/j.ophtha.2008.12.045
57. Folgar FA, Yuan EL, Farsiu S, Toth CA. Lateral and axial measurement differences between spectral-domain optical coherence tomography systems. *J Biomed Opt.* (2014) 19:16014. doi: 10.1117/1.JBO.19.1.016014
58. Kansal V, Armstrong JJ, Pintwala R, Hutnik C. Optical coherence tomography for glaucoma diagnosis: an evidence based meta-analysis. *PLoS ONE.* (2018) 13:e190621. doi: 10.1371/journal.pone.0190621
59. Qu D, Lin Y, Jiang H, Shao Y, Shi Y, Airen S, et al. Retinal nerve fiber layer (RNFL) integrity and its relations to retinal microvasculature and microcirculation in myopic eyes. *Eye Vis.* (2018) 5:25. doi: 10.1186/s40662-018-0120-3

9

Associations Between Diabetic Retinal Microvasculopathy and Neuronal Degeneration Assessed by Swept-Source OCT and OCT Angiography

Bingjie Qiu[1,2†], *Lin Zhao*[1†], *Xinyuan Zhang*[1,2*†], *Yanhong Wang*[3], *Qiyun Wang*[1,2], *Yao Nie*[1,2], *Xiaosi Chen*[1,2] *and Carol Y. L. Cheung*[4]

[1] *Beijing Tongren Eye Center, Beijing Institute of Ophthalmology, Beijing Tongren Hospital, Capital Medical University, Beijing, China,* [2] *Beijing Retinal Choroidal Vascular Diseases Study Group,* [3] *Department of Epidemiology and Biostatistics, Institute of Basic Medical Sciences Chinese Academy of Medical Sciences & School of Basic Medicine Peking Union Medical College, Beijing, China,* [4] *Department of Ophthalmology and Visual Sciences, The Chinese University of Hong Kong, Hong Kong, China*

***Correspondence:**
Xinyuan Zhang
mmzxy2010@163.com

† *These authors have contributed equally to this work*

Purpose: To provide clinical evidence of the associations between retinal neuronal degeneration and microvasculopathy in diabetic retinopathy (DR).

Methods: This case-control study included 76 patients (76 eyes) with type 2 diabetes mellitus (DM), and refraction error between −3.0 and +3.0 D. The eyes were assigned into DM (without DR), non-proliferative DR (NPDR), and proliferative DR (PDR) groups. Age-, sex-, and refractive error-matched normal subjects were enrolled as controls. The mean retinal thickness (mRT), the relative mean thickness of the retinal nerve fiber layer (rmtRNFL, mtRNFL/mRT), ganglion cell layer (rmtGCL), ganglion cell complex (rmtGCC) layer, foveal avascular zone area (FAZa), FAZ perimeter (FAZp), FAZ circularity index (FAZ-CI), and vessel density (VD) in superficial capillary plexus (SCP) and deep capillary plexus (DCP) were assessed by swept-source optical coherence tomography (OCT) and OCT angiography (OCTA). Group comparison and Spearman's partial correlation coefficient analysis were applied to evaluate the correlation between these morphological parameters.

Results: rmtRNFL, FAZa, and FAZp in SCP and DCP increased with the DR severity ($p_{rmtRNFL} < 0.001$; $p_{FAZa,SCP} = 0.001$; $p_{FAZa,\ DCP} = 0.005$; $p_{FAZp,\ SCP} < 0.001$; $p_{FAZp,\ DCP} < 0.001$). The rmtGCL, FAZ-CI in SCP and DCP, and VD in DCP decreased with the DR severity ($p_{rmtGCL} = 0.002$, $p_{FAZ-CI,\ SCP} = 0.002$; $p_{FAZ-CI,DCP} < 0.001$, $p_{VD,\ DCP} < 0.001$). After controlling age, sex, duration of diabetes, and hypertension, the rmtRNFL, FAZa in SCP and DCP, and FAZp in SCP and DCP were correlated with the severity of DR ($p < 0.05$), while VD in SCP and DCP, FAZ-CI, and rmtGCL were negatively correlated with the severity of DR ($p < 0.05$). The rmtGCL was negatively correlated with the FAZa in SCP ($r = -0.34$, $p = 0.002$) and DCP ($r = -0.23$, $p = 0.033$), and FAZp in SCP ($r = -0.37$, $p = 0.001$) and DCP ($r = -0.32$, $p = 0.003$), but positively correlated with VD in SCP ($r = 0.26$, $p = 0.016$), VD in DCP ($r = 0.28$, $p = 0.012$), and FAZ-CI in DCP ($r = 0.31$, $p = 0.006$).

Conclusions: rmtRNFL, FAZ-CI in SCP and DCP, and FAZp in SCP are strong predictors of the severity of DR. The ganglion cell body loss is highly correlated with increased FAZp and FAZa, decreased FAZ-CI, and reduced VD with the severity of DR.

Keywords: diabetic retinopathy, retinal neuronal degeneration, diabetic microvasculopathy, swept source optical coherence tomography, OCT angiography

INTRODUCTION

Diabetic retinopathy (DR) is among the most significant and disabling chronic complications of diabetes mellitus (1, 2). Although cumulative evidence from basic science and clinical research suggested that DR is a neurovascular disease (3, 4), the correlation between diabetic retinal microvasculopathy and neuronal degeneration still remains uncertain, and their synergistic effect is yet to be illustrated in humans.

In previous studies, retinal neuronal degeneration and microvascular dysfunction have been shown to promote the occurrence and development of DR (5–8). We further confirmed that retinal ganglion cell is the most susceptible retinal neuronal cell type in response to hyperglycemia in a diabetic animal model (3). Clinical studies further confirmed that retinal neurons dysfunction occurred before retinal microvasculopathy using electroretinography (ERG) and visual field examinations (9–11). However, the underlying mechanisms and the correlation between diabetic retinal microvasculopathy and neuron degeneration are yet uncertain. In this study, advanced swept-source optical coherence tomography (SS-OCT) and OCT angiography (OCTA) were used to further investigate the correlation between the early and sensitive parameters of retinal microvasculopathy including the foveal avascular zone area (FAZa), FAZ perimeter (FAZp), FAZ circularity index (FAZ-CI), and retinal vessel density (VD) in superficial capillary plexus (SCP) and deep capillary plexus (DCP), and the parameters for evaluation of the early morphological changes of ganglion cells including the relative mean thickness of the retinal nerve fiber layer (rmtRNFL, mtRNFL/mRT), the relative mean thickness of the ganglion cell layer (rmtGCL), and the relative mean thickness of the ganglion cell complex layer (rmtGCC) in DR.

SUBJECTS AND METHODS

Participants

This study followed the Ethical Principles for Medical Research Involving Human Subjects of the Declaration of Helsinki and was approved by the Ethics Committee of Beijing Tongren Hospital, Capital Medical University. All the enrolled subjects signed an informed consent form before participation.

A total of 76 patients (76 eyes) with type 2 diabetes mellitus (T2DM) were enrolled in this study, including 39 males and 37 females, aged 40–71 years (average 58.34 ± 7.47 years), with a refractive error between −3.0 diopter (D) and +3.0 D and registered in the outpatient clinic of Beijing Tongren Hospital from September 2018 to September 2019. Age-, sex-, and refractive error-matched 28 healthy subjects (28 eyes) [aged 43–78 years, median (interquartile, IQR) 53 (48–62) years] constituted the normal control group. If bilateral eyes were diagnosed as DR in patients with T2DM, only the severely affected eye was enrolled in the study.

Sample Size Calculation

Combined with our pilot study results, which enrolled at least 15 subjects per group to show the statistical significance, Cochran's sample size formula was applied and the previous studies were referenced (27). Sample size was calculated at 95% confidence level with a margin of error of ±5%. We determined the minimum sample size to be 20 subjects in each group to detect the difference (0.83) between means of the OCT and OCTA parameters with a significance level of (alpha) 0.05.

Inclusion and Exclusion Criteria

The inclusion criteria were as follows: (1) participants aged 40–70 years with T2DM; (2) refractive errors between −3.00 D and +3.00 D. T2DM was defined according to the American Diabetes Association (ADA) guidelines of DM (28–33), while DR was defined and classified by ophthalmologists according to the 2017 "Diabetic Retinopathy: A Position Statement of Diabetic Retinopathy" by the American Diabetes Association (34). Age-, sex-, and refractive error-matched normal subjects were enrolled as controls.

Abbreviations: ADA, American Diabetes Association; ANOVA, One-way analysis of variance; BCVA, Best-corrected visual acuity; CBF, Cerebral blood flow; D, Diopter; DCP, Deep capillary plexus; DM, Diabetes mellitus; DR, Diabetic retinopathy; ERG, Electroretinography; ETDRS, Early Treatment Diabetic Retinopathy Study Classification; FAZ, Foveal avascular zone; FAZa, Foveal avascular zone area; FAZ-CI, Foveal avascular zone-circularity index; FAZp, Foveal avascular zone perimeter; FFA, Fundus fluorescein angiography; GCC, Ganglion cell complex; GCL, Ganglion cell; ICP, Intracranial pressure; IIH, Idiopathic intracranial hypertension; IQR, Interquartile; mRT, Mean retinal thickness; NPDR, Non-proliferative diabetic retinopathy; NVU, Neurovascular unit; OCT, Optical coherence tomography; OCTA, Optical coherence tomography angiography; PDR, Proliferative diabetic retinopathy; rmtGCC, Relative mean thickness of the ganglion cell complex; rmtGCL, Relative mean thickness of the ganglion cell; rmtRNFL, Relative mean thickness of the retinal nerve fiber; RNFL, Retinal nerve fiber; RNVU, Retinal neuronal vascular unit; SCP, Superficial capillary plexus; SS-OCT, Swept-source optical coherence tomography; T2DM, Type 2 diabetes mellitus; TABS, TOPCON Advanced Boundary Segmentation; VD, Vessel density; VEP, Visual evoked potential.

The exclusion criteria were as follows: (1) cysts detected in the neural retina by OCT; (2) macular edema secondary to any other retinal vascular diseases; (3) patients with other fundus diseases, such as age-related macular degeneration, uveitis, and retinal inherited diseases; (4) eyes with history of posterior surgery within 1 year; (5) eyes that underwent pan-retinal photocoagulation or focal/grid laser treatment; (6) eyes treated with intravitreal anti-vascular endothelial growth factor (VEGF) agent or steroid within one year; (7) patients with glaucoma or ocular hypertension; (8) fundus examination could not be performed due to ocular media opacities; (9) patients could not tolerate examinations due to severe systemic diseases.

Eye Examination

Routine Eye Examinations

The best-corrected visual acuity (BCVA), non-contact intraocular pressure (TX20 Automatic Non-contact Tonometer, Canon Co., Ltd., Tokyo, Japan), slit-lamp microscopic examination (SL-IE Slit Lamp Microscope, Topcon Co., Ltd., Tokyo, Japan), and fundus examination with mydriasis and fundus photography (CR-1 non-mydriatic Fundus Camera, Canon Co., Ltd., Tokyo, Japan) were employed in all the enrolled subjects.

Detection and Quantification of the Morphological Parameters by OCT

Imaging with DRI-Triton OCT: All subjects were examined by SS-OCT (DRI OCT1 Atlantis scanner, Topcon Co., Ltd., Tokyo, Japan). A 9 × 9 mm scanning range mode was selected to obtain B-scan images. The thickness of the retinal nerve fiber layer (RNFL), ganglion cell layer (GCL), and ganglion cell complex (GCC) in nine macular regions was measured automatically using TOPCON Advanced Boundary Segmentation (TABS) software. The nine regions were designed according to the Early Treatment Diabetic Retinopathy Study Classification (ETDRS) system. The ETDRS map was divided into nine parts: one 1 mm diameter circle at the center, outside four inner-quarter annuluses on the outside between the 1 and 3 mm diameter circles, and four outer-quarter annuluses between the 3 and 6 mm diameter circles (**Figure 1**). All images were measured independently by two ophthalmologists. Computer-aided manual correction of OCT segmentation was used for correcting thickness measurements in cases with errors.

Detection and Quantification of the OCTA Parameters

Optical coherence tomography angiography images were obtained using a 6 × 6 mm scanning mode in the macular area. Individual images in SCP, DCP, outer retina, and choriocapillaris plexus were generated by Topcon IMAGEnet® 6 software with the computer-aided manual correction in cases with errors (35). FAZa and FAZp in SCP and DCP were measured by Image J software (version 1.48, available online at http://rsb.info.nih.gov/ij/, National Institutes of Health, Bethesda, MD, USA). Foveal avascular zone circularity index (FAZ-CI) (36) is an indicator and novel biomarker representing disruption of the parafoveal capillary network. The shape of FAZ is closer to a regular circular shape when FAZ-CI is close to 1. The formula of the FAZ-CI is:

$$FAZ - CI = \frac{4\pi \times area}{perimeter^2}$$

OCTA images were binarized with Ostu threshold method using Image J software (37). The VD in superficial and deep capillary networks was measured by calculating the proportion of vessel area with blood flow over the total area measured (38) (**Figure 2**).

To avoid individual differences and other confounding factors, we used the mean value (the average of ETDRS nine subfields) and relative thickness to describe the morphological parameters of retinal ganglion cells determined by SS-OCT. The relative mean thickness of RNFL (rmtRNFL), GCL (rmtGCL), and GCC (rmtGCC) was defined as the mean thickness of RNFL, GCL, or GCC/mean retinal thickness, respectively.

Statistical Analysis

Statistical analysis was performed using SPSS software (SPSS, Inc. 24.0, Chicago, IL, USA). Age of patients, the duration of diabetes, the FAZa, rmtRNFL, rmtGCL, and rmtGCC in each group were described by means ± standard deviation (mean ± SD) or median (interquartile range). The comparisons between the groups were analyzed by one-way analysis of variance (ANOVA) or Kruskal–Wallis test. Spearman's partial correlation analysis was used to analyze the correlation between the parameters of retinal degeneration and microvasculopathy or between various morphological parameters with the severity of DR after controlling the age, gender, duration of diabetes, and hypertension. A value of $P < 0.05$ was considered statistically significant.

RESULTS

Demographic Characteristics of the Enrolled Subjects

The DM group included 10 males (10 eyes) and 11 females (11 eyes) (aged 42–70 years, average: 59.62 ± 7.57 years), while 18 males (18 eyes) and 15 females (15 eyes) (aged 40–71 years, average: 59.76 ± 7.43 years) constituted the non-proliferative diabetic retinopathy (NPDR) group, and 11 males (11 eyes) and 11 females (11 eyes) (aged 43–70 years, average: 55.00 ± 6.63 years) constituted the proliferative diabetic retinopathy (PDR) group. In the control group, 28 patients (28 eyes) with normal age matching were selected, including 11 males (11 eyes) and 17 females (17 eyes) (aged 43–78 years, median (IQR) 53 (12–26) years) (**Table 1**).

No statistically significant difference was found in the gender and age among the four groups ($p_{gender} = 0.633$, $p_{age} = 0.086$). No significant difference was observed in the duration of DM in the DM, NPDR, and PDR groups ($p = 0.171$). Also, no significant difference was noted in the fasting blood glucose in the DM, NPDR, and PDR groups ($p = 0.658$). The glycosylated hemoglobin levels in the DM, NPDR, and PDR groups did not differ significantly ($p = 0.464$). Furthermore, no significant difference was detected in the duration of hypertension among the four groups ($\chi^2 = 2.20$, $p = 0.333$) (**Table 1**).

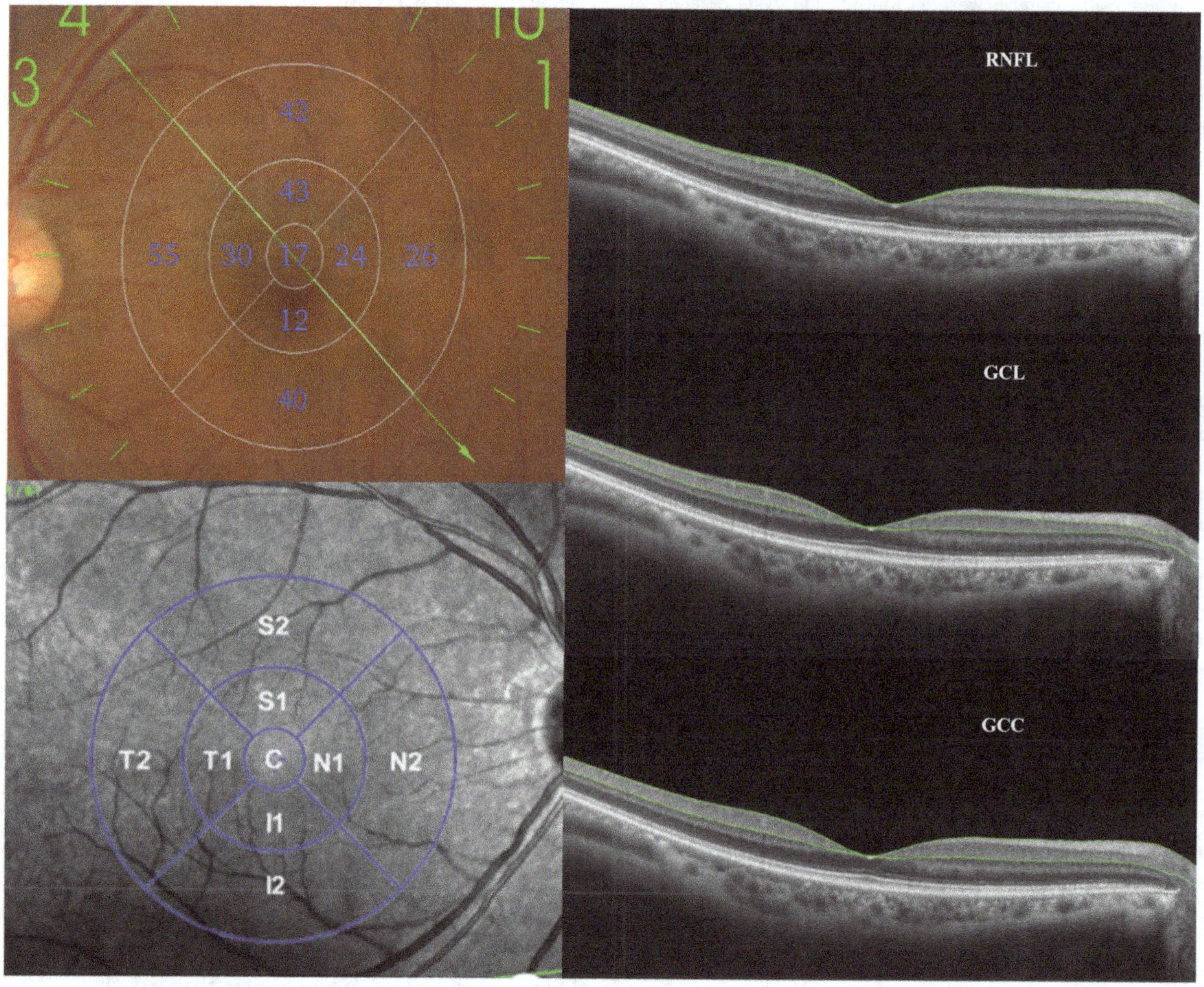

FIGURE 1 | Measurement and analysis of the thickness of RNFL, GCL, and GCC layers. The ETDRS map (nine subfields) was utilized to calculate the average thickness of the RNFL, GCL, and GCC layers. RNFL, retinal nerve fiber layer; GCL, ganglion cell layer; GCC, ganglion cell complex layer; ETDRS, the Early Treatment Diabetic Retinopathy Study.

Correlations of the Mean Macular Thickness With Diabetic Retinopathy Severity

According to the general trend, the mean macular thickness increased with DR severity. However, there was no statistically significant difference observed between the normal (277.60 ± 14.56 μm), DM (282.17 ± 13.31 μm), NPDR (289.05 ± 20.54 μm), and PDR (293.43 ± 34.23 μm) groups (277.60 ± 14.56 μm vs. 282.17 ± 13.31 μm vs. 289.05 ± 20.54 μm vs. 293.43 ± 34.23 μm, $p_{all} = 0.052$) (**Table 1**).

Relative Mean RNFL Thickness Increased With Diabetic Retinopathy Severity

The rmtRNFL thickness (ratio of the mean thickness of RNFL) in the DM group was 0.11 ± 0.01, and that in the NPDR, PDR, and normal control groups was 0.11 (0.11–0.12), 0.13 ± 0.02, and 0.10 (0.10–0.11), respectively. The rmtRNFL thickness in the normal group was significantly lower than that in the NPDR and PDR groups [0.11 (0.11Ű-0.12) vs. 0.10 (0.10Ű-0.11), $p_{NPDRvs.Normal} = 0.007$ and 0.13 ± 0.02 vs. 0.10 (0.10-Ű0.11), $p_{PDRvs.Normal} < 0.001$]. The rmtRNFL thickness in the DM group was significantly lower than that in the PDR group [0.13 ± 0.02 vs. 0.11 ± 0.01, $p_{PDRvs.DM} < 0.001$]. These results indicated that the mean thickness of RNFL/RT increased gradually with an increase in severity of DR (**Figure 3A, Table 2**).

Relative Mean GCL Thickness Decreased With Diabetic Retinopathy Severity

The rmtGCL thickness (GCL/RT) layer was 0.27 ± 0.01 in the DM group, 0.27 ± 0.02 in the NPDR group, 0.25 ± 0.02 in the PDR group, and 0.26 ± 0.02 in the normal control group, respectively. The rmtGCL thickness was significantly lower in the PDR group than that in the normal control, DM, and NPDR

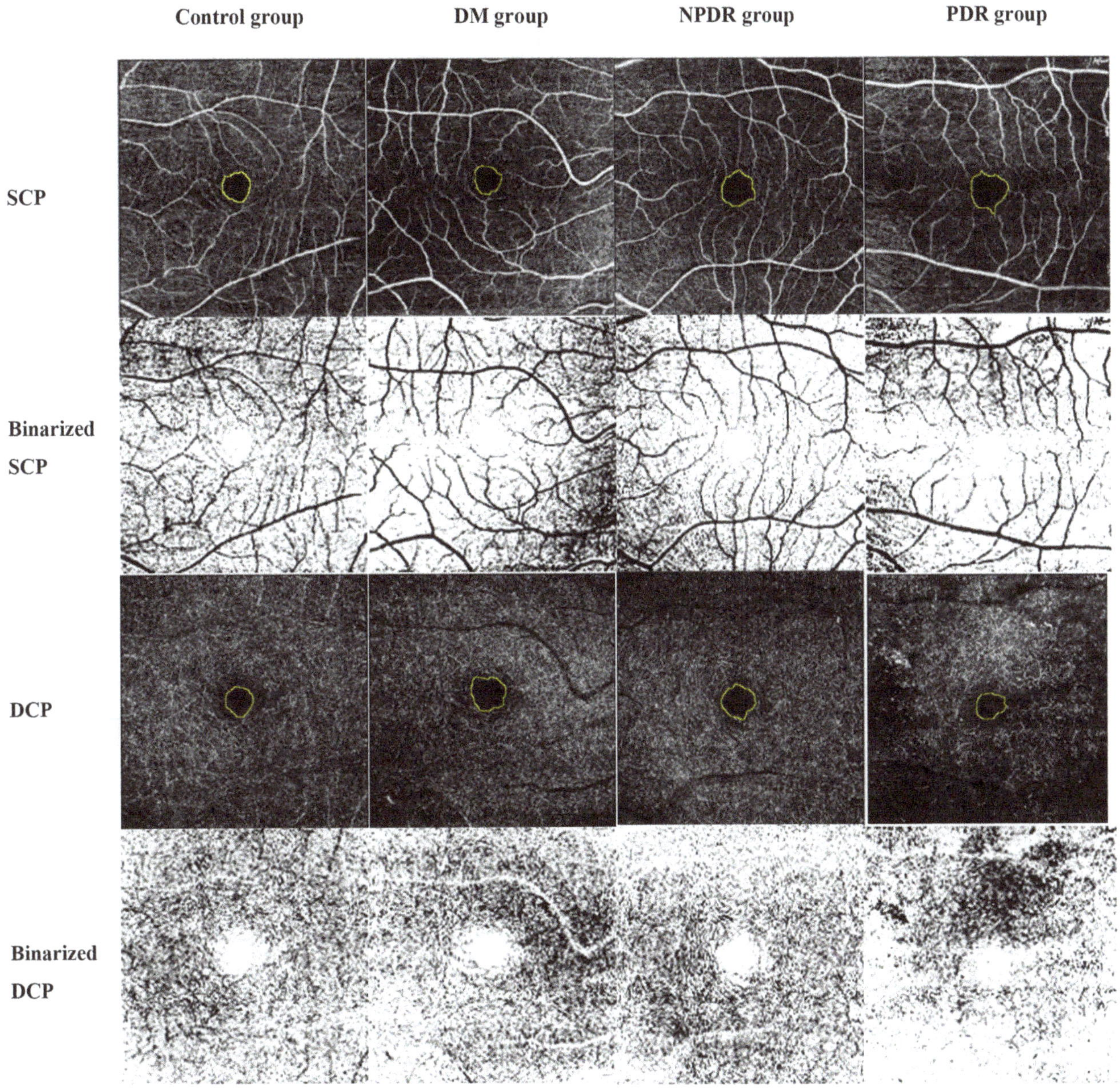

FIGURE 2 | Representative OCTA images illustrate the quantification methods of VD, FAZa, FAZp, and FAZ-CI in SCP and DCP. OCTA images were obtained using a 6 × 6 mm scanning mode in the macular area. Individual images in SCP, DCP, outer retina, and choriocapillaris plexus were generated by Topcon IMAGEnet® 6 software with the computer-aided manual correction in cases with errors in eyes with normal control (healthy subjects), DM (no DR), NPDR, and PDR. The FAZa and perimeter (yellow circle) were quantified by Image J software. Ostu method was applied to calculate the VD using Image J software. OCTA, optical coherence tomography angiography; VD, vessel density; FAZ, foveal avascular zone; FAZ-CI, FAZ circularity index; SCP, superficial capillary plexus; DCP, deep capillary plexus; DM, diabetes mellitus; DR, diabetic retinopathy; NPDR, non-proliferative diabetic retinopathy; PDR, proliferative diabetic retinopathy.

groups (0.25 ± 0.02 vs. 0.26 ± 0.02, $p_{PDRvs.Normal} = 0.040$; 0.25 ± 0.02 vs. 0.27 ± 0.01, $p_{PDRvs.DM} = 0.002$; 0.25 ± 0.02 vs. 0.27 ± 0.02, $p_{PDRvs.NPDR} = 0.009$, respectively) (**Figure 3B, Table 2**).

Correlations of the Mean GCC Thickness With Diabetic Retinopathy Severity

No statistically significant difference was observed in the rmtGCC thickness in the normal control (0.37 ± 0.02), DM (0.38 ± 0.01), NPDR (0.38 ± 0.03), and PDR (0.38 ± 0.03) groups (0.37 ± 0.02 vs. 0.38 ± 0.01 vs. 0.38 ± 0.03 vs. 0.38 ± 0.03, $p = 0.108$) (**Figure 3C, Table 2**).

Vessel Density in SCP and DCP Decreased With Diabetic Retinopathy Severity

Superficial capillary plexus vessel density was 29.12 ± 3.98% in the normal control, 27.88 ± 4.18% in DM, 26.25 ± 4.94%

TABLE 1 | The demographic characteristics and the biochemical indicators of subjects.

	DM (N = 21)	NPDR (N = 33)	PDR (N = 22)	Control (N = 28)	F/χ^2	P value
Age, y [mean ± SD or median (interquartile range)]	59.62 ± 7.57	59.76 ± 7.43	55.00 ± 6.63	53 (48.62)	2.259[a]	0.086
Gender, female (N) (%)	11 (52.4)	15 (44.1)	11 (50.0)	17 (60.7)	1.720[c]	0.633
Duration of Hypertension≥15 years/Duration of Hypertension<15 years	6/10	14/18	5/16	–	2.197[c]	0.333
Duration of DM (mean ± SD)	11.58 ± 5.41	15.24 ± 7.51	14.32 ± 6.50	–	1.808[a]	0.171
Fasting blood glucose, mmol/L (mean ±SD)	8.10 ± 2.36	8.50 (6.35, 10.07)	8.06 ± 2.49	–	0.836[b]	0.658
HbA1c, % (mean ± SD)	8.02 ± 1.81	7.93 ± 1.25	8.46 ± 1.69	–	0.775[a]	0.464
RT, μm (mean ± SD)	282.17 ± 13.31	289.05 ± 20.54	293.43 ± 34.23	277.60 ± 14.56	2.663[a]	0.052

**Statistically significant: $P \leq 0.05$. According to the type of data and the data distribution, [a]one-way ANOVA analysis, Post-hoc Bonferroni's statistic, [b]Kruskal–Wallis test, and [c]Chi-square test were applied.*

SD, standard deviation; HbA1c, hemoglobin a1c; RT, retinal thickness; DM, diabetes mellitus; NPDR, non-proliferative diabetic retinopathy; PDR, proliferative diabetic retinopathy.

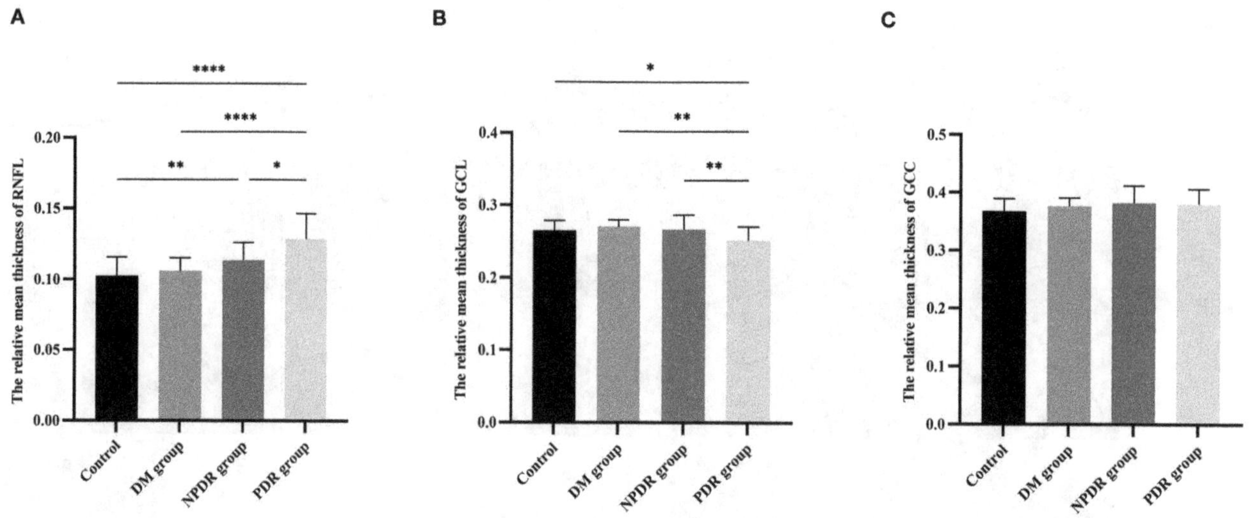

FIGURE 3 | Comparisons of relative mean thickness of RNFL, GCL, and GCC layers among the DM, NPDR, PDR, and normal control groups. The bar charts show the comparison results of the relative mean thickness of RNFL **(A)**, GCL **(B)**, GCC **(C)** in eyes with normal control (healthy subjects), DM (no DR), NPDR, and PDR. RNFL, retinal nerve fiber layer; GCL, ganglion cell layer; GCC, ganglion cell complex layer; DM, diabetes mellitus; DR, diabetic retinopathy; NPDR, non-proliferative diabetic retinopathy; PDR, proliferative diabetic retinopathy. * p<0.05, ** p<0.01, *** p<0.001.

in NPDR, and 26.25 ± 3.72% in PDR, respectively. From these results, we found that the SCP vessel density decreased with diabetic retinopathy severity while there was no significant difference between the four groups (29.12 ± 3.98% vs. 27.88 ± 4.18% vs. 26.25 ± 4.94% vs. 26.25 ± 3.72%, p_{all} = 0.067) (**Figure 4A**, **Table 2**).

Deep capillary plexus vessel density was 30.77 ± 2.94% in the normal control, 30.13 ± 2.81% in DM, 28.58 ± 6.22% in NPDR, and 25.28 ± 2.76% in PDR, respectively. A significant difference was observed between the four groups (30.77 ± 2.94% vs. 30.13 ± 2.81% vs. 28.58 ± 6.22% vs. 25.28 ± 2.76%, p_{all} < 0.001). DCP vessel density is significantly higher than that in the PDR groups (25.28 ± 2.76% vs. 30.77 ± 2.94%, $p_{PDRvs.Normal}$ < 0.001). DCP vessel density in the DM group was significantly larger than that in PDR group (25.28 ± 2.76% vs. 30.13 ± 2.81%, $p_{PDRvs.DM}$ < 0.001), and the value in the NPDR group was significantly larger than that in the PDR group (25.28 ± 2.76% vs. 28.58 ± 6.22%, $p_{PDRvs.NPDR}$ = 0.050) (**Figure 4B**, **Table 2**).

Correlations of FAZ Area in SCP and DCP With Diabetic Retinopathy Severity

The value of FAZa in SCP was 0.36 ± 0.14 mm^2 in the normal control, 0.34 ± 0.10 mm^2 in DM, 0.47 ± 0.17 mm^2 in NPDR, and 0.57 ± 0.25 mm^2 in PDR, respectively. A significant difference was observed between the four groups (0.36 ± 0.14 mm^2 vs. 0.34 ± 0.10 mm^2 vs. 0.47 ± 0.17 mm^2 vs. 0.57 ± 0.25 mm^2, p_{all} = 0.001). The FAZa in the PDR group was significantly enlarged than that in the DM (0.57 ± 0.25 mm^2 vs. 0.34 ± 0.10 mm^2, $p_{PDRvs.DM}$ = 0.006) and normal control (0.57 ± 0.25 mm^2 vs. 0.36 ± 0.14 mm^2, $p_{PDRvs.Normal}$ = 0.002) groups (**Figure 4C**, **Table 2**).

The value of FAZa in DCP was 0.52 ± 0.21 mm^2 in the normal control, 0.59 ± 0.16 mm^2 in DM, 0.69 ± 0.21 mm^2 in NPDR, and

TABLE 2 | Comparisons of the parameters of the ganglion cell degeneration and microvasculopathy in the normal (no DM), DM (no DR), NPDR, and PDR groups.

	Control (N = 28)	DM (N = 21)	NPDR (N = 33)	PDR (N = 22)	$F/\chi2$ (all)	P-value (all)	
rmtRNFL [mean ±SD or median (interquartile range)]	0.10 (0.10, 0.11)	0.11 ± 0.01	0.11 (0.11, 0.12)	0.13 ± 0.02	35.10[b]	<0.001*	
		$p_{DMvs.Normal}$	$p_{NPDRvs.Normal}$	$p_{PDRvs.Normal}$	$p_{NPDRvs.DM}$	$p_{PDRvs.DM}$	$p_{PDRvs.NPDR}$
		1.000	**0.007***	**<0.001***	0.249	**<0.001***	**0.039***
rmtGCL [mean ±SD or median (interquartile range)]	0.26 ± 0.02	0.27 ± 0.01	0.27 ± 0.02	0.25 ± 0.02	5.38[a]	0.002*	
		$p_{DMvs.Normal}$	$p_{NPDRvs.Normal}$	$p_{PDRvs.Normal}$	$p_{NPDRvs.DM}$	$p_{PDRvs.DM}$	$p_{PDRvs.NPDR}$
		1.000	1.000	**0.040***	1.000	**0.002***	**0.009***
rmtGCC [mean ±SD or median (interquartile range)]	0.37 ± 0.02	0.38 ± 0.01	0.38 ± 0.03	0.38 ± 0.03	2.08[a]	0.108	
		$p_{DMvs.Normal}$	$p_{NPDRvs.Normal}$	$p_{PDRvs.Normal}$	$p_{NPDRvs.DM}$	$p_{PDRvs.DM}$	$p_{PDRvs.NPDR}$
		1.000	0.127	0.375	1.000	1.000	1.000
SCP vessel density, % (mean ± SD)	29.12 ± 3.98	27.88 ± 4.18	26.25 ± 4.94	26.25 ± 3.72	2.45[a]	0.067	
		$p_{DMvs.Normal}$	$p_{NPDRvs.Normal}$	$p_{PDRvs.Normal}$	$p_{NPDRvs.DM}$	$p_{PDRvs.DM}$	$p_{PDRvs.NPDR}$
		1.000	0.094	0.161	1.000	1.000	1.000
DCP vessel density, % [mean ± SD or median (interquartile range)]	30.77 ± 2.94	30.13 ± 2.81	28.58 ± 6.22	25.28 ± 2.76	24.846[b]	<0.001*	
		$p_{DMvs.Normal}$	$p_{NPDRvs.Normal}$	$p_{PDRvs.Normal}$	$p_{NPDRvs.DM}$	$p_{PDRvs.DM}$	$p_{PDRvs.NPDR}$
		1.000	0.144	**<0.001***	0.457	**<0.001***	**0.050***
FAZ area in superficial capillary plexus, mm^2 [mean ± SD or median (interquartile range)]	0.36 ± 0.14	0.34 ± 0.10	0.47 ± 0.17	0.57 ± 0.25	17.54[b]	0.001*	
		$p_{DMvs.Normal}$	$p_{NPDRvs.Normal}$	$p_{PDRvs.Normal}$	$p_{NPDRvs.DM}$	$p_{PDRvs.DM}$	$p_{PDRvs.NPDR}$
		1.000	0.095	**0.002***	0.197	**0.006***	0.846
FAZ area in deep capillary plexus, mm^2 (mean ± SD or median (interquartile range)]	0.52 ± 0.21	0.59 ± 0.16	0.69 ± 0.21	0.79 ± 0.31	12.83[b]	0.005*	
		$p_{DMvs.Normal}$	$p_{NPDRvs.Normal}$	$p_{PDRvs.Normal}$	$p_{NPDRvs.DM}$	$p_{PDRvs.DM}$	$p_{PDRvs.NPDR}$
		1.000	**0.040***	**0.007***	0.873	0.227	1.000
FAZ perimeter in superficial capillary plexus, mm [mean ± SD or median (interquartile range)]	2.29 ± 0.49	2.32 ± 0.33	2.86 ± 0.54	3.15 (2.67, 4.07)	23.82[b]	<0.001*	
		$p_{DMvs.Normal}$	$p_{NPDRvs.Normal}$	$p_{PDRvs.Normal}$	$p_{NPDRvs.DM}$	$p_{PDRvs.DM}$	$p_{PDRvs.NPDR}$
		1.000	**0.005***	**<0.001***	0.057	**0.004***	1.000
FAZ perimeter in deep capillary plexus, mm [mean ± SD or median (interquartile range)]	2.67 ± 0.61	3.19 (2.80, 3.31)	3.31 (2.81, 3.94)	4.14 ± 1.34	22.92[b]	<0.001*	
		$p_{DMvs.Normal}$	$p_{NPDRvs.Normal}$	$p_{PDRvs.Normal}$	$p_{NPDRvs.DM}$	$p_{PDRvs.DM}$	$p_{PDRvs.NPDR}$
		0.557	**0.009***	**<0.001***	1.000	**0.023***	0.392
FAZ-CI in superficial capillary plexus [mean ± SD or median (interquartile range)]	0.82 ± 0.10	0.79 ± 0.08	0.71 ± 0.13	0.65 ± 0.21	14.50[b]	0.002*	
		$p_{DMvs.Normal}$	$p_{NPDRvs.Normal}$	$p_{PDRvs.Normal}$	$p_{NPDRvs.DM}$	$p_{PDRvs.DM}$	$p_{PDRvs.NPDR}$
		1.000	**0.011***	**0.008***	0.395	0.241	1.000
FAZ-CI in deep capillary plexus [mean ± SD or median (interquartile range)]	0.88 ± 0.04	0.78 ± 0.08	0.75 ± 0.10	0.63 ± 0.19	36.54[b]	<0.001*	
		$p_{DMvs.Normal}$	$p_{NPDRvs.Normal}$	$p_{PDRvs.Normal}$	$p_{NPDRvs.DM}$	$p_{PDRvs.DM}$	$p_{PDRvs.NPDR}$
		0.004*	**<0.001***	**<0.001***	1.000	0.090	0.336

Statistically significant: $P \leq 0.05$. According to the type of data and the data distribution, [a]one-way ANOVA analysis, Post-hoc Bonferroni's statistic, [b]Kruskal–Wallis test, and [c]Chi-square test were applied.

SD, standard deviation; rmtRNFL, relative mean thickness of retinal nerve fiber layer; rmtGCL, relative mean thickness of ganglion cell layer; rmtGCC, relative mean thickness of ganglion cell complex; SCP, superficial capillary plexus; DCP, deep capillary plexus; FAZ, foveal vascular zone; FAZ-CI, circularity index of the foveal avascular zone; DM, diabetes mellitus; NPDR, non-proliferative diabetic retinopathy; PDR, proliferative diabetic retinopathy.

0.79 ± 0.31 mm^2 in PDR, respectively. There was a significant difference between the four groups (0.52 ± 0.21 mm^2 vs. 0.59 ± 0.16 mm^2 vs. 0.69 ± 0.21 mm^2 vs. 0.79 ± 0.31 mm^2, $p_{all} = 0.005$). The FAZa in DCP in the normal control group was significantly smaller than that in the NPDR (0.69 ± 0.21 mm^2 vs. 0.52 ± 0.21 mm^2, $p_{NPDRvs.Normal} = 0.040$) and PDR (0.79 ± 0.31 mm^2 vs. 0.52 ± 0.21 mm^2, $p_{PDRvs.Normal} = 0.007$) groups (**Figure 4D, Table 2**).

Correlations of FAZ Perimeter in SCP and DCP With Diabetic Retinopathy Severity

The FAZp in SCP was 2.29 ± 0.49 mm in the normal control group, 2.32 ± 0.33 mm in DM, 2.86 ± 0.54 mm in NPDR, and 3.15 (2.67–4.07) mm in PDR, respectively. A significant difference was detected between the four groups [2.29 ± 0.49 mm vs. 2.32 ± 0.33 mm vs. 2.86 ± 0.54 mm vs. 3.15 (2.67–4.07) mm, $p_{all} < 0.001$]. The FAZp in SCP layer in the NPDR and PDR groups were significantly enlarged than that in the normal group [2.86 ± 0.54 mm vs. 2.29 ± 0.49 mm, $p_{NPDRvs.Normal} = 0.005$ and 3.15 (2.67–4.07) mm vs. 2.29 ± 0.49 mm, $p_{PDRvs.Normal} < 0.001$, respectively]. The FAZp in SCP layer in the PDR group was significantly enlarged than that in the DM group [3.15 (2.67–4.07) mm vs. 2.32 ± 0.33 mm, $p_{PDRvs.DM} = 0.004$] (**Figure 4E, Table 2**).

The value of FAZp in DCP was 2.67 ± 0.61 mm in the normal control, 3.19 (2.80–3.31) mm in DM, 3.31(2.81–3.94) mm in NPDR, and 4.14 ± 1.34 mm in PDR, respectively. There was a significant difference between the four groups (2.67 ± 0.61 mm vs. 3.19 (2.80–3.31) mm vs. 3.31 (2.81–3.94) mm vs. 4.14 ± 1.34 mm, $p_{all} < 0.001$). The FAZp in DCP in the NPDR and PDR group was significantly enlarged than that in the normal group [3.31(2.81–3.94) mm vs. 2.67 ± 0.61 mm, $p_{NPDRvs.Normal} = 0.009$ and 4.14 ± 1.34 mm vs. 2.67 ± 0.61 mm, $p_{PDRvs.Normal} < 0.001$, respectively]. The FAZp in DCP in the PDR group was significantly enlarged than that in the DM group [4.14 ± 1.34 mm vs. 3.19 (2.80–3.31) mm, $p_{PDRvs.DM} = 0.023$] (**Figure 4F, Table 2**).

FAZ-CI in SCP and DCP Decreased With Diabetic Retinopathy Severity

The value of FAZ-CI in SCP was 0.82 ± 0.10 in the normal control, 0.79 ± 0.08 in DM, 0.71 ± 0.13 in NPDR, and 0.65 ± 0.21 in PDR, respectively. A significant difference was observed between the four groups (0.82 ± 0.10 vs. 0.79 ± 0.08 vs. 0.71 ± 0.13 vs. 0.65 ± 0.21, $p_{all} = 0.002$). The FAZ-CI in SCP in the normal control group was significantly bigger than that in the NPDR (0.71 ± 0.13 vs. 0.82 ± 0.10, $p_{NPDRvs.Normal} = 0.011$) and PDR (0.65 ± 0.21 vs. 0.82 ± 0.10, $p_{PDRvs.Normal} = 0.008$) groups (**Figure 4G, Table 2**).

The value of FAZ-CI in DCP was 0.88 ± 0.04 in the normal control, 0.78 ± 0.08 in DM, 0.75 ± 0.10 in NPDR, and 0.63 ± 0.19 in PDR, respectively. A significant difference was observed between the four groups (0.88 ± 0.04 vs. 0.78 ± 0.08 vs. 0.75 ± 0.10 vs. 0.63 ± 0.19, $p_{all} < 0.001$). The FAZ-CI in DCP in the normal control group was significantly bigger than that in the DM (0.78 ± 0.08 vs. 0.88 ± 0.04, $p_{DMvs.Normal} = 0.004$), NPDR (0.75 ± 0.10 vs. 0.88 ± 0.04, $p_{NPDRvs.Normal} < 0.001$), and PDR (0.63 ± 0.19 vs. 0.88 ± 0.04, $p_{PDRvs.Normal} < 0.001$) groups (**Figure 4H, Table 2**).

Correlation Between Microvasculopathy and Neuronal Degeneration Among Different Groups

After controlling the age, sex, duration of diabetes, and hypertension, Spearman's partial coefficient correlation analysis showed that the rmtRNFL ($r = 0.52$, $p < 0.001$); FAZa in SCP ($r = 0.34$, $p < 0.001$) and in DCP ($r = 0.26$, $p = 0.015$); and FAZp in SCP($r = 0.43$, $p < 0.001$) and in DCP ($r = 0.36$, $p = 0.001$) were positively significantly correlated with the severity of DR. SCP vessel density ($r = -0.24$, $p = 0.027$), DCP vessel density ($r = -0.39$, $p < 0.001$), FAZ-CI in SCP($r = -0.44$, $p < 0.001$), DCP ($r = -0.46$, $p < 0.001$), and rmtGCL ($r = -0.24$, $p = 0.022$) were negatively correlated with the severity of DR.

The rmtGCL was significantly negatively correlated with the FAZa in SCP ($r = -0.34$, $p = 0.002$) and DCP ($r = -0.23$, $p = 0.033$), and with FAZp in SCP ($r = -0.37$, $p = 0.001$) and DCP ($r = -0.32$, $p = 0.003$). However, the rmtGCL was positively correlated with SCP vessel density ($r = 0.26$, $p = 0.016$) and DCP vessel density ($r = 0.28$, $p = 0.012$), and FAZ-CI in DCP ($r = 0.31$, $p = 0.006$) (**Figure 5**).

DISCUSSION

In this study, we found that increased rmtRNFL, FAZa, and FAZp, decreased rmtGCL, VD, and FAZ-CI are correlated with the severity of DR. rmtRNFL, FAZ-CI in SCP and DCP, and FAZp in SCP are stronger predictors of the severity of DR than the FAZa. The ganglion cell body loss (rmtGCL) is highly correlated with increased FAZa and perimeter, decreased FAZ-CI, and reduced VD with the severity of DR. These results indicated that diabetic microvasculopathy is highly correlated with neuronal degeneration, and neuron protection is an essential strategy to improve prevention and management in DR (3).

Neurovascular unit (NVU) is a new concept in neuroscience introduced by the Stroke Progress Review Group (39). The NVU is a complex structural and functional unit that regulates regional cerebral blood flow (CBF) and the delivery of nutrients (40). The dysfunction of NVU has been implicated in several diseases, such as stroke and Alzheimer's disease (41). Based on the concept of brain NVU and the close correlation between the retina and the brain in all aspects of function and anatomy, the concept of retinal neuronal vascular unit (RNVU) was proposed (42, 43). Neurons and endothelial cells are the critical components of RNVU. The interactions between neurons and microvasculature in DR have gained increasing attention in recent years. In this study, we found that the ganglion cell body loss is highly correlated with the retinal vasculature changes (increased FAZp, decreased FAZ-CI, and reduced VD) with the severity of DR, which is consistent with previous reports (44, 45).

A ganglion cell is mainly composed of a cell body (soma), a single axon, and dendrites. The electrical impulses transmitted by neurons mainly depend on axon transport, the process by which nerve cells transfer substances from the cell body to the axon tip. This ATP-dependent process plays an important role in maintaining the physiological activities of neurons and can occur in two delivery directions: anterograde (from the cell body to the axon tips) and retrograde (from the axon tips back to the cell body) transport. The microtubule cytoskeleton and motor proteins are critical for long-range axon transport.

The axons of the GCL constitute RNFL. Increasing evidence speculated that mitochondrial dysfunction and axoplasmic flow stasis in optic neuropathy (44, 45) lead to axonal swelling and contribute to most of the neurodegenerative diseases including DR (46–49). Eyes with early Leber Hereditary Optic Neuropathy (E-LHON) showed a thicker RNFL, but a thinner RNFL was seen in eyes with atrophic LHON (A-LHON) in comparison with the control group, thereby suggesting that the changes in RNFL thickness represent the different course of the disease (50). In a diabetic rat model, expression level of the synaptic proteins including vesicular glutamate transporter-1, syntaxin-1, and synaptotagmin-1 was decreased in the GCL, but the level of dynein motor proteins increased in the GCL after 8 weeks of diabetes, indicating that axonal transport contributes to early signs of neural dysfunction in the diabetic rat retinas (51). Furthermore, the degree of increased thickness of RNFL is closely correlated with visual evoked potential (VEP)

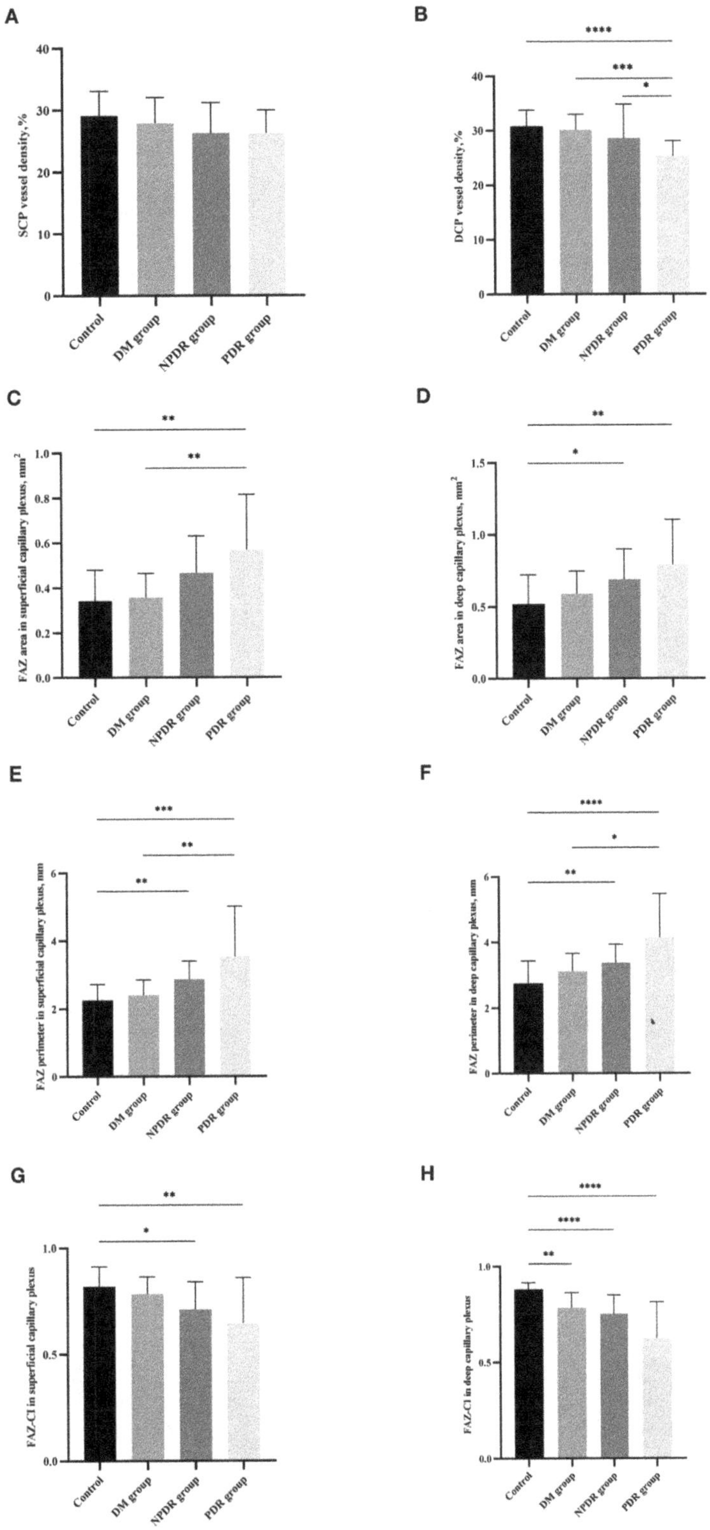

FIGURE 4 | Comparisons of the retinal microvasculopathy (FAZa, FAZp, FAZ-CI, and VD in SCP and DCP) among the normal control (healthy subjects), DM (no DR), NPDR and PDR groups. The bar charts show the comparison results of the VD in SCP **(A)**, VD in DCP **(B)**, FAZa in SCP **(C)**, FAZa in DCP **(D)**, FAZp in SCP **(E)**, FAZp in DCP **(F)**, FAZ-CI in SCP **(G)**, and FAZ-CI in DCP **(H)** in eyes with normal control (healthy subjects), DM (no DR), NPDR, and PDR. FAZ, foveal avascular zone; FAZ-CI, FAZ circularity index; VD, vessel density; SCP, superficial capillary plexus; DCP, deep capillary plexus; DM, diabetes mellitus; DR, diabetic retinopathy; NPDR, non-proliferative diabetic retinopathy; PDR, proliferative diabetic retinopathy.

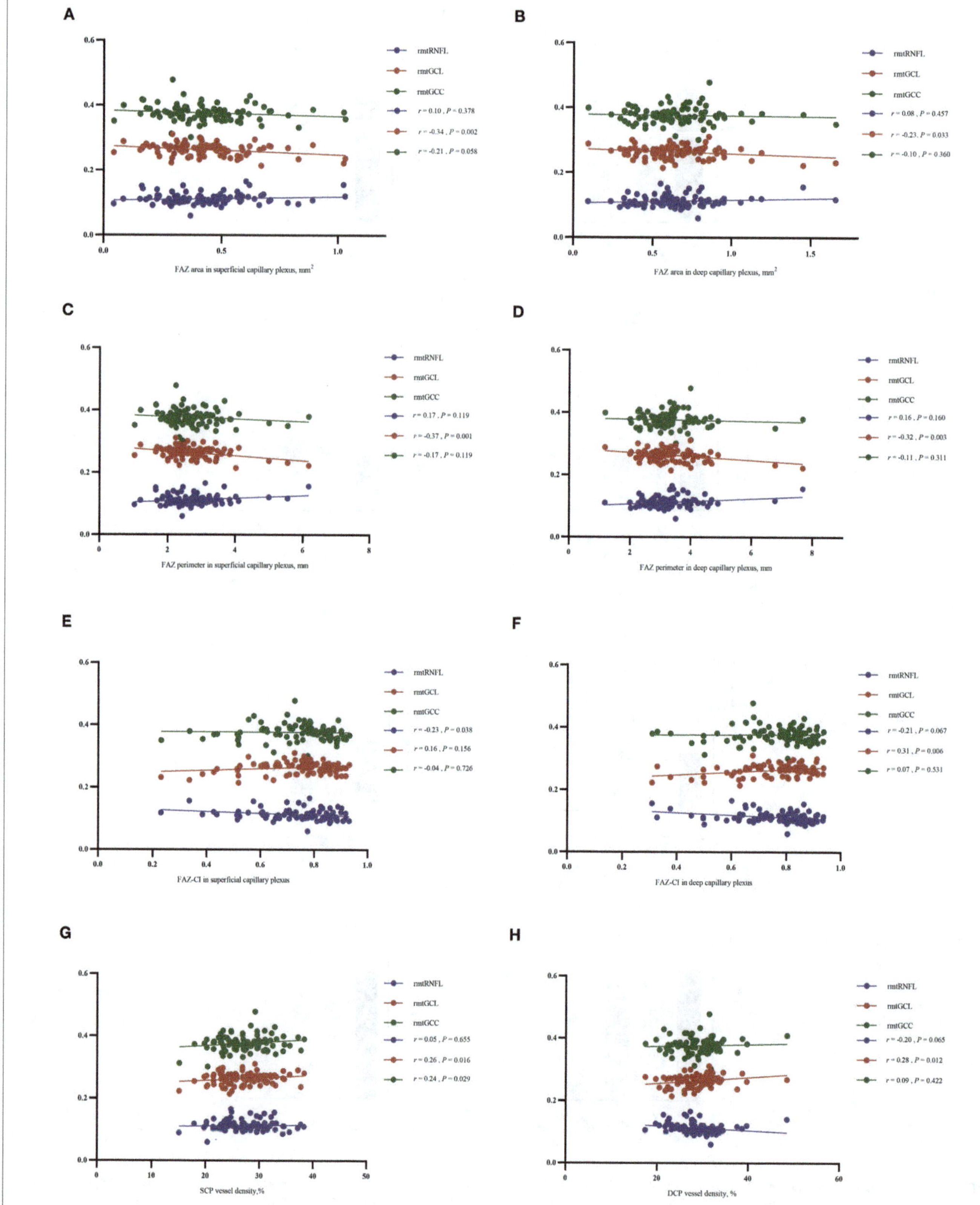

FIGURE 5 | Relationship between the parameters of retinal microvasculopathy (FAZa, FAZp, FAZ-CI, and VD in SCP and DCP) and ganglion cell degeneration (the relative mean thickness of RNFL, GCL, and GCC). After controlling the age, sex, and duration of DM and hypertension with Spearman's partial coefficient

(Continued)

FIGURE 5 | correlation analysis, the rmtGCL was negatively correlated with the FAZa in SCP ($r = -0.34$, $P = 0.002$) and DCP ($r = -0.23$, $P = 0.033$), and FAZp in SCP ($r = -0.37$, $P = 0.001$) and DCP ($r = -0.32$, $P = 0.003$), but positively correlated with VD in SCP ($r = 0.26$, $P = 0.016$) and DCP ($r = 0.28$, $P = 0.012$), and FAZ-CI in DCP ($r = 0.31$, $P = 0.006$). The correlations between rmtRNFL, rmtGCL and rmtGCC with the FAZa in SCP **(A)**, FAZa in DCP **(B)**, FAZp in SCP **(C)**, FAZp in DCP **(D)**, FAZ-CI in SCP **(E)**, FAZ-CI in DCP **(F)**, VD in SCP **(G)** and VD in DCP **(H)** were described. The rmtRNFL was negatively correlated with FAZ-CI in SCP ($r = -0.23$, $P = 0.038$). The rmtGCC was positively correlated with SCP vessel density ($r = 0.24$, $P = 0.029$). FAZ, foveal avascular zone; FAZ-CI, FAZ circularity index; VD, vessel density; SCP, superficial capillary plexus; DCP, deep capillary plexus; rmtRNFL, relative mean thickness of retinal nerve fiber layer; rmtGCL, relative mean thickness of ganglion cell layer; rmtGCC, relative mean thickness of ganglion cell complex; DM, diabetes mellitus.

amplitude loss and degree of optic atrophy, indicating that during the progression of DR, a thinner RNFL is a sign of optic atrophy following the swelling stage of axons of ganglion cells (52), and the degree of thickened RNFL may be an indicator of optic atrophy for patients with DR. Furthermore, in a primate model of human non-arteritic anterior ischemic optic neuropathy, RNFL swelling is confirmed as a strong and independent predictor of optic nerve atrophy, which agrees with our results (52). In this study, we have shown that the relative thickness of RNFL increased with DR severity concomitant with the decreased thickness of the GCL layer. This phenomenon suggested that the swelling of the GCL axon preceded the GCL cell body loss under hyperglycemia, thereby reflecting the unique hypoglycemia-mediated pathological damage of GCL. The pathological evidence, either in animal models or humans, is consistent with the findings of the current study (53–57).

Furthermore, FAZp, FAZ-CI, and VD are good sensors of retinal ischemia and have been implicated in several clinical studies to predict disease progression (58–60). Increased FAZp, FAZ-CI, and VD have been found to be an earlier sign of diabetic retinal vasculopathy (60–62) and are highly correlated with the severity of DR (12, 62). In comparison with FAZa, which significantly varies in the population, FAZ-CI is a better measurement index to assess FAZ circularity with a value range from 0 to 1 (13). FAZ-CI has been found to be tightly correlated with visual acuity in patients with DR (13, 14). We also found that enlargement of FAZp in SCP and DCP was correlated with DR severity as well as the duration of diabetes, which is in parallel to the previously published data (15–17). In previous studies, SCP and DCP vessel density was demonstrated to be decreased in DM (18) and highly correlated with DR progression (19), which are consistent with our results. We further demonstrated that microvascular injury is associated with GCL cell body loss in DR, providing the evidence for the first time that there is an interaction between retinal microvasculopathy and neuronal degeneration. Interestingly, we also found that in comparison with RNGL, GCL has a closer relationship with the vasculature ischemic parameters (FAZp, FAZ-CI, VD), indicating that the ganglion cell body is a good sensor for retinal ischemia.

The rapid revolution of OCT and OCTA has provided a powerful weapon for evaluating the morphological and structural changes in the various layers of the retina (20–22). Compared to traditional OCT, SS-OCT provides longer and deeper detection ability, ultra-high image acquisition speed, and a more powerful function of eliminating motion artifacts, thereby providing a distinct retinal microstructure (20, 23–26). OCTA has the advantage of investigating retinal vasculature non-invasively layer-by-layer (**Figure 2**). Automatic quantitative OCTA metrics have provided valuable information for disease progression beyond that could be obtained from fundus fluorescein angiography (FFA) (63).

In this study, to avoid the individual differences, the inter-eye correlation, and the other confounding factors, we used the following: (1) average value of ETDRS nine subfields to describe the thickness of the retina, RNFL, GCL, and GCC (64, 65); (2) all the values were automatically provided by Topton triton SS-OCT TABS software; (3) the relative mean thickness of RNFL, GCL, and GCC was defined as the mean thickness of RNFL, GCL, or GCC/mean retinal thickness. Gabriele et al. described a relative method in which RNFL thickness profiles relative to the distance from the disc center were computed for quadrants and clock hours (66). In our pilot study, a linear trend was established among the four groups, which was similar between the relative mean ETDRS macular thickness and absolute thickness; however, data distribution was based on relative thickness and indicated the differences among the groups.

Although the current study successfully showed the correlation between diabetic retinal vasculopathy and neuronal degeneration, these findings are limited due to the case-control design, and the causal relationship between neuronal degeneration and microvasculopathy cannot be determined, hence future validation using longitudinal data is warranted. Furthermore, the small sample size could not eliminate some confounding factors in the analysis, and so well-designed and large-scale prospective clinical trials are also needed to support the conclusions in the study. Morphological (OCT/OCTA) and functional evaluations (ERG) of neurons in a cohort study could also be considered to further determine the pathological changes in other neuronal cell types under hyperglycemia.

In summary, we found that there was a close correlation between diabetic retinal microvasculopathy and neuronal degeneration with respect to the occurrence and severity of DR in humans. The current results also hinted that neuroprotection is also critical for the prevention and managing of DR. Further, well-designed, large cohort studies are warranted to validate the findings of this study.

ETHICS STATEMENT

The studies involving human participants were reviewed and approved by Beijing Tongren Hospital, Capital Medical University. The patients/participants provided their written informed consent to participate in this study.

AUTHOR CONTRIBUTIONS

XZ contributed to the conception and design of the study and revision of the manuscript. BQ and LZ organized the database and drafted the manuscript. YW and BQ performed the statistical analysis. QW, YN, XC, and CC helped to enroll subjects. All authors contributed to manuscript revision, and read approved the submitted version.

REFERENCES

1. Spaide RF. Measurable aspects of the retinal neurovascular unit in diabetes, glaucoma, and controls. *Am J Ophthalmol.* (2019) 207:395-409. doi: 10.1016/j.ajo.2019.04.035
2. Yau JW, Rogers SL, Kawasaki R, Lamoureux EL, Kowalski JW, Bek T, et al. Global prevalence and major risk factors of diabetic retinopathy. *Diabetes Care.* (2012) 353:556-64. doi: 10.2337/dc11-1909
3. Zhang XY, Lai D, Bao S, Hambly BD, Gillies MC. Triamcinolone acetonide inhibits p38MAPK activation and neuronal apoptosis in early diabetic retinopathy. *Curr Mol Med.* (2013) 136:946-58. doi: 10.2174/1566524011313060007
4. Zhang XY, Wang NL, Barile GR, Bao S, Gillies MC. Diabetic retinopathy: neuron protection as a therapeutic target. *Int J Biochem Cell Biol.* (2013) 457:1525-9. doi: 10.1016/j.biocel.2013.03.002
5. Zafar S, Sachdeva M, Frankfort BJ, Channa R. Retinal neurodegeneration as an early manifestation of diabetic eye disease and potential neuroprotective therapies. *Curr Diab Rep.* (2019) 194:17. doi: 10.1007/s11892-019-1134-5
6. Stem MS, Gardner TW. Neurodegeneration in the pathogenesis of diabetic retinopathy: molecular mechanisms and therapeutic implications. *Curr Med Chem.* (2013) 2026:3241-50. doi: 10.2174/092986731132099 90027
7. Antonetti DA, Barber AJ, Bronson SK, Freeman WM, Gardner TW, Jefferson LS, et al. Diabetic retinopathy: seeing beyond glucose-induced microvascular disease. *Diabetes.* (2006) 559:2401-11. doi: 10.2337/db 05-1635
8. Zhang X, Bao S, Lai D, Rapkins RW, Gillies MC. Intravitreal triamcinolone acetonide inhibits breakdown of the blood-retinal barrier through differential regulation of VEGF-A and its receptors in early diabetic rat retinas. *Diabetes.* (2008) 574:1026-33. doi: 10.2337/db07-0982
9. Pescosolido N, Barbato A, Stefanucci A, Buomprisco G. Role of electrophysiology in the early diagnosis and follow-up of diabetic retinopathy. *J Diabetes Res.* (2015) 2015:319692. doi: 10.1155/2015/319692
10. Tzekov R. Full-field ERG in diabetic retinopathy: a screening tool? *Graefes Arch Clin Exp Ophthalmol.* (2015) 2537:987-8. doi: 10.1007/s00417-015-3037-8
11. Bearse MA, Adams AJ, Ying H, Schneck ME, Ng J, Bronson-Castain K, et al. A multifocal electroretinogram model predicting the development of diabetic retinopathy. *Prog Retinal Eye Res.* (2006) 255:425-48. doi: 10.1016/j.preteyeres.2006.07.001
12. Johannesen SK, Viken JN, Vergmann AS, Grauslund J. Optical coherence tomography angiography and microvascular changes in diabetic retinopathy: a systematic review. *Acta Ophthalmol.* (2019) 971:7-14. doi: 10.1111/aos.13859
13. Tang FY, Ng DS, Lam A, Luk F, Wong R, Chan C, et al. Determinants of quantitative optical coherence tomography angiography metrics in patients with diabetes. *Sci Rep.* (2017) 71:2575. doi: 10.1038/s41598-017-0 2767-0
14. Sim DA, Keane PA, Zarranz-Ventura J, Fung S, Powner MB, Platteau E, et al. The effects of macular ischemia on visual acuity in diabetic retinopathy. *Invest Ophthalmol Vis Sci.* (2013) 543:2353-60. doi: 10.1167/iovs.12-11103
15. Gill A, Cole ED, Novais EA, Louzada RN, de Carlo T, Duker JS, et al. Visualization of changes in the foveal avascular zone in both observed and treated diabetic macular edema using optical coherence tomography angiography. *Int J Retina Vitreous.* (2017) 3:19. doi: 10.1186/s40942-017-0074-y
16. Liu L, Jian G, Bao W, Hu C, Xu Y, Zhao B, et al. Analysis of foveal microvascular abnormalities in diabetic retinopathy using optical coherence tomography angiography with projection artifact removal. *J Ophthalmol.* (2018) 2018:3926745. doi: 10.1155/2018/3926745
17. Krawitz BD, Mo S, Geyman LS, Agemy SA, Scripsema NK, Garcia PM, et al. Acircularity index and axis ratio of the foveal avascular zone in diabetic eyes and healthy controls measured by optical coherence tomography angiography. *Vision Res.* (2017) 139:177-86. doi: 10.1016/j.visres.2016.09.019
18. Lupidi M, Cerquaglia A, Gujar R, Fruttini D, Cardillo Piccolino F, Fiore T, et al. Functional correlation between choroidal and retinal vascularity in low-grade diabetic retinopathy. *Acta Diabetol.* (2020) 578:983-90. doi: 10.1007/s00592-020-01507-7
19. Ryu G, Kim I, Sagong M. Topographic analysis of retinal and choroidal microvasculature according to diabetic retinopathy severity using optical coherence tomography angiography. *Graefes Arch Clin Exp Ophthalmol.* (2021) 2591:61-8. doi: 10.1007/s00417-020-04785-7
20. Vira J, Marchese A, Singh RB, Agarwal A. Swept-source optical coherence tomography imaging of the retinochoroid and beyond. *Expert Rev Med Dev.* (2020) 175:413-26. doi: 10.1080/17434440.2020.1755256
21. Spaide RF, Klancnik JJ, Cooney MJ. Retinal vascular layers imaged by fluorescein angiography and optical coherence tomography angiography. *JAMA Ophthalmol.* (2015) 1331:45-50. doi: 10.1001/jamaophthalmol.2014.3616
22. Jia Y, Tan O, Tokayer J, Potsaid B, Wang Y, Liu JJ, et al. Split-spectrum amplitude-decorrelation angiography with optical coherence tomography. *Optics Exp.* (2012) 204:4710-25. doi: 10.1364/OE.20.004710
23. Miller AR, Roisman L, Zhang Q, Zheng F, Rafael de Oliveira Dias J, Yehoshua Z, et al. Comparison between spectral-domain and swept-source optical coherence tomography angiographic imaging of choroidal neovascularization. *Invest Ophthalmol Vis Sci.* (2017) 583:1499-505. doi: 10.1167/iovs.16-20969
24. Statler B, Kosmorsky G, Rachitskaya A. Swept source OCT angiography of optic nerve head retinal capillary hemangioma. *Ophthalmol Retina.* (2020) 48:822. doi: 10.1016/j.oret.2020.04.004
25. Cicinelli MV, Cavalleri M, Consorte AC, Rabiolo A, Sacconi R, Bandello F, et al. Swept-source and spectral domain optical coherence tomography angiography versus dye angiography in the measurement of type 1 neovascularization. *Retina.* (2020) 403:499-506. doi: 10.1097/IAE.0000000000002452
26. Alibhai AY, Or C, Witkin AJ. Swept source optical coherence tomography: a review. *Curr Ophthalmol Rep.* (2018) 6:7-16. doi: 10.1007/s40135-018-0158-3
27. Liu L, Wang Y, Liu HX, Gao J. Peripapillary region perfusion and retinal nerve fiber layer thickness abnormalities in diabetic retinopathy assessed by

OCT angiography. *Transl Vis Sci Technol.* (2019) 84:14. doi: 10.1167/tvst.8.4.14

28. American Diabetes Association. Standards of medical care in diabetes-2016 abridged for primary care providers. *Clin Diabetes.* (2016) 341:3–21. doi: 10.2337/diaclin.34.1.3
29. American Diabetes A. Standards of medical care in diabetes-2017 abridged for primary care providers. *Clin Diabetes.* (2017) 351:5–26. doi: 10.2337/cd16-0067
30. American Diabetes Association. Standards of medical care in diabetes-2018 abridged for primary care providers. *Clin Diabetes.* (2018) 361:14–37. doi: 10.2337/cd17-0119
31. American Diabetes Association. Standards of medical care in diabetes-2019 abridged for primary care providers. *Clin Diabetes.* (2019) 371:11–34. doi: 10.2337/cd18-0105
32. American Diabetes Association. Standards of medical care in diabetes-2020 abridged for primary care providers. *Clin Diabetes.* (2020) 381:10–38. doi: 10.2337/cd20-as01
33. American Diabetes Association. Standards of medical care in diabetes-2021 abridged for primary care providers. *Clin Diabetes.* (2021) 391:14–43. doi: 10.2337/cd21-as01
34. Solomon SD, Chew E, Duh EJ, Sobrin L, Sun JK, VanderBeek BL, et al. Diabetic retinopathy: a position statement by the American Diabetes Association. *Diabetes Care.* (2017) 403:412–8. doi: 10.2337/dc16-2641
35. Spaide RF, Curcio CA. Evaluation of segmentation of the superficial and deep vascular layers of the retina by optical coherence tomography angiography instruments in normal eyes. *JAMA Ophthalmol.* (2017) 1353:259–62. doi: 10.1001/jamaophthalmol.2016.5327
36. Choi J, Kwon J, Shin JW, Lee J, Lee S, Kook MS. Quantitative optical coherence tomography angiography of macular vascular structure and foveal avascular zone in glaucoma. *PLoS One.* (2017) 129:e0184948. doi: 10.1371/journal.pone.0184948
37. Nicolo M, Rosa R, Musetti D, Musolino M, Saccheggiani M, Traverso CE. Choroidal vascular flow area in central serous chorioretinopathy using swept-source optical coherence tomography angiography. *Invest Ophthalmol Vis Sci.* (2017) 584:2002–10. doi: 10.1167/iovs.17-21417
38. You QS, Chan JCH, Ng ALK, Choy BKN, Shih KC, Cheung JJC, et al. Macular vessel density measured with optical coherence tomography angiography and its associations in a large population-based study. *Invest Ophthalmol Vis Sci.* (2019) 6014:4830–7. doi: 10.1167/iovs.19-28137
39. Stamatovic SM, Keep RF, Andjelkovic AV. Brain endothelial cell-cell junctions: how to "Open" the blood brain barrier. *Curr Neuropharmacol.* (2008) 63:179–92. doi: 10.2174/157015908785777210
40. Cai W, Zhang K, Li PY, Zhu L, Xu J, Yang BY, et al. Dysfunction of the neurovascular unit in ischemic stroke and neurodegenerative diseases: an aging effect. *Ageing Res Rev.* (2016) 34:77–87. doi: 10.1016/j.arr.2016.09.006
41. Shabir O, Berwick J, Francis SE. Neurovascular dysfunction in vascular dementia, Alzhiemers and atherosclerosis. *BMC Neurosci.* (2018) 191:62. doi: 10.1186/s12868-018-0465-5
42. Zhang XY, Zeng H, Bao S, Wang NL, Gillies MC. Diabetic macular edema: new concepts in patho-physiology and treatment. *Cell Biosci.* (2014) 41:27. doi: 10.1186/2045-3701-4-27
43. Gardner TW, Davila JR. The neurovascular unit and the pathophysiologic basis of diabetic retinopathy. *Graefes Arch Clin Exp Ophthalmol.* (2017) 2551:1–6. doi: 10.1007/s00417-016-3548-y
44. Berdahl JP, Ethier CR, Allingham RR. Cerebrospinal fluid pressure and glaucomatous optic disc cupping. *Graefes Arch Clin Exp Ophthalmol.* (2009) 2479:1289–90; author reply 1291–1284. doi: 10.1007/s00417-009-1110-x
45. Hayreh SS. Optic disc edema in raised intracranial pressure. *V. Pathogenesis. Arch Ophthalmol.* (1977) 959:1553–65. doi: 10.1001/archopht.1977.04450090075006
46. Baptista FI, Gaspar JM, Cristovao A, Santos PF, Kofalvi A, Ambrosio AF. Diabetes induces early transient changes in the content of vesicular transporters and no major effects in neurotransmitter release in hippocampus and retina. *Brain Res.* (2011) 1383:257–69. doi: 10.1016/j.brainres.2011.01.071
47. Gaspar JM, Castilho A, Baptista FI, Liberal J, Ambrosio AF. Long-term exposure to high glucose induces changes in the content and distribution of some exocytotic proteins in cultured hippocampal neurons. *Neuroscience.* (2010) 1714:981–92. doi: 10.1016/j.neuroscience.2010.10.019
48. Morgan JE. Circulation and axonal transport in the optic nerve. *Eye.* (2004) 1811:1089–95. doi: 10.1038/sj.eye.6701574
49. Chevalier-Larsen E, Holzbaur EL. Axonal transport and neurodegenerative disease. *Biochim Biophys Acta.* (2006) 176211-12:1094–108. doi: 10.1016/j.bbadis.2006.04.002
50. Barboni P, Savini G, Valentino ML, Montagna P, Cortelli P, De Negri AM, et al. Retinal nerve fiber layer evaluation by optical coherence tomography in Leber's hereditary optic neuropathy. *Ophthalmology.* (2005) 1121:120–6. doi: 10.1016/j.ophtha.2004.06.034
51. Baptista FI, Pinto MJ, Elvas F, Martins T, Almeida RD, Ambrosio AF. Diabetes induces changes in KIF1A, KIF5B and dynein distribution in the rat retina: implications for axonal transport. *Exp Eye Res.* (2014) 127:91–103. doi: 10.1016/j.exer.2014.07.011
52. Johnson MA, Miller NR, Nolan T, Bernstein SL. Peripapillary retinal nerve fiber layer swelling predicts peripapillary atrophy in a primate model of nonarteritic anterior ischemic optic neuropathy. *Invest Ophthalmol Vis Sci.* (2016) 572:527–32. doi: 10.1167/iovs.15-17880
53. Skau M, Yri H, Sander B, Gerds TA, Milea D, Jensen R. Diagnostic value of optical coherence tomography for intracranial pressure in idiopathic intracranial hypertension. *Graefes Arch Clin Exp Ophthalmol.* (2013) 2512:567–74. doi: 10.1007/s00417-012-2039-z
54. Huang-Link YM, Al-Hawasi A, Oberwahrenbrock T, Jin YP. OCT measurements of optic nerve head changes in idiopathic intracranial hypertension. *Clin Neurol Neurosurg.* (2015) 130:122–7. doi: 10.1016/j.clineuro.2014.12.021
55. Soni D, Sagar P, Takkar B. Diabetic retinal neurodegeneration as a form of diabetic retinopathy. *Int Ophthalmol.* (2021) 41:3223–481. doi: 10.1007/s10792-021-01864-4
56. Ng DS, Chiang PP, Tan G, Cheung CG, Cheng CY, Cheung CY, et al. Retinal ganglion cell neuronal damage in diabetes and diabetic retinopathy. *Clin Exp Ophthalmol.* (2016) 444:243–50. doi: 10.1111/ceo.12724
57. Mantelli F, Lambiase A, Colafrancesco V, Rocco M L, Macchi I, Aloe L. NGF and VEGF effects on retinal ganglion cell fate: new evidence from an animal model of diabetes. *Eur J Ophthalmol.* (2014) 242:247–53. doi: 10.5301/ejo.5000359
58. de Carlo TE, Chin AT, Bonini Filho MA, Adhi M, Branchini L, Salz DA, et al. Detection of microvascular changes in eyes of patients with diabetes but not clinical diabetic retinopathy using optical coherence tomography angiography. *Retina.* (2015) 3511:2364–70. doi: 10.1097/IAE.0000000000000882
59. Ishibazawa A, Nagaoka T, Takahashi A, Omae T, Tani T, Sogawa K, et al. Optical coherence tomography angiography in diabetic retinopathy: a prospective pilot study. *Am J Ophthalmol.* (2015) 1601:35–44.e31. doi: 10.1016/j.ajo.2015.04.021
60. Al-Sheikh M, Akil H, Pfau M, Sadda SR. Swept-Source OCT angiography imaging of the foveal avascular zone and macular capillary network density in diabetic retinopathy. *Invest Ophthalmol Vis Sci.* (2016) 578:3907–13. doi: 10.1167/iovs.16-19570
61. Kim K, Kim ES, Yu SY. Optical coherence tomography angiography analysis of foveal microvascular changes and inner retinal layer thinning in patients with diabetes. *Br J Ophthalmol.* (2017) 1029:1226–31. doi: 10.1136/bjophthalmol-2017-311149
62. Inanc M, Tekin K, Kiziltoprak H, Ozalkak S, Doguizi S, Aycan Z. Changes in retinal microcirculation precede the clinical onset of diabetic retinopathy in children with Type 1 diabetes mellitus. *Am J Ophthalmol.* (2019) 207:37–44. doi: 10.1016/j.ajo.2019.04.011
63. Lee H, Lee M, Chung H, Kim HC. Quantification of retinal vessel tortuosity in diabetic retinopathy using optical coherence tomography angiography. *Retina.* (2017) 385:976–85. doi: 10.1097/IAE.0000000000001618
64. Huang JJ, Liu X, Wu ZQ, Xiao H, Dustin L, Sadda S. Macular thickness measurements in normal eyes with time-domain and Fourier-domain optical coherence tomography. *Retina.* (2009) 297:980–7. doi: 10.1097/IAE.0b013e3181a2c1a7
65. Grover S, Murthy RK, Brar VS, Chalam KV. Comparison of retinal thickness in normal eyes using stratus and spectralis optical coherence tomography. *Invest Ophthalmol Vis Sci.* (2010) 515:2644–7. doi: 10.1167/iovs.09-4774

10

Microvascular Changes After Conbercept Intravitreal Injection of PDR with or without Center-Involved Diabetic Macular Edema Analyzed by OCTA

Wei Lin [1†], Meng Feng [1†], Tingting Liu [2,3,4,5†], Qingxu Wang [6], Wenqi Wang [2,3,4,7], Xiao Xie [2,3,4,7], Wenhao Li [8], Jitian Guan [2,3,4,5], Zhongyu Ma [7], Tong Liu [9] and Qingjun Zhou [3,4,5,10]*

[1] School of Basic Medicine, Shandong First Medical University and Shandong Academy of Medical Science, Shandong Provincial Hospital Affiliated to Shandong First Medical University, Jinan, China, [2] Eye Hospital of Shandong First Medical University (Shandong Eye Hospital), Jinan, China, [3] State Key Laboratory Cultivation Base, Shandong Provincial Key Laboratory of Ophthalmology, Qingdao, China, [4] Shandong Eye Institute, Shandong First Medical University and Shandong Academy of Medical Sciences, Qingdao, China, [5] School of Ophthalmology, Shandong First Medical University, Jinan, China, [6] Jinan Mingshui Eye Hospital, Jinan, China, [7] The First Clinical Medical College of Shandong University of Traditional Chinese Medicine, Jinan, China, [8] Computer Department of Southwest University of Science and Technology, Mianyang, China, [9] Department of Medicine, Xizang Minzu University, Xianyang, China, [10] Qingdao Eye Hospital of Shandong First Medical University, Qingdao, China

***Correspondence:**
Tingting Liu
tingtingliu@vip.sina.com

† These authors share first authorship

Purpose: To investigate the intravitreal injection of conbercept as a treatment strategy for proliferative diabetic retinopathy (PDR) with or without center-involved diabetic macular edema (CI-DME) and evaluate its effect on the microvascular changes in the eyes.

Methods: In this prospective study, 43 patients including 29 cases (56 eyes) in CI-DME with PDR patients, and 14 cases (26 eyes) in the non-center involving diabetic macular edema (NCI-DME) with PDR patients were involved in this study. The best corrected visual acuity (BCVA), central retinal thickness (CRT), foveolar avascular zone (FAZ), and macular capillary vessel density (VD) of the superficial retinal capillary plexus (SCP) and deep retinal capillary plexus (DCP) were assessed before and after conbercept treatments for 1, 3, or 6 months.

Results: The BCVA was significantly increased after conbercept treatment in the eyes of CI-DME patients. After 6 months of treatment with the conbercept, microvascular density of the inferior area in SCP and the central fovea area in DCP increased significantly, regardless of the central fovea involvement. The effect of the conbercept treatment on the VD of NCI-DME was higher than that of CI-DME. Then, after 6 months of treatment, the CRT of patients with CI-DME and NCI-DME were decreased significantly.

Conclusions: In this study, an intravitreal injection of conbercept significantly improved vision, alleviated macular edema in patients with DME. Conbercept treatment also altered the microvascular density in the retina.

Keywords: proliferative diabetic retinopathy (PDR), conbercept, foveolar avascular zone (FAZ), central retinal thickness (CRT), best corrected visual acuity (BCVA), optical coherence tomography angiography (OCTA)

INTRODUCTION

Diabetic retinopathy (DR) is the common microvascular complications of diabetes. It is the main cause of visual impairment worldwide. Millions of patients with diabetes may progress to vision-threatening retinopathy, defined as proliferative diabetic retinopathy (PDR) or macular edema (1–4). PDR combined with different degrees of diabetic macular edema (DME) is one of the most common causes of visual impairment.

Intravitreal anti-vascular endothelial growth factor (VEGF) therapy is a first-line treatment for DME (5–11). Ranibizumab is an anti-VEGF inhibitor. Recently, the randomized Diabetic Retinopathy Clinical Research Network (DRCR.net) Protocol S clinical trial showed that ranibizumab intravitreal therapy was effective for treating PDR (12). Conbercept (KH902; Chengdu Kanghong Biotech Co., China) is a recombinant anti-VEGF protein. It has been produced by the expression system of Chinese hamster ovary (CHO) cells (13, 14). Studies proved the efficacy and safety of conbercept injections for the treatment of DME and PDR (15, 16).

It is important to evaluate the macular perfusion of repeated injections that are often required for long-term treatment. Some studies have analyzed macular capillary perfusion by fundus autofluorescence (FFA). But FFA requires manual measurement of macular capillary perfusion, and its analysis results are easily affected by factors, such as leakage, hemorrhage, and image quality (17–21). Optical coherence tomography angiography (OCTA) is a newly developed technology of fundus angiography, which is used to stratify the vessels of the retina and choroid, and has become an important instrument for the diagnosis and treatment of diabetic retinopathy (2, 22). Thus, OCTA can be used to observe the therapeutic effect of anti-VEGF drugs more precisely (10, 11, 15, 23). A few prior studies compared the effect of conbercept on DME by OCTA, and the results were controversial (22–24).

In this study, we aimed to investigate the intravitreal treatment of conbercept for PDR with or without center-involved DME (CI-DME) and evaluated its effect on the microvascular changes in retina.

METHODS

Ethical Approval and Study Registration

Patients with type 2 diabetes were recruited from Eye Center, Shandong Eye Hospital in China, from November 2019 to November 2020. In total, 82 eyes of 43 patients were diagnosed as DME by FFA and optical coherence tomography (OCT). Study approval was obtained from by the Institutional Ethics Committee of Shandong eye hospital (approval No. 2019S001) and the study followed the Declaration of Helsinki. According to whether the central fovea involved patients were divided into two groups: center-involving DME (CI-DME) with PDR patients and non-center involving DME (NCI-DME) with PDR patients. All of them are naive patients who have never been diagnosed and treated. Informed consent was obtained from all patients who received intravitreal conbercept injection (5–7, 25, 26).

Inclusion and Exclusion Criteria

The patients recruitment criteria were as follows: (1) BCVA needed to have a measure of 20/400 or better, and pre-treatment and post-treatment OCTA images needed to be of good quality ($\geq$6/10 quality score). (2) Patients with type 2 diabetes aged $\geq$ 18 years. (3) Patients with PDR, retina neovascularization by FFA. Patients with DME, retinal thickening within two disc diameters of the central fovea and can be either focal or diffuse. Patients with CI-DME, retinal thickening in the macula that involves a central subfield zone is 1 mm in diameter (11, 22, 23). Patients with NCI-DME, retinal thickening in the macula that does not involve a central subfield zone is 1 mm in diameter (5–7). (4) The patients who met the criteria of anti-VEGF treatment guidelines would receive at least 3 months consecutive intravitreal conbercept. (5) No history of ocular trauma and surgery and no history of fundus related diseases or treatment.

Exclusion criteria were as follows: (1) patients who could not tolerate surgery due to poor general condition. (2) Patients with refractive turbid media and poor fixation. (3) Patients who received intrabulbar injection or other ophthalmic surgery. (4) Patients with other diseases causing macular edema. (5) Eyes with low quality OCTA images (image quality index <60) or media opacities, such as vitreous hemorrhage.

Fundus Microvasculature Imaging by OCTA

The AngioVue system (Optovue RTVue XR100 Avanti; Optovue, Inc, Fremont, CA, USA) software (V.2017.1.0.155, Optovue, Fremont, CA, USA) was used for analyzing the OCTA images which were obtained before and after anti-VEGF treatment. The OCTA images were obtained at 7–11 am in the morning. The central fovea can be observed in each 6 × 6 mm image. In addition to the retina and choroid, the device software automatically depicts the structures of the SCP from DCP. The AngioVue software detects the SCP, consisting of a layer extending from 6 mm below the internal limiting membrane (ILM) to 15 μm below the inner plexiform layer (IPL), while the DCP extends from 15 to 70 μm below the IPL. Then, based on the collected images, VD in the SCP and DCP were automatically calculated as the percentage area occupied by blood vessels within 6 × 6 mm area, and the FAZ in the SCP and DCP were automatically calculated using the non-flow function in the software. If the segmentation lines were not correctly aligned according to the parameters defined above, we corrected them by using the manually correction of segmentation error. One expert grader evaluated the segmentation lines of the SCP and DCP (ILM, IPL, outer plexiform layer (OPL), and retinal pigment epithelium) in the registered horizontal OCT B-scan (18, 19). The "Edit Bnd/Propagation" option of the Optovue RTVue XR100 Avanti software (V.2017.1.0.155) was used for manually correction on the segmentation to the registered OCT B-scan and propagates the correction to the adjacent B-scans (18, 19). The segmentation correction was started from inner layers (ILM to OPL) on a single B-scan in the central fovea, and propagation function was automatically applied to correct the entire image for other B-scans. In addition, the measuring and comparing of the FAZ of each patient before and after IVC by automatic after manual correction measurement of OCTA (18, 19).

Conbercept Treatment

Intravitreal injection of conbercept: levofloxacin eye drops were applied to prevent infection. Moreover, we recommend that patients use it 1 day before operation and 1 week after injection, and used it 4 times a day. After the conjunctival sac was flushed under surface anesthesia, a 30 GA syringe was used to inject 0.05 ml (0.5 mg) of conbercept into the vitreous. All patients were examined in the Shandong Eye hospital and received the treatment regime of intravitreal injection of conbercept. Patients initially received intravitreal conbercept injection for 3 months and 3 times a month and followed pro-re nata (PRN) injections treatment. If the patient showed a recurrence of macular edema and the central retinal thickness (CRT) exceeds 300 μm, the patient should be re-treated with conbercept in the 4th, 5th, and 6th month.

Statistical Analyses

Our study was a randomized, single-masked analyze. The patient data included complete medical history and ophthalmic history: CRT, and retinal microvessels (mainly including VD and FAZ) were evaluated by OCTA before conbercept treatment and 1, 3, and 6 months after the conbercept treatment (one treatment per month, three consecutive times). The BCVA were evaluated before conbercept treatment and after the conbercept treatment for 6 months.

The SPSS (version 11.0) was used to calculate the mean and SD (mean ± SD) and p for all statistical data ($^*p < 0.05$ and $^{**}p < 0.01$). The gender differences of all subjects were analyzed by x^2 test. In addition, the age changes of all subjects were analyzed by t-test. When standard normal distribution was satisfied, the paired t-test was used to compare the pre-treatment and post-treatment after the conbercept treatment for 1, 3 months, or 6 months. But when the standard normal distribution was not satisfied, the Wilcoxon signed rank test was used. For analyzing the differences between groups (before 1st, 3rd, and 6th month), if normally distributed, we used ANOVA by ranks test. If it does not fit the normal distribution, we used Friedman's test.

TABLE 1 | Baseline characteristics of participants.

Variables	NCI-DME	CI-DME	*p* value
Number of patients	14 (26 eyes)	30 (56 eyes)	–
Male	8 (16 eyes)	19 (37 eyes)	–
Female	6 (10 eyes)	10 (19 eyes)	–
Age (mean ± SD), years	58.2 ± 5.5 (50–65)	57.8 ± 3 (52–63)	0.239
BCVA (mean ± SD)	0.38 ± 0.07	0.28 ± 0.08	<0.05
CRT (mean ± SD), μm	334.62 ± 12.23	426.46 ± 82.92	<0.05
FAZ (mean ± SD), mm^2	0.40 ± 0.32	0.31 ± 0.06	<0.05

BCVA, best corrected visual acuity; CRT, central retinal thickness; FAZ, foveolar avascular zone. p <0.05, there is statistical difference.

RESULTS

In this prospective study, the information of 30 CI-DME with PDR patients and 30 NCI-DME with PDR patients were collected. However, a total of 17 patients were excluded, including 1 DME patient and 16 other patients with vitreous hemorrhage, macular fibrovascular hyperplasia, or media turbidity that may affect the image quality. Finally, 43 patients (27 men and 16 women) were included in this study. There were 29 cases (56 eyes) in CI-DME with PDR, including 37 eyes in 19 men and 19 eyes in 10 women, aged from 52 to 63 years (mean ± SD: 57.8 ± 3). There were 14 cases (26 eyes) in the NCI-DME with PDR, such as 16 eyes in 8 men and 10 eyes in 6 women, aged from 50 to 65 years (mean ± SD: 58.2 ± 5.5). The age and gender

TABLE 2 | The change vessel density of superficial retinal capillary plexus and deep retinal capillary plexus_after conbercept treated CI-DME for 1, 3, and 6 months, compared to pre-treatment.

CI-DME		Pre-treatment (*n* = 56)	Post-treatment (1) (*n* = 56)	Post-treatment (3) (*n* = 56)	Post-treatment (6) (*n* = 56)	Pre vs. Post -1 *p* value	Pre vs. Post -3 *p* value	Pre vs. Post -6 *p* value	Rank test[#]
SCP	-S	41.23 ± 6.79	43.64 ± 15.00	41.64 ± 5.21	42.27 ± 9.68	0.243	0.680	0.499	0.002**
	-I	41.90 ± 6.70	43.71 ± 15.12	41.06 ± 5.69	47.27 ± 4.89	0.092	0.393	0.002**	0.000***
	-N	42.41 ± 6.18	42.78 ± 16.23	41.67 ± 6.30	44.34 ± 5.08	0.863	0.476	0.179	0.023*
	-T	40.71 ± 6.31	42.87 ± 13.99	41.74 ± 5.33	41.24 ± 6.14	0.271	0.296	0.594	0.060
	-F	21.43 ± 6.83	18.55 ± 7.89	21.48 ± 4.13	21.82 ± 3.78	0.033*	0.624	0.790	0.003**
DCP	-S	42.16 ± 4.94	42.51 ± 4.47	46.13 ± 42.02	42.94 ± 5.08	0.564	0.481	0.374	0.474
	-I	42.03 ± 5.26	42.37 ± 4.63	48.81 ± 38.88	43.21 ± 6.08	0.601	0.196	0.251	0.000***
	-N	42.26 ± 4.87	42.54 ± 4.65	48.70 ± 41.09	43.21 ± 3.61	0.647	0.258	0.256	0.578
	-T	41.60 ± 5.32	41.31 ± 4.86	49.22 ± 37.94	44.36 ± 37.97	0.714	0.153	0.601	0.000***
	-F	28.99 ± 6.97	19.58 ± 9.11	22.96 ± 3.77	23.00 ± 3.64	0.000***	0.000***	0.000***	0.000***
CRT	-F	426.46 ± 82.92	393.39 ± 68.13	392.58 ± 62.94	334.39 ± 96.55	0.000***	0.000***	0.000***	0.000***

*We used the paired t-test and Wilcoxon signed rank test test to analyze the effect of Conbercept intravitreal injection acted on CI-DME before treatment and 1, 3 and 6 months after treatment. And rank test was used to analyze the differences between groups (#, Friedman test). These were tested in SCP, superficial retinal capillary plexus; DCP, deep retinal capillary plexus; CRT, central retinal thickness; S, segmented from superior; I, inferior; N, nasal; T, tempo; F, fovea. Pre-treatment/Pre, before tretment; Post-treatment (1)/Post (1), one month after treatment; Post-treatment (3)/Post (3), three month after treatment; Post-treatment (6)/Post (6), six month after treatment. *p < 0.05, **p < 0.01, ***p < 0.001.*

were not different between the patients with CI-DME and NCI-DME (**Table 1**). The patients with CI-DME had worse vision than NCI-DME (BCVA: 0.28 ± 0.08 vs. 0.38 ± 0.07, $p < 0.05$). The CRT in CI-DME group was thicker (426.46 ± 82.92 vs. 334.62 ± 12.23 μm, $p < 0.05$). The FAZ of NCI-DME was larger (0.31 ± 0.06 vs. 0.40 ± 0.32 mm^2, $p < 0.05$).

Conbercept was applied for intravitreal injection. The average injection times of patients with CI-DME and NCI-DME are 4.23 and 3.3, respectively (the injection times of all patients are between 3 and 5, $p < 0.001$). At the same time, we did not observe any serious complications during or after intravitreal therapy. Moreover, 6 months after intravitreal injections of conbercept, BCVA was increased in CI-DME group (0.28 ± 0.08 vs. 0.45 ± 0.12, $p < 0.001$), indicating that vision improved with conbercept treatment in the CI-DME group. However, conbercept treatment did not improve the vision in NCI-DME group (0.38 ± 0.07 vs.

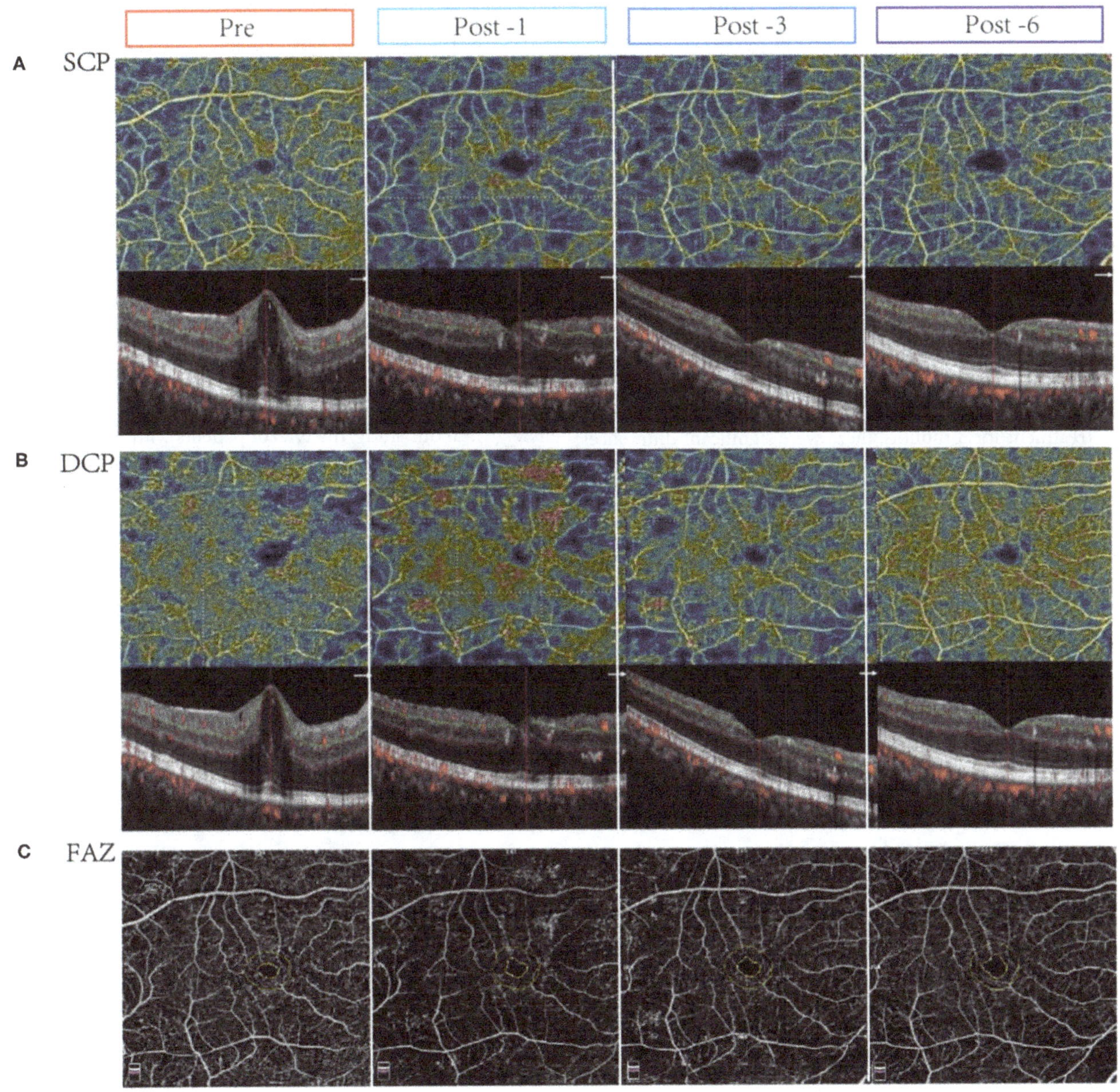

FIGURE 1 | Changes in vessel density and flow area in eyes with center-involved diabetic macular edema (CI-DME) before and after intravitreal conbercept injection. Pre: before treatment; Post -1: 1 month after treatment; Post -3: 3 months after treatment; Post -6: 6 months after treatment. **(A)** The vessel density in the superficial capillary plexus (SCP) in patients with CI-DME before and after treatment for 1, 3, and 6 months: after treatment, the microvascular density in the inferior area of SCP improved. **(B)** The vessel density in the deep capillary plexus (DCP) in patients with CI-DME before and after treatment for 1, 3, and 6 months: there were no significant changes in different areas of DCP before and after treatment. **(C)** The foveolar avascular zone (FAZ) in patients with CI-DME before and after conbercept intravitreal injection: there was no significant difference before and after treatment.

0.42 ± 0.12, $p = 0.058$). After intravitreal injection of conbercept for 6 months, the CRT in the CI-DME and NCI-DME group were significantly lower compared with that in patients before the treatment (CI-DME: 426.46 ± 82.92 vs. 334.39 ± 96.55, $p < 0.001$; NCI-DME: 334.62 ± 12.23 vs. 295.58 ± 19.30, $p < 0.001$). After intravitreal injection of conbercept, there were no statistical differences in the FAZ. However, the reduction of FAZ in CI-DME was higher than that in patients with NCI-DME (0.12 vs. 0.07). Our results showed that the conbercept treatment improved the vision of CI-DME, and decreased the CRT in CI-DME. Therefore, conbercept is effective in the patients with PDR.

Moreover, retinal microvascular changes after conbercept treatment were evaluated by OCTA. In CI-DME group, after treatment for 1 month, the VD of central fovea area in SCP had a slight reduction ($p = 0.033$). After 6 months of treatment, the VD in the inferior area of SCP was significantly increased ($p = 0.002$). There were significant differences in the VD of central fovea area in DCP between pre- and post-treatment ($p < 0.001$). However, there was no significant difference for VD in superior, inferior, nasal, tempo areas of DCP before and after treatment, even when the treatment was continued for 6 months (**Table 2**). **Figures 1A–C** shows the representative OCTA images of retinal VD and FAZ with CI-DME (pre-treatment vs. post-treatment).

However, in NCI-DME group, the VD in inferior area of SCP was increased 6 months after conbercept treatment (**Table 3**). After treatment for 3 months, there were significant differences in the nasal, tempo, and central fovea areas of DCP. All parameters of the VD in the whole images and regions of DCP in NCI-DME group were significantly changes after 6 months conbercept treatment (**Table 3**). Representative OCTA images demonstrating the changes in VD and FAZ with NCI-DME group (pre-treatment vs. post-treatment) are shown in **Figures 2A–C**. Above all, the conbercept treatment affects the DCP of NCI-DME group.

DISCUSSION

Our results suggested that vision has significantly improved before and after intravitreal injection of conbercept in the CI-DME group. Some clinical trials have demonstrated that anti-VEGF therapy has been adopted as the first-line therapy in CI-DME (5–7, 27) and it is more effective in improving the vision and visual acuity in CI-DME compared with focal laser treatment. Anti-VEGF treatment blocked the formation of neovascularization and reduced retinal thickening (5, 26, 27). In addition, multiple intravitreal conbercept in patients with DME may improve macular VD. Our study further showed the effect of conbercept on the SCP and DCP of CI-DME and NCI-DME. Regardless of the central fovea involvement, the conbercept improved microvascular density in DME, which affected VD in retinal capillary plexus which may be the mechanism of the drug. The conbercept treatment improved the microvascular density in multiple regions of NCI-DME, which are more than that of CI-DME. Thus, our results showed that the intravitreal conbercept was effective on PDR and DME. Furthermore, the conbercept treatment can decrease the retinal thickness and reduce the area of macular edema.

As a new non-invasive and high-resolution fundus angiography technology, OCTA is extremely useful in the quantitative analysis of macular VD and segment detection of FAZ (2). In our study, the FAZ of patients with PDR (before and after intravitreal injection of conbercept treatment) was observed by OCTA. This technique is very effective in revealing vascular abnormalities, such as neovascularization on the surface of the retina and optic nerves, and OCTA has also been applied to the diagnosis, treatment, and follow-up of various fundus vascular diseases (22–24). However, it is not capable of visualizing leakage and completely avoiding stepwise segmentation error, which could be construed as limitations (18–21, 28).

TABLE 3 | The change vessel density of superficial retinal capillary plexus and deep retinal capillary plexus after conbercept treated NCI-DME for 1, 3, and 6 months, compared to pre-treatment.

NCI-DME		Pre-treatment ($n = 26$)	Post-treatment (1) ($n = 26$)	Post-treatment (3) ($n = 26$)	Post-treatment (6) ($n = 26$)	Pre vs. Post -1 p value	Pre vs. Post -3 p value	Pre vs. Post -6 p value	Rank test#
SCP	-S	43.69 ± 5.59	47.43 ± 18.64	43.43 ± 7.16	44.76 ± 5.42	0.567	0.852	0.128	0.089
	-I	42.23 ± 4.86	48.19 ± 17.17	44.53 ± 4.75	47.23 ± 4.89	0.014*	0.021*	0.005**	0.000***
	-N	43.76 ± 4.26	47.23 ± 15.87	42.94 ± 6.21	45.33 ± 4.95	0.422	0.970	0.193	0.403
	-T	42.69 ± 5.11	45.69 ± 15.62	43.91 ± 9.50	44.52 ± 4.47	0.193	0.429	0.435	0.009**
	-F	19.53 ± 6.49	19.35 ± 10.14	20.92 ± 5.24	21.23 ± 5.45	0.374	0.394	0.150	0.000***
DCP	-S	42.99 ± 2.94	43.30 ± 3.72	44.16 ± 5.62	40.25 ± 3.68	0.711	0.216	0.000***	0.000***
	-I	43.08 ± 3.46	43.15 ± 4.09	44.46 ± 3.86	40.23 ± 3.21	0.576	0.137	0.000***	0.000***
	-N	42.85 ± 2.57	43.41 ± 3.63	44.31 ± 4.28	40.15 ± 3.28	0.474	0.029*	0.000***	0.000***
	-T	43.09 ± 4.33	43.99 ± 5.56	44.61 ± 3.91	39.81 ± 3.74	0.162	0.013*	0.011*	0.000***
	-F	16.58 ± 7.61	15.91 ± 7.13	22.12 ± 3.75	21.88 ± 3.39	0.567	0.002**	0.000***	0.005**
CRT	-F	334.62 ± 12.23	329.15 ± 19.84	331.34 ± 20.16	295.58 ± 19.30	0.135	0.437	0.000***	0.000***

*We used the paired t-test and Wilcoxon signed rank test test to analyze the effect of Conbercept intravitreal injection acted on NCI-DME before treatment and 1, 3 and 6 months after treatment. And rank test was used to analyze the differences between groups (#, Friedman test). These were tested in SCP, superficial retinal capillary plexus; DCP, deep retinal capillary plexus; CRT, central retinal thickness; S, segmented from superior; I, inferior; N, nasal; T, tempo; F, fovea. Pre-treatment/Pre, before tretment; Post-treatment (1)/Post -1, one month after treatment; Post-treatment (3)/Post -3, three month after treatment; Post-treatment (6)/Post -6, six month after treatment. * $p < 0.05$, ** $p < 0.01$, *** $p < 0.001$.*

In addition, in previous research, anti-VEGF drugs, such as bevacizumab, ranibizumab, aflibercept, and conbercept were effective for DME (14, 29). However, there has been controversy about whether the macular perfusion will get better or worse after anti-VEGF treatment (15, 22–24, 30). Zhao et al. considered that there were no significant changes of macular and papillary VD after either the panretinal photocoagulation or intravitreal conbercept treatment (23). However, with the progress of DR and the decrease of VD, both treatments may prevent the loss of macular and papillary VD in PDR. Although there are normal diurnal variations of macular thickness/perfusion (31, 32), some studies considered that anti-VEGF treatment may have a positive effect on macular perfusion status, such as the improvement of BCVA and the reduction of neovascularization (2, 22, 24). Conbercept treatment was proved to affect the superficial macular VD (15, 23). Our study proved that intravitreal

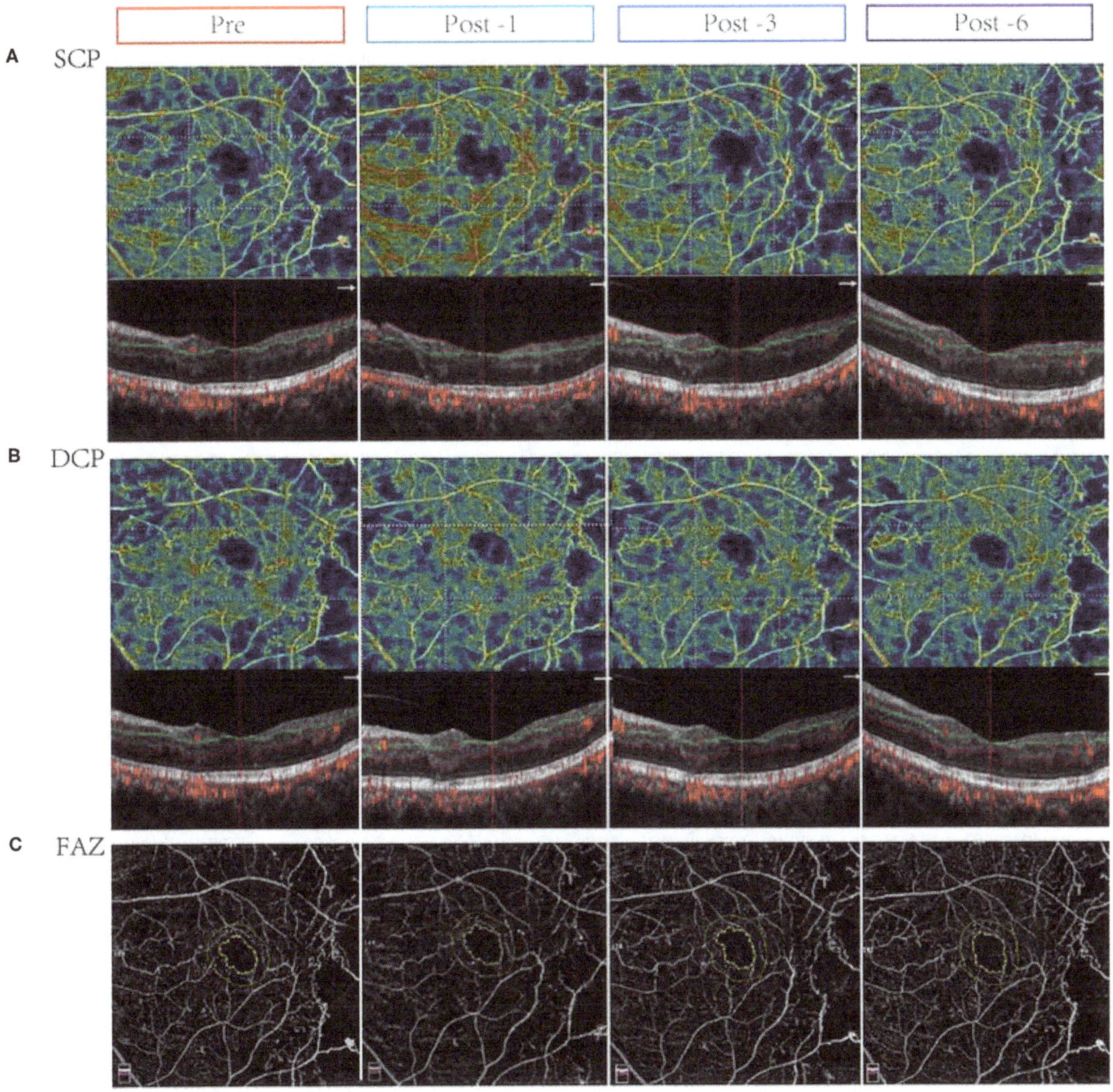

FIGURE 2 | Changes in vessel density (VD) and flow area in eyes with non-center involved DME (NCI-DME) before and after intravitreal conbercept injection. Pre: before treatment; Post -1, 1 month after treatment; Post -3, 3 months after treatment; Post -6, 6 months after treatment. **(A)** The vessel density in the superficial capillary plexus (SCP) before and after treatment for 1, 3, and 6 months with NCI-DME patients: after treatment, the microvascular density in the inferior area of SCP improved. **(B)** The vessel density in the deep capillary plexus (DCP) in patients with NCI-DME before and after treatment for 1, 3, and 6 months: after treatment, the microvascular density in the central fovea area of DCP improved. **(C)** The FAZ in patients with NCI-DME before and after conbercept intravitreal injection: there was no significant difference before and after treatment.

conbercept treatment improved the vision and VD in patients with DME.

However, there are some limitations to our study which are as follows: (1) there were biases in the selection of patients. OCTA was used to observe the fundus, so the patients with poor vision and poor fixation were excluded. (2) Lacking the data on deep FAZ and ignoring diurnal variations in choroidal sublayer perfusion. (3) The number of cases was limited and the follow-up time was short. Therefore, in future studies, we need to increase the sample size, the number, and the follow-up time and prolong the treatment time to support our research.

In conclusion, OCTA is a non-invasive and promising emerging technique, which can be used to obtain quantitative data and more detailed information of the SCP or DCP vascular network in the eyes of patients with CI-DME and NCI-DME. We found that conbercept effectively relieved macular edema and improved vision.

ETHICS STATEMENT

This Human Research was approved by the Institutional Ethics Committee of Shandong Eye Hospital (Approval No. 2019S001) on November 16, 2019. The patients/participants provided their written informed consent to participate in this study. Written informed consent was obtained from the individual(s) for the publication of any potentially identifiable images or data included in this article.

AUTHOR CONTRIBUTIONS

TiL and WLin designed and conducted clinical examinations. TiL, WLin, and MF wrote and revised the manuscript. QW and ZM collated the clinical data. WW, XX, and WLi analyzed and interpreted the data. XX, WW, JG, and ToL collated and drew the figures and tables. QZ gave guidance and put forward suggestions for revision. All authors contributed to the revision steps and approved the final version of the manuscript for submission.

REFERENCES

1. Ding J, Wong TY. Current epidemiology of diabetic retinopathy and diabetic macular edema. *Curr Diab Rep.* (2012) 12:346–54. doi: 10.1007/s11892-012-0283-6
2. Yau JW, Rogers SL, Kawasaki R, Lamoureux EL, Kowalski JW, Bek T et al. Global prevalence and major risk factors of diabetic retinopathy. *Diabetes Care.* (2012) 35:556–64. doi: 10.2337/dc11-1909
3. Debata PP, Mohapatra P. Diagnosis of diabetes in pregnant woman using a Chaotic-Jaya hybridized extreme learning machine model. *J Integr Bioinform.* (2020) 18:81–99. doi: 10.1515/jib-2019-0097
4. Scanlon PH, Aldington SJ, Stratton IM. Epidemiological issues in diabetic retinopathy. *Middle East Afr J Ophthalmol.* (2013) 20:293–300. doi: 10.4103/0974-9233.120007
5. Baker CW, Glassman AR, Beaulieu WT, Antoszyk AN, Browning DJ, Chalam KV, et al. Effect of initial management with aflibercept vs. laser photocoagulation vs. observation on vision loss among patients with diabetic macular edema involving the center of the macula and good visual acuity: a randomized clinical trial. *JAMA.* (2019) 321; 19:1880–94. doi: 10.1001/jama.2019.5790
6. Wong TY, Sun J, Kawasaki R, Ruamviboonsuk P, Gupta N, Lansingh VC, et al. Guidelines on diabetic eye care: the international council of ophthalmology recommendations for screening, follow-up, referral, and treatment based on resource settings. *Ophthalmology.* (2018) 10:1608–22. doi: 10.1016/j.ophtha.2018.04.007
7. Figueira J, Henriques J, Carneiro Â, Marques-Neves C, Flores R, Castro-Sousa JP, et al. Guidelines for the management of center-involving diabetic macular edema: treatment options and patient monitorization. *Clin Ophthalmol.* (2021) 15:3221–30. doi: 10.2147/OPTH.S318026
8. Chatziralli I, Loewenstein A. Intravitreal anti-vascular endothelial growth factor agents for the treatment of diabetic retinopathy: a review of the literature. *PHARMACEUTICS.* (2021) 8:1137. doi: 10.3390/pharmaceutics13081137
9. Boyer DS, Hopkins JJ, Sorof J, Ehrlich JS. Anti-vascular endothelial growth factor therapy for diabetic macular edema. *Ther Adv Endocrinol Metab.* (2013) 4:151–69. doi: 10.1177/2042018813512360
10. Elnahry AG, Abdel-Kader AA, Raafat KA, Elrakhawy K. Evaluation of changes in macular perfusion detected by optical coherence tomography angiography following 3 intravitreal monthly bevacizumab injections for diabetic macular edema in the IMPACT study. *J Ophthalmol.* (2020) 2020:5814165. doi: 10.1155/2020/5814165
11. Alagorie AR, Nittala MG, Velaga S, Zhou B, Rusakevich AM, Wykoff CC, et al. Association of intravitreal aflibercept with optical coherence tomography angiography vessel density in patients with proliferative diabetic retinopathy: a secondary analysis of a randomized clinical trial. *JAMA Ophthalmol.* (2020) 8:851–857. doi: 10.1001/jamaophthalmol.2020.2130
12. Mansour SE, Browning DJ, Wong K, Flynn HJ, Bhavsar AR. The evolving treatment of diabetic retinopathy. *Clin Ophthalmol.* (2020) 14:653–678, doi: 10.2147/OPTH.S236637
13. Li X, Xu G, Wang Y, Xu X, Liu X, Tang S et al. Safety and efficacy of conbercept in neovascular age-related macular degeneration: results from a 12-month randomized phase 2 study: AURORA study. *Ophthalmology.* (2014) 121:1740–7. doi: 10.1016/j.ophtha.2014.03.026
14. Lu X, Sun X. Profile of conbercept in the treatment of neovascular age-related macular degeneration. *Drug Des Devel Ther.* (2015) 9:2311–20. doi: 10.2147/DDDT.S67536
15. Elnahry AG, Elnahry GA. Optical coherence tomography angiography of macular perfusion changes after Anti-VEGF Therapy for diabetic macular edema: a systematic review. *J Diabetes Res.* (2021) 2021:6634637. doi: 10.1155/2021/6634637
16. Sorour OA, Elsheikh M, Chen S, et al. Mean macular intercapillary area in eyes with diabetic macular oedema after anti-vascular endothelial growth factor

therapy and its association with treatment response. *Clin Exp Ophthalmol.* (2021) 49; 7:714–23. doi: 10.1111/ceo.13966

17. Akil H, Karst S, Heisler M, Etminan M, Navajas E, Maberley D. Application of optical coherence tomography angiography in diabetic retinopathy: a comprehensive review. *CAN J OPHTHALMOL.* (2019) 54:519–28. doi: 10.1016/j.jcjo.2019.02.010
18. Ghasemi Falavarjani K, Habibi A, Anvari P, Ghasemizadeh S, Ashraf Khorasani M, Shenazandi H, et al. Effect of segmentation error correction on optical coherence tomography angiography measurements in healthy subjects and diabetic macular oedema. *Br J Ophthalmol.* (2020) 2:162–6. doi: 10.1136/bjophthalmol-2019-314018
19. Ghasemi Falavarjani K, Mirshahi R, Ghasemizadeh S, Sardarinia M. Stepwise segmentation error correction in optical coherence tomography angiography images of patients with diabetic macular edema. *Ther Adv Ophthalmol.* (2020) 12:2515841420947931. doi: 10.1177/2515841420947931
20. Lauermann JL, Woetzel AK, Treder M, Alnawaiseh M, Clemens CR, Eter N, et al. Prevalences of segmentation errors and motion artifacts in OCT-angiography differ among retinal diseases. *Graefes Arch Clin Exp Ophthalmol.* (2018) 10:1807–16. doi: 10.1007/s00417-018-4053-2
21. Bontzos G, Kabanarou SA, Garnavou-Xirou C, Gkizis I, Kontou E, Triantafyllou D, et al. Segmentation errors and motion artifacts in OCT-A associated with epiretinal membranes. *Can J Ophthalmol.* (2020) 4:293–300. doi: 10.1016/j.jcjo.2019.12.007
22. He F, Yang J, Zhang X, Yu W. Efficacy of conbercept combined with panretinal photocoagulation in the treatment of proliferative diabetic retinopathy. *Sci Rep.* (2020) 1:8778. doi: 10.1038/s41598-020-65833-0
23. Zhao H, Yu M, Zhou L, Li C, Lu L, Jin C. Comparison of the effect of pan-retinal photocoagulation and intravitreal conbercept treatment on the change of retinal vessel density monitored by optical coherence tomography angiography in patients with proliferative diabetic retinopathy. *J Clin Med.* (2021) 19:4484. doi: 10.3390/jcm10194484
24. Zhu Z, Liang Y, Yan B, Meng Z, Long K, Zhang Y, et al. Clinical effect of conbercept on improving diabetic macular ischemia by OCT angiography. *BMC Ophthalmol.* (2020) 1:382. doi: 10.1186/s12886-020-01648-x
25. Vaz-Pereira S, Morais-Sarmento T, Esteves MR. Optical coherence tomography features of neovascularization in proliferative diabetic retinopathy: a systematic review. *Int J Retina Vitreous.* (2020) 6:26. doi: 10.1186/s40942-020-00230-3
26. Lee J, Moon BG, Cho AR, Yoon YH. Optical coherence tomography angiography of dme and its association with anti-vegf treatment response. *Ophthalmology.* (2016) 123:2368–2375. doi: 10.1016/j.ophtha.2016.07.010
27. Hodzic-Hadzibegovic D, Sander BA, Lund-Andersen H. Diabetic macular oedema quantified with spectral-domain optical coherence tomography–evaluation of boundary line artefacts and the effect on retinal thickness. *Acta Ophthalmol.* (2015) 93:74–82. doi: 10.1111/aos.12494
28. Podkowinski D, Beka S, Mursch-Edlmayr AS, Strauss RW, Fischer L, Bolz M. A Swept source optical coherence tomography angiography study: imaging artifacts and comparison of non-perfusion areas with fluorescein angiography in diabetic macular edema. *PLoS One.* (2021) 4:e0249918. doi: 10.1371/journal.pone.0249918
29. Cui J, Sun D, Lu H, Dai R, Xing L, Dong H et al. Comparison of effectiveness and safety between conbercept and ranibizumab for treatment of neovascular age-related macular degeneration. a retrospective case-controlled non-inferiority multiple center study. *Eye. (Lond).* (2018) 32:391–9. doi: 10.1038/eye.2017.187
30. Elnahry AG, Abdel-Kader AA, Habib AE, Elnahry GA, Raafat KA, Elrakhawy K. Review on recent trials evaluating the effect of intravitreal injections of anti-vegf agents on the macular perfusion of diabetic patients with diabetic macular edema. *Rev Recent Clin Trials.* (2020) 15:188–98. doi: 10.2174/1574887115666200519073704
31. Diabetic Retinopathy Clinical Research Network, Danis RP, Glassman AR, Aiello LP, Antoszyk AN, Beck RW, et al. Diurnal variation in retinal thickening measurement by optical coherence tomography in center-involved diabetic macular edema. *Arch Ophthalmol.* (2006) 124:1701–7. doi: 10.1001/archopht.124.12.1701
32. Rommel F, Siegfried F, Sochurek JAM, Rothe M, Brinkmann MP, Kurz M, et al. Mapping diurnal variations in choroidal sublayer perfusion in patients with idiopathic epiretinal membrane: an optical coherence tomography angiography study. *Int J Retina Vitreous.* (2019) 5:12. doi: 10.1186/s40942-019-0162-2

11

Observation of Peripapillary Choroidal Vascularity in Natural Disease Course and After Gene Therapy for Leber's Hereditary Optic Neuropathy

Jingwen Jiang [1†], Gongpeng Sun [1†], Qingmei Miao [1], Bin Li [2,3], Dan Wang [2], Jiajia Yuan [1] and Changzheng Chen [1*]*

[1] Eye Center, Renmin Hospital of Wuhan University, Wuhan, China, [2] Department of Ophthalmology, Tongji Hospital, Tongji Medical College, Huazhong University of Science and Technology, Wuhan, China, [3] Neurophth Biotechnology Co., Ltd. Wuhan, China

***Correspondence:**
Jiajia Yuan
yuanjj911@163.com
Changzheng Chen
whuchenchzh@163.com

† These authors have contributed equally to this work and share first authorship*

Purpose: To compare peripapillary choroidal vascularity among Leber's Hereditary Optic Neuropathy (LHON) patients at different stages of natural course and healthy controls using optical coherence tomography (OCT), and to evaluate peripapillary choroidal vascularity changes in LHON patients before and after gene therapy.

Methods: 57 LHON patients and 15 healthy controls were enrolled in this prospective clinical study. LHON patients were divided into three duration groups based on stage of disease progression. Both patients and healthy controls underwent OCT scans focused on the optic disc at baseline with Heidelberg Spectralis, and patients underwent OCT at 1, 3, and 6 months after gene therapy. OCT images were converted and binarized using ImageJ software. Choroidal thickness (CT), total choroidal area (TCA), and choroidal vascularity index (CVI) in each quadrant of OCT images were measured to evaluate peripapillary choroidal vascularity.

Results: At baseline, the average CT was not significantly different between LHON patients at different stages and between healthy controls ($P = 0.468$). Although average TCA and average CVI were slightly higher in LHON patients at different stages than in healthy controls, the difference was not statistically significant ($P = 0.282$ and 0.812, respectively). After gene therapy, The average TCA at 1 month after gene therapy was significantly higher than that before gene therapy ($P = 0.003$), while no significant differences were found in the average CT or average CVI in LHON patients before and 1,3 and 6 months after gene therapy using pairwise comparisons (all $P > 0.05$).

Conclusions: No significant difference was found in choroidal vascularity of LHON patients at different stages and healthy controls. Choroidal vascularity seems to stay stable after gene therapy.

Keywords: Leber's hereditary optic neuropathy, choroidal thickness, choroidal vascularity, blood flow, gene therapy

INTRODUCTION

Leber's hereditary optic neuropathy (LHON) is a maternally-inherited mitochondrial disease that leads to acute bilateral loss of visual acuity (VA) and visual field in young adulthood (1). LHON patients with the most common mutation site 11778G >A show the worst VA prognosis, and, nowadays, gene therapy targeting this mutation has proven to be the most promising treatment in our previous studies (2, 3).

Along with mutations in mitochondrial DNA (mtDNA), the dysfunction of the mitochondrial respiratory chain complex 1 leads to impairment of ATP production and increased production of reactive oxygen species (ROS), resulting in loss of retinal ganglion cells (RGC) and, eventually, optic nerve atrophy (4). The advent of optical coherence tomography (OCT) has enabled the visualization of structural features in the eyes of LHON patients, such as the progression of retinal nerve fiber layer (RNFL) and ganglion cell complex (GCC) pathology at different stages of the disease (5–8). Furthermore, retinal and peripapillary retinal capillaries were found to be abnormal in LHON patients using OCT angiography (OCTA) (9, 10).

There have been few investigations focused on choroidal vascularity in LHON even though studies have confirmed that choroidal vessels play an important role in the pathogenesis of other optic nerve diseases such as anterior ischemic optic neuropathy (AION) and glaucoma (11–14). Recent research has shed some light on changes in choroidal thickness (CT) in the eyes of LHON patients (15, 16). Nevertheless, as reported previously, the reproducibility of CT is not ideal due to its significant variation with gender, age, and refractive error. Choroidal vascularity index (CVI) is a novel and stable parameter in evaluating the choroidal vascular system and is defined as the ratio of the luminal area (LA) of the choroid to the total choroidal area (TCA) in binarized OCT images (17). In previous studies, CVI has been applied in normal subjects and patients with various ocular pathologies including AION and glaucoma (11–14). So far, CVI has not been studied in LHON patients along the natural disease course or before and after gene therapy.

The aim of the present study was to determine peripapillary CVI in the eyes of LHON patients at different stages of the disease and to explore the possible changes of CVI before and after gene therapy. Our findings help to improve our understanding of whether the choroidal vasculature is involved in the mechanisms underlying LHON pathology or gene therapy.

METHODS

Study Subjects

This prospective multicenter clinical study (NCT03153293) was approved by the ethics committees at Tongji Hospital of Wuhan (TJ-IRB20180316), Taihe Hospital of Shiyan (2017-01), and Ezhou Central Hospital (2017-K-05) in strict accordance with the regulations of the Declaration of Helsinki. Each subject provided written informed consent prior to the examination. Participants received unilateral intravitreal injection of 0.05 mL rAAV2-ND4 ($1.0 \times 1{,}010$ vg/μL) and were followed up for 6 months with complete ophthalmic and general system evaluation.

LHON patients between ages of 6 and 65 years old with confirmed genetic diagnosis of mtDNA 11,778 (G > A) mutation and binocular best-corrected VA (BCVA) worse than 0.3 logMAR were recruited at Tongji Hospital (Tongji Medical College of Huazhong University of Science and Technology). Exclusion criteria: Systemic and other ocular diseases that may affect the patient's cisual function, use of any drug or therapy that may interfere the gene therapy within 6 months (such as idebenone), heavy smokers or drinkers and pregnant women. For each subject, the eye with poorer BCVA was selected for intravitreal rAAV2-ND4 injection, while the right eye was selected if the BCVA was the same bilaterally. The BCVA improvement ≥ 0.3 logMAR was considered clinically significant.

Patients with LHON were divided into three groups based on the international consensus statement (18) and clinical practice: group 1 (active stage), disease duration ≤ 12 months; group 2 (early chronic stage), disease duration 12–24 months; group 3 (late chronic stage), disease duration ≥ 24 months. Fifteen age-matched and sex-matched healthy individuals were also recruited as healthy controls and underwent OCT examination at baseline.

Ophthalmologic Examinations

LHON patients underwent full ophthalmologic examinations including intraocular pressure (IOP), BCVA testing, visual field, visual evoked potentials (VEP), electroretinography (ERG), and OCT examination before treatment and 1, 3, and 6 months after intravitreal injection.

OCT Analysis

All subjects were imaged using a 3.4-mm-diameter 360-degree-circle scan centered on the optic nerve head on OCT equipment (Spectralis, Heidelberg Engineering GmbH, Heidelberg, Germany) by experienced operators. CT in each quadrant was manually determined by measuring the vertical distance between the Bruch membrane interface and the choroid-sclera interface using the built-in software.

To measure the CVI, the OCT images were binarized and segmented using ImageJ (version 1.53c, http://fiji.sc/) as described previously (19). First, the image was opened in ImageJ and converted to an 8-bit image. Then, Niblack's auto local threshold adjustment was applied to binarize the image and the LA was determined using the threshold tool, with light pixels representing stromal area and dark pixels representing LA. Manual segmentation of TCA was done using the polygon tool after applying the pixel to mm conversion. The upper boundary of the TCA was along the Bruch membrane interface and the lower boundary was along the choroidal-scleral interface. Finally, the image was equally divided into four quadrants (superior, inferior, temporal, and nasal), and TCA, LA, stromal area, and CVI in each quadrant were then automatically calculated and recorded (**Figure 1**). The analysis of OCT images was conducted by two independent investigators, and the images that were judged to be of poor quality by both investigators were excluded.

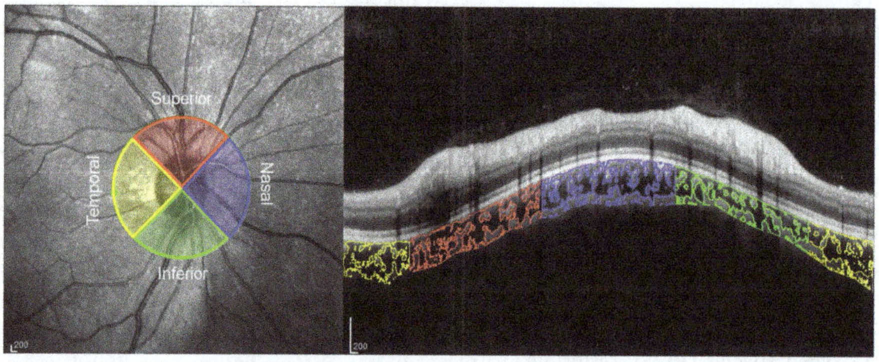

FIGURE 1 | Peripapillary choroidal vascularity index (CVI) in 4 quadrants on an optical coherence tomography (OCT) image. The choroidal luminal areas in the temporal, superior, nasal, and inferior quadrants are outlined in yellow, red, blue, and green, respectively.

TABLE 1 | Demographic and clinical characteristics of LHON Patients in different disease courses.

Characteristic	Group 1 (*N* = 16)	Group 2 (*N* = 24)	Group 3 (*N* = 17)
Sex (m:f)	12:4	22:2	13:4
Age (years)	14.81 ± 5.11	17.17 ± 3.56	22.17 ± 8.80
BCVA (LogMar)	1.60 ± 0.42	1.68 ± 0.46	1.68 ± 0.44
Disease duration (months)	6.38 ± 1.12	17.42 ± 3.35	86.53 ± 73.34

LHON, leber hereditary optic neuropathy; BCVA, best-corrected visual acuity.

Statistical Analysis

Statistical analysis was performed using SPSS 23.0 software (SPSS Inc, Chicago, Illinois, USA). A Shapiro–Wilk test was used to evaluate the normal distribution of the variables. CT, TCA, and CVI in different duration groups at baseline were compared using one-way ANOVA. CT, TCA, and CVI at baseline and 1, 3, and 6 months after gene therapy were compared using one-way ANOVA for repeated measurements. A Bonferroni *post hoc* test was performed for pairwise comparisons. $P < 0.05$ was considered statistically significant.

RESULTS

Study Population

159 LHON patients (159 Eyes) with the G11778A mutation were recruited for this study. 85 LHON patients were excluded on the basis of incomplete follow-up after 6 Months and 17 LHON patients were excluded on the basis of vague scleral junction in low-quality OCT images. Overall, 57 LHON patients were included in this study. among the 57 LHON patients, 47 (82.46%) were male, and the average age Was 16.97 ± 6.52 Years (Range: 8–41 Years). The mean BCVA was 1.66 ± 0.44 (Range: 0.7–2.3 LogMAR) and the mean IOP Was 18.93 ± 3.9 MmHg (Range: 12–28 MmHg). The mean disease duration was 34.93 ± 52.12 Months (Range: 1–312 Months). The demographic data of difference of LHON patients at different stages are shown in **Table 1**.

Peripapillary CT, TCA, and CVI Within Each Group at Baseline

Table 2, **Figure 2** show the peripapillary CT, TCA, and CVI of each quadrant based on OCT imaging of the eyes of patients with LHON and healthy controls. No significant difference was found in average CT between LHON patients at different stages and healthy controls ($P = 0.468$). For each quadrant, values of nasal CT in group 1–3 were significantly higher than that of healthy controls (P = 0.015, 0.007, and 0.004, respectively), while no significant difference was found in the superior, nasal, and inferior quadrants ($P = 0.835$, 0.835, and 0.747, respectively)

As for TCA, no significant difference was found in the values of average TCA between LHON patients at different stages and healthy controls ($P = 0.282$). For each quadrant, no significant difference was found in superior, temporal and inferior quadrants between LHON patients at different stages and healthy controls ($P = 0.547$, 0.697 and 0.425, respectively), whereas nasal TCA in groups 1–3 was significantly higher than that in healthy controls ($P = 0.010$, 0.010, and 0.003, respectively).

Although average CVI was slightly higher in LHON patients than in healthy controls, no significant difference was found in average and nasal, superior, temporal and inferior quadrants between LHON patients at different stages and healthy controls ($P = 0.812$, 0.224, 0.660, 0.346, and 0.736, respectively).

Peripapillary CT, TCA, and CVI in LHON Patients Before and After Gene Therapy

Among the 57 LHON patients, 30 (52.6%) had clinically significantly improved BCVA 6 months after gene therapy compared with baseline BCVA. **Table 3**, **Figure 3** show the peripapillary CT, TCA, and CVI of each quadrant in LHON patients before and 1, 3, and 6 months after gene therapy. The average TCA at 1 month after gene therapy was significantly higher than that before gene therapy ($P = 0.003$), while no significant difference was found in the average CT or average CVI in LHON patients before and 1,3 and 6 months after gene therapy analyzed using pairwise comparisons (all $P > 0.05$). For each quadrant, the temporal CT at baseline was significantly lower than that at 1 and 6 months after gene therapy ($P < 0.001$ and

TABLE 2 | Peripapillary CT, TCA and CVI in LHON patients of different duration groups and healthy controls at baseline.

	Group 1 (*N* = 16)	Group 2 (*N* = 24)	Group 3 (*N* = 17)	Control (*N* = 15)	*P*-value
CT (μm)					
Temporal	210.27 ± 63.47	221.17 ± 71.29	222.22 ± 59.36	203.72 ± 79.30	0.835
Superior	204.41 ± 61.67	209.33 ± 61.79	209.16 ± 54.40	193.27 ± 46.90	0.835
Nasal	212.66 ± 51.75	214.08 ± 70.44	221.03 ± 48.56	161.58 ± 45.92	0.017*
Inferior	157.96 ± 50.80	169.67 ± 67.68	172.48 ± 48.46	153.19 ± 63.45	0.409
Average	196.30 ± 52.53	203.56 ± 64.24	206.22 ± 47.23	177.94 ± 52.22	0.468
TCA (mm²)					
Temporal	0.60 ± 0.11	0.60 ± 0.17	0.65 ± 0.13	0.59 ± 0.19	0.697
Superior	0.59 ± 0.15	0.60 ± 0.17	0.62 ± 0.12	0.54 ± 0.13	0.547
Nasal	0.57 ± 0.14	0.56 ± 0.17	0.59 ± 0.12	0.43 ± 0.11	0.014*
Inferior	0.47 ± 0.12	0.51 ± 0.17	0.52 ± 0.13	0.45 ± 0.14	0.425
Average	0.56 ± 0.12	0.57 ± 0.15	0.59 ± 0.11	0.50 ± 0.13	0.282
CVI (%)					
Temporal	61.40 ± 3.81	63.27 ± 3.19	62.11 ± 4.41	61.26 ± 4.35	0.346
Superior	62.93 ± 4.06	62.48 ± 3.86	61.66 ± 4.13	61.48 ± 2.98	0.660
Nasal	64.77 ± 3.98	64.27 ± 5.02	65.42 ± 4.96	62.06 ± 4.59	0.224
Inferior	61.67 ± 4.07	60.35 ± 4.55	61.84 ± 4.94	61.08 ± 5.18	0.736
Average	62.80 ± 3.61	62.68 ± 3.56	62.65 ± 4.05	61.67 ± 3.39	0.812

*LHON, Leber hereditary optic neuropathy; CT, choroidal thickness; TCA, total choroidal area; CVI, choroidal vascularity index. All data are presented as mean ± SD. One-way ANOVA analysis, *P < 0.05 indicates statistically significance.*

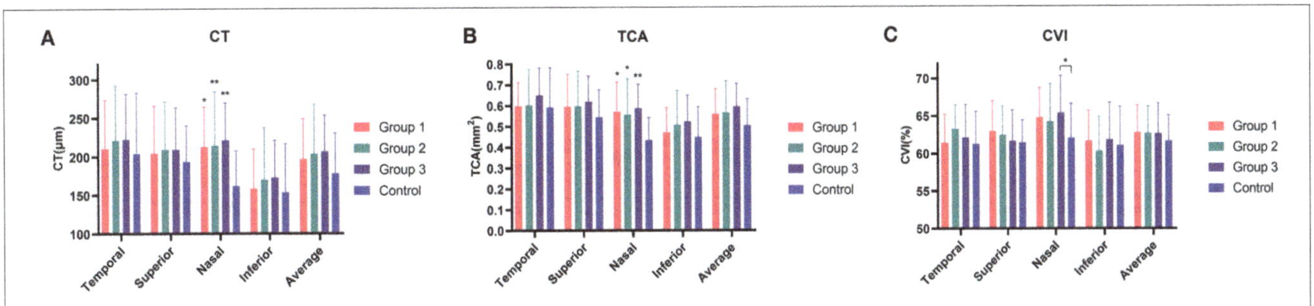

FIGURE 2 | The peripapillary choroidal thickness (CT), total choroidal area (TCA) and CVI in Leber's hereditary optic neuropathy (LHON) patients in three duration groups and in normal controls **(A–C)**. Note that the CT, TCA and CVI in LHON patients were slightly higher than those in controls, especially in nasal quadrant **(A–C)**. *$P < 0.05$ and **$P < 0.01$ indicate statistically significant difference.

0.033, respectively). The temporal TCA at baseline was lower than that at 1 and 6 months after gene therapy (both $P < 0.001$) and the nasal TCA at 1 month after gene therapy was higher than that at 3 and 6 months after gene therapy ($P = 0.006$ and 0.003, respectively). The superior CVI at 1 month after gene therapy was significantly higher than that at 3 months after gene therapy ($P = 0.036$). Furthermore, no significant difference was found in the maximum value of the change of average CVI between patients with improved and unimproved BCVA ($P = 0.197$).

DISCUSSION

LHON is the most common inherited optic neuropathy and is mainly caused by mitochondrial mutations (1). Numerous mitochondria are required in the prelaminar and laminar optic nerve axons to conduct electrical signals. Consequently, the decline of ATP synthesis function caused by mitochondrial changes can result in damage to the optic nerve. The blood supply to the prelaminar and laminar optic nerve axons relies on the posterior short ciliary artery, which also provides the choroidal blood supply. It has been proposed that mitochondrial damage can affect the peripapillary vascularity through a direct effect on viability of endothelial cells and vascular smooth muscle cells (20, 21). OCTA has been used to observe the characteristics of optic nerve microvasculature in LHON. Kousal et al. (10) witnessed the dropout of peripapillary capillaries, and Balducci et al. (9) found that the microvascular changes in the temporal optic disc of LHON patients precede the changes in RNFL. Unfortunately, the choroidal vasculature was not observed in these studies.

Based on OCT imaging, previous studies have shown that CT differs in the eyes between patients at different stages of LHON progression and healthy controls (15, 16). Conversely, no

TABLE 3 | Peripapillary CT, TCA and CVI in LHON Patients Before and After Gene Therapy.

	Baseline	1 m after gene therapy	3 m after gene therapy	6 m after gene therapy	*P*-value
CT (μm)					
Nasal	215.75 ± 58.66	217.01 ± 52.65	212.42 ± 47.79	209.32 ± 45.90	0.343
Superior	207.90 ± 58.63	216.5 ± 43.57	211.78 ± 41.12	210.81 ± 40.79	0.205
Temporal	218.39 ± 64.81	240.27 ± 59.94	231.19 ± 53.23	230.38 ± 49.76	0.001*
Inferior	167.22 ± 57.50	175.71 ± 50.55	178.11 ± 46.33	177.54 ± 45.21	0.016*
Average	201.45 ± 55.67	211.17 ± 45.85	208.43 ± 42.29	206.07 ± 39.61	0.850
TCA (mm²)					
Nasal	0.57 ± 0.15	0.60 ± 0.14	0.57 ± 0.13	0.57 ± 0.13	0.026*
Superior	0.60 ± 0.15	0.63 ± 0.13	0.61 ± 0.13	0.62 ± 0.13	0.610
Temporal	0.61 ± 0.15	0.68 ± 0.15	0.65 ± 0.14	0.66 ± 0.15	0.001*
Inferior	0.50 ± 0.14	0.53 ± 0.14	0.54 ± 0.13	0.54 ± 0.13	0.022*
Average	0.57 ± 0.13	0.61 ± 0.13	0.59 ± 0.12	0.60 ± 0.12	0.003*
CVI (%)					
Nasal	64.76 ± 4.67	64.46 ± 4.22	63.32 ± 4.90	64.08 ± 4.69	0.118
Superior	62.36 ± 3.96	62.41 ± 3.59	61.22 ± 3.60	61.84 ± 3.41	0.024*
Temporal	62.40 ± 3.78	61.39 ± 4.84	60.02 ± 3.58	61.69 ± 3.95	0.107
Inferior	61.16 ± 4.52	61.56 ± 4.11	60.56 ± 3.57	60.85 ± 3.81	0.301
Average	62.70 ± 3.66	62.61 ± 3.31	61.58 ± 3.56	62.23 ± 3.64	0.038*

*LHON, Leber hereditary optic neuropathy; CT, choroidal thickness; TCA, total choroidal area; CVI, choroidal vascularity index. One-way ANOVA repeated measurement analysis, *P < 0.05 indicates statistically significance.*

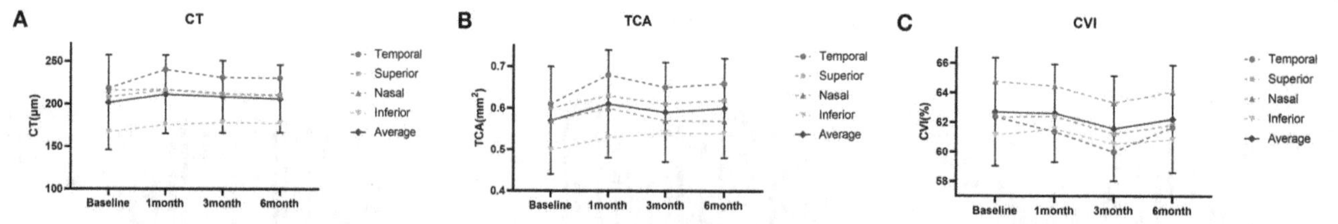

FIGURE 3 | The peripapillary CT, TCA and CVI of different quadrants in LHON patients before and 1, 3, and 6 months after gene therapy **(A–C)**. Bar charts represent mean and error bars represent standard deviation. The average CT, TCA and CVI showed slight changes before and after gene therapy **(A–C)**.

significant difference in average CT was observed in our analysis. One possible reason for this discrepancy is that CT can be easily affected by various physiological factors. Current evidence indicates that compared with CT, CVI is a novel and relatively stable parameter that enables more accurate quantification of choroidal vascularity (22). In the present study, although no statistically significant difference was found in the average peripapillary TCA or CVI within the three duration groups of LHON patients and the healthy controls, the average TCA and CVI were slightly higher in LHON patients in each stage than in healthy controls. A possible reason for this result could be the relatively small sample size of patients in this study. Therefore, a follow-up with more LHON patients from across the natural course of disease progression, especially those in the subacute or dynamic stages, is essential for further research. Additionally, whether there is a difference in CVI between NA-AION patients and healthy controls still remains controversial (11, 12), indicating that CVI in optic nerve diseases has not been fully understood and more investigations are essential.

In LHON patients, the 11778G > A mutation impacts a crucial amino acid in the NADH dioxygenase subunit 4 complex 1 (ND4) gene, and therefore, intravitreal injection of rAAV2/2-ND4 is an effective method for the treatment of LHON (3). Both our previous and the current studies have shown the remarkable effectiveness of gene therapy (2, 3), while the anatomical effect of gene therapy on LHON has not been fully described yet. John et al. (23) witnessed that the temporal RNFL was thicker in treated than in fellow eyes at month 12, but due to the small sample size, more evidence is needed to further confirm whether gene therapy can reduce RNFL loss. Studies focused on choroid in LHON patients have shown that choroidal vascularity may be used as a follow-up indicator of the effectiveness of treatment (15, 16). Recent studies have demonstrated that changes in CVI can serve as a potential indicator for evaluation of treatment for various diseases (17). In our study, both CT and TCA in nasal or inferior quadrant increased after gene therapy, while CVI did not show significant changes. The possible reason for the changes of CT and TCA could be that choroidal stromal and luminal area may have a similar increase to some extent after gene therapy, but since CVI is the more stable parameter that tells the choroidal vascularity more accurately, the result may still indicate that there is no significant change in peripapillary choroidal vascularity after gene therapy. In addition, there was also no significant difference in the maximum value of the change in average CVI between patients with improved and unimproved BCVA. Our findings raise the possibility that choroidal vascularity may not be highly involved in the mechanisms underlying the gene therapy of LHON, but larger scale research is still required to confirm this hypothesis in the future.

The present study has some limitations. The sample size was limited due to the low incidence of the disease, and the follow-up time for patients after gene therapy was relatively short. Studies with larger sample sizes and longer follow-up time are still essential. Considering the loss of follow-up and the low-quality images caused by poor VA in some patients, there is still population bias in our study. The relationship between macular CT and anatomical changes in LHON patients at different stages of disease progression has been described in previous research. The observation on macular CVI is therefore also of great value and will be carried out in future work. Furthermore, the investigation of the relationship between peripapillary CVI, retinal capillaries, and choroidal capillaries (CC) observed by OCTA, as well as the exploration of the possible correlation between CVI and the visual prognosis of LHON patients are promising avenues for future study.

Overall, to our knowledge, our study is the first to investigate CVI in LHON patients. No significant difference was found in peripapillary choroidal vascularity within LHON patients at different stages and healthy controls, and choroidal vascularity seems to stay stable after gene therapy. Still, future studies at a larger scale are still necessary.

ETHICS STATEMENT

The studies involving human participants were reviewed and approved by the Ethics Committee at Tongji Hospital of Wuhan, Taihe Hospital of Shiyan, and Ezhou Central Hospital. Written informed consent to participate in this study was provided by the participant's legal guardian/next of kin.

AUTHOR CONTRIBUTIONS

JY and CC: conceptualization and study design. JJ and GS: data collection, methodology, and writing. QM and DW: data collection and analysis. BL and JY: data provisiong. CC: review and editing. All authors contributed to the article and approved the submitted version.

REFERENCES

1. Yu-Wai-Man P, Griffiths PG, Chinnery PF. Mitochondrial optic neuropathies - disease mechanisms and therapeutic strategies. *Prog Retin Eye Res.* (2011) 30:81–114. doi: 10.1016/j.preteyeres.2010.11.002
2. Zhang Y, Li X, Yuan J, Tian Z, Liu H, Wang D, et al. Prognostic factors for visual acuity in patients with Leber's hereditary optic neuropathy after rAAV2-ND4 gene therapy. *Clin Exp Ophthalmol.* (2019) 47:774–8. doi: 10.1111/ceo.13515
3. Yuan J, Zhang Y, Liu H, Wang D, Du Y, Tian Z, et al. Seven-year follow-up of gene therapy for Leber's hereditary optic neuropathy. *Ophthalmology.* (2020) 127:1125–7. doi: 10.1016/j.ophtha.2020.02.023
4. Coussa RG, Merat P, Levin LA. Propagation and selectivity of axonal loss in Leber hereditary optic neuropathy. *Sci Rep.* (2019) 9:6720. doi: 10.1038/s41598-019-43180-z
5. Huang S, Chen Q, Ma Q, Liu X, Lu F, Shen M, et al. G11778A MUTATION WITH LEBER'S HEREDITARY OPTIC NEUROPATHY. *Retina.* (2016) 36:2409–18. doi: 10.1097/IAE.0000000000001111
6. Akiyama H, Kashima T, Li D, Shimoda Y, Mukai R, Kishi S. Retinal ganglion cell analysis in Leber's hereditary optic neuropathy. *Ophthalmology.* (2013) 120:1943–4. doi: 10.1016/j.ophtha.2013.05.031
7. Balducci N, Savini G, Cascavilla ML, La Morgia C, Triolo G, Giglio R, et al. Macular nerve fibre and ganglion cell layer changes in acute Leber's hereditary optic neuropathy. *Br J Ophthalmol.* (2016) 100:1232–7. doi: 10.1136/bjophthalmol-2015-307326
8. Moster SJ, Moster ML, Scannell Bryan M, Sergott RC. Retinal ganglion cell and inner plexiform layer loss correlate with visual acuity loss in LHON: a longitudinal, segmentation OCT analysis. *Invest Ophthalmol Vis Sci.* (2016) 57:3872–83. doi: 10.1167/iovs.15-17328
9. Balducci N, Cascavilla ML, Ciardella A, La Morgia C, Triolo G, Parisi V, et al. Peripapillary vessel density changes in Leber's hereditary optic neuropathy: a new biomarker. *Clin Exp Ophthalmol.* (2018) 46:1055–62. doi: 10.1111/ceo.13326
10. Kousal B, Kolarova H, Meliska M, Bydzovsky J, Diblik P, Kulhanek J, et al. Peripapillary microcirculation in Leber hereditary optic neuropathy. *Acta Ophthalmol.* (2019) 97:e71–e6. doi: 10.1111/aos.13817
11. Pellegrini M, Giannaccare G, Bernabei F, Moscardelli F, Schiavi C, Campos EC. Choroidal vascular changes in arteritic and nonarteritic anterior ischemic optic neuropathy. *Am J Ophthalmol.* (2019) 205:43–9. doi: 10.1016/j.ajo.2019.03.028
12. Guduru A, Abdul Rasheed M, Goud A, Ashik M, Kumar VK, Chhablani J, et al. Choroidal vascularity in non-arteritic anterior ischaemic optic neuropathy. *Neuroophthalmology.* (2019) 43:305–9. doi: 10.1080/01658107.2019.1566384
13. Park Y, Cho KJ. Choroidal vascular index in patients with open angle glaucoma and preperimetric glaucoma. *PLoS ONE.* (2019) 14:e0213336. doi: 10.1371/journal.pone.0213336
14. Park JW, Suh MH, Agrawal R, Khandelwal N. Peripapillary choroidal vascularity index in glaucoma-a comparison between spectral-domain OCT and OCT angiography. *Invest Ophthalmol Vis Sci.* (2018) 59:3694–701. doi: 10.1167/iovs.18-24315

15. Borrelli E, Triolo G, Cascavilla ML, La Morgia C, Rizzo G, Savini G, et al. Changes in choroidal thickness follow the RNFL changes in leber's hereditary optic neuropathy. *Sci Rep.* (2016) 6:37332. doi: 10.1038/srep37332
16. Darvizeh F, Asanad S, Falavarjani KG, Wu J, Tian JJ, Bandello F, et al. Choroidal thickness and the retinal ganglion cell complex in chronic Leber's hereditary optic neuropathy: a prospective study using swept-source optical coherence tomography. *Eye.* (2020) 34:1624–30. doi: 10.1038/s41433-019-0695-5
17. Agrawal R, Ding J, Sen P, Rousselot A, Chan A, Nivison-Smith L, et al. Exploring choroidal angioarchitecture in health and disease using choroidal vascularity index. *Prog Retin Eye Res.* (2020) 77:100829. doi: 10.1016/j.preteyeres.2020.100829
18. Carelli V, Carbonelli M, de Coo IF, Kawasaki A, Klopstock T, Lagrèze WA, et al. International consensus statement on the clinical and therapeutic management of Leber hereditary optic neuropathy. *J Neuroophthalmol.* (2017) 37:371–81. doi: 10.1097/WNO.0000000000000570
19. Tan KA, Laude A, Yip V, Loo E, Wong EP, Agrawal R. Choroidal vascularity index - a novel optical coherence tomography parameter for disease monitoring in diabetes mellitus? *Acta Ophthalmol.* (2016) 94:e612–e6. doi: 10.1111/aos.13044
20. Chiong M, Cartes-Saavedra B, Norambuena-Soto I, Mondaca-Ruff D, Morales PE, García-Miguel M, et al. Mitochondrial metabolism and the control of vascular smooth muscle cell proliferation. *Front Cell Dev Biol.* (2014) 2:72. doi: 10.3389/fcell.2014.00072
21. Goveia J, Stapor P, Carmeliet P. Principles of targeting endothelial cell metabolism to treat angiogenesis and endothelial cell dysfunction in disease. *EMBO Mol Med.* (2014) 6:1105–20. doi: 10.15252/emmm.201404156
22. Iovino C, Pellegrini M, Bernabei F, Borrelli E, Sacconi R, Govetto A, et al. Choroidal vascularity index: an in-depth analysis of this novel optical coherence tomography parameter. *J Clin Med.* (2020) 9:595. doi: 10.3390/jcm9020595
23. Guy J, Feuer WJ, Davis JL, Porciatti V, Gonzalez PJ, Koilkonda RD, et al. Gene therapy for Leber hereditary optic neuropathy: low- and medium-dose visual results. *Ophthalmology.* (2017) 124:1621–34. doi: 10.1016/j.ophtha.2017.05.016

12

Characteristics of Silicone Oil Emulsification After Vitrectomy for Rhegmatogenous Retinal Detachment: An Ultrasound Biomicroscopy Study

Hongmei Zhao[1,2,3,4,5†], *Jian Yu*[1,2,3,4,5†], *Yuan Zong*[1,2,3,4,5], *Chunhui Jiang*[1,2,3,4,5*], *Haohao Zhu*[6*] and *Gezhi Xu*[1,2,3,4,5]

[1] *Department of Ophthalmology and Vision Science, Eye and Ear, Nose and Throat Hospital, Fudan University, Shanghai, China,* [2] *Key Laboratory of Myopia of State Health Ministry, Shanghai, China,* [3] *Key Laboratory of Visual Impairment and Restoration of Shanghai, Shanghai, China,* [4] *National Health Commission (NHC) Key Laboratory of Myopia, Fudan University, Shanghai, China,* [5] *Key Laboratory of Myopia, Chinese Academy of Medical Sciences, Shanghai, China,* [6] *Department of Ophthalmology, Shanghai Fifth People's Hospital, Fudan University, Shanghai, China*

Correspondence:
Chunhui Jiang
chhjiang70@163.com
Haohao Zhu
haohao700315@163.com

† These authors have contributed equally to this work and share first authorship

Purpose: To investigate the characteristics of silicone oil (SO) emulsification after vitrectomy for rhegmatogenous retinal detachment (RRD) and possible correlations with clinical factors.

Methods: Patients who underwent primary pars plana vitrectomy with SO injection for RRD followed by SO removal at the Eye and ENT Hospital of Fudan University between January 2016 and January 2020 were included. Ultrasound biomicroscopy (UBM) images of the anterior segment were taken before SO removal. Eight signs of SO emulsification in the UBM images were graded as 1 (present) or 0 (not present) and the grades for all signs in each eye were summed. Correlations between SO emulsification grade and clinical factors were determined.

Results: A total of 118 patients (118 eyes) were enrolled in this study. Emulsified SO particles were found in all 118 eyes (100%). The eight signs were more frequently detected in the superior part of the eye. The mean total SO emulsification grade was 19.99 ± 12.98 (range: 1–36). Younger age and male (both $P < 0.05$) were associated with higher total SO emulsification grade. Patients with intraocular pressure (IOP) > 21 mmHg or the use of antiglaucoma medications at the time of SO removal had a higher total SO emulsification grade, were younger, and were more frequently male (all $P < 0.05$) than patients without ocular hypertension.

Conclusions: UBM could play an important role in the diagnosis and grading of SO emulsification. Younger patients and males are more prone to SO emulsification, which may lead to elevated IOP.

Keywords: silicone oil, emulsification, ultrasound biomicroscopy, vitrectomy, rhegmatogenous retinal detachment

INTRODUCTION

Silicone oil (SO), first introduced by Cibis et al. in the 1960s (1), is now widely used in the management of complicated retinal detachment. However, complications of this procedure have been reported, the most frequent of which are SO emulsification and glaucoma (2, 3). The incidence of glaucoma following SO tamponade was reported to range from 11 to 56% (4, 5), exceeding the frequency in cases without SO tamponade (6). SO emulsification was proposed as a major reason for this complication (3). Many methods have been used to detect and evaluate SO emulsification, including ultrasound biomicroscopy (UBM). UBM can be used to take high-resolution images of the anterior segment and has improved our understanding of many ocular diseases, especially glaucoma. Azzolini et al. (7) and Grigera et al. (8) described the UBM findings of SO emulsification in the anterior segment. However, those studies did not fully explore the correlations between UBM findings and other clinical characteristics, such as glaucoma. Therefore, we used UBM to study SO emulsification in the anterior segment in a group of patients who underwent vitrectomy and SO tamponade for rhegmatogenous retinal detachment. We also explored the potential correlations between UBM and the clinical findings.

MATERIALS AND METHODS

Study Subjects and Ethics Statement

This was a single-center, observational, cross-sectional study. Patients who underwent primary pars plana vitrectomy (PPV) with SO injection for rhegmatogenous retinal detachment (RRD), followed by SO removal, at the Eye and ENT Hospital of Fudan University between January 2016 and January 2020 were enrolled in the study. The study was approved by the Institutional Review Board of the Eye and ENT Hospital of Fudan University, and conformed to the tenets of the Declaration of Helsinki. All of the patients signed an informed consent form.

Standard three-port, 23-gauge PPV was performed in all patients by a single surgeon (CH Jiang) using the Alcon Constellation system (Alcon Laboratories, Inc., Fort Worth, TX, USA). After central vitreous removal, triamcinolone acetonide was injected to visualize the residual posterior hyaloid, which was then removed. Additional procedures such as membrane peeling, perfluorocarbon liquid injection (DK-line), relaxing retinotomy, and inferior peripheral iridectomy were performed depending on the state of the retina. After fluid–air exchange and endophotocoagulation, SO (5700 cSt; Bausch & Lomb Inc., Rochester, NY, USA) was injected.

Patients with a history of trauma, SO injection, or intraocular surgery other than PPV or cataract surgery, an intraocular disease other than RRD or cataract (e.g., glaucoma, uveitis), elevated intraocular pressure (IOP > 21 mmHg) before PPV, diabetes, or age < 18 years at the time of primary PPV were excluded from the study.

Main Ophthalmic Measurements

Before SO removal, each patient underwent a thorough ophthalmic examination, which included assessment of best-corrected visual acuity [BCVA, logarithm of the minimal angle of resolution (logMAR)], calculation of spherical equivalent power (calculated as one-half of the cylindrical dioptric plus the spherical diopter), slit-lamp microscopy, dilated fundus examination with a non-contact lens (Maxfield 84 Diopter; Ocular, USA), measurement of IOP by non-contact tonometry, measurement of axial length (AL) using an IOLmaster (version 3.01; Carl Zeiss Meditec, Jena, Germany), and UBM (MD-300L, 50-MHz probe transducer; Meda Co., Ltd, Tianjin, China). We also collected demographic and clinical histories, including the presence of choroidal detachment, whether or not combined phacoemulsification was performed during PPV, history of intraocular operation, duration of SO *in situ*, lens status (aphakic, pseudophakic, or phakic), and the usage and number of antiglaucoma medications before SO removal.

Examination Methods

UBM was performed by experienced ophthalmologists using the protocol described by Grigera et al. (8) and Avitabile et al. (9) UBM was performed with the patients lying in a supine position. The gain was set at 81 dB. Tetracaine 1% was applied for topical anesthesia. An eye cup with a diameter of 18–24 mm was placed into the conjunctival sac according to the size of the eye, and was then filled with care solution or normal saline. A central scan in the horizontal axis and additional scans in eight clock directions (12:00, 1:30, 3:00, 4:30, 6:00, 7:30, 9:00, and 10:30) were taken.

Image Analysis Methods

All UBM images were analyzed by two independent readers. The extent of SO emulsification detected by UBM was classified according to the method described by Grigera et al. (8). The following five signs were considered to indicate SO emulsification. (1) Floating droplets: tiny reflective particles (droplets) with definite outlines, floating in AC (**Figure 1A**). (2) Endothelial deposits with a fixed status (**Figure 1B**). (3) Ghost images (**Figure 1C**): multiple echoes of SO particles adjacent to the corneal endothelium that may be visible as needle-shaped images hanging from the endothelium. (4) Hyperoleon: a massive collection of emulsified particles (**Figure 1D**). (5) Impregnation or impregnation of tissues (**Figure 1D**): increased reflectivity in the anterior chamber angle (ACA) filtration area, the anterior/posterior iris surface, or the ciliary body, as compared with that in normal eyes.

Using the horizontal central scan image, floating droplets, endothelial deposits with a fixed status, ghost images, and hyperoleon were graded as 1 (present) or 0 (not present) (8). The area of hyperoleon was measured using ImageJ software (National Institute of Health, Bethesda, MD, USA) (**Figure 2**). Impregnation of tissue at four locations (ACA, anterior iris surface, posterior iris surface, and ciliary body) was graded as 1 (present) or 0 (not present) on the images acquired in the eight clock directions, as reported by Grigera et al. (8). If the grades determined by both graders were identical, they were used as the final grades. If the grades differed, the final grade was determined by a senior specialist (Qian Chen). The grades for all signs in each eye were summed (**Supplementary Figure 1**). Intraobserver repeatability and interobserver reproducibility were evaluated for 20 central scan images by two observers, who each measured the same scan from each eye twice. The intraclass correlation (ICC)

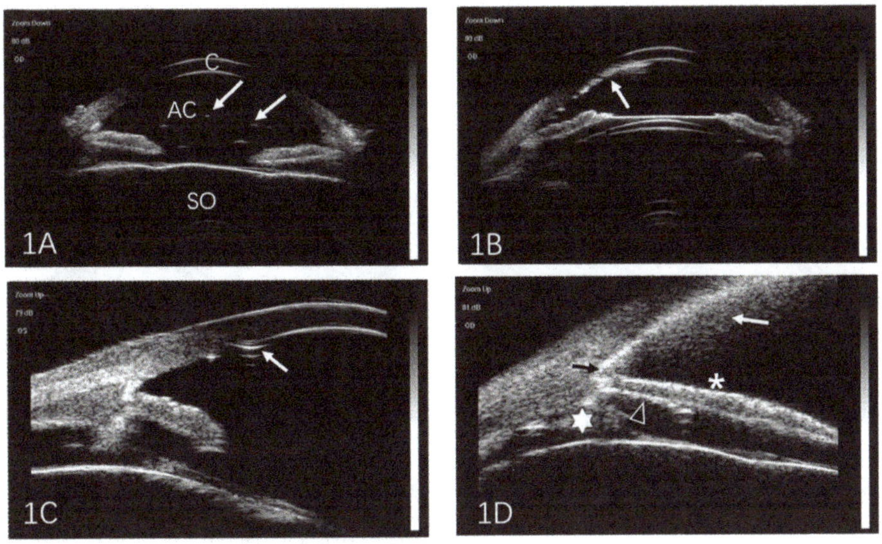

FIGURE 1 | Representative ultrasound biomicroscopic images of silicone oil (SO) emulsification. **(A)** Individual SO particles floating in the anterior chamber (arrows). **(B)** SO particles adjacent to the cornea (arrow). **(C)** Ghost images. Multiple echoes from SO particles adjacent to the corneal endothelium may be seen as needle-shaped artifacts hanging from the endothelium (arrow). **(D)** Hyperoleon. A massive collection of emulsified SO particles (white arrow), and impregnation of the anterior chamber angle (black arrow), anterior surface of the iris (asterisk), posterior surface of the iris (triangle), and ciliary body (star). C, cornea; AC, anterior chamber; SO, silicone oil.

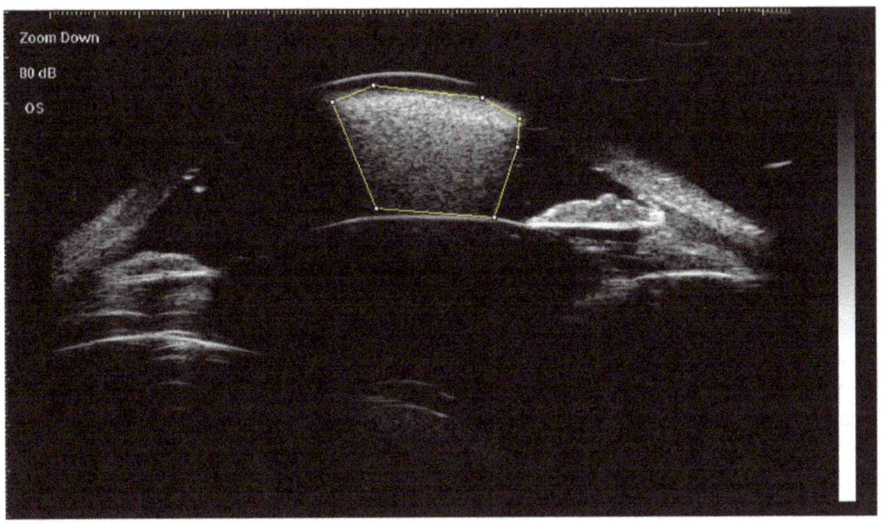

FIGURE 2 | Measurement of the area of hyperoleon (indicated with the yellow border) in the anterior chamber using ImageJ software.

coefficient was used to assess repeatability and reproducibility. The mean of three measurements of the area of hyperoleon was used as the final value.

Data and Statistical Analysis

All analyses were performed using SPSS software version 20.0 (SPSS, Inc., Chicago, IL, USA). The K–S test was used to determine the normality of data. The χ^2 test, independent-samples t-test, Spearman's correlation coefficient, Mann–Whitney U test and multiple linear regression were used to assess correlations between clinical characteristics and SO emulsification. The independent sample t-test, χ^2 test or Mann–Whitney U test were used to assess the differences between patients with/without elevated IOP (IOP > 21 mmHg) or the use of antiglaucoma medications. Continuous data are expressed as the mean $\pm$ standard deviation. Statistical significance was defined as a P value of < 0.05. ICC coefficients were used to assess repeatability and reproducibility; an ICC coefficient of 0.81–1.00 indicates almost perfect agreement between repeated measurements and values < 0.40 indicate poor to fair agreement.

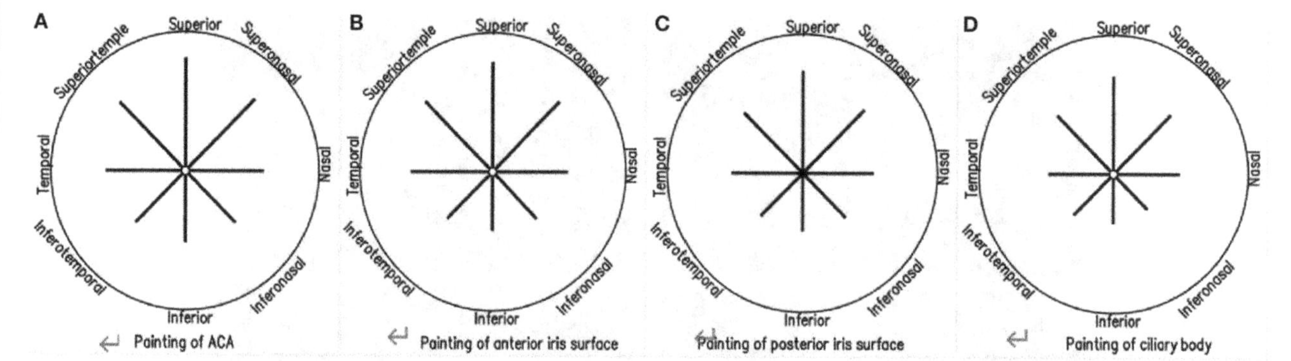

FIGURE 3 | Ultrasound biomicrosopic findings of emulsified silicone oil in eight directions, showing impregnation of the anterior chamber angle **(A)**, the anterior iris surface **(B)**, the posterior iris surface **(C)**, and the ciliary body **(D)**.

TABLE 1 | Associations between clinical characteristics and total SO emulsification grade.

Characteristic	Total grade/correlation coefficient	*U* value	*P* value
Gender: female/male	15.80 ± 12.85 vs. 24.194 ± 11.79	1094.5	0.001*
Combined phacoemulsification with PPV+SO injection: yes/no	25.73 ± 11.05 vs. 18.37 ± 13.08	773.55	0.006*
Choroidal detachment: yes/no	22.23 ± 13.93 vs. 19.71 ± 12.90	583.0	0.392
Lens status: phakic/non-phakic	27.67 ± 9.77 vs. 18.61±13.04	508.5	0.003*
Age	$r = -0.313$	-	0.001*
AL	$r = 0.230$	-	0.012*
BCVA before PPV + SO injection (logMAR)	$r = 0.153$	-	0.098
Duration of SO *in situ*	$r = 0.192$	-	0.037*

**P* < 0.05 was considered statistically significant. Mann-Whitney U test or Spearman's correlation coefficients were used to assess correlations between clinical characteristics and total SO emulsification grade.*
SO, silicone oil; PPV, pars plana vitrectomy; AL, axial length; BCVA, best-corrected visual acuity; logMAR, logarithm of the minimum angle of resolution.

RESULTS

A total of 118 eyes (69 right) in 118 patients (59 males) were included in this study. The mean age of the sample was 55.76 ± 10.76 years (range 24–78 years), the mean duration of SO *in situ* was 23.72 ± 14.53 weeks (range 2–96 weeks), and the mean AL was 26.68 ± 2.92 mm (range 22–37 mm). Thirteen patients had choroidal detachment at the time of PPV. Fifty-two eyes were highly myopic (AL ≥ 26 mm). Combined phacoemulsification, without intraocular lens implantation, was performed in 51 eyes (**Supplementary Table 1**).

Before SO removal, signs of SO emulsification were detected in all 118 eyes (100%). Floating droplets were found in 100%, hyperoleon in 20.33%, endothelial deposits in 28.81%, ghost images in 37.29%, impregnation of the ACA in 83.90%, impregnation of the anterior iris surface in 81.36%, impregnation of the posterior iris surface in 79.66%, and impregnation of the ciliary body in 77.97% of eyes. The mean ICC coefficient for measurement of the area of hyperoleon was 0.998 for intra-observer repeatability and 0.997 for interobserver reproducibility. When different directions were involved, tissue impregnation was most frequently detected in the superior part (**Supplementary Table 2; Figure 3**).

The mean total SO emulsification grade was 19.99 ± 12.98 (range:1–36). Age (negatively), duration of SO *in situ* (positively), AL (positively), combined phacoemulsification (positively), and male (positively) were significantly correlated with the total SO emulsification grade (all $P < 0.05$; **Table 1**). Multiple linear regression revealed that younger age and male (both $P < 0.05$) were associated with higher total SO emulsification grade (**Table 2**).

At the time of SO removal, 69 patients had an IOP of > 21 mmHg or were using antiglaucoma medications. These patients had a higher SO emulsification grade, a larger area of hyperoleon, were younger, and were more frequently males than patients without ocular hypertension (all $P < 0.05$) (**Table 3**).

DISCUSSION

In this study, we used UBM to assess the presence of and to grade SO emulsification in a group of patients with RRD. SO emulsification was more commonly found in the superior direction, and was more severe in younger patients and in males. Furthermore, the SO emulsification grade was higher in patients with IOP > 21 mmHg or patients using antiglaucoma medications.

TABLE 2 | Results of multiple linear regression of factors associated with the total SO emulsification grade.

Clinical factor	β coefficient (95%CI)	P value
Gender: female/male	11.173 (5.142, 17.203)	0.000*
Age	−0.364 (0.669, −0.060)	0.019*
Duration of SO *in situ*	0.164 (−0.047, 0.375)	0.127
AL	0.902 (0.181, 1.984)	0.102
Combined phacoemulsification with PPV + SO injection: yes/no	−5.207 (−13.622, 3.208)	0.223
Lens status: non-phakic/phakic	3.899 (−4.465, 16.2279)	5.881
Choroidal detachment: yes/no	1.924 (−8.287 12.135)	0.710
BCVA before PPV + SOI (logMAR)	1.417 (−0.766, 3.601)	0.201

$^{*}P < 0.05$ was considered statistically significant.
SO, silicone oil; AL, axial length; pars plana vitrectomy; BCVA, best-corrected visual acuity; logMAR, logarithm of the minimum angle of resolution.

TABLE 3 | Comparison of clinical factors between patients with and without ocular hypertension (IOP > 21 mmHg or use of antiglaucoma medications).

Clinical factor	Ocular hypertension		P value
	Yes (n = 69)	No (n = 49)	
Total grade	22.70 ± 12.64	16.18 ± 12.62	0.005*
Duration of SO *in situ* (weeks)	24.30 ± 15.71	22.90 ± 12.80	0.778
Age (years)	52.83 ± 10.11	59.91 ± 10.36	0.000*
AL (mm)	27.03 ± 2.94	26.18 ± 2.86	0.105
BCVA before PPV + SO injection (logMAR)	2.17 ± 1.06	2.08 ± 1.00	0.450
Male/female (n)	40/29	19/30	0.040* $\chi^2 = 4.223$
Choroidal detachment, yes/no (n)	60/9	45/4	0.404 $\chi^2 = 0.696$
Combined phacoemulsification with PPV + SO injection: yes/no (n)	51/18	41/8	0.207 $\chi^2 = 1.589$
Lens status: non-phakic/phakic (n)	14/55	4/45	0.071 $\chi^2 = 3.259$

$^{*}P < 0.05$ was considered statistically significant.
Independent-samples t-tests, χ^2 tests and Mann–Whitney U tests were used to compare clinical factors between patients with without ocular hypertension (IOP > 21 mmHg or the use of antiglaucoma medications). Values are expressed as the number of patients or as the mean ± standard deviation.
IOP, intraocular pressure; SO, silicone oil; AL, axial length; BCVA, best-corrected visual acuity; log MAR, logarithm of the minimal angle of resolution; PPV, pars plana vitrectomy.

Several studies have observed SO emulsification using UBM. Avitabile et al. (9) determined the height of SO emulsification in the AC, and Grigera et al. (8) described various signs of SO emulsification. However, the correlations between signs of SO emulsification on UBM and clinical factors have not been well-studied. In our study, signs of SO emulsification in different directions were recorded by UBM and analyzed semi-quantitatively, and we explored their potential correlations with clinical factors (**Supplementary Table 3**). We found that the grade of SO emulsification was correlated with younger age and male gender. Previous studies (4, 10) also reported a correlation between SO emulsification and age. Aqueous proteins and eye movement, which facilitate SO emulsification and are greater in younger eyes, might be contributing factors (11). Greater activity may have contributed to the higher grade of SO emulsification in males in our study. Patients who underwent combined phacoemulsification during PPV possibly experienced more severe postoperative reactions or inflammation, which could contribute to their higher grade of SO emulsification. In addition, AL was significantly and positively correlated with the grade of SO emulsification. The reason for this is not fully understood, but it is possible that eyes with a longer AL were injected with a greater volume of SO, thus increasing the interface between SO and intraocular fluid. With a greater interface, the surfactants (surface active agents) have more opportunity to interact with SO, thus increasing the risk of emulsification (4). These factors might contribute to the higher grading observed in this study. In our study, UBM focused on the anterior segment. Weakened zonular laxity in highly myopic eyes (12) might permit emulsified SO droplets to enter the posterior and anterior chambers more easily.

Our study found the correlation between SO emulsification and elevated IOP, which was also observed in prior studies (9, 13). Wickham et al. used transmission electron microscopy and detected SO in the trabecular meshwork (14). In addition, Rentsch et al. (15) reported SO-laden macrophages within the trabecular meshwork of three human eyes, which were enucleated due to glaucoma following SO injection. It has also been proposed that SO might initiate localized inflammation in the trabecular meshwork (14, 16). Formerly Federman and Schubert (2) reported that 100% of eyes injected with SO showed some degree of emulsification. And this time, SO emulsification was observed in every eye included in our study. Here, we found that impregnation of the ACA was more frequent in patients with IOP > 21 mmHg or using antiglaucoma medications (**Supplementary Table 4**). As a result, SO emulsification seemed to be almost inevitable, also as it is closely associated with high IOP or the usage of antiglaucoma medications, so in these cases, emulsified SO droplets should be removed as thorough as possible. On the other hand, our result here reminds us that though presently most attention was paid to removing the SO droplets in the vitreous cavity, the anterior segment should also be taken care. Anterior chamber irrigation should be performed during silicone oi removal, especially in cases with high IOP.

Here, some of our findings were in accordance with former reports, this accordance suggested the UBM method used here a useful and reliable tool to evaluate the situation of SO emulsification. Compared to other ways like a Coulter Counter (10, 17, 18) and B-scan ultrasonography (19–21), UBM was non-invasive and cost effective, furthermore it could be used before SO removal, while the other two only postoperatively. On the other hand, slit-lamp microscopy, which could also be used before SO removal, was rather subjective and difficult to be quantified. Using the method described here, the situation of SO emulsification could be properly evaluated, and for those with higher sore, special attention should be paid to the removal of the SO droplets, and longer irrigation and multiple air-fluid exchange should be performed (18). Other methods including the recently introduced F4H5 (19), which is believed to dissolve the emulsified SO droplets, could also be considered.

Our study was limited by its single-center, cross-sectional design and we only included patients with RRD who were treated with one type of SO. On the other hand, we followed the standard described by Grigera DE, these are possibility that signs like impregnation of tissues could also result from reasons other than emulsified SO droplets.

In conclusion, UBM might play an important role in the diagnosis and quantification of SO emulsification. Younger patients and males may be more prone to SO emulsification and at increased risk of elevated IOP. SO should be removed as soon as possible in these patients. The method used to evaluate SO emulsification could be used in future studies in this field.

ETHICS STATEMENT

The studies involving human participants were reviewed and approved by the Institutional Review Board of the Eye and ENT Hospital of Fudan University. The patients/participants provided their written informed consent to participate in this study.

AUTHOR CONTRIBUTIONS

CJ performed the surgery. HZha and JY analyzed the patient data and made major contributions for writing the manuscript. YZ performed the literature review for similar topics and made major contributions to acquisition and interpretation of data. HZhu and GX made substantial contributions to conception and design this study. All authors have read and approved the final manuscript.

ACKNOWLEDGMENTS

We thank Dr. Qian Chen for the clinical help.

REFERENCES

1. Cibis PA, Becker B, Okun E, Canaan S. The use of liquid silicone in retinal detachment surgery. *Arch Ophthalmol.* (1962) 68:590–9. doi: 10.1001/archopht.1962.00960030594005
2. Federman JL, Schubert HD. Complications associated with the use of silicone oil in 150 eyes after retina-vitreous surgery. *Ophthalmology.* (1988) 95:870–6. doi: 10.1016/S0161-6420(88)33080-0
3. Honavar SG, Goyal M, Majji AB, Sen PK, Naduvilath T, Dandona L. Glaucoma after pars plana vitrectomy and silicone oil injection for complicated retinal detachments. *Ophthalmology.* (1999) 106:169–77. doi: 10.1016/S0161-6420(99)90017-9
4. Miller JB, Papakostas TD, Vavvas DG. Complications of emulsified silicone oil after retinal detachment repair. *Semin Ophthalmol.* (2014) 29:312–8. doi: 10.3109/08820538.2014.962181
5. Al-Jazzaf AM, Netland PA, Charles S. Incidence and management of elevated intraocular pressure after silicone oil injection. *J Glaucoma.* (2005) 14:40–6. doi: 10.1097/01.ijg.0000145811.62095.fa
6. Koreen L, Yoshida N, Escariao P, Niziol LM, Koreen IV, Musch DC, et al. Incidence of, risk factors for, and combined mechanism of late-onset open-angle glaucoma after vitrectomy. *Retina.* (2012) 32:160–7. doi: 10.1097/IAE.0b013e318217fffb
7. Azzolini C, Pierro L, Codenotti M, Bandello F, Brancato R. Ultrasound biomicroscopy following the intraocular use of silicone oil. *Int Ophthalmol.* (1995) 19:191–5. doi: 10.1007/BF00133737
8. Grigera DE, Zambrano A, Cazon GP, Cavanagh E, Girado SG. Ultrasound biomicroscopy in silicone oil-filled eyes. *Retina.* (2000) 20:524–31. doi: 10.1097/00006982-200009000-00015
9. Avitabile T, Bonfiglio V, Cicero A, Torrisi B, Reibaldi A. Correlation between quantity of silicone oil emulsified in the anterior chamber and high pressure in vitrectomized eyes. *Retina.* (2002) 22:443–8. doi: 10.1097/00006982-200208000-00008
10. Yu J, Zong Y, Jiang C, Zhu H, Deng G, Xu G. Silicone oil emulsification after vitrectomy for rhegmatogenous retinal detachment. *J Ophthalmol.* (2020) 2020:6940625. doi: 10.1155/2020/6940625
11. Chan YK, Ng CO, Knox PC, Garvey MJ, Williams RL, Wong D. Emulsification of silicone oil and eye movements. *Invest Ophthalmol Vis Sci.* (2011) 52:9721–7. doi: 10.1167/iovs.11-8586
12. Dureau P. Pathophysiology of zonular diseases. *Curr Opin Ophthalmol.* (2008) 19:27–30. doi: 10.1097/ICU.0b013e3282f29f01
13. Valone J, McCarthy M. Emulsified anterior chamber silicone oil and glaucoma. *Ophthalmology.* (1994) 101:1908–12. doi: 10.1016/S0161-6420(94)31084-0
14. Wickham L, Asaria RH, Alexander R, Luthert P, Charteris DG. Immunopathology of intraocular silicone oil: enucleated eyes. *Br J Ophthalmol.* (2007) 91:258–62. doi: 10.1136/bjo.2006.103564
15. Rentsch FJ, Atzler P, Liesenhoff H. Histological and electron microscopy studies of a human eye several years after an intravitreous silicone implant. *Ber Zusammenkunft Dtsch Ophthalmol Ges.* (1978) 75:70–4. doi: 10.1007/978-3-642-47090-5_16
16. Ni C, Wang WJ, Albert DM, et al. Intravitreous silicone injection. Histopathologic findings in a human eye after 12 years. *Arch Ophthalmol.* (1983) 101:1399–401. doi: 10.1001/archopht.1983.01040020401013
17. Chan YK, Cheung N, Chan WS, Wong D. Quantifying silicone oil emulsification in patients: are we only seeing the tip of the iceberg? *Graefes Arch Clin Exp Ophthalmol.* (2015) 253:1671–5. doi: 10.1007/s00417-014-2866-1
18. Yu J, Zong Y, Tan Y, et al. Comparison of repeated fluid-air exchange and passive drainage for removing residual emulsified silicone oil droplets. *J Ophthalmol.* (2020) 2020:6940625. doi: 10.1155/2020/8184607
19. Stalmans P, Pinxten A-M, Wong DS. Cohort safety and efficacy study of Siluron2000 emulsification-resistant silicone oil and F4h5 in the treatment of full-thickness macular hole. *Retina.* (2015) 35:2558–66. doi: 10.1097/IAE.0000000000000647
20. Shiihara H, Sakamoto T, Terasaki H, Yamashita T, Yoshihara N, Okamoto F, et al. Effect of fluid-air exchange on reducing residual silicone oil after silicone oil removal. *Graefes Arch Clin Exp Ophthalmol.* (2017) 255:1697–704. doi: 10.1007/s00417-017-3701-2
21. Shiihara H, Terasaki H, Yoshihara N, Shirasawa M, Otsuka H, Yamashita T, et al. Amount of residual silicone oil in vitreous cavity is significantly correlated with axial length. *Retina.* (2016) 36:181–7. doi: 10.1097/IAE.0000000000000656

13

Association of Myopia with Microvascular Alterations in Patients with Type 2 Diabetes: An Optical Coherence Tomography Angiography Study

Xin Wen†, Zijing Li†, Jianhui Xiao, Xuane Liu, Yichi Zhang‡ and Yuqing Lan‡*

Guangdong Provincial Key Laboratory of Malignant Tumor Epigenetics and Gene Regulation, Department of Ophthalmology, Sun Yat-sen Memorial Hospital, Sun Yat-sen University, Guangzhou, China

***Correspondence:**
Yuqing Lan
lanyq@mail.sysu.edu.cn

†These authors share first authorship

‡These authors share senior authorship

Purpose: To determine the association of myopia with peripapillary and macular microvasculature in eyes with type 2 diabetes using optical coherence tomography angiography (OCTA).

Methods: Diabetic patients with and without diabetic retinopathy (DR) were recruited and grouped according to myopic status in this cross-sectional study. Axial length, refractive error, and OCTA parameters were measured. OCTA parameters were analyzed with adjustment of confounding factors and further Bonferroni analysis was performed to determine the differences in multiple group comparisons.

Results: Compared with the diabetic eyes without myopia, those with myopia had lower rate of DR (21.82 vs. 35.90%, $\chi^2 = 6.190$, $P = 0.013$), longer axial lengths (24.94 ± 0.75 vs. 23.16 ± 0.64, $F = 311.055$, $P < 0.001$) and reduced whole vessel density (VD) of optic nerve head (ONH) (45.89 ± 5.76 vs. 49.14 ± 4.33, $F = 19.052$, $P < 0.001$), peripapillary VD (48.75 ± 6.56 vs. 50.76 ± 4.51, $F = 7.600$, $P = 0.006$), and reduced thickness of the retinal nerve fiber layer (RNFL) (95.50 ± 12.35 vs. 100.67 ± 13.68, $F = 5.020$, $P = 0.026$). In eyes without myopia, the superficial vessel density (SVD) (46.58 ± 4.90 vs. 43.01 ± 4.25; 95% CI, 1.80–4.61; $P < 0.001$), deep vessel density (DVD) (45.64 ± 6.34 vs. 42.15 ± 6.31; 95% CI, 1.07–5.00; $P < 0.001$), and FD300 area density (50.31 ± 5.74 vs. 44.95 ± 6.96; 95% CI, 2.88–7.27; $P < 0.001$) were significant reduced in eyes with DR(DR eyes) comparing to those without DR (NoDR eyes). In eyes with myopia, only SVD were significantly reduced in DR eyes comparing to NoDR eyes (41.68 ± 3.34 vs. 45.99 ± 4.17; 95% CI, 1.10–7.22; $P = 0.002$). In NoDR eyes, both whole VD of ONH and Peripapillary VD demonstrated a significant decrease in eyes with myopia comparing to those without myopia (49.91 ± 4.36 vs. 45.61 ± 6.32; 95% CI, 1.95–6.27; $P < 0.001$ and 51.36 ± 4.24 vs. 48.52 ± 6.99; 95% CI, 0.56–5.11; $P = 0.006$, respectively).

Conclusions: In diabetic patients, myopic eyes exhibited lower prevalence of DR and thinner thickness of RNFL. The refractive status could possibly impact the retinal microvascular changes from NoDR to DR stage.

Keywords: microvascular alterations, myopia, diabetic retinopathy, axial length, optical coherence tomography angiography, vessel density

INTRODUCTION

Diabetic retinopathy (DR) was a leading global cause of preventable blindness in working-age population (1). Various clinical studies showed that myopia was a protective factor against the onset and progression of DR (2–4). The preventive effect was closely related to the degree of DR, axial length, and refractive error. The speculated cause was that the elongation of axial length thinned the retina or retinal nerve fiber layer (RNFL) and enlarge the peripapillary atrophy (5), resulting in reduced retinal oxygen demand and lower risk of DR. Nevertheless, the specific mechanism remained unknown. Using optical coherence tomography angiography (OCTA), a recently introduced non-invasive vascular imaging technology, it was possible to detect microvascular alterations layer by layer in retinal pathologies such as diabetes and myopia (6, 7). Despite conflicting results of myopia on the retinal vessel density (VD), myopia appeared to decrease the VD in either the macula or the optic nerve head (ONH), or in both regions in healthy adults (8–10). Because decreased VD in macula and ONH had also been reported in DR (11–14), the actual blood perfusion in diabetic patients with myopia was ambiguous. To our knowledge, quantitative OCTA analysis of microvasculature in diabetic patients with and without myopia had not yet been reported. Therefore, in the present study, we analyzed the OCTA parameters in diabetic eyes with and without myopia in order to determine the correlation between myopia and microvasculature in diabetic patients.

MATERIALS AND METHODS

Participants

This cross-sectional retrospective study recruited type 2 diabetes mellitus (T2DM) patients with and without myopia from September 1, 2018 to September 1, 2019. The inclusion criteria were diagnosis of T2DM and disease duration >1 year. Exclusion criteria included ocular diseases with severe opacity of refractive media that would influence fundus examination or any other ocular diseases that would affect retinal circulation, including glaucoma, age-related macular degeneration, and retinal artery/vein occlusion. Because DR could cause cataract and affect the results of refractive error, and DR of any stage were closely related to mild myopia (15), for the purpose of minimizing the interference, we defined myopia as a spherical equivalent of <-3.0 diopters(D) or axial length of >24.00 mm and non-myopic eyes as a spherical equivalent of −2.75 to 0.5 D, with axial length of <24.00 mm (16).

Clinical Examinations

All participants underwent comprehensive ophthalmic examinations, including best-corrected visual acuity (BCVA) (LogMAR visual acuity), intraocular pressure (IOP), slit-lamp biomicroscopy, and dilated fundus examination using a non-contact slit lamp lens, color fundus photographs, OCTA, and fundus fluorescein angiography (only in patients with DR).

OCTA

The OCTA images were obtained using an RTVue XR Avanti spectral domain OCT device (Optovue, Inc., Fremont, CA, USA). A 3 × 3 mm area of macula and a 4.5 × 4.5 mm area of ONH were scanned at 70,000 A-scans/second with a wavelength of 840 nm. A split-spectrum amplitude-decorrelation angiography algorithm was used to detect erythrocyte movement in OCTA. The retinal vascular networks and nerve fibers of macula and ONH were analyzed.OCTA images with scan quality ≥ 6 were included. OCTA images with poor quality or large motion artifacts or shadow artifacts or segmentation errors were excluded.

OCTA Image Analysis

Using prototype AngioVue software 2.0, the parameters of the macula and ONH were automatically measured and analyzed without any attempts at manual alteration. Macula-associated parameters included whole VD of superficial capillary plexus (SCP) and deep capillary plexus (DCP), foveal vessel density in a 300-μm region around FAZ (FD300). VD were defined as the percentage of the area occupied by blood vessels. The area of vessels was calculated using software by extracting a binary image from the grayscale OCTA image, and then calculating the percentage of pixels occupied by blood vessels in the defined region. The SCP slab was segmented from ILM to inner plexiform layer (IPL). The DCP slab was segmented from 15 μm posterior to the IPL to the outer plexiform layer (OPL). Other macula-associated parameters such as FAZ perimeter (PERIM), acircularity index (AI), foveal VD, parafoveal VD, and perifoveal VD in the SCP and DCP were not included, because the high correlation between any two of the above parameters would interfere the results of the statistical model. ONH-associated parameters included VD of the whole 4.5 × 4.5 mm area, peripapillary area as well as the average RNFL thickness of the entire peripapillary area. The peripapillary area was defined as a 1.0 mm-wide round annulus extending from the 2.0-mm circle of ONH.

Statistical Analysis

SPSS 22.0 (SPSS Inc. Chicago, IL, USA) were used for statistical analyses. All variables were calculated as means ± standard deviation. Categorical variables were analyzed using the Chi-square test. OCTA parameters were analyzed using univariate general linear analysis and further Bonferroni analysis was used to assess the differences in multiple group comparisons. Analysis of OCTA parameters were performed with adjustment for confounding factors including age and signal strength (SS) of OCTA images. $P < 0.05$ were considered statistically significant.

RESULTS

Study Population

We enrolled 250 eyes of 156 patients, including 55 eyes (15 bilateral eyes, 25 unilateral eyes including 10 right eyes and 15 left eyes) with myopia of 40 diabetic patients (mean ± SD age, 53.66 ± 12.58 years) and 195 eyes (79 bilateral eyes, 37 unilateral eyes, including 22 right eyes and 15 left eyes) without myopia

TABLE 1 | Clinical and demographic characteristics of non-myopic and myopic eyes.

Characteristics	No. (%) or mean ± SD			
	Non-myopic (n = 195)	Myopic eyes (n = 55)	F/χ^2	P-value
Age, y (range)	53.66 ± 12.58 (18 to 89)	49.09 ± 17.21 (25–85)	4.761	0.030*
Female	86(86/195, 44.10%)	15(15/55, 27.27%)	4.372	0.037*
Axial length, mm (range)	23.16 ± 0.64 (21.61–24.00)	24.94 ± 0.75 (24.11–27.40)	311.055	<0.001*
Signal strength of OCTA images	7.33 ± 1.11 (6–10)	7.07 ± 1.02 (6–9)	2.356	0.126
Refractive error, D (range)	−0.88 ± 0.70 (−2.75 to 0.50)	−2.76 ± 2.70 (−12.00 to −0.25)	20.227	<0.001*
BCVA logMAR (range)	0.09 ± 0.41 (−0.20 to 4.00)	0.09 ± 0.30 (−0.10 to 1.20)	<0.001	0.992
IOP, mmHg (range)	15.57 ± 2.78 (11–26)	16.09 ± 2.61 (11–23)	1.520	0.219
Duration of DM, y (range)	6.10 ± 3.13 (1–15)	6.33 ± 2.66 (2–15)	0.236	0.628
HbA1c, % (range)	8.65 ± 1.59 (5.90–14.30)	8.19 ± 1.75 (6.20–15.40)	3.397	0.067
DR	70 (70/195, 35.90%)	12 (12/55, 21.82%)	6.190	0.013*
Mild NPDR	6 (6/70, 8.57%)	1 (1/12, 8.33%)	1.360	0.715
Moderate NPDR	50 (50/70, 71.43%)	9 (9/12, 75.00%)		
Severe NPDR	12 (12/70, 17.14%)	1 (1/12, 8.33%)		
PDR	2 (2/70, 2.86%)	1 (1/12, 8.33%)		

*BCVA, best corrected visual acuity; IOP, intraocular pressure; HbA1c, glycosylated hemoglobin. DR, diabetic retinopathy; NPDR, non-proliferative diabetic retinopathy. *Indicates statistically significant difference between the groups. P < 0.05 were considered statistically significant.*

of 116 diabetic patients (mean ± SD age, 49.09 ± 17.21 years). The myopic group included 43 eyes without DR and 12 eyes with DR. The non-myopic group included 125 eyes without DR and 70 eyes with DR. There were significant differences between the myopic and non-myopic groups with respect to age, gender, axial length, spherical equivalent refractive error, and the rate of DR (**Table 1**).

The comparison of the RNFL and the VD between eyes of diabetic patients with and without myopia were displayed in **Table 2**. Reduced thickness of the RNFL were observed in myopic eyes comparing to non-myopic ones(95.50 ± 12.35 vs. 100.67 ± 13.68, F = 5.020, P = 0.026), especially in the nasal (68.56 ± 10.27 vs. 75.04 ± 16.11, F = 6.037, P = 0.015) and inferior (119.97 ± 23.28 vs. 127.65 ± 20.52, F = 4.298, P = 0.039) sections. Accordingly, diabetic eyes with myopia exhibited decreased whole VD of ONH (45.89 ± 5.76 vs. 49.14 ± 4.33, F = 19.052, P < 0.001) and peripapillary VD (48.75 ± 6.56 vs. 50.76 ± 4.51, F = 7.600, P = 0.006), comparing to eyes without myopia (**Figure 1**). However, no significant differences were found in terms of macula-associated parameters such as SVD, DVD, or FD300 area density between diabetic eyes with and without myopia (**Table 2**).

In intergroup comparisons within diabetic eyes without DR (NoDR eyes), those with myopia demonstrated reduced whole VD of ONH comparing to those without myopia(45.61 ± 6.32 vs. 49.91 ± 4.36; 95% CI, 1.95–6.27; P < 0.001). Peripapillary VD demonstrated a similar decrease while comparing NoDR eyes with myopia to those without myopia (48.52 ± 6.99 vs. 51.36 ± 4.24; 95% CI, 0.56–5.11; P = 0.006) (**Figure 1**).

In intragroup comparison of eyes without myopia, DR eyes showed significant reduction in SVD (43.01 ± 4.25 vs. 46.58 ± 4.90; 95% CI, 1.80–4.61; P < 0.001), DVD (42.15 ± 6.31 vs. 45.64 ± 6.34; 95% CI, 1.07–5.01; P < 0.001), and FD300 area density (44.95 ± 6.96 vs. 50.31 ± 5.74; 95% CI, 2.88–7.27; P < 0.001) while comparing to NoDR eyes. However, in intragroup comparison of diabetic eyes with myopia, only SVD demonstrated decrease (41.68 ± 3.34 vs. 45.99 ± 4.17; 95% CI, 1.10–7.22; P = 0.002) in DR eyes while comparing to NoDR ones (**Figures 2, 3**).

DISCUSSION

The effect of myopia on VD was complicated. In healthy adults, myopia were reported to decrease the VD in either peripapillary (10, 17), the macula (8), or in both regions (6, 9). The possible mechanism was that excessive elongation of the globe would cause thinning of the retina and result in reduced oxygen demand. Alternatively, the elongation of globe would mechanically stretch retinal tissue, resulting in decreased vascular endothelial growth factor production (18, 19). Both mechanisms would possibly result in reduced retinal microvascular density. The fact that myopic changes were mainly located in the peripapillary area compared to the parafoveal area (20) made

TABLE 2 | Differences of RNFL and VD between non-myopic and myopic eyes of diabetes.

	Non-myopic eyes (n = 195)	Myopic eyes (n = 55)	F	P-value
Thickness of RNFL (μm) (range)	100.67 ± 13.68 (40.80–148.00)	95.50 ± 12.35 (63.70–116.90)	5.020	0.026*
Superior (μm)	121.72 ± 20.85 (34.30–180.00)	120.43 ± 19.71 (66.50–155.10)	0.132	0.716
Nasal (μm)	75.04 ± 16.11 (43.60–163.50)	68.56 ± 10.27 (45.10–85.10)	6.037	0.015*
Inferior (μm)	127.65 ± 20.52 (34.00–217.10)	119.97 ± 23.28 (51.80–206.50)	4.298	0.039*
Temporal (μm)	77.23 ± 13.47 (36.80–131.20)	73.81 ± 12.85 (39.80–95.80)	3.054	0.082
Whole VD of ONH (%) (range)	49.14 ± 4.33 (36.97–65.65)	45.89 ± 5.76 (29.71–53.05)	19.052	<0.001*
Peripapillary VD (%) (range)	50.76 ± 4.51 (33.43–61.39)	48.75 ± 6.56 (28.15–58.44)	7.600	0.006*
SVD (%) (range)	45.30 ± 4.97 (29.34–55.87)	45.05 ± 4.36 (35.19–53.24)	0.037	0.847
DVD (%) (range)	44.38 ± 6.53 (18.21–62.83)	44.61 ± 6.16 (31.05–59.96)	0.956	0.329
FD300 area density (%) (range)	48.39 ± 6.70 (27.06–60.74)	48.88 ± 7.19 (30.80–61.93)	1.448	0.230

*RNFL, retinal nerve fiber layer; ONH, optic nerve head; VD, vessel density; SVD, superficial vessel density; DVD, deep vessel density. *Indicates statistically significant difference between the groups. $P < 0.05$ were considered statistically significant.*

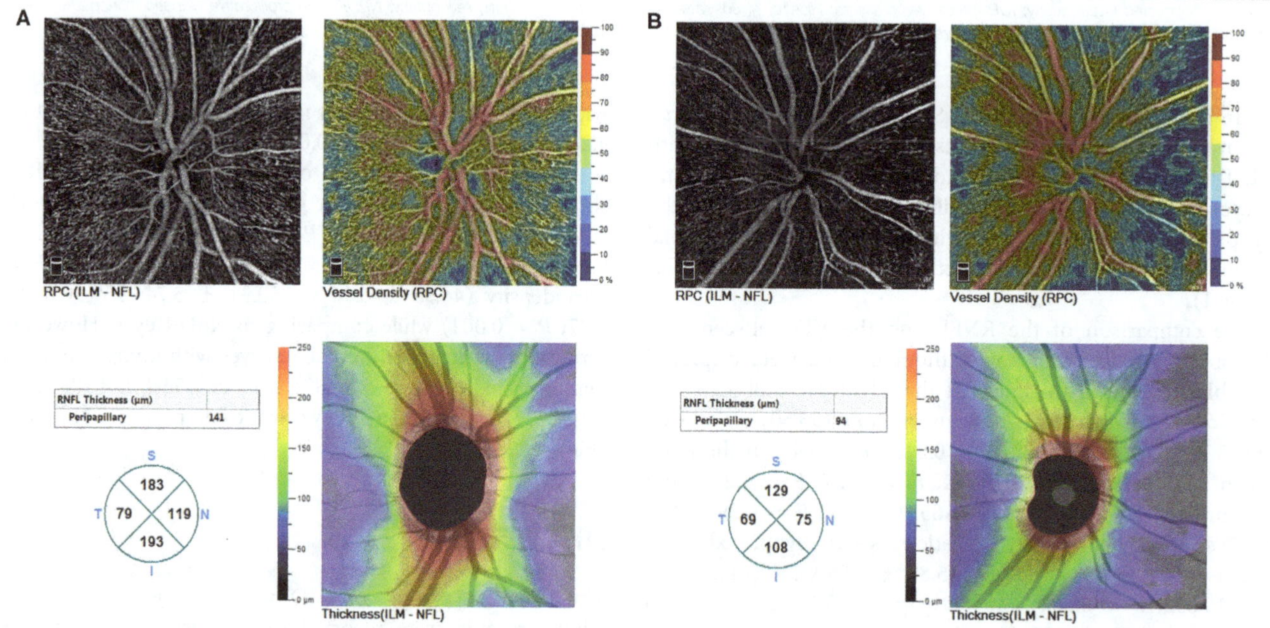

FIGURE 1 | (A) A non-myopic eye without DR (a right eye of a male patient aged 47). **(B)** A myopic eye without DR (a right eye of a male patient aged 21). Whole VD of ONH, peripapillary VD, and thickness of RNFL demonstrated a decreased trend from non-myopic to myopic eyes. DR, diabetic retinopathy; VD, vessel density; ONH, optic nerve head; RNFL, the retinal nerve fiber layer.

peripapillary area more vulnerable to the elongating effect of myopia in healthy controls. In diabetic eyes of our study, only reduced VD of ONH, but not VD of macula, were observed in myopic eyes compared to non-myopic ones. The reason could be that compared to normal individuals, diabetic patients had thinner RNFL (21) which might required less regional oxygen and blood supply in the peripapillary area, resulting in the reduction of VD in peripapillary region via autoregulatory

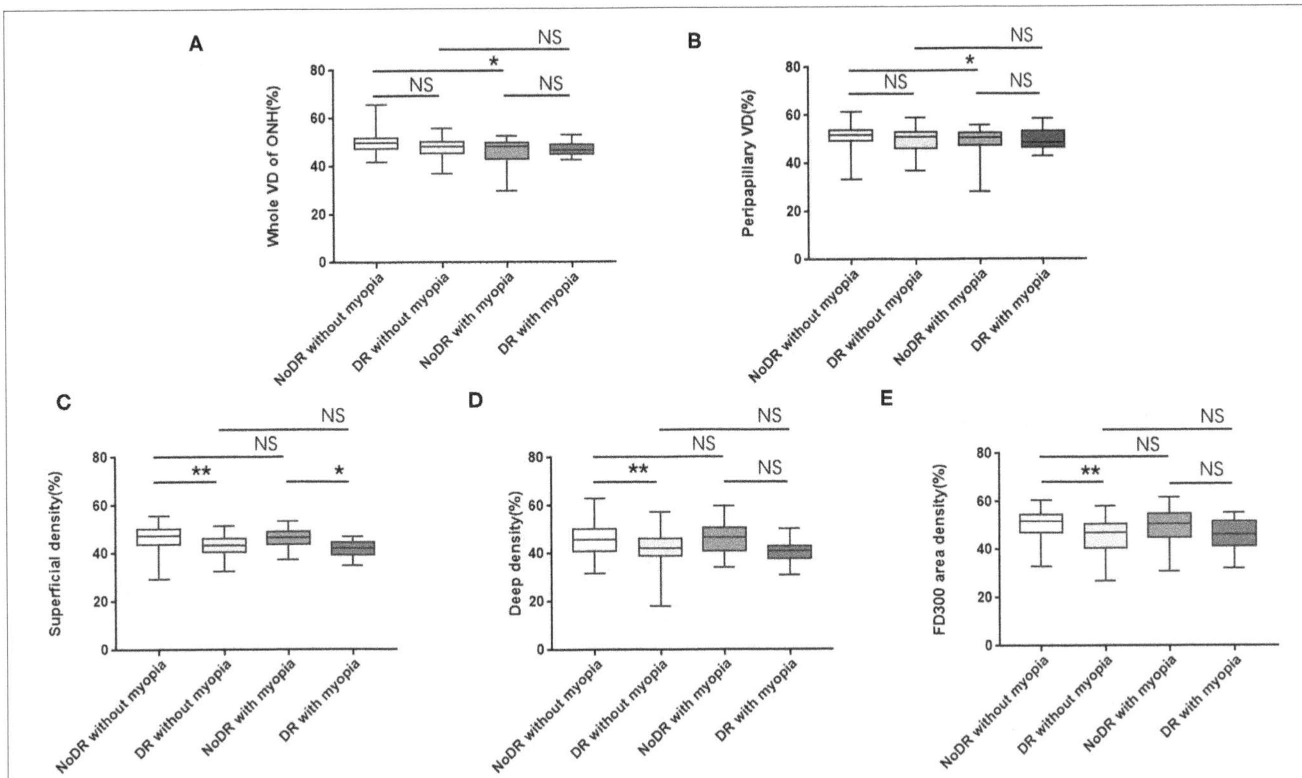

FIGURE 2 | Differences in VD of ONH and macula among subgroups **(A–E)**. VD, vessel density; ONH, optic nerve head; NoDR, diabetic eyes without diabetic retinopathy; DR, eyes with diabetic retinopathy; NS, no significant. $^*P < 0.05$; $^{**}P < 0.001$. $P < 0.05$ were considered statistically significant.

mechanisms (20). The superimposed effect of myopia and diabetes on the reduced RNFL thickness would make the VD of ONH more susceptive than the VD in macular region in diabetic patients.

As demonstrated in our further subgroup analysis, the association of myopia with reduction of VD in ONH were only significant in NoDR eyes, but not in DR eyes. It was suggested that, in NoDR eyes, myopia probably played an independent role in the reduction of VD apart from the effect of diabetes. However, in eyes with DR, myopia played a minor role compared to that of DR, or the deteriorated effect of DR on the VD overwhelmed the protective effect of myopia. The result was consistent with other study, although the researchers did not take myopia or axial length into consideration (22). There were also several studies reporting different results that peripapillary VD of both NoDR and DR patients were lower comparing to VD of normal controls. These discrepancies could be explained by the fact that there were no significant differences in axial length among NoDR, DR, and control groups in the study (23) or that myopia and axial length were not considered while analyzing the OCTA parameters (24–26).

In diabetic eyes with and without DR, the microvascular alterations in macular region varied while considering myopia. Our results suggested that DR were closely associated with decreased SVD, DVD, and FD300 area density in non-myopic eyes; however, in myopic eyes, only SVD exhibited reduction while comparing DR eyes to NoDR eyes. The change of DVD between DR and NoDR eyes in myopic group was not so dramatic as that in non-myopic group, probably implying that myopia could protect the retinal microvasculature from severe damage of DR via DVD. The possible mechanism was that the axial elongation caused retinal neurodysfunction particularly in the outer retina (27), resulting in reduced metabolic demand and consequent decrease in the VD particularly in outer retina. Degenerative changes in the outer retina would therefore increase the facility of oxygen acquisition in inner retina to partly alleviate the hypoxic assaults in outer retina (28) and therefore alleviated the reduction of SVD in diabetes. However, even in myopic eyes, DR were closely related the decrease of SVD, indicating that in myopic eyes, SVD could alternatively serve as a sensitive indicator of microvascular alterations of DR. The effect of myopia could partly explain the conflicting results of other studies in which either SVD or DVD (or both) were decreased in DR (29, 30). Therefore, we also suggested that when analyzing the VD in macular region, axial length, and myopia should be considered.

This study had several limitations. First, a relatively high proportion of younger patients were included in the group of diabetic patients with myopia. Based on a recent study indicating that VD did not change significantly with age (31), the difference between myopic and non-myopic patients was not considered interfering in the study. However, considering other studies showed a significant decrease in VD with age in Chinese population (32), we speculated that the effect of myopia was underestimated. Second, our study shared the limitations

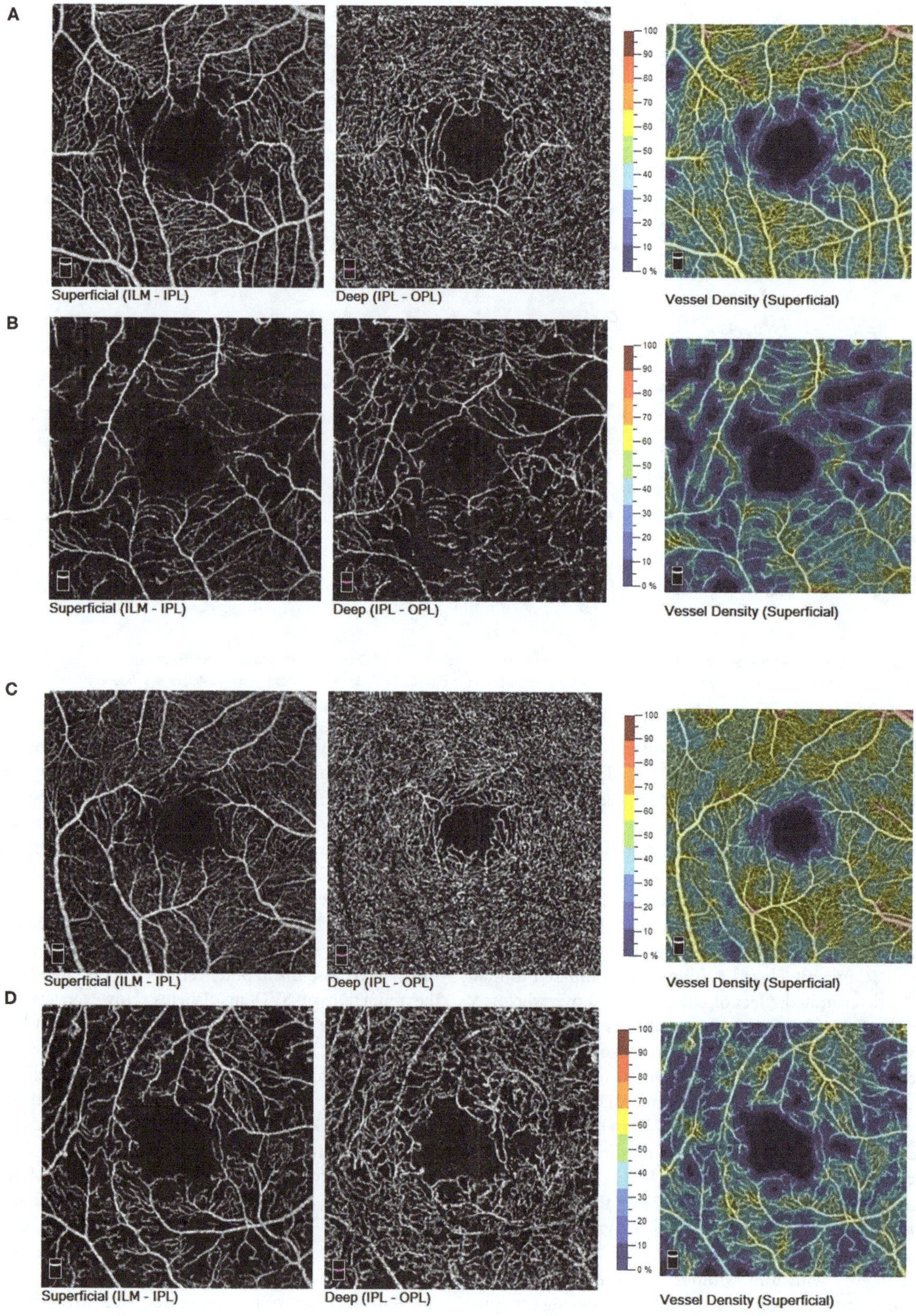

FIGURE 3 | In non-myopic eyes of diabetic patients, both SVD and DVD showed decreased trend from NoDR eyes **(A)** to DR eyes **(B)**. In myopic eyes of diabetic patients, only SVD demonstrated a decreased trend from NoDR eyes **(C)** to DR eyes **(D)**. SVD, superficial vessel density; DVD, deep vessel density; NoDR, diabetes without diabetic retinopathy; DR, diabetic retinopathy.

of cross-sectional studies that could not confirm causation. The question regarded to whether microvascular alterations in myopic eyes occurred before or after RD remained uncertain. Further prospective longitudinal studies were needed. Third, the SVD would superimpose on the DVD. The artifact was called "projection artifact." Additionally, the OCTA software could introduce artifacts such as loss of detail, doubling of vessels, stretching defects, or false flow artifact (33). In the present study, we excluded OCTA images with significant projection artifacts and other software-induced artifacts to minimize the interference. Nevertheless, it was impossible to completely avoid artifacts which might inevitably exert some confounding effects on the analyses.

In summary, our findings suggested that in diabetic patients, myopic eyes showed lower DR prevalence and thinner RNFL thickness at the nasal and inferior region. In NoDR period, myopia were closely related to the reduction of whole VD of ONH and peripapillary VD. DR were closely related to the reduction of SVD and DVD in non-myoptic eyes, but were closely related to the reduction of SVD in myopic eyes. When analyzing microvascular alterations in diabetic eyes, axial length, and myopia should be taken into consideration.

ETHICS STATEMENT

The study was approved by the research Ethics Committee of Sun Yat-sen Memorial Hospital, Sun Yat-sen University. The patients/participants provided their written informed consent to participate in this study. Written informed consent was obtained from the individual(s) for the publication of any potentially identifiable images or data included in this article.

AUTHOR CONTRIBUTIONS

XW, YZ, and YL: design. XW and ZL: conduct of the study and analysis. XW and XL: collection and preparation. XW, XL, and JX: management. XW, YZ, and JX: interpretation of data. XW, ZL, YZ, and YL: review. XW, ZL, YZ, JX, XL, and YL: approval of the manuscript. All authors contributed to the article and approved the submitted version.

REFERENCES

1. Jee D, Lee WK, Kang S. Prevalence and risk factors for diabetic retinopathy: the Korea National Health and Nutrition Examination Survey 2008-2011. *Invest Ophthalmol Vis Sci.* (2013) 54:6827–33. doi: 10.1167/iovs.13-12654
2. Moss SE, Klein R, Klein BE. Ocular factors in the incidence and progression of diabetic retinopathy. *Ophthalmology.* (1994) 101:77–83. doi: 10.1016/S0161-6420(94)31353-4
3. Dogru M, Inoue M, Nakamura M, Yamamoto M. Modifying factors related to asymmetric diabetic retinopathy. *Eye.* (1998) 12:929–33. doi: 10.1038/eye.1998.241
4. Wang X, Tang L, Gao L, Yang Y, Cao D, Li Y. Myopia and diabetic retinopathy: a systematic review and meta-analysis. *Diabetes Res Clin Pract.* (2016) 111:1–9. doi: 10.1016/j.diabres.2015.10.020
5. Ng DS, Cheung CY, Luk FO, Mohamed S, Brelen ME, Yam JC, et al. Advances of optical coherence tomography in myopia and pathologic myopia. *Eye.* (2016) 30:901–16. doi: 10.1038/eye.2016.47
6. Sung MS, Lee TH, Heo H, Park SW. Association between optic nerve head deformation and retinal microvasculature in high myopia. *Am J Ophthalmol.* (2018) 188:81–90. doi: 10.1016/j.ajo.2018.01.033
7. Spaide RF, Fujimoto JG, Waheed NK, Sadda SR, Staurenghi G. Optical coherence tomography angiography. *Prog Retin Eye Res.* (2018) 64:1–55. doi: 10.1016/j.preteyeres.2017.11.003
8. Fan H, Chen HY, Ma HJ, Chang Z, Yin HQ, Ng DS, et al. Reduced macular vascular density in myopic eyes. *Chinese Med J.* (2017) 130:445–51. doi: 10.4103/0366-6999.199844
9. He J, Chen Q, Yin Y, Zhou H, Fan Y, Zhu J, et al. Association between retinal microvasculature and optic disc alterations in high myopia. *Eye.* (2019) 33:1494–503. doi: 10.1038/s41433-019-0438-7
10. Wen C, Pei C, Xu X, Lei J. Influence of axial length on parafoveal and peripapillary metrics from swept source optical coherence tomography angiography. *Curr Eye Res.* (2019) 44:980–6. doi: 10.1080/02713683.2019.1607393
11. Bhanushali D, Anegondi N, Gadde SG, Srinivasan P, Chidambara L, Yadav NK, et al. Linking retinal microvasculature features with severity of diabetic retinopathy using optical coherence tomography angiography. *Invest Ophthalmol Vis Sci.* (2016) 57:519–25. doi: 10.1167/iovs.15-18901
12. Khadamy J, Abri Aghdam K, Falavarjani KG. An update on optical coherence tomography angiography in diabetic retinopathy. *J Ophthalmic Vis Res.* (2018) 13:487–97. doi: 10.4103/jovr.jovr_57_18
13. Li Z, Wen X, Zeng P, Liao Y, Fan S, Zhang Y, et al. Do microvascular changes occur preceding neural impairment in early-stage diabetic retinopathy? Evidence based on the optic nerve head using optical coherence tomography angiography. *Acta Diabetol.* (2019) 56:531–9. doi: 10.1007/s00592-019-01288-8
14. Li Z, Alzogool M, Xiao J, Zhang S, Zeng P, Lan Y. Optical coherence tomography angiography findings of neurovascular changes in type 2 diabetes mellitus patients without clinical diabetic retinopathy. *Acta Diabetol.* (2018) 55:1075–82. doi: 10.1007/s00592-018-1202-3
15. He J, Xu X, Zhu J, Zhu B, Zhang B, Lu L, et al. Lens power, axial length-to-corneal radius ratio, and association with diabetic retinopathy in the adult population with type 2 diabetes. *Ophthalmology.* (2017) 124:326–35. doi: 10.1016/j.ophtha.2016.10.041
16. Shin JW, Kwon J, Lee J, Kook MS. Choroidal microvasculature dropout is not associated with myopia, but is associated with glaucoma. *J Glaucoma.* (2018) 27:189–96. doi: 10.1097/IJG.0000000000000859
17. Sung MS, Lee TH, Heo H, Park SW. Clinical features of superficial and deep peripapillary microvascular density in healthy myopic eyes. *PLoS ONE.* (2017) 12:e0187160. doi: 10.1371/journal.pone.0187160
18. Chen W, Song H, Xie S, Han Q, Tang X, Chu Y. Correlation of macular choroidal thickness with concentrations of aqueous vascular endothelial growth factor in high myopia. *Curr Eye Res.* (2015) 40:307–13. doi: 10.3109/02713683.2014.973043
19. Shin YJ, Nam WH, Park SE, Kim JH, Kim HK. Aqueous humor concentrations of vascular endothelial growth factor and pigment epithelium-derived factor in high myopic patients. *Mol Vis.* (2012) 18:2265–70.
20. Wang X, Kong X, Jiang C, Li M, Yu J, Sun X. Is the peripapillary retinal perfusion related to myopia in healthy eyes? A prospective comparative study. *BMJ Open.* (2016) 6:e010791. doi: 10.1136/bmjopen-2015-010791
21. Mehboob MA, Amin ZA, Islam QU. Comparison of retinal nerve fiber layer thickness between normal population and patients with diabetes

mellitus using optical coherence tomography. *Pak J Med Sci.* (2019) 35:29–33. doi: 10.12669/pjms.35.1.65

22. Feng K, Hu YT, Ma Z. Prognostic indicators for no light perception after open-globe injury: eye injury vitrectomy study. *Am J Ophthalmol.* (2012) 153:777. doi: 10.1016/j.ajo.2011.12.003
23. Shin YI, Nam KY, Lee SE, Lee MW, Lim HB, Jo YJ, et al. Peripapillary microvasculature in patients with diabetes mellitus: an optical coherence tomography angiography study. *Sci Rep.* (2019) 9:15814. doi: 10.1038/s41598-019-52354-8
24. Cao D, Yang D, Yu H, Xie J, Zeng Y, Wang J, et al. Optic nerve head perfusion changes preceding peripapillary retinal nerve fibre layer thinning in preclinical diabetic retinopathy. *Clin Experiment Ophthalmol.* (2019) 47:219–25. doi: 10.1111/ceo.13390
25. Rodrigues TM, Marques JP, Soares M, Dolan MJ, Melo P, Simão S, et al. Peripapillary neurovascular coupling in the early stages of diabetic retinopathy. *Retina.* (2019) 39:2292–302. doi: 10.1097/IAE.0000000000002328
26. Vujosevic S, Muraca A, Gatti V, Masoero L, Brambilla M, Cannillo B, et al. Peripapillary microvascular and neural changes in diabetes mellitus: an OCT-Angiography study. *Invest Ophthalmol Vis Sci.* (2018) 59:5074–81. doi: 10.1167/iovs.18-24891
27. Man REK, Gan ATL, Gupta P, Fenwick EK, Sabanayagam C, Tan NYQ, et al. Is myopia associated with the incidence and progression of diabetic retinopathy? *Am J Ophthalmol.* (2019) 208:226–33. doi: 10.1016/j.ajo.2019.05.012
28. Sawada O, Miyake T, Kakinoki M, Sawada T, Kawamura H, Ohji M. Negative correlation between aqueous vascular endothelial growth factor levels and axial length. *Jpn J Ophthalmol.* (2011) 55:401–4. doi: 10.1007/s10384-011-0027-1
29. Al-Sheikh M, Akil H, Pfau M, Sadda SR. Swept-source OCT angiography imaging of the foveal avascular zone and macular capillary network density in diabetic retinopathy. *Invest Ophthalmol Vis Sci.* (2016) 57:3907–13. doi: 10.1167/iovs.16-19570
30. Carnevali A, Sacconi R, Corbelli E, Tomasso L, Querques L, Zerbini G, et al. Optical coherence tomography angiography analysis of retinal vascular plexuses and choriocapillaris in patients with type 1 diabetes without diabetic retinopathy. *Acta Diabetol.* (2017) 54:695–702. doi: 10.1007/s00592-017-0996-8
31. Gadde SG, Anegondi N, Bhanushali D, Chidambara L, Yadav NK, Khurana A, et al. Quantification of vessel density in retinal optical coherence tomography angiography images using local fractal dimension. *Invest Ophthalmol Vis Sci.* (2016) 57:246–52. doi: 10.1167/iovs.15-18287
32. Yu J, Jiang C, Wang X, Zhu L, Gu R, Xu H, et al. Macular perfusion in healthy Chinese: an optical coherence tomography angiogram study. *Invest Ophthalmol Vis Sci.* (2015) 56:3212–7. doi: 10.1167/iovs.14-16270
33. Spaide RF, Fujimoto JG, Waheed NK. Image artifacts in optical coherence tomography angiography. *Retina.* (2015) 35:2163–80. doi: 10.1097/IAE.0000000000000765

14

Change of Retinal Vessels in Different Sectors of the Parapapillary Area in Primary Open-Angle Glaucoma

Jingyi Cheng [1,2,3†], Hongmei Zhao [1,2,3†], Chunhui Jiang [1,2,3], Xiangmei Kong [1,2,3] and Xinghuai Sun [1,2,3,4*]*

[1] Department of Ophthalmology and Visual Science, Eye, Ear, Nose and Throat Hospital, Fudan University, Shanghai, China, [2] Key Laboratory of Myopia, Ministry of Health, Fudan University, Shanghai, China, [3] Shanghai Key Laboratory of Visual Impairment and Restoration, Fudan University, Shanghai, China, [4] State Key Laboratory of Medical Neurobiology, Institutes of Brain Science, Fudan University, Shanghai, China

***Correspondence:**
Chunhui Jiang
chhjiang70@163.com
Xinghuai Sun
xhsun@shmu.edu.cn

†These authors have contributed equally to this work and share first authorship

Purpose: To investigate the changes in the retinal vessels (RVs) in different sectors in patients with primary open-angle glaucoma (POAG), and their possible correlations with retinal nerve fiber layer thickness (RNFLT) and visual-field defects in the temporal parapapillary region.

Methods: The RV diameters, RNFLTs, and visual-field parameters were measured. The temporal parapapillary region was divided into the temporal (T, 315°-45°), temporal superior (TS, 45°-90°), and temporal inferior sectors (TI, 270°-315°). The changes in the RV diameters in each sector were determined, and their relationships with RNFLT, the mean deviation (MD), and visual field sensitivity (VFS) were examined.

Results: Fifty POAG patients (50 eyes) and 50 healthy subjects (50 eyes) were included. Compared with the healthy subjects, the POAG group had a significantly smaller accumulated parapapillary RV diameter ($P < 0.001$), which was positively correlated with the MD and RNFLT. When the different temporal sectors were examined, the accumulated RV diameters were significantly smaller in the POAG group than in the healthy controls in the TI and T sectors, but not in the TS sector. The accumulated diameters in the TI and T sectors were correlated with the corresponding RNFLTs (all $P < 0.05$), but only the accumulated diameter in the TI sector was correlated with the VFS.

Conclusions: In POAG, the changes in the RVs differed between different temporal sectors, with the most prominent changes occurring in the TI and T sectors.

Keywords: retinal vessel, retinal nerve fiber layer thickness, visual field, primary open-angle glaucoma, parapapillary area

INTRODUCTION

The retinal vascular caliber is a structural marker of microvascular changes in the fundus, and studies have shown that a smaller retinal vascular caliber is correlated with thinner neuroretinal rim tissue (1), a larger vertical cup-to-disc ratio (2, 3), greater nerve fiber layer visibility (1), and the presence of glaucoma (4–6). Previous studies have examined the relationship between the retinal vessel (RV) diameter and the retinal nerve fiber layer thickness (RNFLT) in patients with primary open-angle glaucoma (POAG), but the results were contradictory (7–12). It has also been reported that the RVs in different sectors respond differently in POAG. The main manifestation of glaucomatous visual field (VF) damage is the nasal VF defect (13), including arcuate scotoma in superior or/and inferior visual field, paracentral scotomas, arcs, or nasal steps, and the main blood vessels are in the temporal region (14–16). Therefore, in this study, the RV diameters in subjects with POAG were measured by optical coherence tomography (OCT), together with the RNFLTs, VF parameters, and more attention was paid on the differences in the RVs in different sectors of the temporal parapapillary region, which was corresponding to the nasal VF.

MATERIALS AND METHODS

Ethics Statement

This study was performed in accordance with the tenets of the Declaration of Helsinki and was approved by the Medical Ethics Committee of the Eye and ENT Hospital, Fudan University, Shanghai, China. All subjects provided written informed consent to their inclusion in the study after being provided an explanation of the study.

Study Subjects

All subjects underwent a routine ophthalmic examination that included assessment of medical history, best-corrected visual acuity (BCVA), slit-lamp biomicroscopy, gonioscopy (only patients with glaucoma), Goldmann applanation tonometry (Haag Streit AG, Bern, Switzerland), central corneal thickness (CCT; EM-3000, Tomey, Japan), axial length (AL; IOLMaster 500, Carl Zeiss Meditech, Inc., Dublin, CA), and VF testing with Humphrey automated perimetry (SITA 24-2, Carl Zeiss Meditech, Inc., Dublin, CA). The Spectralis OCT+HRA system (Heidelberg Engineering, Heidelberg, Germany) was used to measure RNFLT and RV diameters.

POAG Group

Patients with POAG who visited the Ophthalmology Department of the Eye and ENT Hospital, Fudan University, Shanghai, between January and June 2014 were recruited. The inclusion criteria for the POAG group were: (1) age $\geq$ 30 years old; (2) glaucomatous damage to the optic disc, defined as the presence of at least two of the following characteristics: cup/disc ratio $\geq$ 0.6, cup/disc asymmetry $>$ 0.2, diffuse or focal neural rim thinning, disc hemorrhage, localized rim loss, or nerve fiber layer defects indicative of glaucoma; (3) typical and reliable VF defects, defined as the presence of at least two of the following: a cluster of $\geq$3 non-edge points detected with Humphrey automated perimetry, all of which were depressed on the pattern deviation plot at the $P < 5\%$ level and one of which was depressed at the $P < 1\%$ level, or a glaucoma hemifield test result outside the normal limits, together with a pattern standard deviation of $<$5% of normal fields, fixation losses of $\leq$20%; or $\leq$15% false-positive or false-negative responses; and (4) a normal anterior chamber and open angle based on slit-lamp and gonioscopic examinations.

Patients were excluded if one or more of the following was present: (1) any other ophthalmic disease, such as trauma, inflammation, or retinal or neurological problems that could result in optic-nerve or VF defects; (2) patients with a shallow anterior chamber, narrow angle, or angle closure based on slit-lamp and gonioscopic examinations; (3) diopters < -6 D or $>$ $+1$ D; or (4) AL $>$ 26 mm or $<$ 20 mm; (5) smokers, or those with excessive alcohol consumption, hypertension, diabetes mellitus, or any other circulatory system disease; and (6) patients deemed unsuitable for the study by the researchers.

Control Group

Healthy, non-smoking volunteers were recruited. The inclusion criteria were: (1) BCVA $>$ 0.8; (2) diopters between $+1$ and -6 D; (3) intraocular pressure (IOP) $\leq$ 21 mmHg; and (4) AL of 20–26 mm. Individuals with an ocular disease, excessive alcohol consumption, hypertension, diabetes mellitus, any other circulatory system disease, or those with VF test results outside the normal limits were excluded.

Main Ophthalmic Measurements and Analysis

The VF was tested and different sectors were divided by the method described by Kanamori and Akiyasu (17). Among those sectors, three sectors were evaluated: temporal (T; 315°-45°), temporal superior (TS; 45°-90°), and temporal inferior (TI; 270°-315°) sectors (**Figure 1**). The regional VF sensitivity (VFS) was calculated as the sum of the pattern deviations in the corresponding sector.

A circular scan with a 3.4 mm diameter centered on the optic nerve head was performed through undilated pupils with the Spectralis OCT + HRA system. The automatic real time was set to 100 for maximal quality and resolution of the OCT images. Near-infrared reflectance (IR) images were obtained simultaneously. The average parapapillary RNFLT and the average RNFLTs in the T (315°-45°), TS (45°-90°), and TI (270°-315°) sectors were determined using the Spectralis software (Heidelberg Eye Explorer, version 1.0.10.0) (**Figure 2**).

The RVs were identified on the OCT images based on the near-infrared images. The method used to measure the RV diameters on spectral domain OCT has been described (18). Briefly, the brightness and contrast settings used for the IR images were: "black on white" for the color table, "medium" for sharpening, and "none" for noise reduction. The RV diameter was measured as the maximum reflectance shadowing width on the retinal pigment epithelium (RPE) layer. The RV diameter obtained from IR images was measured vertically to the vessel axis with the caliber tool from the Spectralis software at the crossing point of vessel and OCT scanning line. The overall sums of the parapapillary RV diameters and the sums for the T (315°-45°), TS (45°-90°), and TI (270°-315°) sectors were calculated (**Figure 3**) and listed as the accumulated RV diameters of the parapapillary and different sectors.

Data and Statistical Analysis

One eye from each of the eligible POAG subjects and the healthy subjects was randomly selected for the study using a web-based research randomization tool (19). Statistical analyses were performed using SPSS for Mac, version 23.0. Categorical variables were described as frequencies and constituent ratios, and were

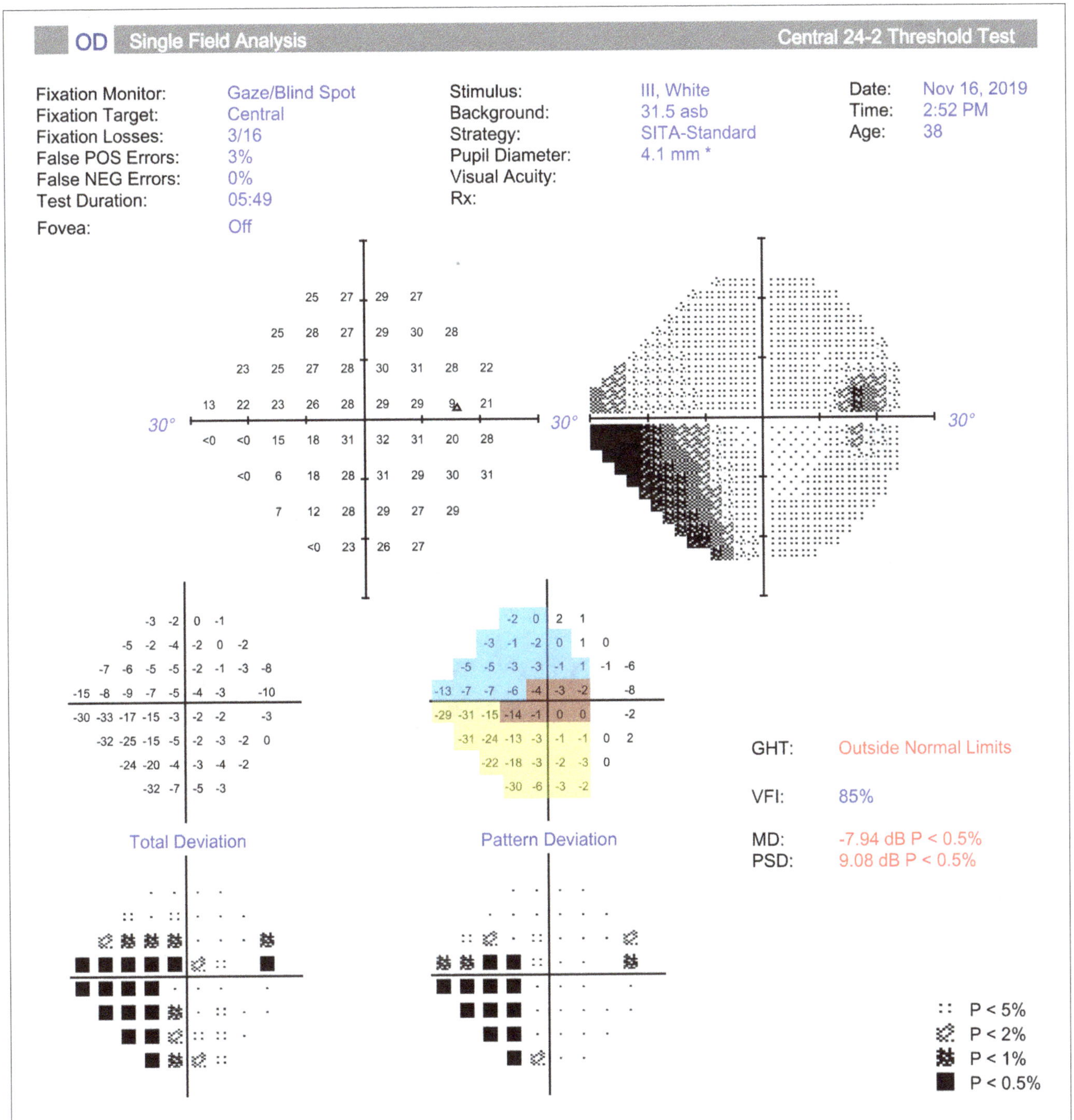

FIGURE 1 | Measurement and regionalized of the visual field (VF) were demonstrated. The VF was tested (Humphrey automated perimetry SITA 24-2), and regionalized into the temporal (T) (315°-45°, red area), temporal superior (TS) (45°-90°, yellow area), and temporal inferior (TI) (270°-315°, blue area) sectors according to previous study. Regional visual field sensitivity (VFS) was calculated as the sum of the pattern deviations in a specific sector.

analyzed with χ^2 tests. Continuous variables were described as means and standard deviations (SD). Statistical comparisons between the POAG patients and healthy subjects were made using independent-samples two-tailed *t*-tests. The correlations between the accumulated parapapillary RV diameter and RNFLT or VFS were determined using Pearson's correlation coefficient. A *P*-value < 0.05 was defined as statistically significant.

RESULTS

Demographic and Ophthalmic Characteristics of the Participants

In total, 50 POAG patients (50 eyes) and 50 healthy subjects (50 eyes) were included in the study. The POAG group had a higher IOP than the control group ($P < 0.001$) and all of the

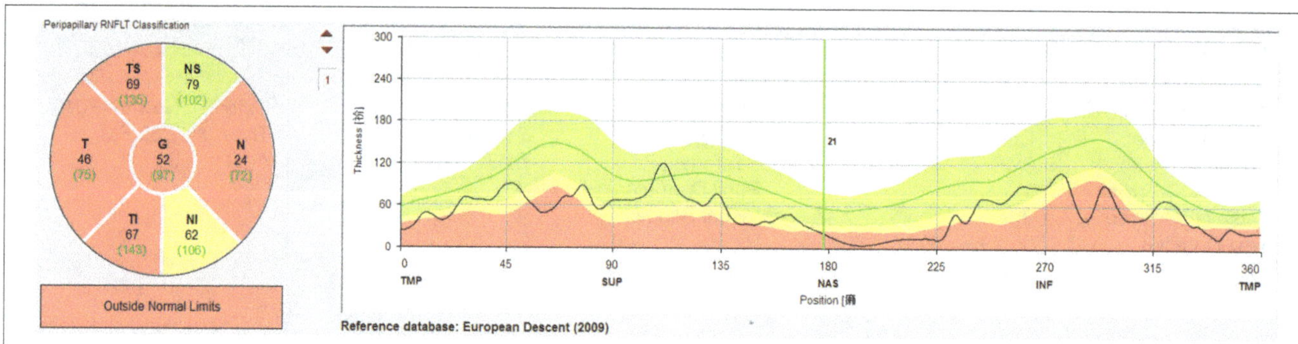

FIGURE 2 | Measurement and regionalized of the retinal nerve fiber layer thickness (RNFLT) were demonstrated. A circular scan with a 3.4 mm diameter centered on the optic nerve head was performed through undilated pupils with the Spectralis OCT + HRA system. The average parapapillary RNFLT(G) and the average RNFLTs in the T (315°-45°), TS (45°-90°), and TI (270°-315°) sectors were obtained with the Spectralis viewing software (Heidelberg Eye Explorer, version 1.0.10.0).

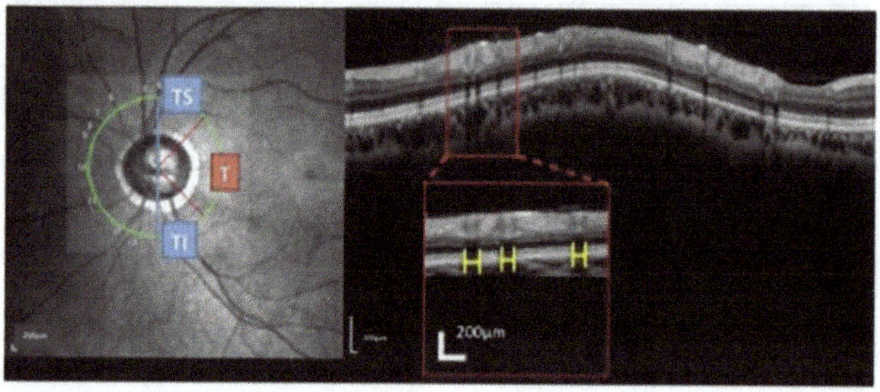

FIGURE 3 | Measurement and regionalized of the retinal vessels (RV) diameter were demonstrated. Using the Spectralis OCT + HRA system, a circular scan with a 3.4 mm diameter centered on the optic nerve was performed through natural pupils. Near-infrared reflectance images were obtained simultaneously. The retinal vessel (RV) diameter was measured as the maximum reflectance shadowing width on the retinal pigment epithelium layer. Using Spectralis software (Heidelberg Eye Explorer, version 1.0.10.0), scales (yellow bar) were drawn and measured. The sums of the overall parapapillary RV diameters, and the average parapapillary RNFLTs were determined for the entire region and for the T (315°-45°), TS (45°-90°), and TI sectors (270°-315°) individually.

enrolled POAG patients used only one antiglaucoma medication, a prostaglandin analog. The sex and age distributions and other characteristics of both groups were similar (**Table 1**).

Accumulated RVs and RNFLTs in the POAG Group

The POAG group had significantly smaller accumulated parapapillary RV diameters and thinner parapapillary RNFLTs ($P < 0.001$) than the control group (**Table 2**). For the individual temporal sectors, the RNFLTs in the T, TS, and TI sectors were significantly thinner (all $P < 0.001$), and the accumulated RV diameters in the T and TI sectors were significantly smaller ($P = 0.001$ and $P = 0.002$, respectively) in the POAG group than the control group.

Correlations Among Accumulated RVs, RNFLT, and VFS

In the POAG group, the accumulated parapapillary RV diameter was positively correlated with the MD value ($r = 0.30$, $P = 0.02$) and the RNFLT ($r = 0.40$, $P = 0.004$). For the individual sectors, the accumulated RV diameter in the TI sector was correlated with the corresponding VFS ($r = 0.28$, $P = 0.03$) and RNFLT ($r = 0.45$, $P = 0.001$). The accumulated RV diameter in the T sector was correlated with the corresponding RNFLT ($r = 0.49$, $P < 0.001$) but not with VFS ($r = 0.18$, $P = 0.15$). No significant correlations were detected in the TS sector (**Table 3**).

DISCUSSION

To analyze the differences in the change or damage of RVs in the parapapillary areas in POAG eyes, especially in the temporal side, a group of patients with POAG and healthy controls were recruited. The accumulated parapapillary RV diameter was significantly smaller in the POAG group, and the reductions were most prominent in the TI and T sectors in the studied area. The accumulated parapapillary RV diameter was correlated with both RNFLT and the MD, but when the sectors were analyzed individually, the accumulated RV diameter was only significantly correlated with both RNFLT and VFS in the TI sector.

TABLE 1 | Demographics and ophthalmic characteristics of the POAG and control groups.

	POAG group $N = 50$	Control group $N = 50$	t	P-value
Age	43.50 ± 13.36	38.92 ± 10.75	1.889	0.06
Sex (n, %)			2.966	0.23
Male (n, %)	28 (56%)	28 (56%)		
Female (n, %)	22 (44%)	22 (44%)		1.00
IOP (mmHg)	22.03 ± 5.75	14.76 ± 4.97	5.537	<0.001*
BCVA	0.88 ± 0.21	0.96 ± 0.22	−0.773	0.45
Diopters	−3.54 ± 2.52	−2.46 ± 3.00	−0.977	0.34
CCT (μm)	527.17 ± 42.53	540.92 ± 37.89	0.188	0.09
AL (mm)	24.67 ± 1.22	24.22 ± 1.18	1.895	0.06
MD	−8.27 ± 4.99	−1.44 ± 1.14	−5.053	<0.001*
PSD	8.44 ± 4.31	1.58 ± 0.29	5.932	<0.001*

Statistical comparisons between the POAG and control groups were made with a χ^2 test or an independent-samples two-tailed t-test.
POAG, primary open-angle glaucoma; IOP, intraocular pressure; BCVA, best corrected visual acuity; CCT, central corneal thickness; AL, axial length; MD, mean deviation; PSD, pattern standard deviation.
**Significantly different between the POAG and control groups at $P < 0.05$.*

TABLE 2 | Comparisons of RVs and RNFLT between the POAG and control groups.

	POAG group $N = 50$	Control group $N = 50$	t	P-value
Vessel diameter				
Parapapillary	1096.08 ± 158.62	1280.08 ± 156.01	−5.848	<0.001**
TS	247.58 ± 75.35	262.50 ± 71.25	−1.017	0.31
TI	217.64 ± 59.21	264.12 ± 71.88	−3.529	0.001**
T	126.28 ± 68.31	173.70 ± 83.12	−3.117	0.002*
RNFLT				
Parapapillary	65.46 ± 14.42	101.26 ± 13.32	−12.897	<0.001**
TS	91.76 ± 30.84	140.66 ± 21.20	−9.239	<0.001**
TI	63.72 ± 30.25	158.68 ± 28.54	−16.147	<0.001**
T	63.54 ± 20.11	88.24 ± 17.34	−6.578	<0.001**

Continuous variables are given as means ± SD. Statistical comparisons of the POAG and control groups were made with an independent-samples two-tailed t-test.
RV, retinal vessel; RNFLT, retinal nerve fiber thickness; POAG, primary open-angle glaucoma; T, temporal; TS, temporal superior; TI, temporal inferior.
**Significantly different between the POAG and control groups at $P < 0.05$.*
***Significantly different between the POAG and control groups at $P < 0.001$.*

TABLE 3 | Correlations between RV diameters and VFS or RNFLT within the parapapillary region and individual temporal sectors.

		Parapapillary	Temporal	Temporal superior	Temporal Inferior
VFS	r	0.30	0.18	−0.04	0.28
	P-value	0.02*	0.15	0.77	0.03*
RNFLT	r	0.40	0.49	0.27	0.45
	P-value	0.004*	<0.001**	0.06	0.001*

Pearson's correlation coefficient was used to determine correlations between the regional/sector RV diameters and VFS or RNFLT.
RV, retinal vessel; RNFLT, retinal nerve fiber layer thickness; VFS, visual-field sensitivity.
**Significant correlation at $P < 0.05$.*
***Significant correlation at $P < 0.001$.*

Consistent with previous studies that analyzed the changes in RV in glaucomatous eyes (6, 20, 21), this study shows that the accumulated parapapillary RV diameter was significantly smaller in the POAG group than in the control group. More importantly, we found that, whereas RNFLT was significantly reduced in all three temporal sectors, the RV diameter was significantly reduced in the TI ($P = 0.001$) and T ($P = 0.002$) sectors, but not in the TS sector ($P = 0.31$) (**Table 2**). Previously, Jonas et al. (7) reported that the RV diameter was significantly smaller in glaucomatous eyes, and that the difference was greatest for the TI artery. The more-severe damage to the vessels in the TI sector is consistent with the clinical observation of more frequent and more-severe damage to the neuroretinal rims in TI (22, 23) and the more-pronounced VF changes in the upper nasal quadrant (8, 13). The reason for this is not fully understood, but might be explained as follows. In healthy subjects, Shahidi et al. (24) found that the retinal oxygen saturation was significantly greater in the TS arterioles and venules than in the TI vessels. Moreover, the TI sector of the parapapillary retina was less responsive to vasodilation and more responsive to vasoconstriction than the TS sector (25). When Gazzard and Gus (13) compared the characteristics of the VF defects between patients with primary angle-closure glaucoma (PACG) and patients with POAG, they found that POAG occurs more frequently in the superior hemifield compared with PACG. The authors speculated that under certain conditions, such as glaucoma, the responses of the vessels in the TS and TI quadrants differ and contributes to the different susceptibilities of VF defects or vascular dysfunction in these sectors. This might indeed reflect non-pressure-related optic neuropathy. In this study, the RVs in the TI sector were most frequently impaired in the POAG eyes. Because IOP should be the same throughout the eye, and IOPs of some patients were in the normal range, the more-damaged vessels in the TI sector support the non-pressure-related reason in another way. Therefore, the RVs in different sectors may differ or be affected differently under different pathological conditions, so it is important to compare vessels within the same region.

The accumulated parapapillary RV diameter was correlated positively with MD and RNFLT, but when the sectors were examined individually, only the accumulated RV diameter in the TI sector was correlated with both the corresponding RNFLT and VFS. The relationship between the glaucomatous structural and functional changes is complex and the relationship between the reduced retinal blood flow and glaucoma remains controversial (7–12). For example, using fundus photographs, Zheng et al. (10) found a significant association between a narrower RV caliber and RNFL thinning in the healthy population, but not in patients with glaucoma. Although blood vessels themselves account for ~9% of the total RNFL area, studies had found that blood vessel locations outside the optic nerve head are sufficiently stable over glaucoma severity to represent individual eye anatomy and confirmed close relationship of blood vessel locations and RNFL thickness since arteries having lower diameters (14, 16).

Consistent with our results, Jonas et al. (7) showed that the retinal arteries were significantly wider where the rim area was larger, the rim notch was more distinct, and the RNFL score was higher. Radcliffe et al. (15) found a retinal blood vessel shifts in those eyes with functionally progressive glaucoma, as a result of adjacent neural tissue damage. Hall et al. (8) found a strong association between a reduced peripapillary arteriole diameter and VF defects in the corresponding hemifield in eyes with POAG. This also indicates a spatial correlation between a reduction in the vessel diameter and the glaucomatous damage in the corresponding region. The discrepancies in these findings may be attributable to the different instruments or analytical methods used, the different populations, or the severity of the disease.

It is interesting to note that the accumulated RV diameter in the T sector was correlated with the corresponding RNFLT, but not with the corresponding VFS. Many studies have presented evidence that structural damage often precedes detectable functional changes, and that the association between structure and function increases with increasing disease severity (26). It has been reported that VF abnormalities do not develop until a certain number (at least 25–35%) of retinal ganglion cells are lost (26, 27). The T sector includes the macular area, and has more ganglion cells than the other sectors. It was speculated that the neighboring retinal ganglion cells compensate for neighboring dead or dying cells until most of the cells in a region are no longer functional (26). This might partly explain our findings.

This study was limited by the relatively small sample and its cross-sectional design. Further research with more patients is required. A prospective study is still necessary to investigate the relationship between the vascular structure and the functional damage in glaucoma patients.

In conclusion, the RVs in different parapapillary regions change differently in POAG patients, and the vessels in the TI and T sectors seem to be most susceptible to damage.

ETHICS STATEMENT

The studies involving human participants were reviewed and approved by the Medical Ethics Committee of the Eye and ENT Hospital, Fudan University, Shanghai, China. The patients/participants provided their written informed consent to participate in this study.

AUTHOR CONTRIBUTIONS

JC collected data, performed analyses, and wrote the manuscript. HZ collected data and revised the manuscript. CJ revised the manuscript, gained the fund, and supervised the process. XK provided patients' information. XS gained the fund and supervised the process. All authors contributed to the article and approved the submitted version.

ACKNOWLEDGMENTS

The samples used for the analyses described in this manuscript were obtained from the EENT Biobank. We would like to thank all the participants and staff for their valuable contributions to this research.

REFERENCES

1. Jonas JB, Schiro D. Visibility of the normal retinal nerve fiber layer correlated with rim width and vessel caliber. *Graefes Arch Clin Exp Ophthalmol.* (1993) 231:207-11. doi: 10.1007/BF00918842
2. Lee KE, Klein B, Klein R, Meuer SM. Association of retinal vessel caliber to optic disc and cup diameters. *Invest Ophthalmol Vis Sci.* (2007) 48:63-7. doi: 10.1167/iovs.05-1203
3. Cheung N, Tong L, Tikellis G, Saw SM, Mitchell P, Wang JJ, et al. Relationship of retinal vascular caliber with optic disc diameter in children. *Invest Ophthalmol Vis Sci.* (2007) 48:4945-8. doi: 10.1167/iovs.07-0472
4. Frisén L, Claesson M. Narrowing of the retinal arterioles in descending optic atrophy - ophthalmology. *Ophthalmology.* (1984) 91:1342-6. doi: 10.1016/S0161-6420(84)34144-6
5. Amerasinghe N, Aung T, Cheung N, Fong CW, Wang JJ, Mitchell P, et al. Evidence of retinal vascular narrowing in glaucomatous eyes in an Asian population. *Invest Ophthalmol Vis Sci.* (2008) 49:5397-402. doi: 10.1167/iovs.08-2142
6. Mitchell P, Leung H, Wang JJ, Rochtchina E, Klein R. Retinal vessel diameter and open-angle glaucoma: the Blue Mountains Eye Study. *Ophthalmology.* (2005) 112:245-50. doi: 10.1016/j.ophtha.2004.08.015
7. Jonas JB, Nguyen XN, Naumann GO. Parapapillary chorioretinal atrophy in normal and glaucoma eyes. I. Morphometric data. *Invest Ophthalmol Vis Sci.* (1989) 30:908-18.
8. Hall JK, Andrews AP, Walker R, Piltz-Seymour JR. Association of retinal vessel caliber and visual field defects in glaucoma. *Am J Ophthalmol.* (2001) 132:855-9. doi: 10.1016/S0002-9394(01)01200-4
9. Schmidl D, Resch H, Rensch F, Hommer A, Vass C, Luksch A, et al. Correlation of optic disc morphology and ocular perfusion parameters in patients with primary open angle glaucoma. *Acta Ophthalmol.* (2008) 86. doi: 10.1111/j.1755-3768.2008.4457.x
10. Zheng Y, Cheung N, Aung T, Mitchell P, He M, Wong TY. Relationship of retinal vascular caliber with retinal nerve fiber layer thickness: the Singapore malay eye study. *Invest Ophthalmol Vis Sci.* (2009) 50:4091-6. doi: 10.1167/iovs.09-3444
11. Wolfs R. Changing views on open-angle glaucoma: definitions and prevalences–The Rotterdam Study. *Invest Ophthalmol Vis Sci.* (2000) 41:3309-21. doi: 10.1007/s004170000166
12. Jonas JB, Martus P, Horn FK, Jünemann A, Korth M, Budde WM. Predictive factors of the optic nerve head for development or progression of glaucomatous visual field loss. *Invest Ophthalmol Vis Sci.* (2004) 45:2613-8. doi: 10.1167/iovs.03-1274
13. Gazzard, Gus. The severity and spatial distribution of visual field defects in primary glaucoma: a comparison of primary open-angle glaucoma and

primary angle-closure glaucoma. *Arch Ophthalmol.* (2002) 120:1636-43. doi: 10.1001/archopht.120.12.1636
14. Elze T, Baniasadi N, Jin Q, Hui W, Wang M. Ametropia, retinal anatomy, and OCT abnormality patterns in glaucoma. 1. Impacts of refractive error and interartery angle. *J Biomed Opt.* (2017) 22:1. doi: 10.1117/1.JBO.22.12.121713
15. Radcliffe NM, Smith SD, Syed ZA, Park SC, Ehrlich JR, Moraes CD, et al. Retinal blood vessel positional shifts and glaucoma progression. *Ophthalmology.* (2014) 121:842-8. doi: 10.1016/j.ophtha.2013.11.002
16. Wang M, Jin Q, Wang H, Li D, Baniasadi N, Elze T. The interrelationship between refractive error, blood vessel anatomy, and glaucomatous visual field loss. *Transl Vis Sci Technol.* (2018) 7:4. doi: 10.1167/tvst.7.1.4
17. Kanamori, Akiyasu. Regional relationship between retinal nerve fiber layer thickness and corresponding visual field sensitivity in glaucomatous eyes. *Arch Ophthalmol.* (2008) 126:1500-6. doi: 10.1001/archopht.126.11.1500
18. Ouyang Y, Shao Q, Scharf D, Joussen AM, Heussen FM. Retinal vessel diameter measurements by spectral domain optical coherence tomography. *Graefes Arch Clin Exp Ophthalmol.* (2015) 253:1-11. doi: 10.1007/s00417-014-2715-2
19. Urbaniak GC, Plous S. *Research Randomizer (Version 4.0) [Computer Software]* (2013). Retrieved from: http://www.randomizer.org/ (accessed June 22, 2013).
20. Jonas JB, Fernández MC, Naumann GO. Parapapillary atrophy and retinal vessel diameter in nonglaucomatous optic nerve damage. *Invest Ophthalmol Vis Sci.* (1991) 32:2942-7.
21. Shuang W, Liang X, Wang Y, Wang Y, Jonas JB. Retinal vessel diameter in normal and glaucomatous eyes: the Beijing eye study. *Clin Exp Ophthalmol.* (2007) 35:800-7. doi: 10.1111/j.1442-9071.2007.01627.x
22. Jonas JB, Budde WM, Lang P. Neuroretinal rim width ratios in morphological glaucoma diagnosis. *Br J Ophthalmol.* (1999) 82:1366-71. doi: 10.1136/bjo.82.12.1366
23. Hart WM, Becker B. The onset and evolution of glaucomatous visual field defects. *Ophthalmology.* (1982) 89:268-79. doi: 10.1016/S0161-6420(82)34798-3
24. Shahidi AM, Patel SR, Flanagan JG, Hudson C. Regional variation in human retinal vessel oxygen saturation. *Exp Eye Res.* (2013) 113:143-7. doi: 10.1016/j.exer.2013.06.001
25. Chung HS, Harris A, Halter PJ, Kagemann L, Martin BJ. Regional differences in retinal vascular reactivity. *Invest Ophthalmol Vis Sci.* (1999) 40:2448-53.
26. Lucy KA, Wollstein G. Structural and functional evaluations for the early detection of glaucoma. *Expert Rev Ophthalmol.* (2016) 11:367-76. doi: 10.1080/17469899.2016.1229599
27. Kerrigan-Baumrind LA, Quigley HA, Pease ME, Kerrigan DF, Mitchell RS. Number of ganglion cells in glaucoma eyes compared with threshold visual field tests in the same persons. *Invest Ophthalmol Vis Sci.* (2000) 41:741-8. doi: 10.1097/00004397-200004000-00015

15

Macular Vascular Geometry Changes with Sex and Age in Healthy Subjects: A Fundus Photography Study

Ziqing Feng [1†], Gengyuan Wang [1†], Honghui Xia [2†], Meng Li [1], Guoxia Liang [2], Tingting Dong [2], Peng Xiao [1] and Jin Yuan [1*]*

[1] State Key Laboratory of Ophthalmology, Guangdong Provincial Key Laboratory of Ophthalmology and Visual Science, Guangdong Provincial Clinical Research Center for Ocular Diseases, Zhongshan Ophthalmic Center, Sun Yat-sen University, Guangzhou, China, [2] Department of Ophthalmology, Zhaoqing Gaoyao People's Hospital, Zhaoqing, China

***Correspondence:**
Peng Xiao
xiaopengaddis@hotmail.com
Jin Yuan
yuanjincornea@126.com

† These authors have contributed equally to this work

Purpose: To characterize the sex- and age-related alterations of the macular vascular geometry in a population of healthy eyes using fundus photography.

Methods: A cross-sectional study was conducted with 610 eyes from 305 healthy subjects (136 men, 169 women) who underwent fundus photography examination and was divided into four age groups (G1 with age $\leq$ 25 years, G2 with age 26–35 years, G3 with age 36–45 years, and G4 with age $\geq$ 46 years). A self-developed automated retinal vasculature analysis system allowed segmentation and separate multiparametric quantification of the macular vascular network according to the Early Treatment Diabetic Retinopathy Study (ETDRS). Vessel fractal dimension (D_f), vessel area rate (VAR), average vessel diameter (D_m), and vessel tortuosity (τ_n) were acquired and compared between sex and age groups.

Results: There was no significant difference between the mean age of male and female subjects (32.706 $\pm$ 10.372 and 33.494 $\pm$ 10.620, respectively, $p > 0.05$) and the mean age of both sexes in each age group ($p > 0.05$). The D_f, VAR, and D_m of the inner ring, the D_f of the outer ring, and the D_f and VAR of the whole macula were significantly greater in men than women ($p < 0.001$, $p < 0.001$, $p < 0.05$, respectively). There was no significant change of τ_n between males and females ($p > 0.05$). The D_f, VAR, and D_m of the whole macula, the inner and outer rings associated negatively with age ($p < 0.001$), whereas the τ_n showed no significant association with age ($p > 0.05$). Comparison between age groups observed that D_f started to decrease from G2 compared with G1 in the inner ring ($p < 0.05$) and D_f, VAR, and D_m all decreased from G3 compared with the younger groups in the whole macula, inner and outer rings ($p < 0.05$).

Conclusion: In the healthy subjects, macular vascular geometric parameters obtained from fundus photography showed that D_f, VAR, and D_m are related to sex and age while τ_n is not. The baseline values of the macular vascular geometry were also acquired for both sexes and all age groups.

Keywords: macular vascular geometry, fundus photography, vascular quantification, Early Treatment Diabetic Retinopathy Study (ETDRS), normative baseline

INTRODUCTION

The retina is one of the few tissues in the human body where the blood circulatory system can be non-invasively observed (1, 2). Retinal vascular characteristics can reflect the status of the microcirculation affected by ocular, cardiovascular, and systemic diseases, such as age-related macular degeneration, diabetic retinopathy, Alzheimer's disease, hypertension, etc. (3–11). Since early vascular alterations induced by diseases typically happened in microvasculature (12, 13), changes of the capillaries in the retinal macula are thought to be more sensitive to the early stage of disease progression and could provide significant information for the early diagnosis and monitoring of pathologic changes of related diseases (14–16).

Retinal blood vessels can be observed by imaging techniques such as fundus photography (17), optical coherence tomography angiography (OCTA) (18), fundus fluorescein angiography (FFA) (19), providing abundant retinal vascular structure and perfusion information. While OCTA and FFA could show the more detailed structure and functional changes of microvasculature, FFA is an invasive examination that may induce anaphylactic reactions (20), OCTA provides vascularity of both superficial and deep plexus but is prone to generate artifacts with a scanning imaging regime and its widespread in clinical use and disease screening is limited by the high cost, high patient cooperation and operation difficulties (18, 21). Currently, fundus photography is still the most widely used imaging technique for retinal examination and disease screening due to its advantages of non-invasiveness, relatively low cost, and ease to use the property.

The use of digital image analysis and machine learning techniques for fundus photography has become increasingly common over the past decades (22, 23), offering sophisticated techniques to acquire minute details and quantify the geometry of retinal vascular network (24, 25). Semiautomatic methods developed with Image J (26) and computer-assisted software such as Interactive Vessel Analysis (IVAN), Singapore I Vessel Assessment (SIVA), and Quantitative Analysis of Retinal Vessel Topology and Size (QUARTZ) (25, 27–29) could offer retinal vascular parameters such as vascular length, diameter, tortuosity, and so on. Clinical applications have been conducted showing these parameters may be important indicators of microvascular diseases that can be used in risk prediction (13, 15, 16). Nevertheless, most of the studies focused only on the larger blood vessels around the optic disc (5, 30).

Our former studies have developed a multiparametric retinal vascular network analysis method with a vessel segmentation algorithm based on dense block generative adversarial network (D-GAN) and automated vascular geometry quantification (14, 31). The method has been applied to explore the macular vascular geometry characteristics of fundus photography of patients with diabetes mellitus, showing microvascular morphological parameters may be indicators of the early retinal vessel changes for diabetic retinopathy (14). Though searching for disease-related potential vascular biomarkers is of great importance, the vascular geometry could be different between gender and changes could also be introduced during the normal aging process. While only a few studies have examined the potential sex and age interactions with retinal vasculatures (32, 33), no detailed research has been conducted to quantify the sex- and age-related changes of the microvascular network with fundus photography. In this study, we demonstrated a cross-sectional study aiming to explore the macular vascular geometry variations between sexes and characterized the age-related morphological changes with our multiparametric fundus photography analysis method, finding sensitive indicators of macular vascular geometry changes. Moreover, normative baseline data of both genders in different age groups was provided that can be used as references in identifying progressive macular vascular changes due to different pathologies.

METHODS

Study Subjects

This study was approved by the Medical Ethics Committee, Zhongshan Ophthalmic Center, Sun Yat-sen University (2017KYPJ104), and adhered to the tenets of the Declaration of Helsinki. All the subjects were informed about the data collection and signed informed consent forms. A total of 610 eyes from 305 healthy patients (136 males, 169 females) were recruited from the Zhongshan Ophthalmic Center, Sun Yat-sen University and Zhaoqing Gaoyao People's Hospital, Guangdong province, China between January 1, 2019 and May 15, 2021.

The inclusion criteria were as follows: age 18–70 years old, spherical equivalent within 6.0 diopters (D), no refractive interstitial opacities that affect fundus imaging, intraocular pressure 21 mmHg or less. Ocular examinations included uncorrected and best-corrected visual acuity (BCVA) measurements, digital retinal fundus photography examination with a 50° digital fundus camera (RetiCam 3100, SYSEYE, China) without mydriasis, slit-lamp examination, and intraocular pressure measurement.

The exclusion criteria were BCVA worse than 20/25, history of ocular disease, inflammation, trauma, and any intraocular surgery. Subjects were also excluded if they had any systemic disease, such as diabetes or hypertension that could affect, or are regularly taking any medication.

The subjects were divided into four groups: Group 1 (G1) aged $\leq$ 25 years, Group 2 (G2) aged from 26 to 35 years, Group 3 (G3) aged from 36 to 45 years, and Group 4 (G4) aged $\geq$ 46 years.

Macular Vascular Geometry Multiparametric Measurements

With the color fundus photographs acquired from all the enrolled subjects, multiparametric measurements of the macular vascular geometry were performed with our self-developed fundus photography analysis software. Details of the method could refer to former publications (31). In brief, the fundus image (**Figure 1A**) is first processed by adaptive histogram equalization and bilateral filtering to enhance the contrast between the blood vessels and the background. The enhanced image is then input into a D-GAN-based retinal vascular segmentation algorithm, exporting a binarized retinal vascular network map (**Figure 1B**). The introduction of the dense blocks into the GAN enables more efficient processing between separated spatial regions of

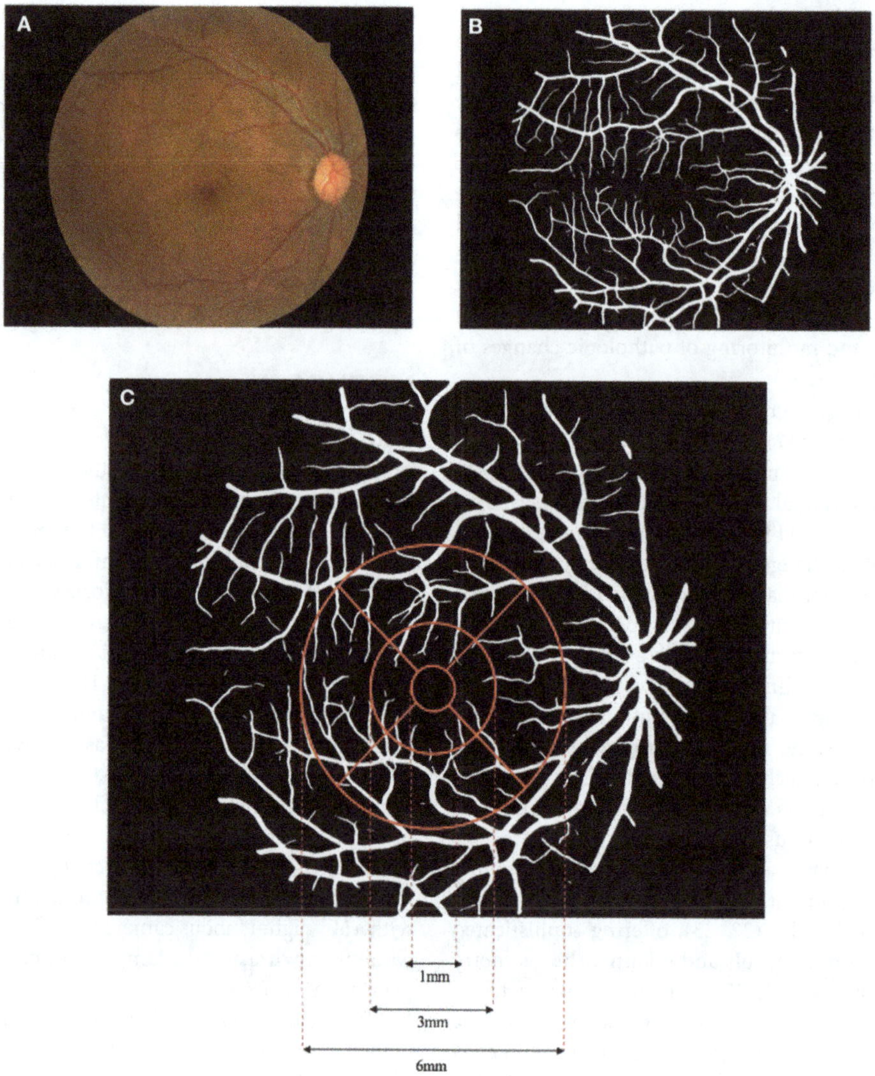

FIGURE 1 | Flowchart of the macular vascular geometry assessment according to Early Treatment Diabetic Retinopathy Study (ETDRS). The fundus photograph **(A)** was pre-processed and input to the dense block generative adversarial network (D-GAN) segmentation system, exporting a binarized retinal vascular network map **(B)**, and further analyzed to quantify the macular vascular geometry based on ETDRS **(C)**.

fundus images, building a more powerful generator to segment smooth, clear, and detailed blood vessels. The segmented vessel network binary image is then further analyzed by our software to quantify the macular vascular geometry based on Early Treatment Diabetic Retinopathy Study (ETDRS), separating the macular area into nine sectors (**Figure 1C**). The diameter of the concentric circles centered at the fovea centers are 1, 3, and 6 mm, respectively, with the inner and outer rings both evenly split into four parts (superior, inferior, nasal, and temporal). Since the innermost circle around the fovea avascular zone seldom has vessels in fundus photographs, this area is excluded for further data analysis. Vascular geometric parameters including fractal dimension (D_f), vessel area rate (VAR), average vessel diameter (D_m), and vessel tortuosity (τ_n) were calculated for both the inner and outer ring as well as their sub-sectors. Note that, D_f is a statistic value calculated with vessel skeletons that describes the space-filling degree of a fractal, measuring the spatial availability of a complex shape, which to some extent can reflect the density and complexity of the selected microvascular network (34–36). VAR is the ratio of the vascular area to the total area of the selected region, which could comprehensively reflect vascular density while D_m is the mean vessel diameter of the vessels in the region. τ_n is defined by multiple subdivision-based algorithms calculating the maximum of the accumulated absolute tangent angle difference of the sub-segments of the blood vessels multiplied by a transformed sigmoid learning curve function of the inflection point numbers of the vessel segment curvature sign, emphasizing the human tortuosity assessment nature focusing not only global but also on local vascular features (31).

Statistical Analysis

Statistical analysis was performed using Statistical Package for Social Sciences software (SPSS for Mac, version 26.0; IBM SPSS, Inc., Chicago, Illinois, USA). Age and sex were analyzed as classification variables while retinal vascular geometry parameters as continuous variables. Normally or approximately normal distributed variables were summarized as mean ± SD. Retinal vascular geometry parameters were assessed by the Shapiro–Wilk test.

Differences in clinical characteristics between sex at each age group were evaluated using the Independent *t*-test. The ratio of men and women in each group was analyzed by Chi-squared test. Due to the correlation nature of the included binocular data, a generalized estimating equation (GEE) procedure analysis was used with an exchangeable correlation structure to account for the inclusion of both eyes from the same participant. The final GEE model was used to calculate the β coefficients and their 95% CIs. Retinal vascular geometry parameters between the male and female subjects were evaluated through the GEE model. The association of age with D_f, VAR, D_m, and τ_n was examined using a linear GEE model. The differences in age group outcomes were analyzed, gender was included as a covariate. All the *p*-values were 2-sided and considered statistically significant when the values were <0.05.

TABLE 1 | Age and gender characteristics of the studied subjects.

Parameters	Male	Female	*t*-statistic	*p*
Subjects, *n* (eyes)	136 (272)	169 (338)		
Age, Mean ± SD, years	32.706 ± 10.372	33.494 ± 10.620	−0.914	0.361
Age group, Mean ± SD, years				
Group 1 (<25)	22.896 ± 1.525 (*n* = 48)	22.778 ± 1.278 (*n* = 54)	0.601	0.548
Group 2 (26–35)	30.488 ± 2.848 (*n* = 43)	30.904 ± 2.851 (*n* = 52)	−1.000	0.318
Group 3 (36–45)	40.083 ± 3.560 (*n* = 24)	41.121 ± 2.847 (*n* = 33)	−1.669	0.099
Group 4 (>46)	51.238 ± 4.808 (*n* = 21)	52.167 ± 5.063 (*n* = 30)	−0.931	0.354

RESULTS

The general age and gender characteristics of the studied subjects are shown in **Table 1**. There were no significant differences between the mean age of all the male and female subjects (32.706 ± 10.372 and 33.494 ± 10.620, respectively, $p > 0.05$) and the mean ages of both sexes in each age group ($p > 0.05$). Sex ratios were also equally represented in each age group.

Table 2 shows the comparison of macular vascular geometric parameters between all the male and female subjects. **Figure 2** shows the mean ETDRS retinal vascular geometric parameters maps with gender differences. The D_f, VAR, and D_m of the inner ring, the D_f of the outer ring, and the D_f and VAR of the whole macular were significantly greater in males than females (**Table 2**; $p < 0.001$, $p < 0.001$, and $p < 0.05$, respectively), especially in the inferior quadrants (**Figure 2**; $p < 0.001$). There was no significant

TABLE 2 | Generalized estimating equation analysis of the differences of macular vascular geometric parameters between the sex.

	Males	Female	β	95%CI		*p*
				Lower	Upper	
Fractal dimension, Mean ± SD, Df						
Whole	1.397 ± 0.033	1.387 ± 0.036	0.010	0.004	0.017	**0.002****
Inner ring	1,118 ± 0.075	1.087 ± 0.085	0.030	0.015	0.045	**<0.001****
Outer ring	1.318 ± 0.028	1.312 ± 0.031	0.008	0.002	0.013	**0.009****
Vessel area rate, Mean ± SD, VAR						
Whole	0.0141 ± 0.0018	0.0135 ± 0.0021	5.270E−4	1.462E−4	9.081E−4	**0.007****
Inner ring	0.0022 ± 0.0005	0.0020 ± 0.0005	2.391E−4	1.431E−4	3.364E−4	**<0.001****
Outer ring	0.0119 ± 0.0015	0.0116 ± 0.0017	2.850E−4	−3.248E−5	6.023E−4	0.079
Average vessel diameter, Mean ± SD, Dm						
Whole	0.146 ± 0.011	0.146 ± 0.013	4.383E−4	−1.806E−3	2.683E−3	0.702
Inner ring	0.120 ± 0.015	0.115 ± 0.016	0.005	0.002	0.007	**0.001****
Outer ring	0.150 ± 0.012	0.151 ± 0.014	−4.312E−4	−2.850E−3	1.987E−3	0.727
Tortuosity, Mean ± SD, τn						
Whole	2.742 ± 0.147	2.765 ± 0.152	−0.023	−0.051	0.005	0.101
Inner ring	2.945 ± 0.357	2.938 ± 0.359	0.007	−0.052	0.066	0.825
Outer ring	2.688 ± 0.158	2.707 ± 0.171	−0.019	−0.048	0.009	0.189

*p-value was based on GEE analysis using an exchangeable correlation structure for the difference between means, accounting for the correlation between eyes of the same participant. CI, 95% Walder confidence interval; **p < 0.01, bold.*

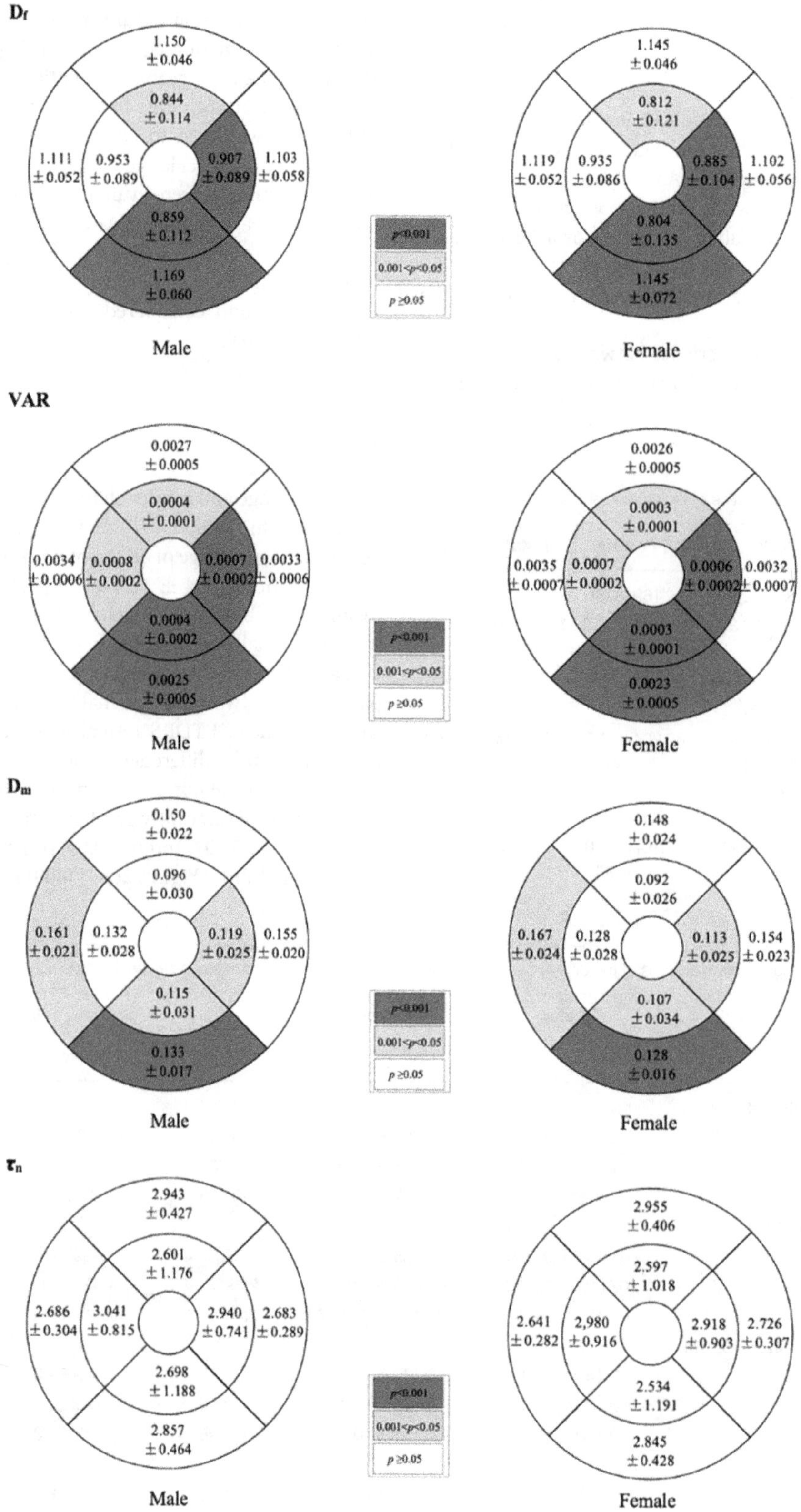

FIGURE 2 | Mean ETDRS retinal vascular geometric parameters maps showing gender differences. Shaded subfields indicate those in which there was a significant difference in macular vascular geometry between the male and female ($p < 0.05$). p-value was based on GEE analysis accounting for the correlation between eyes of the same participant.

TABLE 3 | Generalized estimating equation analysis of the association between macular vascular geometric parameters and age.

	Age			
	β	CI		p
		Lower	Upper	
Fractal dimension, D_f				
Whole	−9.812E−4	−1.276E−3	−6.873E−4	**<0.001****
Inner ring	−2.069E−3	−2.781E−3	−1.357E−3	**<0.001****
Outer ring	−7.904E−4	−1.043E−3	−5.372E−4	**<0.001****
Vessel area rate, VAR				
Whole	−6.179E−5	−7.804E−5	−4.555E−5	**<0.001****
Inner ring	−1.299E−5	−1.772E−5	−8.264E−5	**<0.001****
Outer ring	−4.873E−5	−6.195E−5	−3.551E−5	**<0.001****
Average vessel diameter, D_m				
Whole	−2.710E−4	−3.741E−4	−1.693E−4	**<0.001****
Inner ring	−2.652E−4	−3.861E−4	−1.440E−4	**<0.001****
Outer ring	−2.684E−4	−3.812E−4	−1.562E−4	**<0.001****
Tortuosity, τ_n				
Whole	7.202E−4	−6.023E−4	2.042E−3	0.286
Inner ring	3.764E−4	−2.734E−3	1.981E−3	0.754
Outer ring	5.203E−4	−7.752E−4	1.815E−3	0.432

p-value was based on GEE analysis using an exchangeable correlation structure for the difference between means, accounting for the correlation between eyes of the same participant.
*CI, 95% Walder confidence interval; **$p < 0.01$, bold.*

difference of τ_n between males and females (**Table 2**; **Figure 2**; $p > 0.05$).

Table 3 shows the association results between macular vascular geometric parameters and age. The D_f, VAR, and D_m of the whole macular, inner and outer rings all negatively associated with age (**Table 3**; **Figure 3**; $p < 0.001$), whereas the τ_n of the macular did not correlate with age (**Table 3**; **Figure 3**; $p > 0.05$).

The comparison of macular vascular geometric parameters of the whole, the inner and the outer rings among the different age groups are shown in **Figure 4**. It is resolved that, in the inner ring, G2 showed a significant decrease of the D_f compared with G1 (**Figure 4**; $p < 0.05$), while D_f, VAR, and D_m all decreased from G3 compared with the younger groups in the whole, inner and outer rings (**Figure 4**; $p < 0.05$). τn also has no significant differences (**Figure 4**; $p > 0.05$).

Table 4 shows the baseline values of D_f, VAR, D_m, and τ_n of both sexes in 4 age groups.

DISCUSSION

This is the first study that quantifies the sex- and age-related macular vascular geometry alterations in healthy populations with fundus photography using our customized automatic multiparametric vascular analysis software. We demonstrated that macular vascular D_f, VAR, and average vessel diameter D_m were all significantly lower in the female than male and all decrease with the increase of age, while vessel tortuosity τ_n showed no statistical difference, revealing the physiological variations of macular vascular geometry induced by sex and age. Normative baseline data of macular vascular geometric parameters for both the genders in different age groups were acquired that can potentially be used as references in identifying progressive macular vascular changes due to different pathologies.

In the analysis of the macular vascular geometric difference between male and female healthy subjects, we found that D_f and VAR in the macular area and D_m in the inner area of the macula were significantly greater in men than in women, indicating that male has more complex retinal vascular structures and larger vessel occupation and diameter in the macular area as compared with female. While no studies have demonstrated macular vascular structure analysis with fundus photography between genders, our results showing more abundant vascular network in men are in consistent with the former studies. Using OCTA, Yu et al. (37) reported lower blood flow index in the macula and larger fovea avascular zone in women, and Wang et al. (38) revealed higher superficial retinal vascular density in men than in women. Using fundus photography, Tapp et al. (39) showed that the retinal vascular diameter around the optic disk was larger in male. Since the retina is a tissue with high-oxygen consumption that need to rely on blood perfusion to maintain its metabolic levels, the retinal vascular structure is mainly influenced by the blood perfusion level (37, 40), which is regulated by blood pressure, intraocular pressure (IOP) (41), body mass index (BMI) (42), and hormone (43). Thus, the proven differences in these factors between genders (44) might be the reasons leading to the macular vascular geometry divergence. There were studies exploring gender differences in the epidemiology of ophthalmic diseases that have shown that macular diseases such as age-related macular degeneration (AMD) and macular holes (45, 46) were more likely to happen in females, which could also potentially be related to the macular vascular geometry differences. The detailed mechanisms of the gender-specific differences of macular vascular geometry remain unclear and require further study.

We have described the association between age and macular vascular geometric parameters showing that D_f, VAR, and D_m of the macular area all decrease with the increase of age. The association between age and D_f, VAR, and D_m were significant while the correlation coefficient is relatively low, indicating small age-related macular vascular geometry changes. This is similar to those reported in other studies (47, 48). One possible reason is that the age range of the samples in our study is not wide enough with the fewer elderly samples. The other reason could be that many factors influence macular vessels such as gender, axial length, refractive error (47, 49, 50), while this study limited in exploring only the age-induced changes. In the comparison of macular vascular geometric parameters of different age groups, we have revealed that statistical variation of vascular D_f happened from 26 to 35 age group while VAR and D_m decrease from 36 to 45 age group. These are in accordance with studies demonstrated in exploring retinal vascular alterations with aging (34, 51). Using fundus photography, Azemin et al. (51) and Liew et al. (34) measured the whole retinal and observed a significant decrease

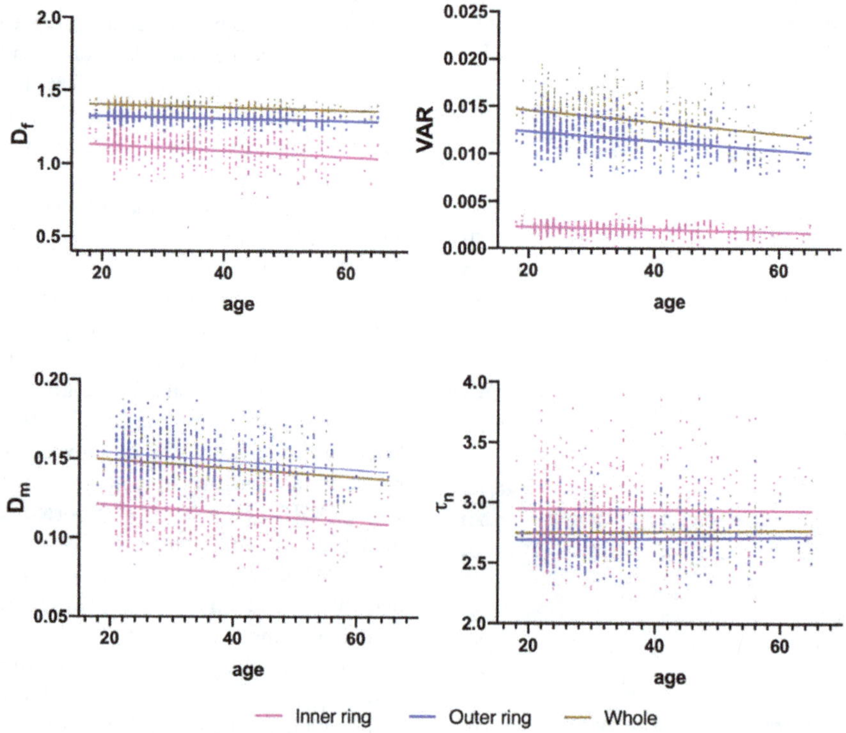

FIGURE 3 | Scatterplots for the associations between macular vascular parameters and age. The significant negative association exists between the D_f, VAR, D_m, and age in the whole macula, inner and outer rings ($p < 0.001$), while τ_n showed no significant association with age ($p > 0.05$).

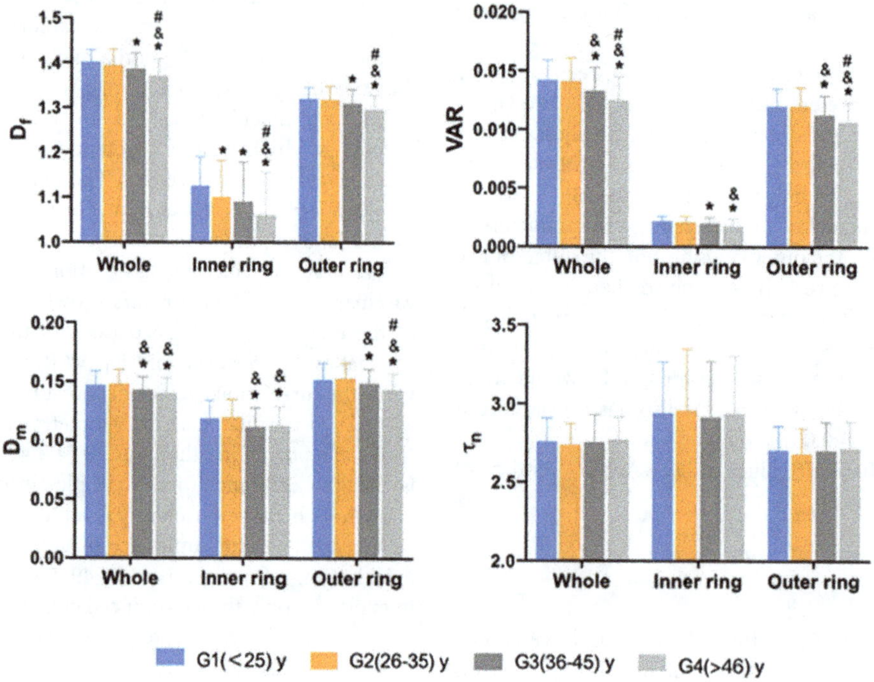

FIGURE 4 | The comparison of macular vascular geometric parameters of the whole, the inner and outer rings among different age groups. Df of the inner ring showed a significant decrease in G2 compared to G1 ($p < 0.05$). D_f, VAR, and D_m all decreased from G3 compared to younger groups in the whole, inner and outer rings ($p < 0.05$). τn has no significant differences ($p > 0.05$). *Compare to G1 $p < 0.05$; [&] compare to G2 $p < 0.05$; #: compare to G3 $p < 0.05$. p value was based on GEE analysis accounting for the correlation between eyes of the same participant and including gender as a covariate.

TABLE 4 | The baseline values of macular vascular geometric parameters of both the sexes in the four age groups.

Age groups	Group 1		Group 2		Group 3		Group 4	
	Male	Female	Male	Female	Male	Female	Male	Female
Fractal dimension, Mean ± SD, D_f								
Whole	1.400 ± 0.027	1.401 ± 0.027	1.399 ± 0.032	1.390 ± 0.038	1.398 ± 0.036	1.378 ± 0.032	1.382 ± 0.038	1.363 ± 0.037
Inner ring	1.128 ± 0.068	1.124 ± 0.061	1.116 ± 0.074	1.088 ± 0.086	1.127 ± 0.081	1.065 ± 0.083	1.090 ± 0.080	1.043 ± 0.099
Outer ring	1.320 ± 0.024	1.322 ± 0.027	1.321 ± 0.027	1.315 ± 0.033	1.318 ± 0.032	1.304 ± 0.029	1.307 ± 0.033	1.290 ± 0.030
Vessel area rate, Mean ± SD, VAR								
Whole	0.0142 ± 0.0016	0.0143 ± 0.0018	0.0144 ± 0.0018	0.0139 ± 0.0020	0.0140 ± 0.0019	0.0129 ± 0.0019	0.0133 ± 0.0021	0.0120 ± 0.0018
Inner ring	0.0023 ± 0.0005	0.0022 ± 0.0004	0.0022 ± 0.0005	0.0020 ± 0.0005	0.0022 ± 0.0005	0.0018 ± 0.0005	0.0021 ± 0.0005	0.0017 ± 0.0006
Outer ring	0.0119 ± 0.0014	0.0121 ± 0.0016	0.0122 ± 0.0015	0.0119 ± 0.0017	0.0117 ± 0.0015	0.0110 ± 0.0016	0.0112 ± 0.0017	0.0103 ± 0.0014
Average vessel diameter, Mean ± SD, D_m								
Whole	0.145 ± 0.011	0.149 ± 0.013	0.149 ± 0.011	0.148 ± 0.012	0.145 ± 0.011	0.142 ± 0.011	0.142 ± 0.011	0.139 ± 0.013
Inner ring	0.121 ± 0.016	0.117 ± 0.014	0.123 ± 0.014	0.117 ± 0.016	0.117 ± 0.014	0.109 ± 0.016	0.115 ± 0.014	0.111 ± 0.017
Outer ring	0.149 ± 0.012	0.154 ± 0.015	0.153 ± 0.012	0.152 ± 0.013	0.151 ± 0.0119	0.147 ± 0.0126	0.146 ± 0.012	0.143 ± 0.014
Tortuosity, Mean ± SD, τ_n								
Whole	2.757 ± 0.144	2.765 ± 0.151	2.729 ± 0.143	2.745 ± 0.134	2.737 ± 0.164	2.769 ± 0.183	2.743 ± 0.141	2.794 ± 0.142
Inner ring	2.921 ± 0.300	2.961 ± 0.343	2.990 ± 0.468	2.930 ± 0.308	2.910 ± 0.291	2.918 ± 0.397	2.945 ± 0.257	2.938 ± 0.425
Outer ring	2.709 ± 0.148	2.701 ± 0.161	2.662 ± 0.158	2.697 ± 0.167	2.694 ± 0.183	2.710 ± 0.180	2.691 ± 0.149	2.735 ± 0.184

in the D_f with aging. Sun et al. (52) found both arterial and venular caliber decrease in the older groups using IVAN software to analyze peripapillary diameter of 3,019 health participants; Pose-Reino et al. (53) analyzed the retinal blood vessel caliber and found that the reduction of retinal arteriole caliber occurs during aging. While the retinal vascular structure is closely related to blood perfusion, measuring by OCTA, Yu et al. (37) have shown that macular perfusion decreased with increasing age in healthy Chinese eyes, and the parafoveal flow index and vessel area density decrease with aging at a rate of 0.6 and 0.4% per year. You et al. also reported that higher superficial and deep capillary densities were significantly associated with younger age and a general negative association between macular vessel density and age (47). Similar results have been reported in several other studies (48). Similar to other human organs, the physiological function of the eye decreases with aging. Since maintaining normal function of the retina depends on normal metabolism level (54), aging causes tissue loss and a corresponding reduction in oxygen demand, altering vascular system, and declining the perfusion of macular, resulting in a reduction in vascular structure and complexity. Studies have also determined that aging could cause thickening of the vascular wall, reducing vascular elasticity (55), and the rigidity of the vessel wall would lead to the decrease of the vessel diameter (56). The reduction in the macular vascular structure might potentially account for some ocular diseases related to age such as age-related macular degeneration (AMD), proliferative diabetic retinopathy (PDR), retinal vein occlusion (RVO), and so on (57, 58).

In this study, we also found that the macular vascular tortuosity τ_n has no variation between gender and across aging. Many studies have shown that retinal vascular tortuosity variation is one of the earliest indicators of a number of relevant diseases such as diabetes, cerebrovascular disease, stroke, ischemic heart disease (14, 59, 60). Our observation indicates no statistical difference of macular vascular tortuosity in healthy individuals of different gender and age further enhancing the feasibility of using tortuosity as a sensitive indicator for the early diagnosis of related diseases.

There are several limitations of this study. First, the number of subjects in the elderly age group was relatively small due to the fact that the healthy subjects we have collected tend to be young since older people are more likely to suffer from systemic diseases such as hypertension, heart disease, and diabetes or cloudy refractive interstitium affecting the fundus image quality (6, 9, 14, 34, 50). Future collection of more healthy elderly subjects to balance the sample size of all the age groups would be beneficial. Second, while this study is limited in exploring macular vascular geometry changes with age and gender, there are many other factors that affect the macular vasculature, such as axial length, refractive error, IOP, blood pressure, and so on (34, 41, 49, 50, 61), it is worth further in-depth study considering these factors. Third, since this is a cross-sectional study without temporal information, future prospective investigation with systematic clinical information acquired could provide more detailed support of the vascular alteration mechanisms. Moreover, with the binocular data acquired in this study, analyzing the intereye correlation and difference of the macular vasculature with fundus photography and comparing it to those acquired with OCTA would be interesting (62). Finally, with the baseline data from the healthy subjects gained, the vascular geometric variation induced by different diseases could be further explored. Improvement of our current vascular analysis software to distinguish the retinal arteries and veins would also provide more functional information to study the retinal vascular circulation.

In conclusion, findings from this study reveal the sex- and age-related macular vascular geometry alterations in healthy human subjects and provide the normative baseline data for both genders in different age groups. The application of our automatic retinal vascular analysis system could provide a useful approach for detecting subtle macular vessels change with fundus photography.

ETHICS STATEMENT

The studies involving human participants were reviewed and approved by Guangzhou, China 2017KYPJ104, Medical Ethics Committee of Zhongshan Ophthalmic Center, Sun Yat-sen University (Guangzhou, China). Written informed consent to participate in this study was provided by the participants' legal guardian/next of kin.

AUTHOR CONTRIBUTIONS

JY and PX conceived and planned the research and reviewed and modified the manuscript. ZF, GW, and HX carried out the studies and wrote the first draft of the manuscript. GL and TD conducted the fundus imaging. GW, PX, and ML processed the images and organized the database. ZF and GL performed the statistical analysis. All the authors provided critical feedback and helped to shape the research, analysis, and manuscript.

REFERENCES

1. Flammer J, Konieczka K, Bruno RM, Virdis A, Flammer AJ, Taddei S. The eye and the heart. *Eur Heart J.* (2013) 34:1270–8. doi: 10.1093/eurheartj/eht023
2. Liew G, Wang JJ, Mitchell P, Wong TY. Retinal vascular imaging: a new tool in microvascular disease research. *Circ Cardiovasc Imaging.* (2008) 1:156–61. doi: 10.1161/CIRCIMAGING.108.784876
3. Parisi V, Ziccardi L, Costanzo E, Tedeschi M, Barbano L, Manca D, et al. Macular functional and morphological changes in intermediate age-related maculopathy. *Invest Ophthalmol Vis Sci.* (2020) 61:11. doi: 10.1167/iovs.61.5.11
4. Ozcaliskan S, Artunay O, Balci S, Perente I, Yenerel NM. Quantitative analysis of inner retinal structural and microvascular alterations in intermediate age-related macular degeneration: a swept-source OCT angiography study. *Photodiagnosis Photodyn Ther.* (2020) 32:102030. doi: 10.1016/j.pdpdt.2020.102030
5. Liew G, Benitez-Aguirre P, Craig ME, Jenkins AJ, Hodgson LAB, Kifley A, et al. Progressive retinal vasodilation in patients with type 1 diabetes: a longitudinal study of retinal vascular geometry. *Invest Ophthalmol Vis Sci.* (2017) 58:2503–09. doi: 10.1167/iovs.16-21015
6. Lim LS, Chee ML, Cheung CY, Wong TY. Retinal vessel geometry and the incidence and progression of diabetic retinopathy. *Invest Ophthalmol Vis Sci.* (2017) 58:200–5. doi: 10.1167/iovs.17-21699
7. Berisha F, Feke GT, Trempe CL, McMeel JW, Schepens CL. Retinal abnormalities in early Alzheimer's disease. *Invest Ophthalmol Vis Sci.* (2007) 48:2285–9. doi: 10.1167/iovs.06-1029
8. Golzan SM, Goozee K, Georgevsky D, Avolio A, Chatterjee P, Shen K, et al. Retinal vascular and structural changes are associated with amyloid burden in the elderly: ophthalmic biomarkers of preclinical Alzheimer's disease. *Alzheimers Res Ther.* (2017) 9:13. doi: 10.1186/s13195-017-0239-9
9. Chua J, Chin CWL, Hong J, Chee ML, Le TT, Ting DSW, et al. Impact of hypertension on retinal capillary microvasculature using optical coherence tomographic angiography. *J Hypertens.* (2019) 37:572–80. doi: 10.1097/HJH.0000000000001916
10. Liu M, Lycett K, Moreno-Betancur M, Wong TY, He M, Saffery R, et al. Inflammation mediates the relationship between obesity and retinal vascular calibre in 11-12 year-olds children and mid-life adults. *Sci Rep.* (2020) 10:5006. doi: 10.1038/s41598-020-61801-w
11. Ong YT, De Silva DA, Cheung CY, Chang HM, Chen CP, Wong MC, et al. Microvascular structure and network in the retina of patients with ischemic stroke. *Stroke.* (2013) 44:2121–7. doi: 10.1161/STROKEAHA.113.001741
12. Durham JT, Herman IM. Microvascular modifications in diabetic retinopathy. *Curr Diab Rep.* (2011) 11:253–64. doi: 10.1007/s11892-011-0204-0
13. Witt N, Wong TY, Hughes AD, Chaturvedi N, Klein BE, Evans R, et al. Abnormalities of retinal microvascular structure and risk of mortality from ischemic heart disease and stroke. *Hypertension.* (2006) 47:975–81. doi: 10.1161/01.HYP.0000216717.72048.6c
14. Li M, Wang G, Xia H, Feng Z, Xiao P, Yuan J. Retinal vascular geometry detection as a biomarker in diabetes mellitus. *Eur J Ophthalmol.* (2021) 20:11206721211033488. doi: 10.1177/11206721211033488
15. Chen Q, Tan F, Wu Y, Zhuang X, Wu C, Zhou Y, et al. Characteristics of retinal structural and microvascular alterations in early type 2 diabetic patients. *Invest Ophthalmol Vis Sci.* (2018) 59:2110–8. doi: 10.1167/iovs.17-23193
16. Jiang H, Wei Y, Shi Y, Wright CB, Sun X, Gregori G, et al. Altered macular microvasculature in mild cognitive impairment and Alzheimer disease. *J Neuroophthalmol.* (2018) 38:292–8. doi: 10.1097/WNO.0000000000000580
17. Sinthanayothin C, Boyce JF, Cook HL, Williamson TH. Automated localisation of the optic disc, fovea, and retinal blood vessels from digital colour fundus images. *Br J Ophthalmol.* (1999) 83:902–10. doi: 10.1136/bjo.83.8.902
18. Spaide RF, Fujimoto JG, Waheed NK, Sadda SR, Staurenghi G. Optical coherence tomography angiography. *Prog Retin Eye Res.* (2018) 64:1–55. doi: 10.1016/j.preteyeres.2017.11.003
19. Manivannan A, Plskova J, Farrow A, Mckay S, Sharp PF, Forrester JV. Ultra-wide-field fluorescein angiography of the ocular fundus. *Am J Ophthalmol.* (2005) 140:525–7. doi: 10.1016/j.ajo.2005.02.055
20. Kornblau IS, El-Annan JF. Adverse reactions to fluorescein angiography: a comprehensive review of the literature. *Surv Ophthalmol.* (2019) 64:679–93. doi: 10.1016/j.survophthal.2019.02.004
21. Chalam KV, Sambhav K. Optical coherence tomography angiography in retinal diseases. *J Ophthalmic Vis Res.* (2016) 11:84–92. doi: 10.4103/2008-322X.180709
22. Silva PS, Cavallerano JD, Sun JK, Noble J, Aiello LM, Aiello LP. Nonmydriatic ultrawide field retinal imaging compared with dilated standard 7-field 35-mm photography and retinal specialist examination for evaluation of diabetic retinopathy. *Am J Ophthalmol.* (2012) 154:549–559.e2. doi: 10.1016/j.ajo.2012.03.019
23. Gulshan V, Peng L, Coram M, Stumpe MC, Wu D, Narayanaswamy A, et al. Development and validation of a deep learning algorithm for detection of diabetic retinopathy in retinal fundus photographs. *JAMA.* (2016) 316:2402–10. doi: 10.1001/jama.2016.17216

24. Thomas GN, Ong SY, Tham YC, Hsu W, Lee ML, Lau QP, et al. Measurement of macular fractal dimension using a computer-assisted program. *Invest Ophthalmol Vis Sci.* (2014) 55:2237–43. doi: 10.1167/iovs.13-13315
25. Zheng Y, Cheung N, Aung T, Mitchell P, He M, Wong TY. Relationship of retinal vascular caliber with retinal nerve fiber layer thickness: the Singapore Malay eye study. *Invest Ophthalmol Vis Sci.* (2009) 50:4091–6. doi: 10.1167/iovs.09-3444
26. Olga GS, Svetlana F, Mikhail S, Igor Z. Evaluation of vascular system of the retina using ImageJ software. *Invest Ophthalmol Vis Sci.* (2011) 52:1281.
27. Lim LS, Cheung CY, Sabanayagam C, Lim SC, Tai ES, Huang L, et al. Structural changes in the retinal microvasculature and renal function. *Invest Ophthalmol Vis Sci.* (2013) 54:2970–6. doi: 10.1167/iovs.13-11941
28. Welikala RA, Fraz MM, Foster PJ, Whincup PH, Rudnicka AR, Owen CG, et al. UK Biobank Eye and Vision Consortium. Automated retinal image quality assessment on the UK Biobank dataset for epidemiological studies. *Comput Biol Med.* (2016) 71:67–76. doi: 10.1016/j.compbiomed.2016.01.027
29. Bankhead P, Scholfield CN, McGeown JG, Curtis TM. Fast retinal vessel detection and measurement using wavelets and edge location refinement. *PLoS One.* (2012) 7:e32435. doi: 10.1371/journal.pone.0032435
30. Cheung CY, Sabanayagam C, Law AK, Kumari N, Ting DS, Tan G, et al. Retinal vascular geometry and 6 year incidence and progression of diabetic retinopathy. *Diabetologia.* (2017) 60:1770–81. doi: 10.1007/s00125-017-4333-0
31. Wang G, Li M, Yun Z, Duan Z, Ma K, Luo Z, et al. novel multiple subdivision-based algorithm for quantitative assessment of retinal vascular tortuosity. *Exp Biol Med.* (2021) 246:2222–9. doi: 10.1177/15353702211032898
32. Benitez-Aguirre P, Craig ME, Cass HG, Sugden CJ, Jenkins AJ, Wang JJ, et al. Sex differences in retinal microvasculature through puberty in type 1 diabetes: are girls at greater risk of diabetic microvascular complications? *Invest Ophthalmol Vis Sci.* (2014) 56:571–7. doi: 10.1167/iovs.14-15147
33. Huang QF, Wei FF, Zhang ZY, Raaijmakers A, Asayama K, Thijs L, et al. Reproducibility of retinal microvascular traits decoded by the Singapore I vessel assessment software across the human age range. *Am J Hypertens.* (2018) 31:438–49. doi: 10.1093/ajh/hpx202
34. Liew G, Wang JJ, Cheung N, Zhang YP, Hsu W, Lee ML, et al. The retinal vasculature as a fractal: methodology, reliability, and relationship to blood pressure. *Ophthalmology.* (2008) 115:1951–6. doi: 10.1016/j.ophtha.2008.05.029
35. Azemin MZ, Kumar DK, Wong TY, Kawasaki R, Mitchell P, Wang JJ. Robust methodology for fractal analysis of the retinal vasculature. *IEEE Trans Med Imaging.* (2011) 30:243–50. doi: 10.1109/TMI.2010.2076322
36. Masters BR. Fractal analysis of the vascular tree in the human retina. *Annu Rev Biomed Eng.* (2004) 6:427–52. doi: 10.1146/annurev.bioeng.6.040803.140100
37. Yu J, Jiang C, Wang X, et al. Macular perfusion in healthy Chinese: an optical coherence tomography angiogram study. *Invest Ophthalmol Vis Sci.* (2015) 56:3212–7. doi: 10.1167/iovs.14-16270
38. Wang Q, Chan S, Yang JY, You B, Wang YX, Jonas JB, et al. Vascular density in retina and choriocapillaris as measured by optical coherence tomography angiography. *Am J Ophthalmol.* (2016) 168:95–109. doi: 10.1016/j.ajo.2016.05.005
39. Tapp RJ, Owen CG, Barman SA, Welikala RA, Foster PJ, Whincup PH, et al. UK Biobank Eye, Vision Consortium. Retinal vascular tortuosity and diameter associations with adiposity and components of body composition. *Obesity.* (2020) 28:1750–60. doi: 10.1002/oby.22885
40. Yu DY, Cringle SJ. Oxygen distribution and consumption within the retina in vascularised and avascular retinas and in animal models of retinal disease. *Prog Retin Eye Res.* (2001) 20:175–208. doi: 10.1016/S1350-9462(00)0 0027-6
41. Alagoz G, Gurel K, Bayer A, Serin D, Celebi S, Kukner S, et al. comparative study of bimatoprost and travoprost: effect on intraocular pressure and ocular circulation in newly diagnosed glaucoma patients. *Ophthalmologica.* (2008) 222:88–95. doi: 10.1159/000112624
42. Hughes AD, Wong TY, Witt N, Evans R, Thom SA, Klein BE, et al. Determinants of retinal microvascular architecture in normal subjects. *Microcirculation.* (2009) 16:159–66. doi: 10.1080/10739680802353868
43. Nuzzi R, Scalabrin S, Becco A, Panzica G. Gonadal hormones and retinal disorders: a review. *Front Endocrinol.* (2018) 9:66. doi: 10.3389/fendo.2018.00066
44. Schmidl D, Schmetterer L, Garhöfer G, Popa-Cherecheanu A. Gender differences in ocular blood flow. *Curr Eye Res.* (2015) 40:201–12. doi: 10.3109/02713683.2014.906625
45. Rudnicka AR, Jarrar Z, Wormald R, Cook DG. Fletcher A, Owen CG. Age and gender variations in age-related macular degeneration prevalence in populations of European ancestry: a meta-analysis. *Ophthalmology.* (2012) 119:571–80. doi: 10.1016/j.ophtha.2011.09.027
46. McCannel CA, Ensminger JL, Diehl NN, Hodge DN. Population-based incidence of macular holes. *Ophthalmology.* (2009) 116:1366–9. doi: 10.1016/j.ophtha.2009.01.052
47. You QS, Chan JCH, Ng ALK, Choy BKN, Shih KC, Cheung JJC, et al. Macular vessel density measured with optical coherence tomography angiography and its associations in a large population-based study. *Invest Ophthalmol Vis Sci.* (2019) 60:4830–7. doi: 10.1167/iovs.19-28137
48. Wei Y, Jiang H, Shi Y, Qu D, Gregori G, Zheng F, et al. Age-related alterations in the retinal microvasculature, microcirculation, and microstructure. *Invest Ophthalmol Vis Sci.* (2017) 58:3804–17. doi: 10.1167/iovs.17-21460
49. Fernández-Vigo JI, Kudsieh B, Shi H, Arriola-Villalobos P, Donate-López J, García-Feijóo J, et al. Normative database and determinants of macular vessel density measured by optical coherence tomography angiography. *Clin Exp Ophthalmol.* (2020) 48:44–52. doi: 10.1111/ceo.13648
50. Cheung CY, Thomas GN, Tay W, Ikram MK, Hsu W, Lee ML, et al. Retinal vascular fractal dimension and its relationship with cardiovascular and ocular risk factors. *Am J Ophthalmol.* (2012) 154:663–74. doi: 10.1016/j.ajo.2012.04.016
51. Azemin MZ, Kumar DK, Wong TY, Wang JJ, Mitchell P, Kawasaki R, et al. Age-related rarefaction in the fractal dimension of retinal vessel. *Neurobiol Aging.* (2012) 33:194.e1–4. doi: 10.1016/j.neurobiolaging.2010.04.010
52. Sun C, Liew G, Wang JJ, Mitchell P, Saw SM, Aung T, et al. Retinal vascular caliber, blood pressure, and cardiovascular risk factors in an Asian population: the Singapore Malay Eye Study. *Invest Ophthalmol Vis Sci.* (2008) 49:1784–90. doi: 10.1167/iovs.07-1450
53. Pose-Reino A, Gomez-Ulla F, Hayik B, Rodriguez-Fernández M, Carreira-Nouche MJ, Mosquera-González A, et al. Computerized measurement of retinal blood vessel calibre: description, validation and use to determine the influence of ageing and hypertension. *J Hypertens.* (2005) 23:843–50. doi: 10.1097/01.hjh.0000163154.35577.8e
54. Vandewalle E, Abegão Pinto L, Olafsdottir OB, De Clerck E, Stalmans P. Van Calster J, et al. Oximetry in glaucoma: correlation of metabolic change with structural and functional damage. *Acta Ophthalmol.* (2014) 92:105–10. doi: 10.1111/aos.12011
55. Meixner E, Michelson G. Measurement of retinal wall-tolumen ratio by adaptive optics retinal camera: a clinical research. *Graefes Arch Clin Exp Ophthalmol.* (2015) 253:1985–95. doi: 10.1007/s00417-015-3115-y
56. Wong TY, Klein R, Klein BE, Tielsch JM, Hubbard L, Nieto FJ. Retinal microvascular abnormalities and their relationship with hypertension, cardiovascular disease, and mortality. *Surv Ophthalmol.* (2001) 46:59–80. doi: 10.1016/S0039-6257(01)00234-X
57. Kromer R, Glusa P, Framme C, Pielen A, Junker B. Optical coherence tomography angiography analysis of macular flow density in glaucoma. *Acta Ophthalmol.* (2019) 97:e199–206. doi: 10.1111/aos.13914
58. Seknazi D, Coscas F, Sellam A, Rouimi F, Coscas G, Souied EH, et al. Optical coherence tomography angiography in retinal vein occlusion: correlations between macular vascular density, visual acuity, and peripheral nonperfusion area on fluorescein angiography. *Retina.* (2018) 38:1562–70. doi: 10.1097/IAE.0000000000001737
59. Cheung CY, Zheng Y, Hsu W, Lee ML, Lau QP, Mitchell P, et al. Retinal vascular tortuosity, blood pressure, and cardiovascular risk factors. *Ophthalmology.* (2011) 118:812–8. doi: 10.1016/j.ophtha.2010.08.045
60. Sasongko MB, Wong TY, Nguyen TT, Cheung CY, Shaw JE, Wang JJ. Retinal vascular tortuosity in persons with diabetes and diabetic retinopathy. *Diabetologia.* (2011) 54:2409–16. doi: 10.1007/s00125-011-2200-y
61. Zhang J, Tang FY, Cheung CY, Chen H. Different effect of media opacity on vessel density measured by different optical coherence tomography angiography algorithms. *Transl Vis Sci Technol.* (2020) 9:19. doi: 10.1167/tvst.9.8.19
62. Fang D, Tang FY, Huang H, Cheung CY, Chen H. Repeatability, interocular correlation and agreement of quantitative swept-source optical coherence tomography angiography macular metrics in healthy subjects. *Br J Ophthalmol.* (2019) 103:415–20. doi: 10.1136/bjophthalmol-2018-311874

16

A Quantitative Comparison of Multispectral Refraction Topography and Autorefractometer in Young Adults

Yunru Liao [1,2†]*, Zhenlan Yang* [1†]*, Zijing Li* [1]*, Rui Zeng* [1]*, Jing Wang* [1]*, Yichi Zhang* [1*‡] *and Yuqing Lan* [1*‡]

[1] *Department of Ophthalmology, Sun Yat-sen Memorial Hospital, Sun Yat-sen University, Guangzhou, China,* [2] *Department of Glaucoma, Zhongshan Ophthalmic Center, Sun Yat-sen University, Guangzhou, China*

Correspondence:
Yichi Zhang
zhangych46@mail.sysu.edu.cn
Yuqing Lan
lanyq@mail.sysu.edu.cn

[†] *These authors have contributed equally to this work and share first authorship*

[‡] *These authors have contributed equally to this work*

Purpose: Purpose of this study is to evaluate the measuring consistency of central refraction between multispectral refraction topography (MRT) and autorefractometry.

Methods: This was a descriptive cross-sectional study including subjects in Sun Yat-sen Memorial Hospital from September 1, 2020, to December 31, 2020, ages 20 to 35 years with a best corrected visual acuity of 20/20 or better. All patients underwent cycloplegia, and the refractive status was estimated with autorefractometer, experienced optometrist and MRT. We analyzed the central refraction of the autorefractometer and MRT. The repeatability and reproducibility of values measured using both devices were evaluated using intraclass correlation coefficients (ICCs).

Results: A total of 145 subjects ages 20 to 35 (290 eyes) were enrolled. The mean central refraction of the autorefractometer was -4.69 ± 2.64 diopters (D) (range -9.50 to $+4.75$ D), while the mean central refraction of MRT was -4.49 ± 2.61 diopters (D) (range -8.79 to $+5.02$ D). Pearson correlation analysis revealed a high correlation between the two devices. The intraclass correlation coefficient (ICC) also showed high agreement. The intrarater and interrater ICC values of central refraction were more than 0.90 in both devices and conditions. At the same time, the mean central refraction of experienced optometrist was -4.74 ± 2.66 diopters (D) (range -9.50 to $+4.75$D). The intra-class correlation coefficient of central refraction measured by MRT and subjective refraction was 0.939.

Conclusions: Results revealed that autorefractometry, experienced optometrist and MRT show high agreement in measuring central refraction. MRT could provide a potential objective method to assess peripheral refraction.

Keywords: consistency, multispectral refraction topography, autorefractometer, refraction, multispectral imaging

INTRODUCTION

Myopia is by far the most common refractive error and a dominant reason of visual impairment globally (1), with a prevalent rate of 10–30% of adults in many countries and 80–90% of young people in some parts of East and South-East Asia (2, 3). Myopia of −6.00 diopters (D) or more severe is called high myopia and is often causes visual impairment due to complications such as posterior uveioma, choroidal new vascularization, retinal detachment and so on (4). Reducing the high myopia incidence rate and improving the quality of life are the goal of prevention and treatment of myopia.

Animal experiments have provided details about myopia: hyperopic defocus increases axial elongation, while myopic defocus decreases axial elongation (4–11). Retinal peripheral visual signals, which are basically the sum of regions, can contral central refractive development independent of central visual experience. The effectiveness of optical defocus in changing axial elongation depends on retinal defocus degree (12, 13). However, there are generally four methods to evaluate eccentric refractive errors (14): subjective eccentric refraction (15), wavefront measurements with an aHS sensor (16), streak retinoscopy (17), and photo refraction with a power refractor (14). However, these methods can only detect a small area of the retina and cannot accurately detect the peripheral defocus of each region of the retina. Further, the process has high requirements for patient cooperation, and it is cumbersome, time-consuming, and difficult to adapt to clinical practice (18, 19).

MRT is a new instrument using multispectral imaging technology (MSI). MSI is an emerging technology based on imaging and spectroscopy. It is the result of remote sensing technology as a kind of analysis tool and can obtain information on the measured target simultaneously from the spectral and spatial dimensions. MRT can detect the refraction of each part of the retina within a range of 30° at the posterior pole of the retina, especially the refraction of the fovea of the macula.

The usage of different technologies in the MRT and other devices above talking about may result in differences in measurements. Because treatment centers use different topographic devices, differences in such measurements might lead to differences between diagnostic or treatment centers.

Therefore, we evaluated agreement between MRT and autorefractometer to see whether they could be interchangeable used or not. The data offered by each device should be maintained consistent at different measurements so that results can be used in research. Hence, we evaluated the repeatability of the devices' measurements to decide their effectiveness and availability.

METHODS

The present research was a descriptive cross-sectional study, and it was conducted in accordance with the tenets of the 1964 Declaration of Helsinki and its later amendments or comparable ethical standards. Local ethical approval (SYSEC-KY-KS-2021-061) was obtained from the Ethics Committee of Sun Yat-sen Memorial Hospital at Sun Yat-sen University, Guangzhou, China. The medical records of consecutive patients in Sun Yat-sen Memorial Hospital from September 1, 2020 to December 31, 2020 were reviewed. The inclusion criteria were as follows: (1) subjects ages 20 to 35 years, (2) subjects with a best corrected visual acuity of 20/20 or better, (3) subjects with MRT results, (4) subjects with the refraction results of autorefractometer and experienced optometrists. Exclusion criteria were as follows: (1) intraocular pressure higher than 21 mmHg, (2) a history of ocular diseases or previous ocular surgery that may influence refraction or axial length, such as corneal and lens diseases, and (3) a history of corneal contact lens, such as orthokeratology.

TABLE 1 | Baseline characteristics of the participants.

Characteristics			Value
Subjects (eye)			145 (290)
Sex	Female		105
	Male		40
Age	Mean		26.23(SD2.62)
	Range		20–35
Emmetropia			3
Ametropia	Myopia	Low(−0.25∼−3.00D)	61
		Medium(−3.25∼−6.00D)	121
		High(< −6.00D)	93
	Hyperopia	Low(+0.25∼+3.00D)	10
		Medium(+3.25∼+5.00D)	2
		High(> +5.00D)	0

SD, standard deviation.

The refractive errors of all eyes were measured by both an autorefractometer (AR-360A, NIDEK Co., Ltd, Japan), an experienced optometrist, and MRT (version 1.0.5T05C; Thondar, Inc.) Thirty minutes before examination, a cycloplegic agent (one drop of 0.5% tropicamide along with 0.5%) phenylephrine hydrochloride (Sinqi Pharmaceutical Co. Ltd., Shenyang, China) was applied 3 times (with 5 min between each application). The mean of three consecutive autorefraction readings was collected as the refractive error value measured by the autorefractometer. MRT measurements use MSI technology for central refraction measurements. To compare the two devices, the central refraction values from the two devices were analyzed. All examinations were performed by the same experienced doctor.

Statistical analysis was performed using SPSS (version 23). Intra-class correlation coefficient (ICC) and repeated measurement analysis of variance (ANOVA) were used to evaluate the repeatability of the equipment. Pearson's correlation coefficient, paired t-test, and Bland-Altman plots were used to compare the two devices. A value of $P < 0.05$ was taken to indicate statistical significance.

RESULTS

This study enrolled 290 eyes of 145 subjects. Baseline characteristics of the subjects are shown in **Table 1**.

All 290 eyes were measured by one technician, and all values were collected for further analysis. The mean central refraction

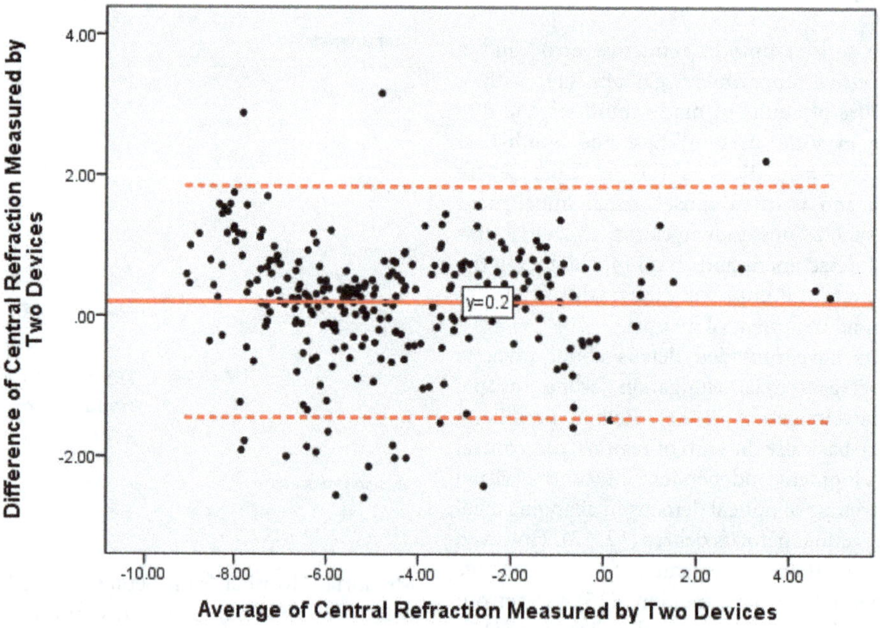

FIGURE 1 | The Bland-Altman plots of central refraction measured by multispectral refraction topography (MRT) and autorefractometer.

measured by an autorefractometer was −4.69 ± 2.64 diopters (D) (range −9.50 to +4.75 D), while the mean central refraction measured by MRT was −4.49 ± 2.61 diopters (D) (range −8.79 to +5.02 D). Pearson correlation analysis revealed a high correlation between MRT and autorefractometer results ($R = 0.950$, $P < 0.001$). **Figure 1** showed the difference values of central refraction between MRT and autorefractometer vs. the average of these two results. The mean difference value was 0.20 D while the 95% confidence interval was −1.43 to +1.83 D.

The correlations of central refraction of the two devices were shown in **Figure 2** ($R = 0.947$, $P < 0.001$).

Tables 2, 3 showed the description and intraclass correlation coefficient (ICC) for central refraction of autorefractometer and multispectral refraction topography. The intrarater and interrater ICC values were 0.947 and 0.973, respectively.

Then we analyzed the result of MRT measurement and subjective refraction. The mean subjective refraction was −4.74 ± 2.66D, its range was −9.50 to +4.75D. The mean of the difference between the central refraction obtained by the MRT measurement and the experienced optometrist was 0.26 ± 0.87D, and its 95% confidence interval was −1.44 to +1.95 (**Figure 3**). The intra-class correlation coefficient of central refraction measured by MRT and subjective refraction was 0.939 (**Figure 4**, $P < 0.001$).

DISCUSSION

The study demonstrates that the central refraction obtained by autorefractometer devices, experienced optometrists, and MRT shows high repeatability and reproducibility. Our results indicate that MRT is a valid and safe method for measuring central refraction error in healthy eyes, particularly for mild myopia. Furthermore, the values showed a high correlation between the two devices. Comparing with autorefractometer or experienced optometrist, measured values by MRT showed a statistically significant shift toward hyperopia. This difference is about 0.20 D (comparing with autorefractometer) to 0.26D (comparing with subjective refraction). It suggests that the accommodation reflex may still have played a role in these participants. We consider the MRT test a more powerful tool to measure the full hyperopic refractive error.

To date, current research suggests that the surrounding area of the eye also plays an important role in controlling the growth of the eye and the development of refractive errors. Peripheral hyperopic defocus of the retina is one of the causes of myopia. If the defocus degree of the retina, especially the peripheral defocus, can be measured effectively and accurately, it will be helpful in preventing myopia. The reason for using objective methods to test peripheral defocus is to try to find the "gold standard" compared with how conventional subjective refraction is used. An ideal screening test should be perfect in specificity, sensitivity, and positive predictive value, but we still can't find any screening method that achieves this level of accuracy. The current methods used to measure peripheral refraction are more difficult to evaluate due to poor retinal image quality, optical aberration and low retinal resolution, which may result in insufficient retinal image sampling (14).

MRT is a new instrument using MSI that can accurately measure the refraction of each part of the retina, and in a sense, it can replace the role of autorefractometer measurement. However,

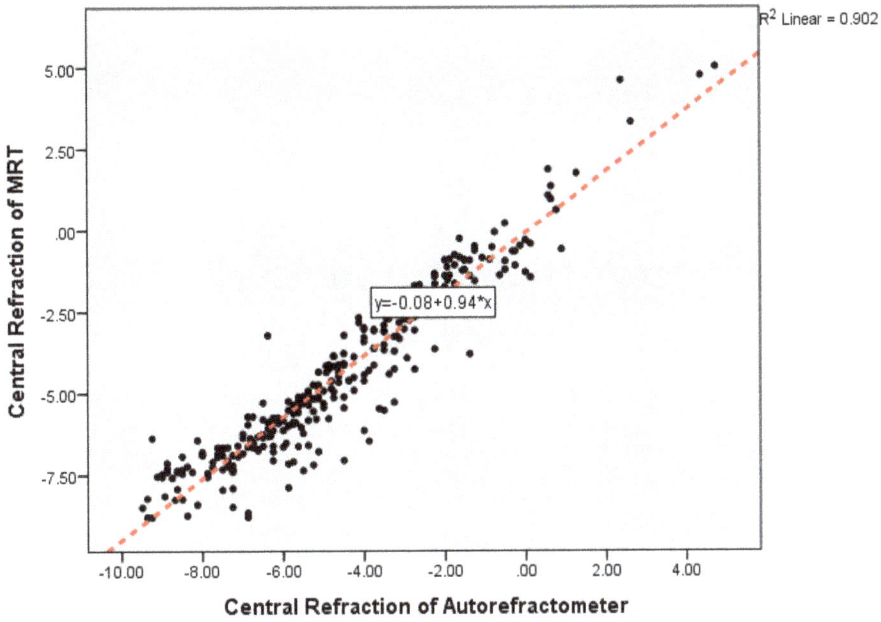

FIGURE 2 | The correlations of central refraction between multispectral refraction topography (MRT) and autorefractometer.

TABLE 2 | Measured Values and Paired *T*-test Results by Autorefractometer and Multispectral Refraction Topography (MRT).

	Mean	Standard deviation	Range	*p*-value(2-tailed) (paired samples test)
Central refraction of MRT	−4.49D	2.61	−8.79D to +5.02D	0.000
Central refraction of autorefractometer	−4.69D	2.64	−9.50D to +4.75D	

TABLE 3 | Intraclass Correlation Coefficient.

	Intraclass	95% confidence interval		F test with true value 0	
	Correlation[b]	Lower bound	Upper bound	Value	Sig
Single measures	0.947[a]	0.931	0.959	38.740	0.000
Average measures	0.973	0.964	0.979	38.740	0.000

Two-way random effects model where both individual effects and measure effects are random. [a]The estimator is the same whether the interaction effect is present or not. [b]Type An intraclass correlation coefficients using an absolute agreement definition.

because the device is a new technology, its accuracy must be compared with the traditional gold standard. Autorefractometers have been used for several decades. They are used in optometric practice all around the world, primarily as a starting point for ophthalmologists or optometrists to assess subjective refraction (20). Autorefractometers are currently the gold standard for testing refration of the central retina. In young adults, most of the time, we would use cycloplegic refraction to detect refractive errors, which is also the gold standard now. Hence, if the central refraction measured by MRT and autorefractometers is consistent in cycloplegic cases, we can assume that the MRT accurately reflects the level of refraction of each part of the retina. MRT is a rapid, accurate, and noninvasive refractometer, and it has excellent specificity and sensitivity. The data of our experiment, under cycloplegic conditions, confirmed that compared with traditional refractometers, MRT can accurately measure central refraction, and the results are closely related to those of autorefractometers. There was no significant difference between the two devices (Pearson correlation coefficient test, $P < 0.001$). To our knowledge, this is the first report of the consistency between MRT and the autorefractometer.

Nevertheless, our experiment has limitations. The subjects of this experiment were Asian individuals ages 20–35 who were treated at Sun Yat-sen Memorial Hospital, and no other ethnic groups were involved. Therefore, further experiments are needed to prove whether this instrument is suitable for other populations. The results included in our study were mostly myopic patients and a few hyperopic patients; there were no patients with high hyperopia, because the greatest proportion of

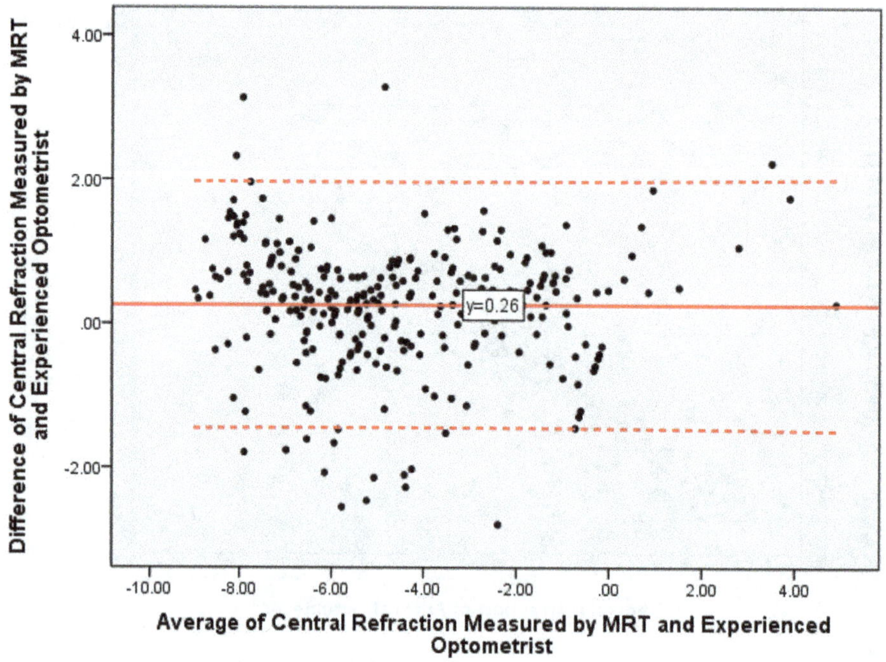

FIGURE 3 | The Bland-Altman plots of central refraction obtained by MRT and experienced optometrist.

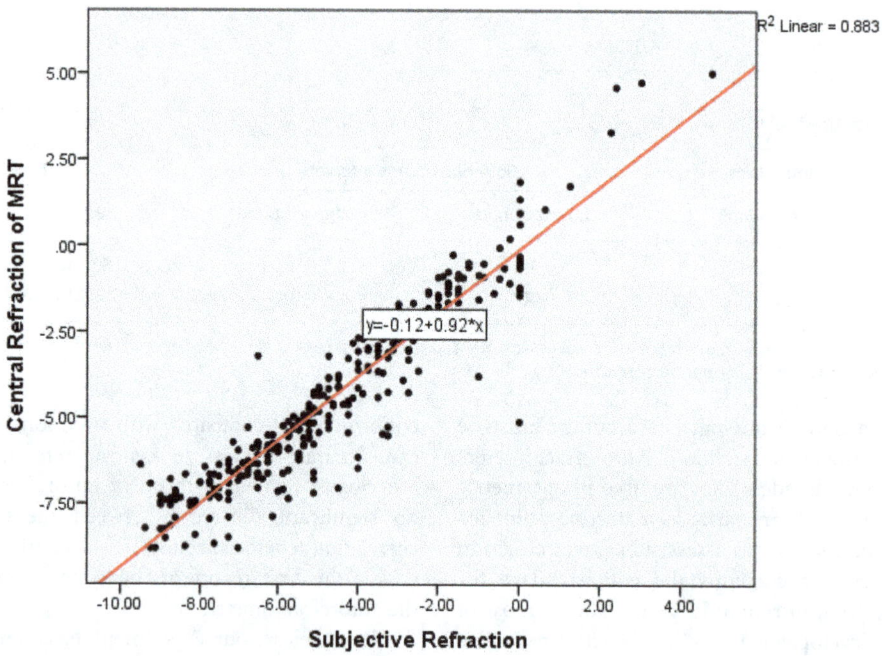

FIGURE 4 | The correlations of central refraction obtained by MRT and experienced optometrist.

myopic patients in China. In the future, we will collect the results of hyperopic patients, especially those with high hyperopia, to clarify the accuracy of the instrument.

In conclusion, results revealed that autorefractometry and MRT show high agreement in measuring central refraction. MRT can accurately reflect the refraction of the retina. It can therefore be used as a potential objective method to measure peripheral defocus of the retina.

ETHICS STATEMENT

The studies involving human participants were reviewed and approved by the Ethics Committee of Sun Yat-sen Memorial Hospital at Sun Yat-sen University. Written informed consent for participation was not required for this study in accordance with the national legislation and the institutional requirements.

AUTHOR CONTRIBUTIONS

YLi, ZY, and YZ contributed to conception and design of the study. ZY, RZ, and JW organized the database. YLi and ZL performed the statistical analysis. YLi wrote the first draft of the manuscript. RZ, ZY, ZL, and YZ wrote sections of the manuscript. All authors contributed to manuscript revision, read, and approved the submitted version.

REFERENCES

1. Dolgin E. The myopia boom. *Nature.* (2015) 519:276–8. doi: 10.1038/519276a
2. Baird PN, Saw SM, Lanca C, Guggenheim JA, Smith EL III, Zhou X, et al. Myopia. *Nat Rev Dis Primers.* (2020) 6:99. doi: 10.1038/s41572-020-00231-4
3. Ding BY, Shih YF, Lin LLK, Hsiao CK, Wang IJ. Myopia among schoolchildren in East Asia and Singapore. *Surv Ophthalmol.* (2017) 62:677–97.
4. Grossniklaus HE, Green WR. Pathologic findings in pathologic myopia. *Retina.* (1992) 12:127–33. doi: 10.1097/00006982-199212020-00009
5. Diether S, Schaeffel F. Local changes in eye growth induced by imposed local refractive error despite active accommodation. *Vision Res.* (1997) 37:659–68. doi: 10.1016/S0042-6989(96)00224-6
6. Irving EL, Sivak JG, Callender MG. Refractive plasticity of the developing chick eye: a summary and update. *Ophthalmic Physiol Opt.* (2015) 35:600–6. doi: 10.1111/opo.12253
7. Smith EL III, Kee CS, Ramamirtham R, Qiao-Grider Y, Hung LF. Peripheral vision can influence eye growth and refractive development in infant monkeys. *Invest Ophthalmol Vis Sci.* (2005) 46:3965–72. doi: 10.1167/iovs.05-0445
8. Benavente-Perez A, Nour A, Troilo D. Axial eye growth and refractive error development can be modified by exposing the peripheral retina to relative myopic or hyperopic defocus. *Invest Ophthalmol Vis Sci.* (2014) 55:6765–73. doi: 10.1167/iovs.14-14524
9. McFadden SA, Howlett MH, Mertz JR. Retinoic acid signals the direction of ocular elongation in the guinea pig eye. *Vision Res.* (2004) 44:643–53. doi: 10.1016/j.visres.2003.11.002
10. Mutti DO, Gwiazda J, Norton TT, Smith EL III, Schaeffel F. To CH: Myopia—yesterday, today, and tomorrow. *Optom Vis Sci.* (2013) 90:1161–4. doi: 10.1097/OPX.0000000000000117
11. Smith EL III, Hung LF, Huang J, Arumugam B. Effects of local myopic defocus on refractive development in monkeys. *Optom Vis Sci.* (2013) 90:1176–86. doi: 10.1097/OPX.0000000000000038
12. Koumbo Mekountchou IO, Conrad F, Sankaridurg P, Ehrmann K. Peripheral eye length measurement techniques: a review. *Clin Exp Optom.* (2020) 103:138–47. doi: 10.1111/cxo.12892
13. Atchison DA, Pritchard N, Schmid KL, Scott DH, Jones CE, Pope JM. Shape of the retinal surface in emmetropia and myopia. *Invest Ophthalmol Vis Sci.* (2005) 46:2698–707.
14. Lundstrom L, Gustafsson J, Svensson I, Unsbo P. Assessment of objective and subjective eccentric refraction. *Optom Vis Sci.* (2005) 82:298–306. doi: 10.1097/01.OPX.0000159366.61943.62
15. Wang YZ, Thibos LN, Lopez N, Salmon T, Bradley A. Subjective refraction of the peripheral field using contrast detection acuity. *J Am Optom Assoc.* (1996) 67:584–9.
16. Liang J, Grimm B, Goelz S, Bille JF. Objective measurement of wave aberrations of the human eye with the use of a Hartmann-Shack wave-front sensor. *J Opt Soc Am A Opt Image Sci Vis.* (1994) 11:1949–57. doi: 10.1364/JOSAA.11.001949
17. Jackson DW, Paysse EA, Wilhelmus KR, Hussein MA, Rosby G, Coats DK. The effect of off-the-visual-axis retinoscopy on objective refractive measurement. *Am J Ophthalmol.* (2004) 137:1101–4. doi: 10.1016/j.ajo.2004.02.012
18. Rosen R, Lundstrom L, Unsbo P. Influence of optical defocus on peripheral vision. *Invest Ophthalmol Vis Sci.* (2011) 52:318–23. doi: 10.1167/iovs.10-5623
19. Atchison DA, Mathur A, Varnas SR. Visual performance with lenses correcting peripheral refractive errors. *Optom Vis Sci.* (2013) 90:1304–11. doi: 10.1097/OPX.0000000000000033
20. Stoor K, Karvonen E, Liinamaa J, Saarela V. Evaluating refraction and visual acuity with the Nidek autorefractometer AR-360A in a randomized population-based screening study. *Acta Ophthalmol.* (2018) 96:384–9. doi: 10.1111/aos.13636

17

Vitrectomy with Peeling the Internal Limiting Membrane for the Treatment of Macular Hole Following Ruptured Retinal Arterial Macroaneurysm

Zhigao Liu[1], *Shuya Wang*[1], *Yu Wang*[2], *Aihua Ma*[3] *and Bojun Zhao*[1,4*]

[1] *First Clinical Medical College, Shandong University of Traditional Chinese Medicine, Jinan, China,* [2] *Department of Ophthalmology, Jinan Aier Eye Hospital, Jinan, China,* [3] *Department of Pediatrics, Shandong Provincial Hospital Affiliated to Shandong First Medical University, Jinan, China,* [4] *Department of Ophthalmology, Shandong Provincial Hospital Affiliated to Shandong First Medical University, Jinan, China*

***Correspondence:**
Bojun Zhao
xiaoyuxinsheng@163.com

Background: This study aimed to report a case of vitrectomy with peeling the internal limiting membrane for the treatment of macular hole (MH) following ruptured retinal arterial macroaneurysm (RAMA).

Case Presentation: A 65-year-old woman noticed a sudden decrease in vision in the left eye. She had no other ocular problems apart from a mild cataract in both eyes before. Her best-corrected visual acuity (BCVA) was 20/33 in the right eye, and 6/100 in the left eye. Fluorescein angiography (FFA) showed a retinal arterial macroaneurysm with telangiectatic retinal vascular changes in the inferior temporal macular region. Optical coherence tomography (OCT) examination demonstrated the presence of subretinal hemorrhage extending into the foveal area and incomplete posterior vitreous detachment. Because of the presence of submacular hemorrhage, some medicine was administrated and the patient was followed up. Then, 5 months later, the hemorrhage was absorbed. OCT examination exhibited a full-thickness MH with a macular epiretinal membrane. The size of the MH was 722 μm in diameter. She was then given a standard three-port pars plana vitrectomy (PPV), along with peeling of the internal limiting membrane (ILM) and filling the vitreous cavity with air. Anatomic closure of the MH was achieved after 4 weeks of the surgery by the examination of OCT. The BCVA was improved to 15/100.

Conclusions: This case expanded our knowledge of the association of MH secondary to ruptured RAMA. We reported a case with successful surgical closure of the MH and improvement of BCVA.

Keywords: retinal arterial macroaneurysm, macular hole (MH), vitrectomy, visual acuity, ILM peeling

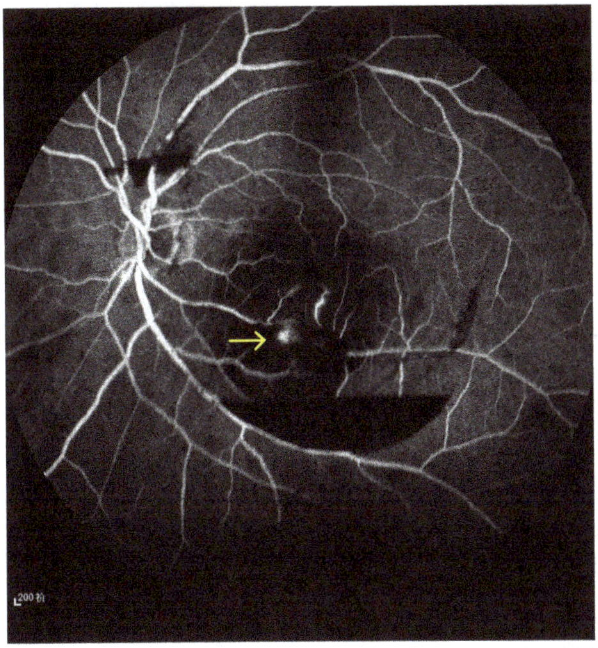

FIGURE 1 | A retinal arterial macroaneurysm with telangiectatic retinal vascular changes in the inferior temporal macular region (yellow arrow shows).

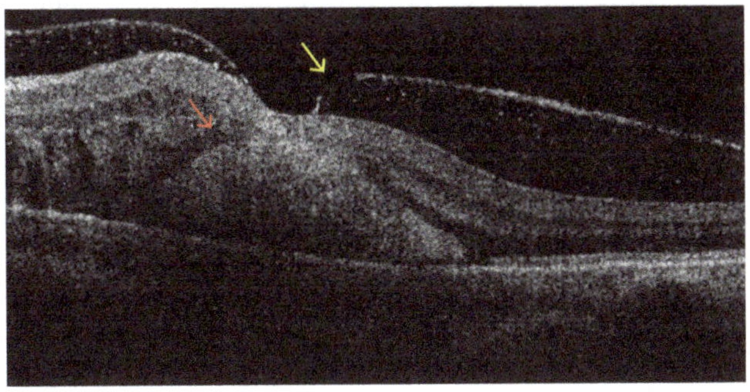

FIGURE 2 | The presence of subretinal hemorrhage which extending into the foveal area (red arrow shows) and incomplete posterior vitreous detachment (yellow arrow shows).

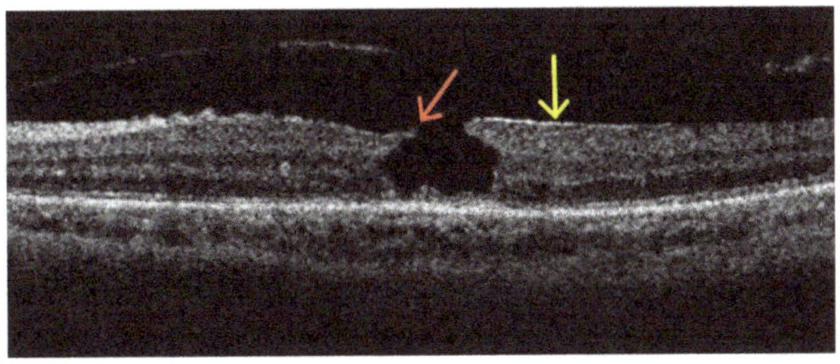

FIGURE 3 | A full-thickness macular hole (MH) (red arrow shows) with macular epiretinal membrane (yellow arrow shows).

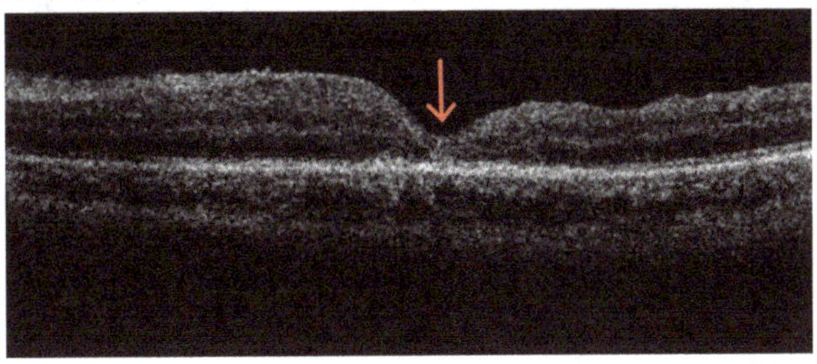

FIGURE 4 | Anatomic closure of the MH (red arrow shows) was achieved after 4 weeks of the surgery. The BCVA was improved to 15/100.

BACKGROUND

Macular holes (MHs) are usually idiopathic and occur most commonly in healthy, middle-aged women. In rare cases, MHs have been associated with retinal vascular diseases such as proliferative diabetic retinopathy (1), hypertensive retinopathy (2), congenital retinal arteriovenous communication (3), and retinal arterial macroaneurysm (4). The onset of MH after the rupture of a retinal arterial macroaneurysm (RAMA) is a sight-threatening complication (5, 6). Previous reports have suggested that 5.9–12.5% of RAMA ruptures result in MH and that anatomic successful rate of surgical intervention for MH secondary to RAMA is between 57.1 and 75%(7, 8). Which is lower than that of surgical intervention for idiopathic MH (9). Moreover, there are limited effective surgical procedures for the treatment of MH after RAMA rupture.

Several studies have reported the efficacy of autologous transplantation of ILM (10, 11) and the inverted ILM flap technique (12) for the treatment of MH. In our report, we described the application of vitrectomy with peeling the Internal limiting membrane for the treatment of stage IV MH caused by RAMA rupture.

CASE PRESENTATION

A 65-year-old woman with a longstanding history of hypertension noticed a sudden decrease in vision in her left eye.

Abbreviations: MH, macular holes; RAMA, rupture of a retinal arterial macroaneurysm.

She had no other ocular problems apart from a mild cataract in both eyes before. Her best-corrected visual acuity was 20/33 in her right eye, and 6/100 in her left eye. Fluorescein angiography showed a retinal arterial macroaneurysm with telangiectatic retinal vascular changes in the inferior temporal macular region (**Figure 1**). Optical coherence tomography (OCT) examination demonstrated the presence of subretinal hemorrhage which extends into the foveal area, and incomplete posterior vitreous detachment (**Figure 2**). Because of the presence of submacular hemorrhage, some medicine was administrated and the patient was followed up. Then, 5 months later, the hemorrhage was absorbed. OCT examination exhibited a full-thickness MH with a macular epiretinal membrane (**Figure 3**). The size of the

MH was 722 μm in diameter. She was then given a standard three-port pars plana vitrectomy, along with peeling of the internal limiting membrane and filling the vitreous cavity with air. Anatomic closure of the MH was achieved after 4 weeks of the surgery by the examination of OCT (**Figure 4**). The BCVA was improved to 15/100.

Pars plana vitrectomy (PPV) method:

Standard three-port vitrectomy was performed, followed by surgical separation of the posterior cortical vitreous from the optic nerve and posterior retina. About 1% indocyanine green (ICG) was injected over the macula region after temporarily stopping the infusion. The ILM with 2 disk diameters of the fovea was removed. The vitreous cavity was filled with air. The patient was asked to remain face down for a week following the surgery.

DISCUSSION

The formation of MH following a ruptured RAMA is not entirely uncommon. Colucciello and Nachbar (5) reported a 67-year-old female patient who developed a full-thickness MH at 5 months after being diagnosed with a ruptured RAMA. A thickened, taut posterior vitreous cortex was observed during vitrectomy. Ciardella and Gaetano (13) reported a patient who developed a stage IV MH in association with a retinal arterial macroaneurysm combined with a total posterior vitreous detachment. In our case, a possible reason for the formation of the MH was that a posterior vitreous detachment induced by the submacular hemorrhage. Another possibility was that acute subretinal hemorrhage might elevate the pressure in the subretinal space which led to the dehiscence of the fovea. The anatomic successful rate of surgical intervention for MH secondary to RAMA is lower than that of idiopathic MH (4, 8, 9). Thus, it is very important to explore surgical methods for the treatment of MH secondary to RAMA. Kumagai et al. (14) reported a retrospective, non-randomized, comparative trial which showed that Internal limiting membrane peeling in MH surgery achieved high closure and low reopening rates. Brooks (9) reported that ILM peeling significantly improved vision and anatomic recovery in all stages of recent and chronic MHs.

In conclusion, this case expanded our knowledge of the association of MHs secondary to ruptured RAMA. We reported a case with successful surgical closure of the MH and improvement of BCVA. Large-scale, randomized, comparative, and prospective studies are needed to further warrant this method.

ETHICS STATEMENT

The studies involving human participants were reviewed and approved by the Ethics Committee of Jinan Aier Eye Hospital. The patients/participants provided their written informed consent to participate in this study. Written informed consent was obtained from the individual(s) for the publication of any potentially identifiable images or data included in this article.

AUTHOR CONTRIBUTIONS

ZL contributed to writing the manuscript. YW and SW contributed to the literature research and preparation of the manuscript and figures. AM and BZ are responsible for the design of the case report. All authors read and approved the final manuscript.

REFERENCES

1. Flynn HW. Macular hole surgery in patients with proliferative diabetic retinopathy. *Arch Ophthalmol.* (1994) 112:877–8. doi: 10.1001/archopht.1994.01090190021011
2. Cohen SM, Gass JDM. Macular hole following severe hypertensive retinopathy. *Arch Ophthalmol.* (1994) 112:878–9. doi: 10.1001/archopht.1994.01090190022012
3. Munoz FJ, Rebolleda G, Cores FJ, Bertrand J. Congenital retinal arteriovenous communication associated with a full thickness macular hole. *Acta Ophthalmol.* (1991) 69:117–20. doi: 10.1111/j.1755-3768.1991.tb02007.x
4. Mitamura Y, Terashima H, Taheuchi S. Macular hole formation following rupture of retinal arterial macroaneurysm. *Retina.* (2002) 22:113–5. doi: 10.1097/00006982-200202000-00023
5. Coucciello M, Nachbar JG. Macular hole following ruptured retinal arterial macroaneurysm. *Retina.* (2000) 20:94–6. doi: 10.1097/00006982-200001000-00018
6. Bakri SJ, Sears JE, Lewis H. Management of macular hole and submacular hemorrhage in the same eye. *Graefes Arch Clin Exp Ophthalmol.* (2007) 245:609–11. doi: 10.1007/s00417-006-0349-8
7. Tashimo A, Mitamura Y, Ohtsuka K, Okushiba U, Imaizumi H, Takeda M. Macular hole formation following ruptured retinal arterial macroaneurysm. *Am J Ophthalmol.* (2003) 135:487–92. doi: 10.1016/S0002-9394(02)02084-6
8. Sagara N, Kawaji T, Koshiyama Y, Inlmata Y, Fukushima M, Tanihara H. Macular hole formation after macular haemorrhage associated with rupture of retinal arterial macroaneurysm. *Br J Ophthalmol.* (2009) 93:1337–40. doi: 10.1136/bjo.2008.149195
9. Brooks HL. Macular hole surgery with and without internal limiting membrane peeling. *Ophthalmology.* (2000) 107:1939–48. doi: 10.1016/S0161-6420(00)00331-6
10. Dai Y, Dong F, Zhang X, Yang Z. Internal limiting membrane transplantation for unclosed and large macular holes. *Graefes Arch Clin Exp Ophthalmol.* (2016) 254:2095–9. doi: 10.1007/s00417-016-3461-4
11. Kumase F, Morizane Y, Kimura S, Toshima S, Shiraga F. Autologous internal limiting membrane transplants successfully close a large parafoveal retinal hole. *Acta Med Okayama.* (2017) 71:255–7. doi: 10.18926/AMO/55209
12. Michalewska Z, Michalewski J, Dulczewska-Cichecka K, Adelman RA, Mrwrocki J. Temporal inverted internal limiting membrane flap technique versus classic inverted interval limiting membrane flap technique: a comparative study.

Retina. (2015) 35:1844–50. doi: 10.1097/IAE.0000000000000555

13. Ciardella A, Barile G, Schiff W. Ruptured retinal arterial macroaneurysm associated with a stage IV macular hole. *Am J Ophthalmol.* (2003) 135:907–9. doi: 10.1016/S0002-9394(02)02238-9
14. Kumagai K, Furukawa M, Ogino N, Uemura A, Demizu S, Larson E. Vitreous surgery with and without internal limiting membrane peeling for macular hole repair. *Retina.* (2004) 24:721–7. doi: 10.1097/00006982-200410000-00006

18

Analysis of Primary Iris and Ciliary Body Cysts in Chinese Patients with Primary Angle Closure Disease

Kun Wei†, Chengguo Zuo†, Jinyi Xu, Liming Chen, Dingqiao Wang, Zhongshu Tang and Mingkai Lin**

State Key Laboratory of Ophthalmology, Zhongshan Ophthalmic Center, Sun Yat-sen University, Guangzhou, China

***Correspondence:**
Zhongshu Tang
tangzhsh@mail.sysu.edu.cn
Mingkai Lin
linmk@mail.sysu.edu.cn*

†These authors have contributed equally to this work and share first authorship

Aim: To investigate the incidence and clinical features of primary iris and ciliary body cysts in Chinese primary angle closure disease (PACD). Patients were evaluated by measuring and analyzing the cysts with an ultrasound biomicroscope (UBM).

Methods: The data of patients diagnosed with PACD were reviewed. Demographic data were collected, and the cyst number, size, location, and trabecular-iris angle (TIA) were measured, with the size including the longest diameter (LD) and its corresponding vertical diameter (CVD).

Results: A total of 1,334 cases (2,317 eyes) were reviewed, and 409 cysts were found in 131 cases (168 eyes), with an average of 2.43 ± 3.14 cysts per eye. The ages of the patients with cysts ranged from 25 to 80 years, with an average age of 55.24 ± 12.22 years. The detection rate was 7.3%, and the majority of cysts were located in the iridociliary sulcus. Among the 131 patients, 94 had monocular cysts, while binocular cysts occurred in 37 patients. The locations of the cysts in both eyes were mainly in the inferior and temporal quadrants (42.5 and 34.0%, respectively). The cysts were mainly of medium size (49.9%), followed by small cysts (33.3%), large cysts (14.7%) and giant cysts (2.2%). The average LD was 0.68 ± 0.33 mm, and the average CVD was 0.45 ± 0.23 mm. There were no statistically significant differences in the TIA between the cyst area and unaffected area.

Conclusions: The incidence of cysts is 7.3% in the PACD population. The cysts are mainly monocular, medium in size, and located in the iridociliary sulcus. Additionally, the cysts were located mainly in the inferior and temporal quadrants. These cysts have little effect on the anterior chamber angle.

Keywords: PACD, primary iris and ciliary body cysts, UBM, monocular, glaucoma

INTRODUCTION

Glaucoma ranks among the top three blinding eye diseases in the world, and the number of cases is on the rise, according to recent surveys. Investigators predict that the number of glaucoma patients in China will increase to approximately 25 million by 2050 (1). Primary angle closure disease (PACD) is a major blinding disease in the Asian population, and PACD includes primary angle closure suspect (PACS), primary angle closure (PAC) and primary angle closure glaucoma (PACG). The structure and position of the iris and ciliary body are important anatomical structures in the pathogenesis of PACD (2, 3). The diagnosis and treatment effect may be affected by abnormalities of the iris and ciliary body. One of the most important congenital/primary abnormalities includes primary iris and ciliary body cysts, which are located mainly in the iridociliary sulcus or ciliary body (4–6). However, to the best of our knowledge, there are no relevant systematic studies on primary iris and ciliary body cysts in PACD patients.

The aim of this study was to investigate the incidence and clinical features of iris and ciliary body cysts in Chinese PACD patients by analyzing ultrasound biomicroscope (UBM) data.

MATERIALS AND METHODS

Methods

Patients diagnosed with PACD underwent UBM anterior segment examination at the Zhongshan Ophthalmic Center of Sun Yat-sen University. We recruited patients with PACD who met the following criteria: age over 18 years, diagnosis of PACD, and intraocular pressure (IOP) controlled within the normal range for more than 1 week. The definitions of PACG, PACS and PAC followed those of the International Society of Geographical & Epidemiological Ophthalmology (ISGEO) (7). Patients with corneal disease, previous ocular surgery, ocular trauma, ocular inflammation, or severe systemic disease were excluded. This study was approved by the Ethics Review Committee (NO. 2021KYPJ003).

Diagnostic Classification

Single cyst refers to only one cyst being found in one eye (**Figures 1A,B**). Multiple cysts refers to two or more cysts being found in one eye (**Figure 1C**). Monocular multiple cysts (MMCs) refers to multiple cysts in only one eye with the other having no cysts. Bilateral multiple cysts (BMCs) refers to multiple cysts in both eyes. Monocular single cysts (MSCs) indicates that only one eye had a single cyst with the other having no cysts. Bilateral single cysts (BSC) indicates a single cyst in each eye. Bilateral mix type cysts (BMTC) refers to a single cyst in one eye and multiple cysts in the other eye. The cyst size was determined by calculating its mean size (MS: average of the longest diameter (LD) and its corresponding vertical diameter (CVD) with the UBM); a MS <0.4 mm was defined as a small cyst, a MS ranging from 0.4 to 0.8 mm was defined as a medium cyst, a MS ranging from 0.8 to 1.3 mm was defined as a large cyst, and a MS >1.3 mm was defined as a giant cyst (8).

Examination Methods

The UBM (model SW-3200 L; Tianjin Suowei Electronic Technology Co, Ltd., Tianjin, China) in the Glaucoma Department of Zhongshan Ophthalmic Center of Sun Yat-sen University was used for inspection. During the examination, the examinee was asked to lie in the supine position. After the examinee was fully anesthetized with topical anesthesia (0.5% proparacaine hydrochloride), the eye cup without the fundus

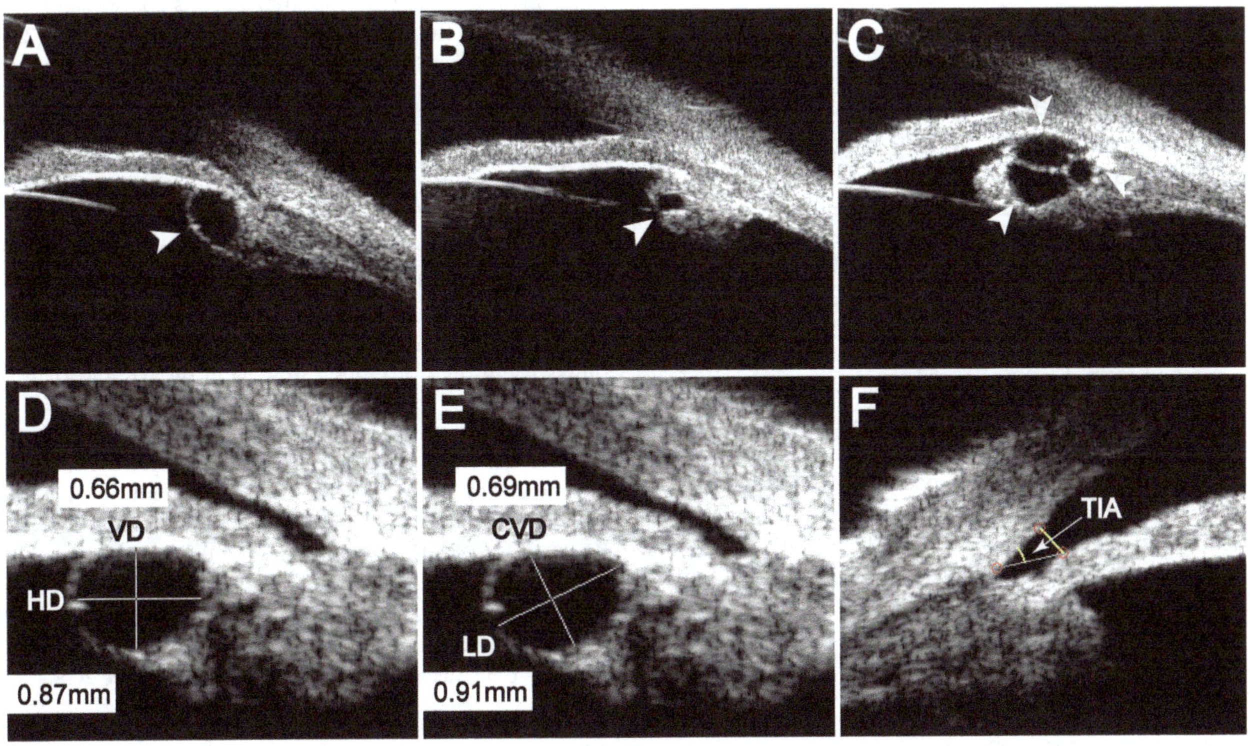

FIGURE 1 | The type and measurement of the cysts. **(A)** Cyst located in the iridociliary sulcus, **(B)** Cyst located in the ciliary body, **(C)** Multiple cysts. **(D)** and **(E)** Different measurement methods for the same cyst; HD, horizontal diameter; VD, vertical diameter; LD, longest diameter; CVD, corresponding vertical diameter of the LD. **(F)** TIA, the trabecular-iris angle.

was placed in the conjunctival sac, and an appropriate amount of sterile normal saline was added. The examiner held the UBM probe on one hand and examined the eye from 12 o'clock clockwise around its entire circumference. Two-dimensional images of the anterior segment of the eyes were recorded, and a clear image was selected for preservation.

Analysis Methods

UBM software was used to measure the cyst, and measurements included the affected eye and the position, LD and CVD of the cyst. The average value and the number of cysts in each eye were also calculated (6, 9). To avoid deviations caused by interobserver error, all measurements were conducted by a single experienced operator. LD represented the longest axis of the cyst, and CVD represented the longest axis perpendicular to the LD (**Figure 1E**). The trabecular-iris angle (TIA) was measured using the ACA/AOD function in the UBM software, with the apex at the scleral spur and the arms of the angle passing through a point on the trabecular meshwork 500 μm from the scleral spur and a perpendicular point on the iris (**Figure 1F**).

Statistical Analysis

All data were analyzed using the statistical software SPSS 23. Differences in mean values were examined using *t*-tests. Categorical data were analyzed using the chi-square test. The incidence of cysts was calculated by means of the odds ratio. A *P*-value of <0.05 was considered to indicate statistical significance. There was no significant difference if the 95% CI of the odds ratio included 1.

RESULT

Detection Rate and General Situation of the Primary Iris and Ciliary Body Cysts

The data of 1,334 patients (2,317 eyes), including 499 males (818 eyes) and 835 females (1,499 eyes), were reviewed. Their ages ranged from 19 to 94 years, with an average age of 60.41 ± 12.07 years. There were 824 cases (1,193 eyes) with PACS, 367 cases (448 eyes) with PAC and 535 cases (676 eyes) with PACG. Of the 1,334 cases (2,317 eyes), 131 cases (168 eyes), aged 25–80 years (average age of 55.24 ± 12.22 years), were found to have primary iris and ciliary body cysts, and the average detection rate accounted for 7.3% of the eyes examined. Of all 131 PACD patients with cysts, 54 (72 eyes) were males, with a 10.8% detection rate in the male population, and 77 (96 eyes) were females, with a 9.2% detection rate in the female population. The odds ratio was 1.195 (95% CI: 0.828–1.724), which indicated that there was no significant difference in the incidences of males and females. Among them, 59 patients (68 eyes) had PACS, 43 patients (46 eyes) had PAC, and 44 patients (54 eyes) had PACG (**Table 1**). There was no significant difference in the proportion of cysts in different diseases ($P = 0.180$).

Distribution of the Cysts

Among the 2,317 eyes reviewed, we found 409 cysts in 168 eyes, with an average of 2.43 ± 3.14 per eye. Among the 409 cysts detected, 199 cysts were found in the right eye, and 210 cysts were found in the left eye. The proportion of cysts was not significantly correlated with the laterality of the eye ($P = 0.475$) (**Table 2**).

TABLE 1 | Demographic features of the population with cysts.

	Disease (eye)				
AGE	PAC	PACG	PACS	Total	Proportion
≤29	2	0	1	3	1.8%
30–39	4	3	8	15	8.9%
40–49	12	14	12	38	22.6%
50–59	10	20	14	44	26.2%
60–69	13	8	23	44	26.2%
≥70	5	9	10	24	14.3%
Total	46	54	68	168	100%

TABLE 2 | The morphology of the cysts.

	Males				Females			
	OD		OS		OD		OS	
	N	%	N	%	N	%	N	%
Small	28	28.6%	34	35.4%	38	37.6%	36	31.6%
Medium	47	48.0%	45	46.9%	48	47.5%	64	56.1%
Large	19	19.4%	15	15.6%	12	11.9%	14	12.3%
Giant	4	4.1%	2	2.1%	3	3.0%	0	0.0%
Total	98	100.0%	96	100.0%	101	100.0%	114	100.0%

Of 409 cysts, 283 (69.2%) were located in the iridociliary sulcus (**Figure 1A**), and 126 (30.8%) were located in the ciliary body (**Figure 1B**). The location of cysts was not significantly related to sex ($P = 0.632$) or the laterality of the eye ($P = 0.479$).

Among the 409 cysts, the most common quadrant was the inferior quadrant (42.5%, 174 cysts), followed by the temporal quadrant (34%, 139 cysts), superior quadrant (12.7%, 52 cysts) and nasal quadrant (10.8%, 44 cysts), indicating that most of the cysts occurred in the inferior and temporal quadrants ($P < 0.001$) (**Figure 2A**). We also found that there was no significant difference in the distribution of cysts in the left and right eyes ($P = 0.221$).

Among 168 eyes with cysts detected, 103 (61.3%) eyes had single cysts, and 65 (38.7%) eyes had multiple cysts. Multiple cysts with 2 to 3 per eye were common, accounting for 22.6% of eyes. Eyes with more than 4 cysts were less frequent, accounting for 16.1% of eyes (**Figure 2B**). Among the 131 patients, 94 had monocular cysts, and 37 had binocular cysts. The incidence of MSCs was significantly higher than that of other types ($P < 0.001$). Additionally, we found that the proportion of females with this type was higher than that of males (**Figure 2C**).

Morphological Analysis of Cysts

Among 409 cysts, the average LD was 0.68 ± 0.33 mm, ranging from 0.18 to 2.07 mm, and the average CVD was 0.45 ± 0.23 mm, ranging from 0.08 to 2.04 mm. There was no statistically

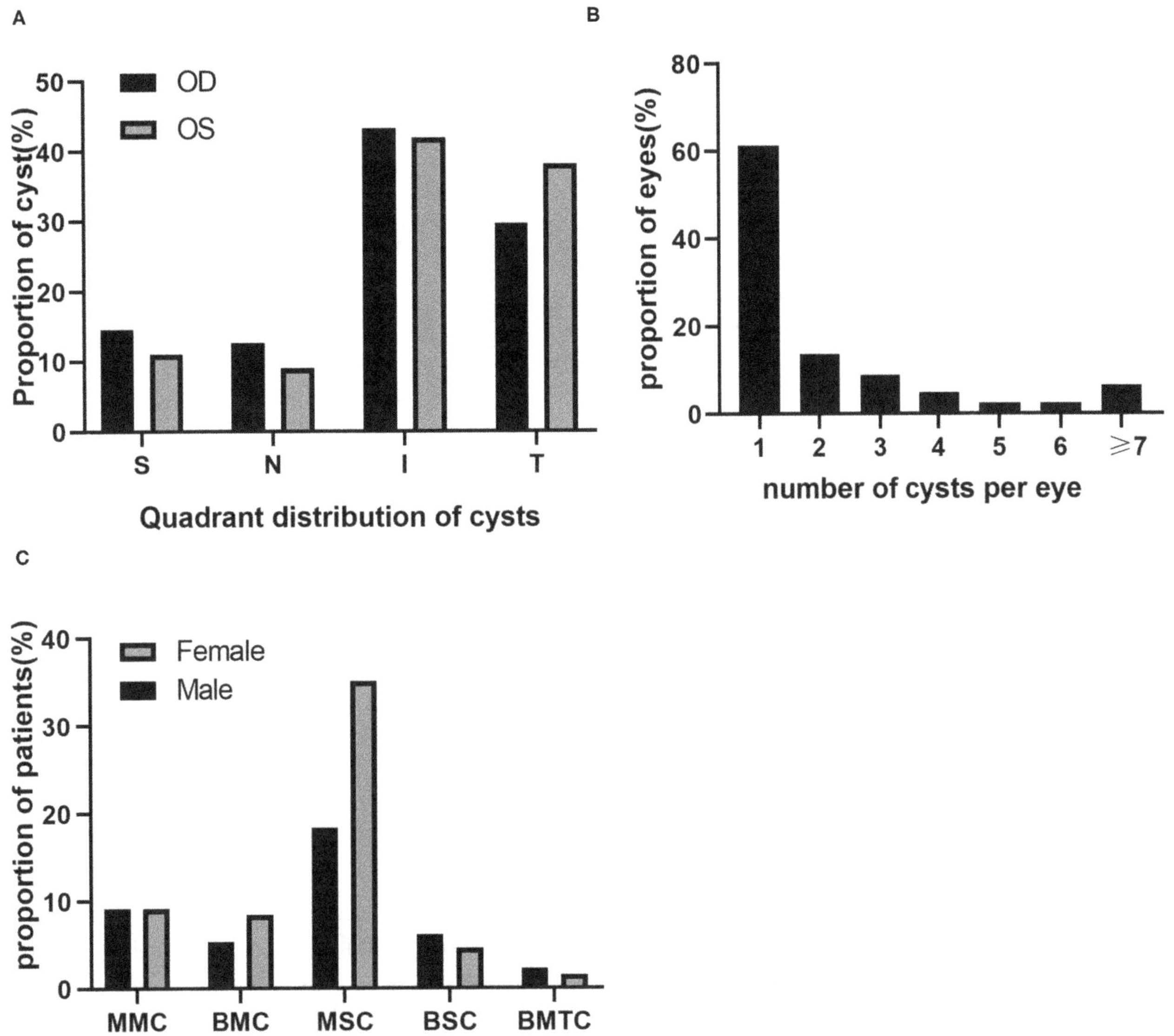

FIGURE 2 | Distribution of cysts. **(A)** Quadrant distribution of cysts; N, nasal; I, inferior; T, temporal; S, superior. **(B)** Number of cysts per eye. **(C)** Type of cysts; MMC, monocular multiple cysts; BMC, bilateral multiple cysts; MSC, monocular single cysts; BSC, bilateral single cysts; BMTC, bilateral mix type cysts.

significant difference between the left and right eyes (P_{LD} = 0.192, P_{CVD} = 0.145).

Among the cysts detected, most were medium cysts, followed by small cysts and large cysts, and the least common were giant cysts. The size distribution of the cysts showed no significant difference between the laterality of eyes (P = 0.312) or between males and females (P = 0.263) (**Table 2**).

TABLE 3 | Analysis of the correlation between cysts and the anterior chamber angle.

Cyst location	Cyst TIA	Baseline TIA	*P*
Ciliary body	13.25 ± 14.51	13.12 ± 12.85	0.896
Iridociliary	10.12 ± 11.81	11.03 ± 10.35	0.145
Total	10.97 ± 12.65	11.60 ± 11.10	0.236

Analysis of the Effect of Cysts on the Anterior Chamber Angle

To analyze the correlation between the cyst and angle more accurately, we measured the TIA of the cysts and the affected eyes. The mean values of TIA at the 3, 6, 9 and 12 o'clock positions were used as the baseline TIA of the affected eye. If there was a cyst at the abovementioned clock position, the average value of the other three clock positions was taken as the baseline TIA. After analyzing the relevant data by means of SPSS software, we found that there was no significant difference in TIA between the area of the cysts and the affected eyes (P = 0.236) (**Table 3**).

DISCUSSION

Using UBM for inspection of 1,334 patients (2,317 eyes) who met our criteria, we found that there were a total of 131 cases (168 eyes) with primary iris and ciliary body cysts. Single cysts accounted for 61.3% of cases, medium cysts accounted for 49.9%, iridociliary sulcus cysts accounted for 69.2%, and inferior quadrant cysts and temporal quadrant cysts accounted for 42.5 and 34.0%, respectively. These results indicate that the incidence of primary iris and ciliary body cysts in Chinese PACD is 7.3% and that the cysts are mainly monocular, medium in size, distributed in the iridociliary sulcus and located in the inferior and temporal quadrants. Additionally, the presence of a cyst does not lead to significant narrowing of the anterior chamber angle.

Despite the critical role of the structure and position of the primary iris and ciliary body in the pathogenesis of PACD, few relevant systematic studies with large samples are currently available. This may be related to the low detection rate of cysts in routine ophthalmic examinations due to iris occlusion (10). In our study, with the application of UBM, ciliary body cysts were observed thoroughly. Since primary iris and ciliary body cysts are mostly congenital (4, 5), the prevalence should be independent of age and eye disease. Nevertheless, the cysts we detected were significantly related to age (89.3% were present in patients over 40 years old). This incidence may be related to the fact that patients with PACD are more likely to come to the hospital for examination due to eye discomfort and thus have a higher probability of cysts screened by UBM. Our data showed that patients with cysts were mainly 40–79 years old, which was also the peak onset age of PACD (11).

With regard to the incidence of cysts, the data obtained by different researchers varied greatly (6, 9, 11). After carefully analyzing the respective research methods and survey populations, we speculated that the differences in incidence may be due to race, age and disease characteristics of the subjects. Different types of UBMs and detection methods would also have an impact. This view is consistent with Kunimatsu, S's article (6).

Our data showed that the cysts were located mainly in the inferior quadrant, followed by the temporal quadrant, superior quadrant and nasal quadrant, which was consistent with the results of other researchers (6, 9, 11). In traditional filtration surgery, antiglaucoma surgery is less affected by the cyst, as the surgical areas are concentrated mostly in the upper area. In the clinic, lens extraction is widely used to treat primary angle closure glaucoma (12, 13). Cysts may have a significant influence on lens extraction, as doctors usually operate in the temporal area (14, 15). Therefore, the presence of cysts in the surgical area may increase the difficulty of an operation when the patient needs lens extraction. For some reasons, a proportion of patients have to undergo antiglaucoma surgery on the inferior and nasal sides due to uncontrolled IOP after the initial antiglaucoma surgery fails (16–18). The presence of cysts may make surgery more difficult. Attention should be given to the situation and type of ocular cysts, especially whether there are cysts in the operation area, which is conducive to reducing the incidence of intraoperative and postoperative complications. A researcher once reported a case in which cyst blockage caused iridotomy failure (19). Another researcher also believes that after precise positioning of the cyst location, selecting a cyst-free area for laser peripheral iridotomy can achieve better surgical results (20).

Some researchers have used horizontal and vertical diameters to measure cyst size (8). In our research, we found that most cysts were irregular in shape and changeable in position. For these cysts, traditional measurements could not accurately reflect the size of the cyst (**Figure 1D**), so we used LD and CVD to measure the cysts (**Figure 1E**). We believe that this new method can more accurately reflect the size of the cyst.

For PACD patients, the degree of narrowing or closure of the anterior chamber angle directly affects the diagnosis and treatment of glaucoma. To further explore the relationship between the cyst and angle, we compared the TIA between the clock position of the cyst and the affected eye, and it turned out that there was no significant correlation between the TIA of the cyst and the baseline TIA of the eye ($P = 0.236$). A few studies have found that cysts might push the iris root closer to the anterior chamber angle, resulting in narrower angles or closure (21, 22). Some researchers believe that cysts can lead to secondary angle closure or even acute secondary glaucoma (23, 24). However, these reports are about large or giant cysts. Since our study identified mainly small and medium cysts, no statistical significance was found in this relatively large cohort, and many studies have shown similar results (8, 25). When PACD coexists with cysts, the possibility of aggravated glaucoma is relatively low.

LIMITATIONS

Bias may exist in hospital-based cross-sectional studies. A larger sample of follow-up observations is essential to verify these results before a more accurate conclusion can be drawn.

Our study shows that the incidence of primary iris and ciliary body cysts in Chinese patients with PACD is 7.3%. Most of them are MSCs. The cysts were mainly medium cysts, with an average size of 0.68 ± 0.33 mm in LD and 0.45 ± 0.23 mm in CVD. Moreover, most of the cysts are located in the inferior and temporal quadrants, which may easily affect an operation on the inferior temporal side. When a patient needs antiglaucoma surgery, the precise positioning of the iris and ciliary body cysts before surgery can help reduce intraoperative and postoperative complications. Additionally, the presence of a cyst does not lead to significant narrowing of the anterior chamber angle. For non-surgical PACD patients, the presence of cysts does not require special treatment.

ETHICS STATEMENT

The studies involving human participants were reviewed and approved by Ethics Review Committee of Zhongshan Ophthalmic Center, Ethical number: 2021KYPJ003. The patients/participants provided their written informed consent to participate in this study.

AUTHOR CONTRIBUTIONS

ML and CZ: design and conduct of the study. LC: collection of the data. KW and ZT: analysis the data. KW, CZ, JX and DW: preparation of the manuscript. KW, CZ, JX, LC, DW, ZT, and ML: review and final approval of the manuscript. All authors contributed to the article and approved the submitted version.

REFERENCES

1. Song P, Wang J, Bucan K, Theodoratou E, Rudan I, Chan KY. National and subnational prevalence and burden of glaucoma in China: a systematic analysis. *J Glob Health.* (2017) 7:020705. doi: 10.7189/jogh.07.020705
2. Li X, Wang W, Huang W, Chen S, Wang J, Wang Z, et al. Difference of uveal parameters between the acute primary angle closure eyes and the fellow eyes. *Eye.* (2018) 32:1174–82. doi: 10.1038/s41433-018-0056-9
3. He N, Wu L, Qi M, He M, Lin S, Wang X, et al. Comparison of ciliary body anatomy between American caucasians and ethnic chinese using ultrasound biomicroscopy. *Curr Eye Res.* (2016) 41:485–91. doi: 10.3109/02713683.2015.1024869
4. SI D. Spontaneous cysts of the ciliary body. *Br J Ophthalmol.* (1960) 44:461–6. doi: 10.1136/bjo.44.8.461
5. Reese AB. Spontaneous cysts of the ciliary body simulating neoplasms*. *Am J Ophthalmol.* (1950) 33:1738–46. doi: 10.1016/0002-9394(50)90597-6
6. Kunimatsu S, Araie M, Ohara K, Hamada C. Ultrasound biomicroscopy of ciliary body cysts. *Am J Ophthalmol.* (1999) 127:48–55. doi: 10.1016/S0002-9394(98)00308-0
7. Foster PJ, Buhrmann R, Quigley HA, Johnson GJ. The definition and classification of glaucoma in prevalence surveys. *Br J Ophthalmol.* (2002) 86:238–42. doi: 10.1136/bjo.86.2.238
8. Wang B-H, Yao Y-F. Effect of primary iris and ciliary body cyst on anterior chamber angle in patients with shallow anterior chamber. *J Zhejiang Univ Sci B.* (2012) 13:723–30. doi: 10.1631/jzus.B1200124
9. Li Z, Xu Z, Wang Y, Liu Q, Chen B. Implantable collamer lens surgery in patients with primary iris and/or ciliary body cysts. *BMC Ophthalmol.* (2018) 18:287. doi: 10.1186/s12886-018-0935-7
10. Aydin A, Kocak I, Sabahyildizi M. Auto-refractometry may assist in discovering asymptomatic iridociliary cysts. *J Fr Ophtalmol.* (2014) 37:e71–2. doi: 10.1016/j.jfo.2013.07.012
11. Cronemberger S, Ferreira DM, Diniz Filho A, Mérula RV, Calixto N. Iridociliary cysts on ultrasound biomicroscopic examinations. *Arq Bras Oftalmol.* (2006) 69:471–5. doi: 10.1590/S0004-27492006000400003
12. Trikha S, Perera SA, Husain R, Aung T. The role of lens extraction in the current management of primary angle-closure glaucoma. *Curr Opin Ophthalmol.* (2015) 26:128–34. doi: 10.1097/ICU.0000000000000128
13. Azuara-Blanco A, Burr J, Ramsay C, Cooper D, Foster PJ, Friedman DS, et al. Effectiveness of early lens extraction for the treatment of primary angle-closure glaucoma (EAGLE): a randomised controlled trial. *Lancet.* (2016) 388:1389–97. doi: 10.1016/S0140-6736(16)30956-4
14. Bayer A, Erdem Ü, Mumcuoglu T, Akyol M. Two-site phacotrabeculectomy versus bimanual microincision cataract surgery combined with trabeculectomy. *Eur J Ophthalmol.* (2009) 19 no. 1:46–54. doi: 10.1177/112067210901900107
15. Vaideanu D, Mandal K, Hildreth A, Fraser SG, Phelan PS. Visual and refractive outcome of one-site phacotrabeculectomy compared with temporal approach phacoemulsification. *Clin Ophthalmol.* (2008) 2:569–74. doi: 10.2147/OPTH.S1764
16. Shao T, Li X, Ge J. Target drug delivery system as a new scarring modulation after glaucoma filtration surgery. *Diagn Pathol.* (2011) 6:64. doi: 10.1186/1746-1596-6-64
17. Choudhary A, Wishart PK. Non-penetrating glaucoma surgery augmented with mitomycin C or 5-fluorouracil in eyes at high risk of failure of filtration surgery: long-term results. *Clin Exp Ophthalmol.* (2007) 35:340–7. doi: 10.1111/j.1442-9071.2007.01483.x
18. Budenz DL, Barton K, Gedde SJ, Feuer WJ, Schiffman J, Costa V, et al. Five-year treatment outcomes in the Ahmed Baerveldt comparison study. *Ophthalmology.* (2015) 122:308–16. doi: 10.1016/j.ophtha.2014.08.043
19. Kun Liu X, Meifeng Cao X, Zhang X. Ultrasound biomicroscopic observation of failed cases of anti-glaucoma surgery. *Chin J Prac Ophthalmol.* (2004) 22:144–6.
20. Ang GS, Bochmann F, Azuara-Blanco A. Argon laser peripheral iridoplasty for plateau iris associated with iridociliary cysts: a case report. *Cases J.* (2008) 1:368. doi: 10.1186/1757-1626-1-368
21. Pathak-Ray V, Ahmed II. Phaco-endocycloplasty: a novel technique for management of ring iridociliary cyst presenting as acute angle closure. *Oman J Ophthalmol.* (2016) 9:63–5. doi: 10.4103/0974-620X.176123
22. Katsimpris J, Petropoulos I, Sunaric-Mégevand G. Ultrasound biomicroscopy evaluation of angle closure in a patient with multiple and bilateral iridociliary cysts. *Klin Monatsbl Augenheilkund.* (2007) 224:324–27. doi: 10.1055/s-2007-962951
23. Viestenz A, Bergua A, Mardin CY, Küchle M. Acute bilateral angle-closure glaucoma secondary to ciliary body epithelial cysts of the pars plicata–correlation with the ultrasound biomicroscope. *Klin Monbl Augenheilkd.* (2000) 217:127–9. doi: 10.1055/s-2000-10396
24. Ispa-Callén MC, Lara-Medina J, Zarco-Tejada JM, López-Mondéjar E, Celis-Sánchez J, González-Del-Valle F. Argon laser iridoplasty as treatment of plateau-like iris configuration secondary to multiple ciliary body cysts: long-term follow-up by ultrasound biomicroscopy. *Arch Soc Esp Oftalmol.* (2009) 84:569–72. doi: 10.4321/S0365-66912009001100006
25. Wang BH, Nie X, Zhou CX, Yao YF. Primary iris-ciliary body cyst and its relevancy with the change of anterior chamber angle. *Zhonghua Yan Ke Za Zhi.* (2008) 44:993–7.

19

Clinical Features of Spontaneous Regression of Retinopathy of Prematurity in China: A 5-Year Retrospective Case Series

Liang Wang [1†], Manhong Li [1†], Jun Zhu [2†], Hongxiang Yan [1], Lei Wu [1], Jing Fan [1], Yi Zhou [1], Kaili Gou [1], Zifeng Zhang [1] and Yusheng Wang [1*]*

[1] Department of Ophthalmology, Eye Institute of Chinese PLA, Xijing Hospital, Fourth Military Medical University, Xi'an, China, [2] State Key Laboratory of Cancer Biology, Institute of Digestive Diseases, Xijing Hospital, Fourth Military Medical University, Xi'an, China

***Correspondence:**
Yusheng Wang
wangys003@126.com
Zifeng Zhang
zzffmmu@163.com

† These authors have contributed equally to this work

Purpose: The aim of this study is to explore the clinical features of spontaneous regression of retinopathy of prematurity (ROP) in China, including fundus appearance, time course, and affecting factors.

Methods: Data of pediatric patients in whom ROP spontaneously regressed without treatment were collected, including general demographics, medical history, zones and stages of ROP, and changes of fundus appearance. The fundus manifestations of spontaneous regression in ROP were systematically summarized. Meanwhile, the time course of spontaneous regression in ROP was further analyzed, including the onset time, completion time, and duration of regression, which were all compared across different ROP zones and stages. The associated factors were analyzed by survival analysis for their correlation with delayed regression for the first time.

Results: Two hundred thirty-seven eyes of 237 pediatric patients were included. The fundus manifestations of regression differed across stages. Lesions gradually subsided, and the retinal vessels gradually vascularized completely. However, despite ROP regression, some abnormalities remained. We observed avascular retina in the temporal periphery (19.0%), increased vascular branching (6.8%), retinal pigmentary changes (6.8%), and smaller angle between the upper and lower temporal retinal vessel trunks (3.0%). Acute ROP started to regress at a median 40 weeks of postmenstrual age (PMA) and completely regressed by median 49.0 weeks of PMA. The median duration for regression was 8.5 weeks. The zone II ROP and stage 3 ROP had a later time for onset and completion of regression, and longer duration. Anemia and retinal hemorrhage (RH) were identified as independent risk factors for delayed regression by survival analysis.

Conclusions: During spontaneous regression, the fundus appearance is diverse, and the retinal vessels gradually vascularized completely. The time course of regression differs depending on the ROP zone and stage. Anemia and RH are independent risk factors for delayed regression. Further research of the natural course of the regression of ROP is needed to help design effective screening and follow-up plans.

Keywords: fundus appearance, infants, regression, retinopathy of prematurity, cox proportional hazard regression model

INTRODUCTION

Retinopathy of prematurity (ROP) is a vasoproliferative retinal disorder frequently seen in infants with low gestational age (GA) and birth weight (BW). Nowadays, it has already been the leading cause of childhood blindness worldwide (1). It is becoming a significant cause of avoidable blindness, especially in developing countries (2, 3). It was estimated that, in 2010, 184,700 patients had ROP worldwide, with 20,000 of them having severe visual impairment (4). Prompt detection of ROP in high-risk infants is crucial for managing severe retinopathy (5). ROP screening is highly heterogeneous globally. In underdeveloped regions, such as Northwest China, the number of medical professionals is insufficient to meet the demands imposed by ROP (6). However, most ROP cases regress spontaneously without treatment, and there were few reports on the clinical characteristics of regression of ROP. A better understanding of the natural course of regression of ROP will support the development of efficient strategies for ROP screening and prevention. A comprehensive investigation of the characteristics of spontaneous regression of ROP is needed. Thus, this retrospective study aimed to explore the clinical features and factors associated with spontaneous regression of ROP in China.

MATERIALS AND METHODS

Data of pediatric patients in whom ROP spontaneously regressed without treatment were collected from January 1, 2016, to December 31, 2019, in the Department of Ophthalmology, Xijing Hospital. This study was approved by the Ethics Committee of Xijing Hospital (KY20202099-C-1) and followed the principles of the Declaration of Helsinki. The infants were screened according to the 2014 Chinese screening guidelines of ROP (7). ROP was classified according to International Classification of Retinopathy of Prematurity revised in 2005 (8). Fundus examination was conducted weekly, fortnightly, or monthly, depending on the severity of the retinal lesions, until the completion of regression or longer. All the patients underwent a thorough fundus examination by RetCam (Clarity Medical Systems, Pleasanton, CA, USA), conducted by the same experienced pediatric ophthalmologist. The infants who were diagnosed as ROP by RetCam examination must be verified by another senior professional pediatric ophthalmologist using indirect ophthalmoscope (Keeler Company, Windsor, UK). Fundus images were recorded using the RetCam system at each follow-up. Fundus appearance, including ROP zones and stages, ridge, "popcorns," retinal hemorrhage (RH), tortuous and dilated retinal vessels, and avascular zone of the peripheral retina, were analyzed.

Since the severity of binocular ROP lesions was identical in 197 of the 237 patients (83.1%), and the binocular eyes could not be considered as independent cases, the eye with more severe ROP was selected for analysis in each patient. If the severity of lesions was identical in both eyes, one eye was randomly selected.

Patients with stage 1–3 ROP, who were followed up until completion of spontaneous regression, were included. Patients with any of the following conditions were excluded: (1) patients who received treatment for ROP; (2) patients in whom ROP had already started to regress before the first examination in our hospital; (3) patients who were not followed up until the completion of regression; and (4) patients with cataract, glaucoma, or other comorbid eye diseases.

According to the research of the Cryotherapy for Retinopathy of Prematurity Cooperative Group (9), meeting any one of the following criteria was enough to define the onset of regression: (1) a decrease of at least two sectors in the number of sectors of the highest stage of acute ROP in a given zone in two consecutive examinations; and (2) recorded completion of vascularization in all sectors of a zone that previously had acute ROP. Meeting any one of the following criteria was enough to define the completion of regression: (1) lesions had faded completely, and complete retinal vascularization (the vessels on the nasal side reached the ora serrata, and the temporal vasculature was separated from the ora serrata by no more than one optic papilla diameter); and (2) despite the presence of abnormal changes, such as increased vascular branching, retinal pigmentary changes, ROP had regressed to a steady state, and the retinal vessels had grown to zone III.

The time of onset of regression was defined as the average time of two consecutive examinations showing acute ROP, without initiation of regression at the first of those examinations, and with a definite onset of regression at the second examination. Similarly, the time for completion of regression was defined as the average time of two consecutive examinations showing ROP at the earlier examination (before regression completion) and a definite regression completion at the next examination.

General demographic data, including sex, GA, BW, singleton or multiple pregnancy, and eutocia or cesarean, were recorded at the first visit. In addition, history of mother's gestational diseases (hypertensive disorders of pregnancy and gestational diabetes mellitus) and the patient's medical history [premature rupture of membranes, placenta previa, placental abruption, asphyxia, apnea, neonatal respiratory distress syndrome (NRDS), pneumonia, anemia (hemoglobin < 110 g/L), blood transfusion, septicemia, hyperbilirubinemia (total bilirubin > 1.5 mg/dl), congenital heart disease, and continuous positive airway pressure (CPAP)] were also recorded in detail. Data were gathered from the hospital medical records of patients. If the patients coming from other hospitals did not carry their medical records when they visited our hospital, we would investigate their medical history *via* telephonic interviews. BW < 1,000 g, GA < 28 weeks, RH, and the abovementioned factors were analyzed for their correlation with delayed regression.

Statistical Analysis

The baseline characteristics of the ROP infants were summarized using descriptive statistics. The onset, completion, and duration times of regression of different ROP zones were analyzed by Wilcoxon rank sum test. The time course in different stages of ROP was investigated using the Kruskal–Wallis test. Related factors for delayed regression were examined by the Kaplan–Meier curve, and the differences were assessed by log-rank test. Cox proportional hazard regression model was further used to perform univariate analysis for the

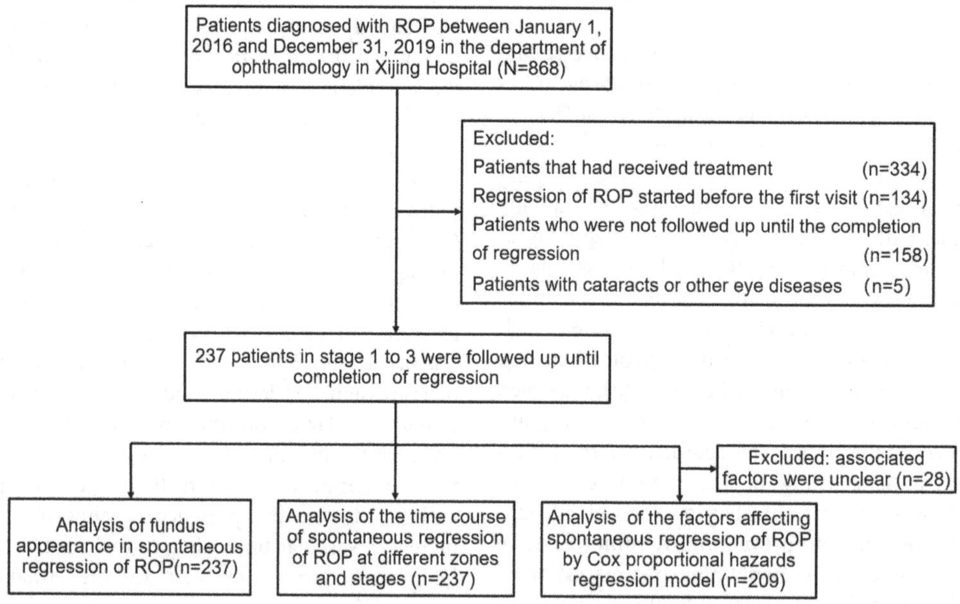

FIGURE 1 | Flowchart of this study. ROP, retinopathy of prematurity.

factors related to delayed regression. Statistically significant factors in the univariate analysis were incorporated into the multivariate Cox proportional hazard regression model to investigate whether these were independent factors affecting delayed regression. All the statistical analyses were performed with R software (Version 3.6.3, The R Foundation for Statistical Computing, Vienna, Austria) (packages: ggplot2, ggpubr, survival, surviminer, and tidyverse). Two-sided $p < 0.05$ was considered statistically significant.

RESULTS

Patients and Data

The clinical data of 4,234 infants who had accepted fundus screening in the Ophthalmology Department of Xijing Hospital were collected, 868 of whom were diagnosed with ROP (20.5%). According to the inclusion and exclusion criteria of this study, 237 eyes of the 237 pediatric patients with ROP, which spontaneously regressed without treatment, were finally included. The flowchart of this study is shown in **Figure 1**. **Table 1** summarizes their baseline characteristics. There were 125 males and 112 females. The mean GA of patients was 30.4 ± 2.15 weeks, and their mean BW was 1,418 ± 358 g. Mothers with multiple pregnancy accounted 22.3% of the cohort, and 59.1% patients were delivered by cesarean section; 210 patients (88.6%) presented bilateral ocular involvement, and 27 (11.4%) showed unilateral anomalies.

TABLE 1 | Baseline characteristics of patients with regression of ROP.

Parameters	Number	Percentage (%)
Sex		
Male	125	52.7
Female	112	47.3
Gestational age (GA)		
<28 weeks	22	9.3
28–32 weeks	171	72.1
>32 weeks	44	18.6
Birth weight (BW)		
<1,000 g	22	9.3
1,000–2,000 g	204	86.1
>2,000 g	11	4.6
Multiple pregnancy	54	22.3
Caesarean	140	59.1
Laterality		
Unilateral ROP	27	11.4
Bilateral ROP	210	88.6
Zone		
II	30	12.7
III	207	87.3
Stage		
1	35	14.8
2	188	79.3
3	14	5.9

ROP, retinopathy of prematurity.

Fundus Appearance of Regression

All the 237 patients with ROP stage 1 to 3 showed spontaneous regression without treatment. During this process, the lesions gradually subsided, and the retinal vessels gradually vascularized completely. In this process of regression, the alleviation of tortuous and dilated retinal vessels may indicate early regression before the ridge acquires a flat appearance and subsides. In the final, 192 patients had complete vascularization. The fundus manifestations of regression changed across stages. The

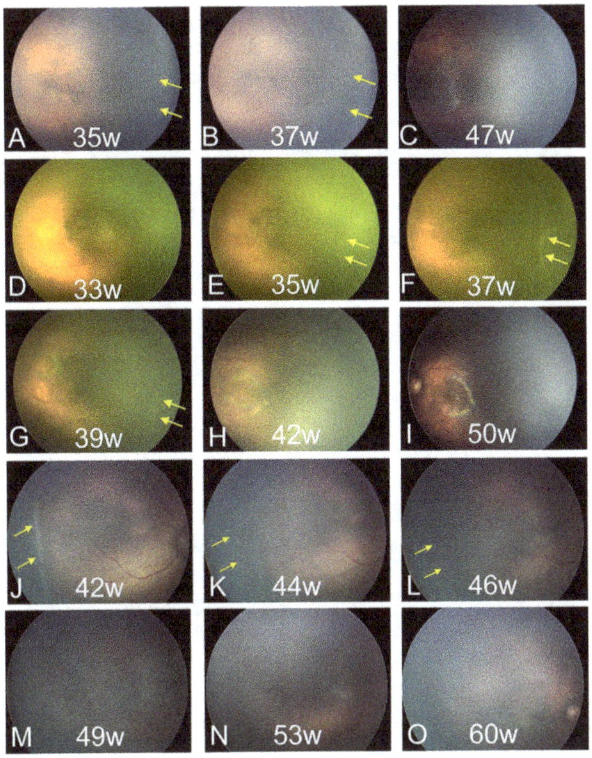

FIGURE 2 | Fundus images of patients with spontaneous regression. **(A–C)** Regression of ROP in stage 1. **(D–I)** Regression of ROP in stage 2. **(J–O)** Regression of ROP in stage 3. ROP, retinopathy of prematurity. The yellow arrow indicates the location of the lesions.

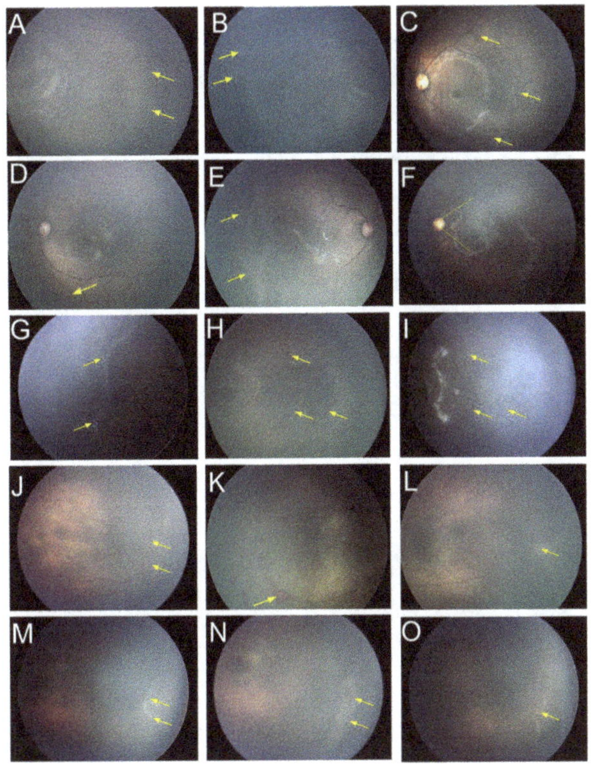

FIGURE 3 | Fundus images of patients with spontaneous regression. **(A)** Increased vascular branching (yellow arrow) in the peripheral retina. **(B)** Gray flaky lesions (yellow arrow). **(C)** Retinal pigmentation and (yellow arrow). **(D)** Punctate retinal hypopigmentation (yellow arrow). **(E)** Ridge-like trace after the regression (yellow arrow). **(F)** Smaller acute angle between the upper and lower temporal retinal vessel trunks (yellow line). **(G)** Vitreous opacity or vitreous condensation (yellow arrow). **(H)** There were no tortuous or dilated retinal vessels (yellow arrow) during the acute phase at a postmenstrual age (PMA) of 41 weeks, **(I)** but the vessels became tortuous and dilated (yellow arrow) after ROP regressed at a PMA of 86 weeks. **(J)** Arteriovenous shunts and the formation of circumferential vessels (yellow arrow) were observed in the vascular–avascular junction. **(K)** Retinal hemorrhage (yellow arrow). **(L)** Irregular ridge (yellow arrow). **(M)** The ridge (yellow arrow) at a PMA of 40 weeks, **(N)** but it turned into a larger flattened patch (yellow arrow) at a PMA of 43 weeks and then disappeared gradually. **(O)** Popcorn (yellow arrow) was observed on the surface of the retina posterior to the ridge. ROP, retinopathy of prematurity; PMA, postmenstrual age.

demarcation line subsided gradually until ROP resolution, and the vessels gradually grew into the avascular peripheral retina in stage 1 ROP (**Figures 2A–C**). ROP regression in stage 2 showed the typical characteristics of gradually flattened ridge and tortuous and dilated retinal vessels, which alleviated gradually (**Figures 2D–I**). Some small, isolated tufts ("popcorn"), which were present in a few cases, also disappeared. In stage 3 ROP, the neovascularization or extraretinal fibrovascular proliferation gradually subsided, and the ridge became flat and disappeared (**Figures 2J–O**).

Despite ROP regression, some fundus abnormalities persisted. Forty-five eyes (19.0%) did not show complete vascularization in the temporal retinal periphery. Sixteen patients (6.8%) showed increased vascular branching in the peripheral retina (**Figure 3A**). Gray, flaky lesions remained in 13 eyes (5.5%, **Figure 3B**). Thirteen eyes showed retinal pigmentary changes (5.5%); among them, seven eyes showed retinal pigmentation, and four eyes had punctate retinal hypopigmentation (**Figures 3C,D**). Nine patients (3.8%) showed ridge-like trace despite ROP regression (**Figure 3E**). A small acute angle between the upper and lower temporal retinal vessel trunks was found in seven eyes (3.0%, **Figure 3F**). Vitreous opacity or vitreous condensation occurred in six eyes (2.5%, **Figure 3G**).

Some special manifestations were observed during the regression. The retinal vessels in some infants did not return to normal despite complete ROP regression. Tortuous and dilated retinal vessels were detected in 25 infants (10.5%) at the beginning, and mildly tortuous or dilated vessels remained despite ROP regression in 15 cases (4.2%). Interestingly, we found no tortuous or dilated retinal vessels at the acute phase in six infants, but the vessels became tortuous and dilated after the ROP regressed (**Figures 3H,I**). Arteriovenous shunts and formation of circumferential vessels were observed in the vascular–avascular junction of 14 patients; they remained in three patients despite ROP regression (**Figure 3J**). RH was detected in 21 cases (8.9%), all of which were absorbed before the completion of regression (**Figure 3K**).

For infants with irregular ridge (13 cases), the ridge gradually became straight and then subsided, with complete regression at a median postmenstrual age (PMA) of 51.0 weeks (**Figure 3L**).

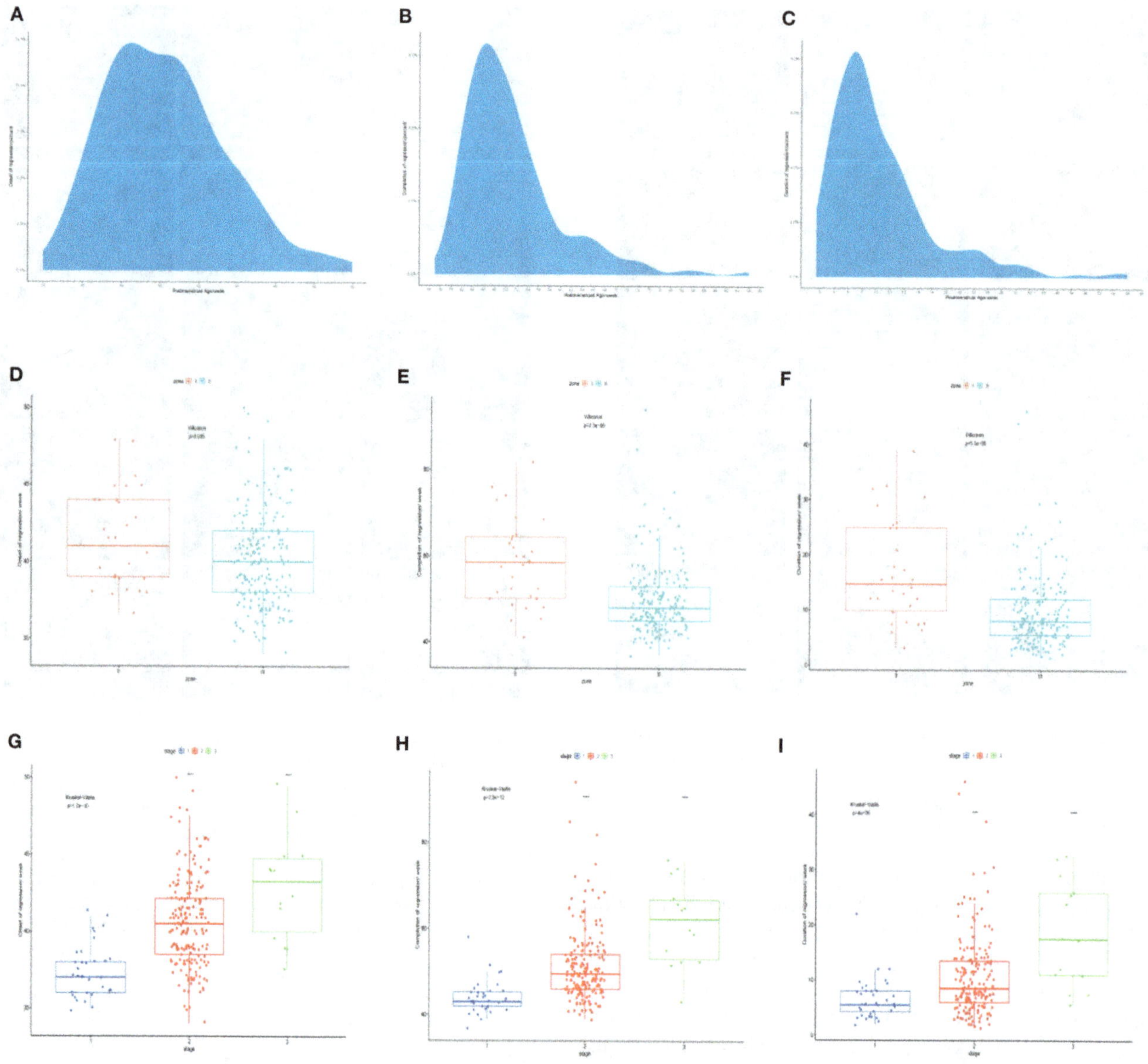

FIGURE 4 | (A–C) The time course for regression onset, completion, and duration. **(D–F)** The comparison of time course of spontaneous regression of ROP among different zones. **(G–I)** The comparison of time course of spontaneous regression of ROP among different stages. ROP, retinopathy of prematurity.

The ridge in some infants did not decrease gradually during the course of regression. Instead, it turned into a larger flatten patch and then disappeared gradually over a longer period (**Figures 3M,N**). The popcorns were observed in seven infants on the retinal surface posterior to the ridge and subsided before the ridge regressed (**Figure 3O**). The regression completed in a median PMA of 56.3 weeks in these infants, longer than that for patients without popcorn.

Time Course of Regression

The time for regression onset ranged between 36.0 and 46.0 weeks of PMA (5–95%), and the peak time ranged between 38.0 and 41.0 weeks, with a median PMA of 40.0 weeks. Furthermore, the time for regression completion varied (PMA range, 41.0–67.3 weeks; 5–95%), and the peak was between 46.0 and 50.0 weeks, with a median PMA of 49.0 weeks. The time for regression duration ranged from 3.0 to 25.1 weeks (5–95%), and the peak was between 6.0 and 10.0 weeks, with a median of 8.5 weeks (**Figures 4A–C**).

There were significant differences in the time course of spontaneous regression of ROP among different zones and stages (**Table 2**). The regression in zone III started at a median PMA of 40.0 weeks, earlier than in zone II (median PMA of 41.0 weeks; $p = 0.035$). ROP in zone III completed regression at a median PMA of 48.0 weeks, much earlier than that in zone II (median PMA of 58.5 weeks; $p < 0.001$). ROP in zone II required more time to complete the regression (median, 14.8

TABLE 2 | Time course of regression for ROP in different zones and stages.

	No. of eyes	Onset of regression (median PMA, W) (5–95%)*	Completion of regression (median PMA, W) (5–95%)*	Duration of regression (median, W) (5–95%)*
Zone				
II	30	41.0 (38.0–46.9)	58.5 (45.2–75.1)	14.8 (6.2–32.3)
III	207	40.0 (36.0–45.9)	48.0 (41.0–65.7)	8.0 (3.0–22.0)
P-value		0.035	<0.001	<0.001
Stage				
1	35	37.0 (35.4–40.7)	43.0 (39.7–50.5)	5.5 (2.9–12.0)
2	188	40.5 (36.5–46.0)	49.5 (42.2–67.0)	8.5 (3.0–24.7)
3	14	43.3 (38.5–48.5)	62.3 (48.6–74.7)	17.5 (6.8–32.2)
P-value		<0.001	<0.001	<0.001

PMA, postmenstrual age; W, weeks.
**The range listed is the fifth to 95th percentile for this cohort.*

weeks) than ROP in zone III (median, 8.0 weeks; $p < 0.001$) (**Figures 4D–F**). In 237 patients, there was no ROP in zone I that regressed spontaneously.

On the other hand, the analysis of regression time based on the stages showed that ROP stage 3 (median, 43.3 weeks) started regression later than ROP stage 2 (median, 40.5 weeks) and ROP stage 1 (median, 37.0 weeks) ($p < 0.001$). ROP stage 1 completed regression first (median, 40.5 weeks), while ROP stage 3 was the last to complete regression (median, 62.3 weeks) ($p < 0.001$). ROP stage 3 required more time to complete regression (median, 17.5 weeks) than ROP stage 2 (median, 8.5 weeks) and stage 1 (median, 5.5 weeks) ($p < 0.001$, in both cases) (**Figures 4G–I**).

Factors Affecting Delayed Regression

Since the ROP-associated factors in 28 infants were unclear, as they were not provided in the medical history or by their parents, only the data of 209 patients with ROP were finally included. In the univariate analyses, a Kaplan–Meier curve was used to screen for factors related to delayed regression, and the differences were assessed by log-rank test. The analysis showed that the patients with apnea, NRDS, anemia, blood transfusion, CPAP, and RH had longer time for completion of regression than those without these conditions (**Figure 5**, all $p < 0.05$). The univariate Cox proportional hazard regression model revealed that apnea (HR = 1.495, 95% CI = 1.087–2.055; $p = 0.013$), NRDS (HR = 1.429, 95% CI = 1.086–1.882; $p = 0.011$), anemia (HR = 1.729, 95% CI = 1.309–2.285; $p < 0.001$), blood transfusion (HR = 1.392, 95% CI = 1.032–1.878; $p = 0.030$), CPAP (HR = 1.803, 95% CI = 1.302–2.495; $p < 0.001$), and RH (HR = 2.114, 95% CI = 1.286–3.475; $p = 0.003$) were closely associated with delayed regression (**Figure 6A**). Multivariate Cox proportional hazard regression model confirmed that anemia (HR = 1.477, 95% CI = 1.075–2.030; $p = 0.016$) and RH (HR = 2.014, 95% CI = 1.218–3.329; $p = 0.006$) were independent factors for delayed regression (**Figure 6B**).

DISCUSSION

The number of infants requiring ROP screening has been increasing in China, which resulted in a prominent contradiction with the shortage of ROP-related medical resources. Excessive fundus examinations during ROP screening and follow-up increased not only the medical costs but also the risk of ocular and systemic adverse events (10). However, most patients with ROP regress spontaneously (11). Maly (12) reported that the incidence of spontaneous regression of ROP was 81.5%. In most cases, it usually occurs at stage 1, stage 2, or mild stage 3 (13). Eighty-five percent of infants with stage 1 ROP completed regression spontaneously, while the proportions of patients with stage 2 and 3 ROP who completed regression spontaneously are 56 and 25%, respectively (13).

ROP gradually disappeared without treatment or retained some traces of involution, achieving a relatively stable state defined as spontaneous regression of ROP (14, 15). It is characterized by lower stage and/or retinal vessel growth into a more peripheral area (9). Although the clinical manifestations of ROP have been clearly described, only few reports have assessed the changes in fundus appearance associated with spontaneous regression. We found that although most of the tortuous and dilated retinal vessels in regressed ROP were reduced, there were still mildly tortuous or dilated vessels in some patients despite ROP regression. These vascular abnormalities possibly occurred due to ROP itself (16, 17). It is worth noting that some vessels, which had not been abnormal previously, became tortuous and dilated eventually. This finding was not reported previously. The most common sequel of ROP regression is incomplete vascularization in the temporal peripheral retina (18). About 84.1% patients with avascular retina present peripheral findings in the future, such as lattice-like changes, retinal holes, and retinal tears (19). Approximately 3% patients in our cohort had popcorn on the retina, and recent research reported that popcorn was generally often indicative of the start of the regression of ROP (20). However, the results showed that regression of ROP with popcorn took longer than that without popcorn. The more acute angle between the upper and lower temporal retinal vessel trunks may be caused by the traction of fibrovascular proliferation. In addition, vitreous condensation and ridge-like traces may increase the risk of retinal holes and retinal detachment (20). Therefore, long-term follow-up of patients with spontaneous regression of ROP is needed.

Understanding the time course of spontaneous regression of ROP, especially the onset and completion of regression, is crucial to design efficient strategies for fundus screening. Although it does not eliminate the need for continuous screening of individual infants, it could provide guidance for doctors to carry out ROP screening and for national public health departments to estimate medical requirements (9). However, there is a lack of research on the time course of regression. Repka et al. (9) reported that the mean time of onset of regression was 38.6 weeks of PMA. In another study, without treatment, acute ROP started to regress at an average PMA of 40.4 weeks, with complete regression by 50.6 weeks (21). Herein, as the regression times were not normally distributed, we used the median as a measure

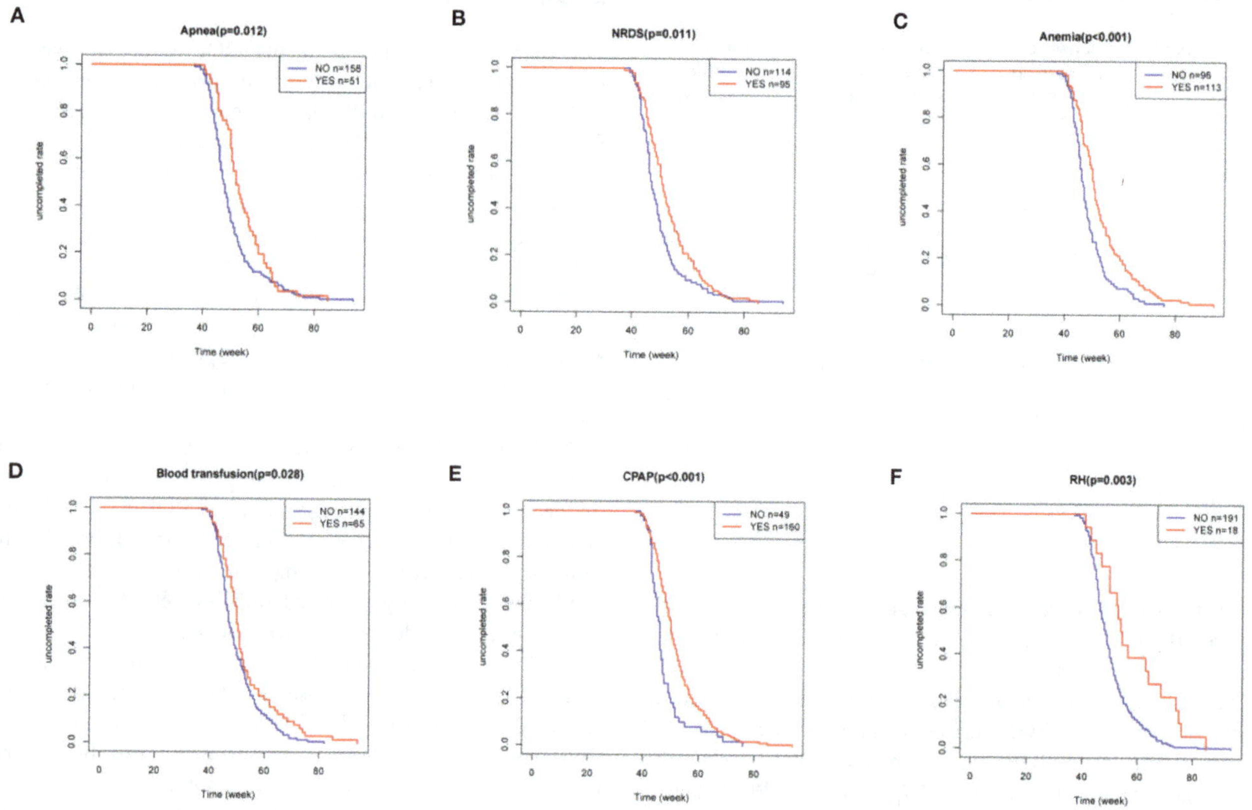

FIGURE 5 | Kaplan–Meier curve was used to screen for factors related to delayed regression, and the differences were assessed by log-rank test. **(A–F)** These six factors were considered statistically significant, all $P < 0.05$. NRDS, neonatal respiratory distress syndrome; CPAP, continuous positive airway pressure; RH, retinal hemorrhage.

of central tendency. Acute ROP started to regress at a median PMA of 40.0 weeks and completed at a median PMA of 49.0 weeks. The median time of duration time was 8.5 weeks. The time course in our study was similar to that reported previously (21). Importantly, our study had a larger sample size and more accurate description of the central tendency.

The time course for regression of different ROP zones and stages was significantly different, which was not quite the same with previous studies (21). The higher stages of ROP had a much later time of onset and completion and a longer duration. ROP in zone II started to regress later than ROP in zone III, and its regression took a longer time. However, a previous study reported no differences between different zones in the onset time of ROP (9, 21). Ninety-five percent of patients in our study started to regress before a PMA of 46 weeks, so the frequency of screening may be reduced after 46 weeks of PMA or after the onset of regression is identified. According to our results, the frequency of follow-up screening might also be reduced in patients who completed the regression in longer periods of time.

Despite numerous reports on the risk factors of ROP (10, 22–24), little is known about the factors affecting its spontaneous regression. Only two small-scale studies have identified the factors influencing ROP regression. Acute ROP in stage 3, anemia, and CPAP might be the factors affecting delayed regression, whereas RH showed an inverse weak correlation with spontaneous regression (11, 21). In our study, the higher stages of ROP tended to complete regression later, and ROP in zone II took longer time to complete regression than did zone III. Furthermore, we used the Kaplan–Meier curve to determine six factors for delayed regression, namely, apnea, NRDS, anemia, blood transfusion, CPAP, and RH. We used univariate and multivariate Cox proportional hazard regression models to analyze independent factors for delayed regression for the first time; and anemia and RH were confirmed as independent factors for delayed regression. Anemia has been regarded as a risk factor for severe ROP and ROP requiring treatment (25). Lower level of hemoglobin may decrease the oxygen-carrying capacity of tissues, and hypoxia might hinder the process of retinal vascularization and spontaneous regression (26, 27). RH was found to occur in 34% of neonates and to be more common in both eyes (28). It may be caused by abnormal retinal arteriovenous shunts and increased vascular fragility in patients with ROP (11). Therefore, it was speculated that RH indirectly reflects the severity of vascular abnormalities that might delay ROP regression.

This study has a few limitations. First, there may exist selection bias, as this was a single-center retrospective study. Our data are not representative of the entire population of

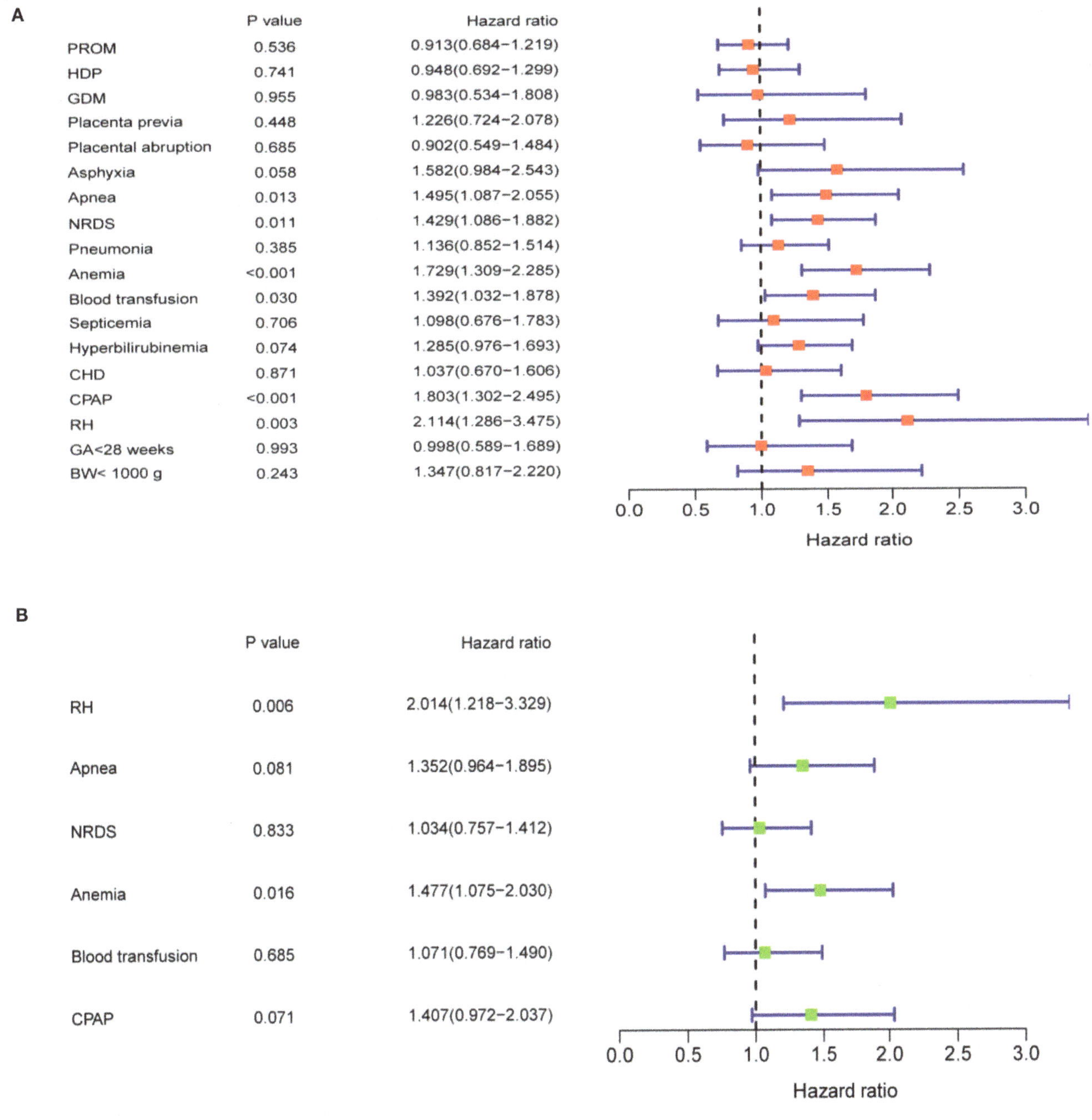

FIGURE 6 | (A) Univariate Cox proportional hazard regression model showed that apnea, NRDS, anemia, blood transfusion, CPAP, and RH were closely associated with delayed regression. **(B)** Multivariate Cox proportional hazard regression model showed that anemia and RH were independent factors affecting delayed regression. BW, birth weight; CHD, congenital heart disease; CPAP, continuous positive airway pressure; GA, gestational age; GDM, gestational diabetes mellitus; HDP, hypertensive disorders of pregnancy; NRDS, neonatal respiratory distress syndrome; PROM, premature rupture of membranes; RH, retinal hemorrhage.

China; although the patients came from a dozen provinces, they were mainly from the underdeveloped northwest regions of China. Further multicenter prospective studies are needed to verify our conclusion. Next, since regression of ROP is a continuous process, it is difficult to determine the exact time. The definition of regression time also affected the calculation of the time course. Then, it is clearer and more accurate to monitor the development of retinal vessels by fundus fluorescein angiography (FFA), while it is an invasive testing especially for premature children. For children with lighter ROP in our study, there were only 19 patients who accepted the FFA examinations. FFA should be used to further study the fundus performance, especially the changes of peripheral vascula in patients with the regression of ROP. Finally, further studies with longer follow-up periods are required for a more complete characterization of the abnormalities in the fundus, and to further understand visual development in these patients.

In conclusion, our study was a large cohort with complete long-term follow-up. We first systematically reported the changes of fundus appearance of spontaneous regression, especially some special manifestations during regression never reported before. Furthermore, we comprehensively described the time course of regression in infants with ROP in different zones and stages and found that ROP in zone II started to regress later than ROP in zone III for the first time. In addition, we found that RH is an independent factor affecting delayed regression for the first time and verified that anemia was also an independent factor. These findings will help understand more about the natural course of regression of ROP and may serve as a reference for developing more reasonable and effective screening and follow-up plans, thereby reducing frequency of the examination and the subsequent follow-up, saving unnecessary medical costs, and alleviating the contradiction between requirements of screening and lack of professionals, so as to promote the screening and prevention of ROP more efficiently.

ETHICS STATEMENT

The studies involving human participants were reviewed and approved by the Ethics Committee of Xijing hospital. Written informed consent for participation was not provided by the participants' legal guardians/next of kin because: This study is a retrospective case series.

AUTHOR CONTRIBUTIONS

ML, ZZ, and YW: performing the screening and diagnosis of ROP. HY, LW, JF, YZ, and KG: collection and assembly of data. LW, JZ, and ZZ: data analysis and interpretation. All authors study conception and design, manuscript writing, and final approval of manuscript.

REFERENCES

1. Hartnett ME, Penn JS. Mechanisms and management of retinopathy of prematurity. *N Engl J Med.* (2012) 367:2515–26. doi: 10.1056/NEJMra1208129
2. Gilbert C, Rahi J, Eckstein M, O'Sullivan J, Foster A. Retinopathy of prematurity in middle-income countries. *Lancet.* (1997) 350:12–4. doi: 10.1016/S0140-6736(97)01107-0
3. Limburg H, Gilbert C, Hon DN, Dung NC, Hoang TH. Prevalence and causes of blindness in children in Vietnam. *Ophthalmology.* (2012) 119:355–61. doi: 10.1016/j.ophtha.2011.07.037
4. Blencowe H, Lawn JE, Vazquez T, Fielder A, Gilbert C. Preterm-associated visual impairment and estimates of retinopathy of prematurity at regional and global levels for 2010. *Pediatr Res.* (2013) 74:35–49. doi: 10.1038/pr.2013.205
5. Fierson WM. Screening examination of premature infants for retinopathy of prematurity. *Pediatrics.* (2018) 142:e20183061. doi: 10.1542/peds.2018-3061
6. Dou G, Li M, Zhang Z, La Y, Zhu Y, Wang H, et al. Demographic profile and ocular characteristics of stage 5 retinopathy of prematurity at a referral center in Northwest China: implications for implementation. *BMC Ophthalmol.* (2018) 18:307. doi: 10.1186/s12886-018-0975-z
7. Li X. Screening guidelines of retinopathy of prematurity in China 2014. *Chin J Ophthalmol.* (2014) 50:933–5.
8. International Committee for the Classification of Retinopathy of Prematurity. The International classification of retinopathy of prematurity revisited. *Arch Ophthalmol.* (2005) 123:991-9. doi: 10.1001/archopht.123.7.991
9. Repka MX, Palmer EA, Tung B. Involution of retinopathy of prematurity. cryotherapy for retinopathy of prematurity cooperative group. *Arch Ophthalmol.* (2000) 118:645–9. doi: 10.1001/archopht.118.5.645
10. Kim SJ, Port AD, Swan R, Campbell JP, Chan RVP, Chiang MF. Retinopathy of prematurity: a review of risk factors and their clinical significance. *Surv Ophthalmol.* (2018) 63:618–37. doi: 10.1016/j.survophthal.2018.04.002
11. Ju R-H, Zhang J-Q, Ke X-Y, Lu X-Y, Liang L-F, Wang W-J. Spontaneous regression of retinopathy of prematurity: incidence and predictive factors. *Int J Ophthalmol.* (2013) 6:475–80. doi: 10.3980/j.issn.2222-3959.2013.04.13
12. Maly E. Frequency and natural history of retinopathy of prematurity (Rop). A prospective study in a Swedish City 1986-1990. *Acta Ophthalmol.* (1993) 210:52–5. doi: 10.1111/j.1755-3768.1993.tb04153.x
13. Quinn GE, Gilbert C, Darlow BA, Zin A. Retinopathy of prematurity: an epidemic in the making. *Chin Med J.* (2010) 123:2929–37.
14. Prost M. [Possibilities of spontaneous regression in active phase of Rop]. *Klin Oczna.* (2003) 105:57–9.
15. Fielder AR. The natural ocular outcome of premature birth and retinopathy: status at 1 year. *Arch Ophthalmol.* (1995) 113:850–1. doi: 10.1001/archopht.1995.01100070020008
16. Vural A, Ekinci DY, Onur IU, Hergunsel GO, Yigit FU. Comparison of fluorescein angiographic findings in type 1 and type 2 retinopathy of prematurity with intravitreal bevacizumab monotherapy and spontaneous regression. *Int Ophthalmol.* (2019) 39:2267–74. doi: 10.1007/s10792-018-01064-7
17. Mansukhani SA. Hutchinson AK, Neustein R, Schertzer J, Allen JC, Hubbard GB. Fluorescein angiography in retinopathy of prematurity: comparison of infants treated with bevacizumab to those with spontaneous regression. *Ophthalmol Retina.* (2019) 3:436–43. doi: 10.1016/j.oret.2019.01.016
18. Preslan MW, Butler J. Regression pattern in retinopathy of prematurity. *J Pediatr Ophthalmol Strabismus.* (1994) 31:172–6. doi: 10.3928/0191-3913-19940501-09
19. Hamad AE, Moinuddin O, Blair MP, Schechet SA, Shapiro MJ, Quiram PA, et al. Late-onset retinal findings and complications in untreated retinopathy of prematurity. *Ophthalmol Retina.* (2020) 4:602–12. doi: 10.1016/j.oret.2019.12.015
20. Xue K. Huang X, Xu S, Zhnag T, Wang X, Zhnag M, et al. The evolution of isolated neovascular tufts ("popcorn") in retinopathy of prematurity. *Retina.* (2020) 40:1353–8. doi: 10.1097/IAE.0000000000002596
21. Ni Y-Q, Huang X, Xue K, Yu J, Ruan L,Shan H-D, et al. Natural involution of acute retinopathy of prematurity not requiring treatment: factors associated with the time course of involution. *Invest Ophthalmol Vis Sci.* (2014) 55:3165–70. doi: 10.1167/iovs.13-13744
22. Wade KC, Ying G-S, Baumritter A, Gong A, Kemper AR, Quinn GE, et al. Factors in premature infants associated with low risk of developing retinopathy of prematurity. *JAMA Ophthalmol.* (2019) 137:160. doi: 10.1001/jamaophthalmol.2018.5520
23. Hellström A, Smith LE, Dammann O. Retinopathy of prematurity. *Lancet.* (2013) 382:1445–57. doi: 10.1016/S0140-6736(13)60178-6

24. Yang Q, Zhou X, Ni Y, Shan H, Shi W, Yin X, et al. Optimised retinopathy of prematurity screening guideline in China based on a 5-year cohort study. *Br J Ophthalmol.* (2020) 105:819-23. doi: 10.1136/bjophthalmol-2020-316401
25. Lundgren P, Athikarisamy SE, Patole S, Lam GC, Smith LE, Simmer K. Duration of anaemia during the first week of life is an independent risk factor for retinopathy of prematurity. *Acta Paediatr.* (2018) 107:759–66. doi: 10.1111/apa.14187
26. Gariano RF, Gardner TW. Retinal angiogenesis in development and disease. *Nature.* (2005) 438:960–6. doi: 10.1038/nature04482
27. Stutchfield CJ, Jain A, Odd D, Williams C, Markham R. Foetal haemoglobin, blood transfusion, and retinopathy of prematurity in very preterm infants: a pilot prospective cohort study. *Eye.* (2017) 31:1451–5. doi: 10.1038/eye.2017.76
28. Emerson MV, Pieramici DJ, Stoessel KM, Berreen JP, Gariano RF. Incidence and rate of disappearance of retinal hemorrhage in newborns. *Ophthalmology.* (2001) 108:36–9. doi: 10.1016/S0161-6420(00)00474-7

20

Associations Between the Choroidal Vascularity Index and Malignant Glaucoma After Trabeculectomy for Primary Angle Closure Glaucoma

Chengguo Zuo [1†], Dingqiao Wang [1†], Xinxing Guo [2], Hui Xiao [1], Shaoyang Zheng [1], Mingkai Lin [1], Lei Fang [1] and Xing Liu [1]*

[1] *State Key Laboratory of Ophthalmology, Zhongshan Ophthalmic Center, Sun Yat-sen University, Guangzhou, China,*
[2] *Wilmer Eye Institute, Johns Hopkins University, Baltimore, MD, United States*

***Correspondence:**
Xing Liu
drliuxing@163.com*

† These authors have contributed equally to this work

Purpose: To compare the choroidal vasculature characteristics by using the choroidal vascularity index (CVI) in eyes with malignant glaucoma (MG), fellow eyes with non-MG, and eyes with uncomplicated primary angle-closure glaucoma (PACG) after trabeculectomy by spectral-domain optical coherence tomography (SD-OCT).

Methods: This case–control study included 53 patients diagnosed with MG after trabeculectomy. Eyes with MG ($n = 53$) and the fellow eyes with non-MG ($n = 50$) were included. Eyes with PACG without MG after trabeculectomy ($n = 60$) were also enrolled as controls. The choroidal parameters, including CVI and the subfoveal choroidal thickness (SFCT), were measured by using SD-OCT images.

Results: Eyes with MG and the fellow eyes showed a significantly lower CVI than eyes with PACG controls ($p < 0.001$). After adjusting for age, sex, axial length (AL), and intraocular pressure (IOP), eyes with the greater CVI [odds ratio (OR), 0.44] were significantly related to MG. The area under the receiver operating characteristic curve of the CVI was greater than that of the SFCT in the diagnosis of MG (0.911 vs. 0.840, $p = 0.034$).

Conclusion: Eyes with MG showed a significantly lower macular CVI than eyes with PACG controls. A higher macular CVI was an associated factor of eyes with MG. The CVI serves as a more stable and sensitive indicator for MG than the SFCT in this group of patients with PACG.

Keywords: choroid, choroidal vascularity index (CVI), choroidal thickness (CT), malignant glaucoma, optical coherence tomography (OCT)

INTRODUCTION

Malignant glaucoma (MG), also known as aqueous misdirection glaucoma or ciliary block glaucoma, was a rare complication mostly seen in penetrating ocular surgery (1). MG may result in optic nerve damage and severe vision loss (2). The pathogenesis of MG has remained elusive. However, the pathogenesis of MG is closely associated with anatomical characteristics such as a relatively large lens, a shallow anterior chamber, and an anterior rotation of the ciliary body (1).

Quigley et al. have proposed that choroidal expansion may play a role in the pathogenesis of primary angle-closure glaucoma (PACG) and even MG (3, 4). Recently, an increasing number of studies, including our previous reports, have demonstrated a thicker choroidal thickness in primary angle-closure diseases than in the non-glaucoma controls (5–7). However, many factors affect the choroidal thickness and it is relatively unstable (8). Therefore, these conclusions are still controversial. Moreover, choroidal thickness does not differentiate vascular vs. stromal changes in the choroid. Thus, choroidal thickness alone does not capture the comprehensive choroidal features.

The choroidal vascularity index (CVI), defined as the proportion of the luminal area (LA) to the total choroidal area (TCA) (9, 10), has been documented to be a more stable and reliable parameter to monitor choroidal vasculature in retinal diseases such as age-related macular degeneration, Vogt–Koyanagi–Harada disease, and in primary open-angle glaucoma (POAG) (11–16) than the subfoveal choroidal thickness (SFCT). However, no studies have investigated the choroidal vascular changes by using the CVI parameter in eyes with MG.

In this study, we evaluated the CVI in eyes with MG, fellow eyes with non-MG, and eyes with uncomplicated PACG controls to investigate the choroidal vasculature changes and compare the stability and sensitivity of the CVI with the parameter of the SFCT.

MATERIALS AND METHODS

Participants

This retrospective study was approved by the Institutional Review Board of Zhongshan Ophthalmic Center. The study was registered at the ClinicalTrials.gov with the registration ID: NCT04220879. This study followed the statements of the Declaration of Helsinki. A total of 53 consecutive patients diagnosed with MG and a total of 60 consecutive patients diagnosed with uncomplicated PACG were included in this study. All the data of the patient were obtained from the Glaucoma Department of Zhongshan Ophthalmic Center of Sun Yat-Sen University (Guangzhou, China) between January 2010 and November 2019.

Patients were diagnosed as having MG after trabeculectomy when they met all of the following criteria: (17, 18) high or normal intraocular pressure (IOP) pretreatment, shallowing of the anterior chamber (by slit-lamp examination), patent iridotomy, absence of signs of overfiltration or bleb leakage, and absence of choroidal effusion or hemorrhage on fundus examination or B-scan ultrasonography. The average duration of MG attacked was 6 months after trabeculectomy. The inclusion criteria for eyes with MG was a diagnosis of MG following trabeculectomy for the treatment of PACG. The fellow eyes of MG patients were also included in this study. The inclusion criteria of the fellow eyes were a diagnosis of suspect primary angle-closure, primary angle-closure, or PACG, and absence of MG disease.

Three eyes without quality optical coherence tomography (OCT) images were excluded due to lens opacity. A total of 60 eyes with uncomplicated PACG from 60 patients who were followed in the same period were included as control subjects. Patient with PACG who met the criteria was enrolled to match the patient with MG recruited in the same year. If both the eyes met the inclusion criteria, the right eye was selected. The inclusion criteria of PACG controls were post-trabeculectomy and absence of MG so far. The exclusion criteria for all the subjects included an axial length (AL) <20 mm, refractive media opacity in eyes affecting the fundus observation, intraocular diseases other than glaucoma (e.g., diabetic retinopathy or non-glaucomatous optic neuropathy), and systemic diseases (hypertension, diabetes, or pituitary tumors). Eyes with a history of ocular trauma or any ocular surgery other than trabeculectomy within the past 3 months were also excluded.

The following ophthalmic evaluations were required in all the patients enrolled in this study: slit-lamp examination, IOP measured with applanation tonometry, AL measured with A- and B-scan ultrasonography (CINESCAN; Quantel Corporation Ltd., Clermont-Ferrand, France, UK), and dilated fundus examination.

Optical Coherence Tomography Image Acquisition

Optical coherence tomography images with enhanced depth imaging (EDI) were obtained by using spectral-domain OCT (SD-OCT) (Spectralis HRA + OCT, Heidelberg Engineering, Heidelberg, Germany, UK) by an experienced ophthalmologist (HX). The EDI-OCT images were performed at the onset of the MG before the further surgical treatment. The scans were horizontal lines of 30° through the central fovea. The scan length was 9 mm. The quality index of each EDI image was no <22 dB. The SFCT was defined as the vertical distance from the outer surface of the retinal pigment epithelium to the inner edge of the choroid–scleral junction (**Figures 1A-C**). The SFCT was measured manually at the foveal center twice by one glaucoma specialist (XL) and the average value was used for analysis.

Choroidal Vascularity Index

The details of the measurement of the CVI were described by Sonoda et al. (9). The EDI-OCT images were binarized by using the ImageJ software (ImageJ Software Inc., MD, USA) (version 1.51; http://imagej.nih.gov/ij/). The TCA was selected with the polygon tool and then converted to an 8-bit format by using Niblack's auto local threshold techniques for image binarization. Then, the image was converted into the red, green, and blue (RGB) image and the luminal and stromal regions were selected with the color threshold tool. In the binarized images (**Figures 1D-F**), dark pixels correspond to the LA and light pixels correspond to the stromal area (SA) (19). The CVI was measured as the ratio of the LA to the TCA. All the image assessments were performed by an experienced investigator (CZ) at two different times. Both the investigator and data collector (SZ) in this study were masked to the clinical histories of the patients.

Data Analysis

Statistical analysis was performed by using the Statistical Package for the Social Sciences (SPSS) software version 25.0 (SPSS Incorporation, Chicago, Illinois, USA). An independent *t*-test

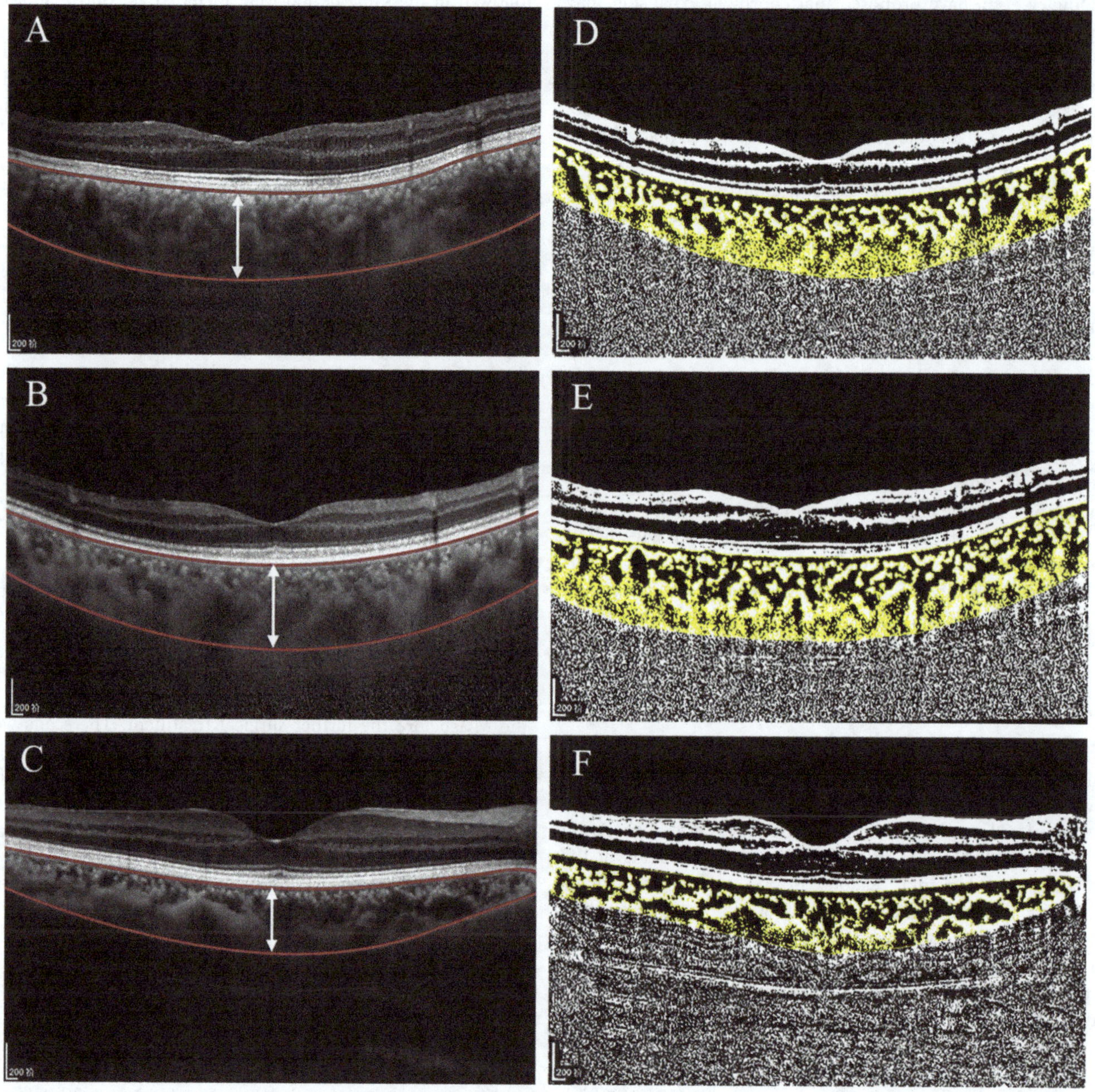

FIGURE 1 | Original spectral-domain optical coherence tomography (SD-OCT) **(A-C)** and binarized SD-OCT images **(D-F)** of this study in eyes with malignant glaucoma (MG) group, the fellow eyes with non-MG group, and control eyes with uncomplicated primary angle-closure glaucoma (PACG) group. **(A-C)** Based on the prebinarized image, two horizontal red lines segment the choroid from Bruch's membrane to the choroidal–scleral interface. The vertical white line at the fovea was used for calculation of the subfoveal choroidal thickness (SFCT), which measured 485, 489, and 330 μm. **(D-F)** Based on the binarized image, the yellow block represents the total choroidal area (TCA), the choroidal vessel lumen area (LA) is represented by dark pixels, and the stromal area (SA) is represented by light pixels. The choroidal vascularity index (CVI) was 61.81, 60.56, and 68.09%.

was applied for normally distributed variables and the chi-squared test was applied for categorical variables to assess the differences in demographic and clinical characteristics between patients with the MG and controls. The Bonferroni test was used for the multiple comparisons of the choroidal parameters among eyes with MG, fellow eyes with non-MG, and eyes with PACG controls. The Pearson correlation analysis was performed to determine the associations of the CVI and the SFCT with demographics and ocular factors, respectively. The multiple logistic regression analysis was performed to determine the factors associated with MG. The receiver operating characteristic (ROC) curve analysis was performed on the choroidal parameters of the CVI and the SFCT to calculate their diagnostic power for MG. The MedCalc statistical software (MedCalc Software Ltd.,

TABLE 1 | Demographic, clinical, and choroidal characteristics of eyes with MG with their fellow eyes and control eyes.

Variables	MG, $n = 53$	Fellow eyes, $n = 50$	Control eyes, $n = 60$	P_1	P_2	P_3
Age (years)	50.3 ± 11.9	-	57.5 ± 7.5	-	**<0.001**†	-
Male sex (*n*, %)	11 (20.8%)	-	34 (56.7%)	-	**<0.001**†	-
Systolic blood pressure (mmHg)	123.0 ± 13.9	-	126.4 ± 16.9	-	0.252†	-
Diastolic blood pressure (mmHg)	77.4 ± 8.3	-	77.3 ± 8.7	-	0.958†	-
IOP (mmHg)	27.1 ± 12.3	19.6 ± 9.9	18.4 ± 8.1	**0.001***	**<0.001***	1*
Axial length (mm)	21.68 ± 1.04	21.74 ± 1.08	22.56 ± 0.73	1*	**<0.001***	**<0.001***
Surgical history						
N/A	0	19	0	-	-	-
Laser iridotomy	0	31	0	-	-	-
Trabeculectomy	53	0	60	-	-	-
SFCT (μm)	471.92 ± 79.64	463.70 ± 81.10	346.05 ± 91.28	1*	**<0.001***	**<0.001***
LA (mm²)	1.35 ± 0.19	1.37 ± 0.26	1.45 ± 0.37	1*	0.211*	0.494*
SA (mm²)	0.90 ± 0.16	0.88 ± 0.26	0.77 ± 0.29	1*	**0.015***	0.050*
TCA (mm²)	2.25 ± 0.33	2.25 ± 0.46	2.22 ± 0.65	1*	1*	1*
CVI (%)	60.13 ± 2.22	61.26 ± 4.83	66.02 ± 3.58	0.314*	**<0.001***	**<0.001***

Values are shown as the mean ± SD.
MG, malignant glaucoma; fellow eyes, fellow eyes of eyes with non-MG; IOP, intraocular pressure; SFCT, subfoveal choroidal thickness; LA, luminal area; SA, stromal area; TCA, total choroidal area; CVI, choroidal vascularity index.
In bold: significant at $p < 0.05$.
P_1 eyes with MG vs. the fellow eyes with non-MG.
P_2 eyes with MG vs. control eyes with PACG.
P_3 fellow eyes with non-MG vs. control eyes with PACG.
†Student's t-test.
**Bonferroni correction.*

Ostend, Belgium) (version 15.2.2, https://www.medcalc.org/) was used to compare the area under the ROC curves between the SFCT and the CVI. Two-sided $p < 0.05$ was considered as statistically significant. Intraobserver reliability was studied by using the Bland–Altman and the intraclass correlation coefficient (ICC) analyses.

RESULTS

A total of 53 MG eyes and 50 fellow non-MG eyes of 53 patients with MG and 60 eyes of 60 PACG controls were enrolled in this study.

The clinical and choroidal characteristics of the patients with MG and control subjects are presented in **Table 1**; **Figure 2**. This study included 53 patients with MG with an average age of 50.3 (±11.9) years and 11 (20.8%) of the patients were male. Of the 60 PACG controls, the average age was 57.5 (±7.5) years and 34 (56.7%) of the patients were male. Patients with MG were younger and more likely to be female than the PACG controls ($p < 0.001$). Eyes with MG had a shorter AL and higher IOP than the eyes of the control group ($p < 0.001$). Fellow eyes with non-MG had a shorter AL than control eyes ($p < 0.001$). No significant differences were detected in the demographic data or choroidal parameters between eyes with MG and the fellow eyes with non-MG, except the IOP (27.1 ± 12.3 vs. 19.6 ± 9.9; $p = 0.001$).

The average macular CVI was lowest in eyes with MG (60.13 ± 2.22%), lower in the fellow eyes with non-MG (61.26 ± 4.83%), and highest in control eyes with PACG (66.02 ± 3.58%). Statistically significant differences were observed in eyes with MG and the fellow eyes with non-MG compared to control eyes with PACG ($p < 0.001$, respectively). The average SFCT was thickest in eyes with MG (471.92 ± 79.64 μm), thicker in the fellow eyes with non-MG (463.70 ± 81.11 μm), and thinnest in control eyes with PACG (346.05 ± 91.28 μm). There were significant differences in the SFCT between eyes with MG and control eyes with PACG ($p < 0.001$) and between the fellow eyes with non-MG and control eyes with PACG ($p < 0.001$). Eyes with MG had a significantly larger SA than control eyes (0.90 ± 0.16 vs. 0.77 ± 0.29 mm², $p = 0.015$).

The Pearson correlation analysis showed that age, AL, and systolic blood pressure were significantly negatively correlated with the SFCT ($r = -0.486$, $p < 0.001$; $r = -0.525$, $p < 0.001$; $r = -0.259$, $p = 0.001$, respectively; **Table 2**). However, none of these factors were significantly correlated with the CVI ($p > 0.05$ for all).

Table 3 shows the results of the multiple logistic regression analysis of the associated factors for eyes with MG in separate models. After adjusting for age, sex, AL, and IOP, eyes with the higher CVI [odds ratio (OR), 0.44; 95% CI, 0.28–0.68] and higher LA (OR, 0.06; 95% CI, 0.01–0.57) were associated factors for MG. Eyes with the thicker SFCT (OR, 1.02; 95% CI, 1.01–1.03) were also related to MG.

We evaluated the ROC curves for the CVI and the SFCT measures in eyes with MG vs. control eyes with uncomplicated PACG (**Table 4**; **Figure 3**). The area under the ROC curve (AUC)

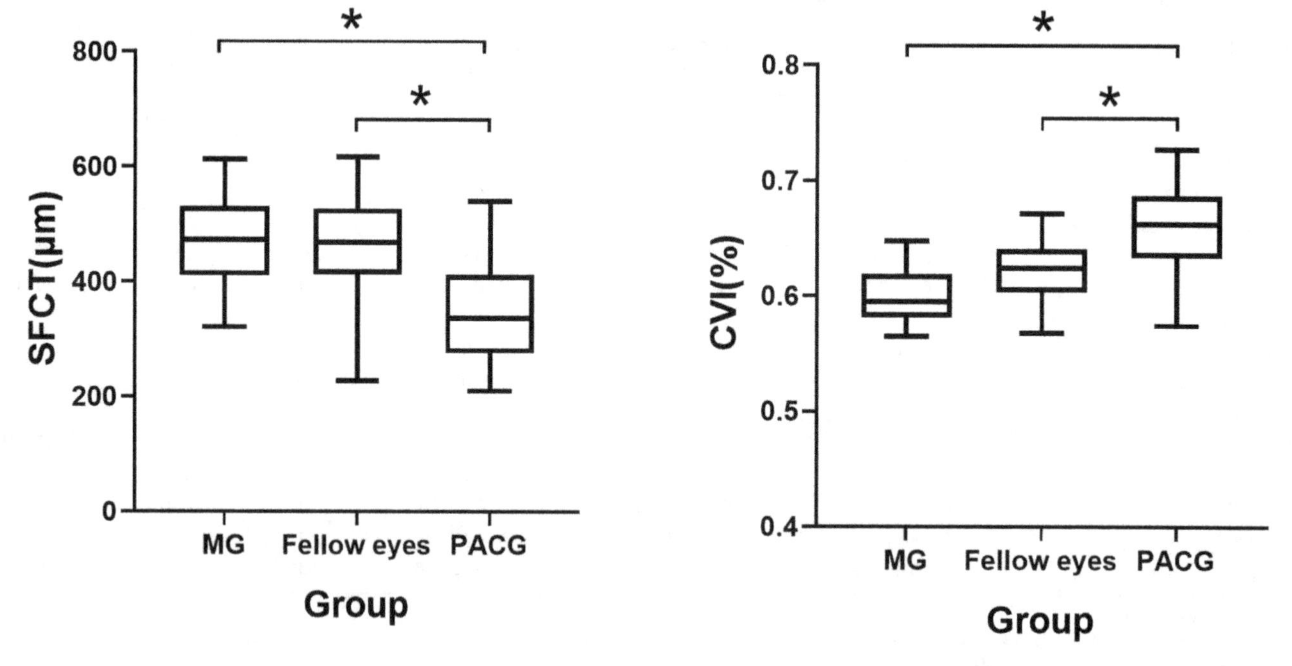

FIGURE 2 | Box chart representing measurements of the CVI and the SFCT across all the groups. *$p < 0.05$. Error bars denote 95% CIs.

TABLE 2 | The Pearson correlations between the SFCT, the CVI, and demographic factors in recruited eyes.

Parameters	Factors	R	P
SFCT	Age (years)	−0.486	**<0.001**
	sex (male)	−0.043	0.582
	Axial length (mm)	−0.525	**<0.001**
	IOP (mmHg)	−0.043	0.591
	Systolic blood pressure (mmHg)	−0.259	**0.001**
	Diastolic blood pressure (mmHg)	−0.129	0.101
CVI	Age (years)	0.133	0.077
	sex (male)	−0.028	0.715
	Axial length (mm)	0.129	0.093
	IOP (mmHg)	−0.018	0.816
	Systolic blood pressure (mmHg)	0.003	0.964
	Diastolic blood pressure (mmHg)	0.048	0.531

R, Pearson's correlation coefficient; SFCT, subfoveal choroidal thickness; CVI, choroidal vascularity index; IOP, intraocular pressure.
In bold: significant at $p < 0.05$.

TABLE 3 | The multiple logistic regression analysis of the associated factors for eyes with MG.

	MG (n = 53) vs. Control eyes (n = 60)		
Parameters	**OR**	**95% CI**	***P***
SFCT (per 1 μm increase)	1.02	1.01–1.03	**<0.001**
LA (per 1 mm^2 increase)	0.06	0.01–0.57	**0.015**
SA (per 1 mm^2 increase)	1.78	0.21–14.90	0.596
TCA (per 1 mm^2 increase)	0.65	0.21–2.00	0.448
CVI (per 1% increase)	0.44	0.28–0.68	**<0.001**

OR, odds ratio; SFCT, subfoveal choroidal thickness; LA, luminal area; SA, stromal area; TCA, total choroidal area; CVI, choroidal vascularity index.
p: Adjusted for age, gender, axial length, and intraocular pressure (IOP) and for each factor in the table.
In bold: significant at $p < 0.05$.

of the CVI was 0.911 (95% CI, 0.859–0.963; $p < 0.001$), showing a better diagnostic power than the SFCT (AUC, 0.840; 95% CI, 0.769–0.912; $p < 0.001$) in separating eyes with MG from control eyes with PACG ($p = 0.034$). The cutoff point of the CVI in the ROC curve analysis was 63.60% for the diagnosis of MG (sensitivity, 96.23%; specificity, 73.33%).

The ICC and the Bland–Altman analysis were used to assess the intraobserver reproducibility for the measurement (**Table 5**). The samples were selected with the random selection subroutine of the SPSS: Random Sample of Cases (version 25; IBM SPSS Corporation, Chicago, Illinois, USA). A total of 40% of the subjects were selected, which included 20 eyes with MG, 19 fellow eyes with non-MG, and 24 control eyes with uncomplicated PACG. The measurements were repeated twice at different times for reproducibility by the same investigator (CZ). The

TABLE 4 | Receiver operating characteristic (ROC) curves of the choroidal vascularity index (CVI) and the subfoveal choroidal thickness (SFCT) parameters to discriminate eyes with MG from control eyes with PACG.

Parameters	AUC	95% CI	*P*	Cutoff point	Sensitivity, %	Specificity, %	*P**
CVI (%)	0.911	0.859–0.963	**<0.001**	<63.60	96.23	73.33	**0.034**
SFCT (μm)	0.840	0.769–0.912	**<0.001**	>431	71.70	85.00	

p: Pairwise comparison of the ROC curves of the SFCT and CVI in the MedCalc software (version 15.2.2).*
Cutoff point: the maximum value at the Youden's index (sensitivity + specificity – 1).
In bold: significant at $p < 0.05$.

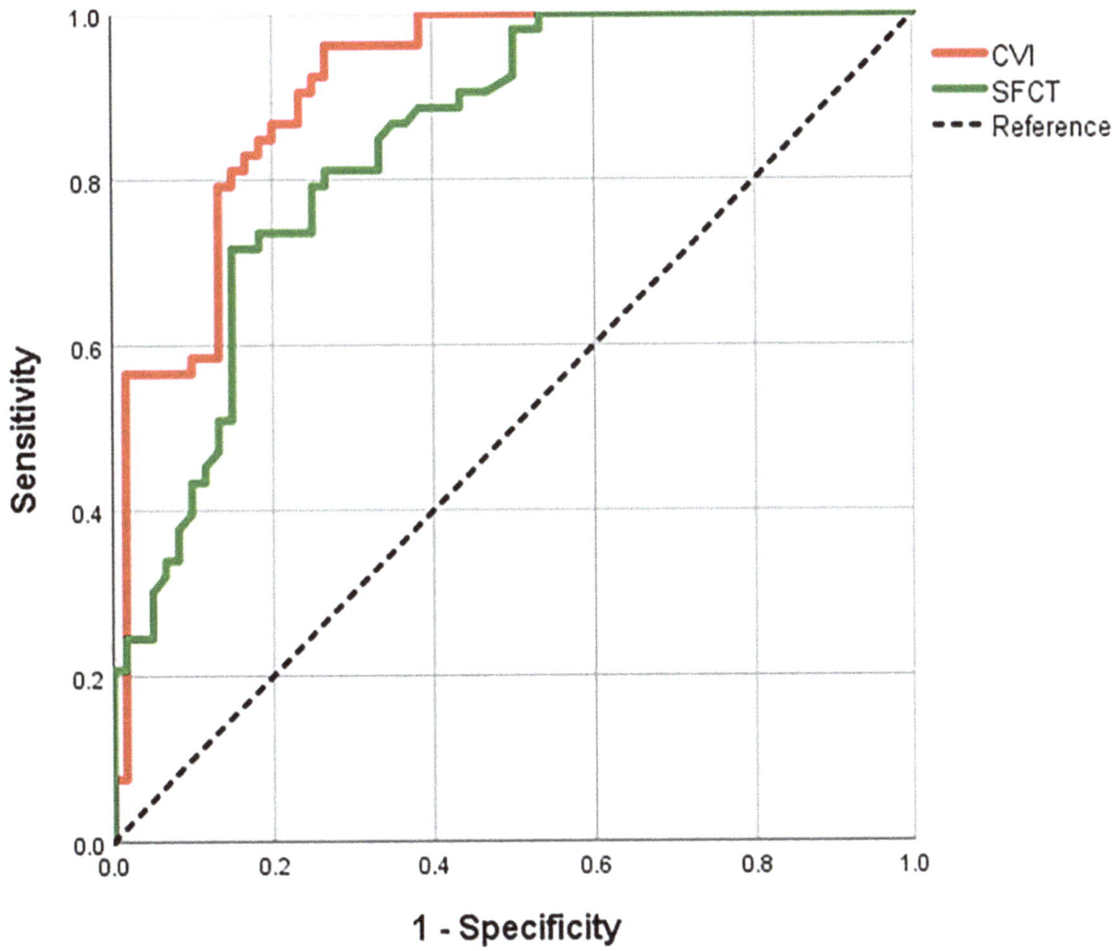

FIGURE 3 | The receiver operating characteristic (ROC) curves for the SFCT and the CVI to separate eyes with MG from control eyes with POCG.

TABLE 5 | Reproducibility of the choroidal parameters in a random subset of eyes.

Parameters	*N*	Mean 1	Mean 2	ICC	*P*	95% LoA
SFCT (μm)	43	405.509	397.190	0.963	**<0.001**	−47.22–63.85
LA (mm^2)	43	1.434	1.372	0.779	**<0.001**	−0.35–0.47
TCA (mm^2)	43	2.263	2.203	0.753	**<0.001**	−0.71–0.83

SFCT, subfoveal choroidal thickness; LA, luminal area; TCA, total choroidal area; ICC, intraclass correlation coefficient; LoA, limits of agreement.
In bold: significant at $p < 0.05$.

annotations were erased after grading each image after the first analysis. The ICC of the SFCT was 0.963 ($p < 0.001$) and the ICCs of the LA and TCA were 0.779 and 0.753, respectively (both $p < 0.001$). The Bland–Altman analysis showed 95% limits of agreement from −47.22 to 63.85 μm with the SFCT, from −0.35 to 0.47 mm^2 with LA, and from −0.71 to 0.83 mm^2 with TCA.

DISCUSSION

This study has highlighted the importance of choroidal thickness in the pathogenesis of MG (8). However, it has been widely reported that choroidal thickness can be influenced by the physiological and ocular variables (8, 20). In this study, a novel index, the CVI, was used to detect the exact changes in the choroidal vascular and stromal components in eyes with MG, the fellow eyes with non-MG, and control eyes with uncomplicated PACG (9, 10). The results showed that eyes with MG eyes and the fellow eyes with non-MG had a significantly lower macular CVI and a thicker SFCT than control eyes with uncomplicated PACG. The greater macular CVI and larger LA appeared to be associated with MG. This study also demonstrated that the CVI was more stable and sensitive than the SFCT and the parameter of the CVI was able to separate eyes with MG from control eyes with uncomplicated PACG significantly.

In this study, significant reductions in the CVI in eyes with MG and the fellow eyes with non-MG were observed compared with control eyes with uncomplicated PACG. The SA was significantly larger in eyes with MG than in control eyes with uncomplicated PACG. This study also showed a significantly thicker SFCT in both the eyes of the patients with MG than in control eyes with uncomplicated PACG. However, there were no significant differences in the CVI, TCA, LA, SA and the SFCT between eyes with MG and the fellow eyes with non-MG. The results indicated that the fellow eyes with non-MG may have a similar anatomic structure of the choroid as eyes with MG, representing a potentially high risk of MG disease (7, 17).

To compare the stability of the CVI and the SFCT, we evaluated factors that may be correlated with the SFCT and the CVI by the Pearson correlation analysis. Our results showed that the SFCT was significantly associated with age, AL, and systolic blood pressure. However, none of these three factors were statistically significantly correlated with the CVI. Our results were consistent with previous studies that observed that the SFCT may be susceptible to the physiological and ocular factors in other diseases (8, 20). Furthermore, several studies have proposed that the SFCT shows variability due to factors such as age, refraction, and AL (21, 22). It has been proposed that the CVI has less variability and is more reliable in diseases such as primary open-angle glaucoma (POAG), polypoidal choroidal vasculopathy, and panuveitis (11, 23–25) than the SFCT. In general, similar to the research of Liu et al. and Adhi et al., our results indicated that the CVI is a more stable surrogate parameter for MG than the SFCT (23, 26). Furthermore, we also investigated the reproducibility of the choroidal parameters. The results revealed a good reproducibility of the SFCT, the LA, and the TCA measurements.

After adjusting for age, sex, AL, and IOP, a greater CVI and greater LA were significantly independently associated with eyes with MG. The CVI was calculated from the binarized images from SD-OCT scans and was described by the ratio of the LA to the TCA. Thus, we speculated that a lower LA was a main contributing factor for a decline in the CVI. The reduction in the LA could be explained by a reduction in the choroidal blood supply. To the best of our knowledge, there was no investigation examining choroidal vascular characteristics in the patients with MG. Park and Cho found a significantly lower CVI and the LA in POAG eyes than healthy eyes (11). They speculated that choroidal ischemia may be related to glaucomatous eyes. Lee et al. and Kim et al. have observed a choroidal microvasculature dropout in POAG eyes on OCT angiography and indocyanine green angiography compared to normal controls (27, 28). Taken together, our findings demonstrated possible choroidal ischemia in patients with MG. Although the difference did not reach statistical significance, we found that eyes with MG had a larger SA than control eyes with uncomplicated PACG. We speculated that the relative increase in the SA may be closely associated with inflammatory factors in the choroid. It has been reported that inflammation may be involved in the pathology of glaucoma (29) and inflammatory cells can target the choroidal stroma, resulting in stromal edema and a lower CVI (30, 31). Therefore, the significant decrease in the LA and the relatively increased SA collectively led to a reduction in the CVI. We speculated that uveal effusion might happen in eyes with MG and lead to the choroidal expansions (4, 32, 33). Consistent with our hypothesis, Sakai et al. proposed that uveal effusion may be associated with eyes with MG and unaffected fellow eyes of PACG or chronic primary angle-closure eyes (34). The uveal effusion might be caused by the inflammation after surgery, which might lead to the destruction of blood–choroid barrier and the exudation of protein in the extravascular choroid. The osmotic force in the choroidal vessels was reduced (4). This could lead to the lower LA, the relatively larger SA, and the lower CVI in eyes with MG. However, uveal effusion in the fellow eyes with MG might be idiopathic. At present, many studies including us cannot explain the reason for the choroidal characteristics of the fellow eyes (34, 35).

Additionally, in this study, a thicker SFCT was found to be an associated factor for eyes with MG after adjusting for age, sex, AL, and IOP. The result of a thicker SFCT was compatible with the findings of our previous study that the choroidal thickness in eyes with MG increased during the onset of MG compared with control eyes with uncomplicated PACG (7). Similarly, Quigley et al. and Zhang et al. provided an assumption that choroidal expansion could play a significant role in the pathogenesis of PACG and even MG, which probably increases pressure in each compartment of the eye, causing a shallow anterior chamber (3, 4, 36). Eyes with MG and the fellow eyes with non-MG had significantly shorter AL values than control eyes with uncomplicated PACG. We also found that MG is more common in younger females among the patients with PACG. These findings were consistent with our previous study and other studies (7, 37).

To compare the sensitivity of the CVI and the SFCT for the diagnosis of MG, the ROC curve analysis was used. In separating eyes with MG from control eyes with uncomplicated PACG, we observed that the CVI displayed a superior diagnostic sensitivity compared to the SFCT. It suggests that the CVI indicator has significantly higher diagnostic potential for MG than the SFCT. Furthermore, the CVI was able to separate eyes with MG from control eyes with uncomplicated PACG significantly and the cutoff point in the ROC curve was 63.60% (sensitivity, 96.23%; specificity, 73.33%). We speculated that a CVI larger than 63.60% may indicate a decreased risk of MG, while a CVI lower than 63.60% may indicate an increased risk of MG. Our results indicated that the CVI could be introduced as a relatively more sensitive parameter for monitoring the choroidal status of MG.

There were some limitations in this study. The sample size of this study was relatively small and may not be representative of other cases with MG or PACG. This was a cross-sectional, observational study and we could not obtain the OCT images of the patients with MG after their treatment of operation.The OCT images in the onset of MG were measured, while images before the onset of MG were not obtained for analysis. The OCT images were only measured once, so it might affect the overall analysis of the pathogenesis of MG (38). Besides, the CVI may not represent the entire status of the global choroidal structure due to its two-dimensional nature. Therefore, the application of the CVI in MG needs to be validated in a prospective and longitudinal clinical trial with a larger sample size.

In conclusion, the macular CVI was significantly lower in both the eyes with MG and the fellow eyes with non-MG than control eyes with uncomplicated PACG. Larger macular CVI and LA were the associated factors for MG. The CVI might be a more stable and sensitive parameter than the SFCT for choroidal evaluation in MG. The CVI is likely a promising indicator for evaluating choroidal vascular changes in patients with MG.

ETHICS STATEMENT

The studies involving human participants were reviewed and approved by the Institutional Review Board of Zhongshan Ophthalmic Center. The study was registered at ClinicalTrials.gov with the registration ID: NCT04220879.

AUTHOR CONTRIBUTIONS

XL and CZ contributed to the design and conduct of the study. DW and HX contributed to the collection of the data. DW and SZ contributed to the analysis of the data. DW and CZ contributed to the preparation of the manuscript. XL, ML, CZ, XG, and LF contributed to the review and final approval of the manuscript. All authors contributed to the article and approved the submitted version.

REFERENCES

1. Ruben S, Tsai J, Hitchings RA. Malignant glaucoma and its management. *Br J Ophthalmol.* (1997) 81:163-7. doi: 10.1136/bjo.81.2.163
2. Kaplowitz K, Yung E, Flynn R, Tsai JC. Current concepts in the treatment of vitreous block, also known as aqueous misdirection. *Surv Ophthalmol.* (2015) 60:229-41. doi: 10.1016/j.survophthal.2014.12.004
3. Quigley HA, Friedman DS, Congdon NG. Possible mechanisms of primary angle-closure and malignant glaucoma. *J Glaucoma.* (2003) 12:167-80. doi: 10.1097/00061198-200304000-00013
4. Quigley HA. Angle-closure glaucoma-simpler answers to complex mechanisms: LXVI Edward Jackson Memorial Lecture. *Am J Ophthalmol.* (2009) 148:657-69.e1. doi: 10.1016/j.ajo.2009.08.009
5. Zhou M, Wang W, Huang W, Gao X, Li Z, Li X, et al. Is increased choroidal thickness association with primary angle closure? *Acta Ophthalmol.* (2014) 92:e514-20. doi: 10.1111/aos.12403
6. Huang W, Wang W, Gao X, Li X, Li Z, Zhou M, et al. Choroidal thickness in the subtypes of angle closure: an EDI-OCT study. *Invest Ophthalmol Vis Sci.* (2013) 54:7849-53. doi: 10.1167/iovs.13-13158
7. Chen X, Guo X, Xu X, Xiao H, Liu X. Is thicker choroid a risk factor for malignant glaucoma? *Ophthalmic Res.* (2018) 60:161-8. doi: 10.1159/000490914
8. Nickla DL, Wallman J. The multifunctional choroid. *Prog Retin Eye Res.* (2010) 29:144-68. doi: 10.1016/j.preteyeres.2009.12.002
9. Sonoda S, Sakamoto T, Yamashita T, Shirasawa M, Uchino E, Terasaki H, et al. Choroidal structure in normal eyes and after photodynamic therapy determined by binarization of optical coherence tomographic images. *Invest Ophthalmol Vis Sci.* (2014) 55:3893-9. doi: 10.1167/iovs.14-14447
10. Agrawal R, Gupta P, Tan KA, Cheung CM, Wong TY, Cheng CY. Choroidal vascularity index as a measure of vascular status of the choroid: measurements in healthy eyes from a population-based study. *Sci Rep.* (2016) 6:21090. doi: 10.1038/srep21090
11. Park Y, Cho KJ. Choroidal vascular index in patients with open angle glaucoma and preperimetric glaucoma. *PLoS ONE.* (2019) 14:e0213336. doi: 10.1371/journal.pone.0213336
12. Agrawal R, Chhablani J, Tan KA, Shah S, Sarvaiya C, Banker A. Choroidal vascularity index in central serous chorioretinopathy. *Retina.* (2016) 36:1646-51. doi: 10.1097/IAE.0000000000001040
13. Agrawal R, Li LK, Nakhate V, Khandelwal N, Mahendradas P. Choroidal vascularity index in vogt-koyanagi-harada disease: an EDI-OCT derived tool for monitoring disease progression. *Transl Vis Sci Technol.* (2016) 5:7. doi: 10.1167/tvst.5.4.7
14. Kinoshita T, Mitamura Y, Shinomiya K, Egawa M, Iwata A, Fujihara A, et al. Diurnal variations in luminal and stromal areas of choroid in normal eyes. Br J Ophthalmol. (2017) 101:360-4. doi: 10.1136/bjophthalmol-2016-308594
15. Yang LH, Jonas JB, Wei WB. Optical coherence tomographic enhanced depth imaging of polypoidal choroidal vasculopathy. *Retina.* (2013) 33:1584-9. doi: 10.1097/IAE.0b013e318285cbb3

16. Cetin EN, Parca O, Akkaya HS, Pekel G. Association of retinal biomarkers and choroidal vascularity index on optical coherence tomography using binarization method in retinitis pigmentosa. *Graefes Arch Clin Exp Ophthalmol.* (2020) 258:23-30. doi: 10.1007/s00417-019-04516-7
17. Wang Z, Huang J, Lin J, Liang X, Cai X, Ge J. Quantitative measurements of the ciliary body in eyes with malignant glaucoma after trabeculectomy using ultrasound biomicroscopy. *Ophthalmology.* (2014) 121:862-9. doi: 10.1016/j.ophtha.2013.10.035
18. Liu X, Li M, Cheng B, Mao Z, Zhong Y, Wang D, et al. Phacoemulsification combined with posterior capsulorhexis and anterior vitrectomy in the management of malignant glaucoma in phakic eyes. *Acta Ophthalmol.* (2013) 91:660-5. doi: 10.1111/j.1755-3768.2012.02451.x
19. Sonoda S, Sakamoto T, Yamashita T, Uchino E, Kawano H, Yoshihara N, et al. Luminal and stromal areas of choroid determined by binarization method of optical coherence tomographic images. *Am J Ophthalmol.* (2015) 159:1123-31.e1. doi: 10.1016/j.ajo.2015.03.005
20. Seidel G, Hausberger S, Herzog SA, Palkovits S, Poschl EM, Wackernagel W, et al. Circadian macular volume changes in the healthy human choroid. *Am J Ophthalmol.* (2015) 159:365-71.e2. doi: 10.1016/j.ajo.2014.11.002
21. Ferrara D, Waheed NK, Duker JS. Investigating the choriocapillaris and choroidal vasculature with new optical coherence tomography technologies. *Prog Retin Eye Res.* (2016) 52:130-55. doi: 10.1016/j.preteyeres.2015.10.002
22. Barteselli G, Chhablani J, El-Emam S, Wang H, Chuang J, Kozak I, et al. Choroidal volume variations with age, axial length, and sex in healthy subjects: a three-dimensional analysis. *Ophthalmology.* (2012) 119:2572-8. doi: 10.1016/j.ophtha.2012.06.065
23. Liu B, Zhang X, Mi L, Peng Y, Wen F. Choroidal structure in subtypes of polypoidal choroidal vasculopathy determined by binarization of optical coherence tomographic images. *Clin Exp Ophthalmol.* (2019) 47:631-7. doi: 10.1111/ceo.13467
24. Bakthavatsalam M, Ng DS, Lai FH, Tang FY, Brelen ME, Tsang CW, et al. Choroidal structures in polypoidal choroidal vasculopathy, neovascular age-related maculopathy, and healthy eyes determined by binarization of swept source optical coherence tomographic images. *Graefes Arch Clin Exp Ophthalmol.* (2017) 255:935-43. doi: 10.1007/s00417-017-3591-3
25. Agrawal R, Salman M, Tan KA, Karampelas M, Sim DA, Keane PA, et al. Choroidal vascularity index (CVI)–a novel optical coherence tomography parameter for monitoring patients with panuveitis? *PLoS ONE.* (2016) 11:e0146344. doi: 10.1371/journal.pone.0146344
26. Adhi M, Ferrara D, Mullins RF, Baumal CR, Mohler KJ, Kraus MF, et al. Characterization of choroidal layers in normal aging eyes using enface swept-source optical coherence tomography. *PLoS ONE.* (2015) 10:e0133080. doi: 10.1371/journal.pone.0133080
27. Lee EJ, Lee KM, Lee SH, Kim TW. Parapapillary choroidal microvasculature dropout in glaucoma: a comparison between optical coherence tomography angiography and indocyanine green angiography. *Ophthalmology.* (2017) 124:1209-17. doi: 10.1016/j.ophtha.2017.03.039
28. Kim JA, Lee EJ, Kim TW. Evaluation of parapapillary choroidal microvasculature dropout and progressive retinal nerve fiber layer thinning in patients with glaucoma. *JAMA Ophthalmol.* (2019) 137:810-6. doi: 10.1001/jamaophthalmol.2019.1212
29. KriŽaj D, Ryskamp DA, Tian N, Tezel G, Mitchell CH, Slepak VZ, et al. From mechanosensitivity to inflammatory responses: new players in the pathology of glaucoma. *Curr Eye Res.* (2014) 39:105-19. doi: 10.3109/02713683.2013.836541
30. Bretz CA, Divoky V, Prchal J, Kunz E, Simmons AB, Wang H, et al. Erythropoietin signaling increases choroidal macrophages and cytokine expression, and exacerbates choroidal neovascularization. *Sci Rep.* (2018) 8:2161. doi: 10.1038/s41598-018-20520-z
31. Liu S, Du L, Zhou Q, Zhang Q, Hu K, Qi J, et al. The choroidal vascularity index decreases and choroidal thickness increases in vogt-koyanagi-harada disease patients during a recurrent anterior uveitis attack. *Ocul Immunol Inflamm.* (2018) 26:1237-43. doi: 10.1080/09273948.2017.1343357
32. Trope GE, Pavlin CJ, Bau A, Baumal CR, Foster FS. Malignant glaucoma. Clinical and ultrasound biomicroscopic features. *Ophthalmology.* (1994) 101:1030-5. doi: 10.1016/S0161-6420(94)31222-X
33. Dugel PU, Heuer DK, Thach AB, Baerveldt G, Lee PP, Lloyd MA, et al. Annular peripheral choroidal detachment simulating aqueous misdirection after glaucoma surgery. *Ophthalmology.* (1997) 104:439-44. doi: 10.1016/S0161-6420(97)30294-2
34. Sakai H, Morine-Shinjyo S, Shinzato M, Nakamura Y, Sakai M, Sawaguchi S. Uveal effusion in primary angle-closure glaucoma. *Ophthalmology.* (2005) 112:413-9. doi: 10.1016/j.ophtha.2004.08.026
35. Zhou M, Wang W, Ding X, Huang W, Chen S, Laties AM, et al. Choroidal thickness in fellow eyes of patients with acute primary angle-closure measured by enhanced depth imaging spectral-domain optical coherence tomography. *Invest Ophthalmol Vis Sci.* (2013) 54:1971-8. doi: 10.1167/iovs.12-11090
36. Zhang X, Wang W, Aung T, Jonas JB, Wang N. Choroidal physiology and primary angle closure disease. *Surv Ophthalmol.* (2015) 60:547-56. doi: 10.1016/j.survophthal.2015.06.005
37. Razeghinejad MR, Amini H, Esfandiari Mh HJ. Lesser anterior chamber dimensions in women may be a predisposing factor for malignant glaucoma. *Med Hypotheses.* (2005) 64:572-4. doi: 10.1016/j.mehy.2004.07.035
38. Zhang X, Cole E, Pillar A, Lane M, Waheed N, Adhi M, et al. The effect of change in intraocular pressure on choroidal structure in glaucomatous eyes. *Invest Ophthalmol Vis Sci.* (2017) 58:3278-85. doi: 10.1167/iovs.17-21598

21

Association of Subregional Quantitative Ultra-Widefield Fluorescence Angiography Characteristics with the Occurrence of Diabetic Macular Edema and Proliferative Diabetic Retinopathy

Gongpeng Sun[†], Xiaoling Wang[†], Jingwen Jiang, Zuohuizi Yi, Mei Fu, Xueying Yang, Hongmei Zheng and Changzheng Chen[*]

Eye Center, Renmin Hospital of Wuhan University, Wuhan, China

Correspondence:
Changzheng Chen
whuchenchzh@163.com

[†]These authors have contributed equally to this work and share first authorship

Purpose: To explore the relationships of region-specific properties of ultra-widefield fluorescence angiography (UWFFA) images with two adverse outcomes, diabetic macular edema (DME) and proliferative diabetic retinopathy (PDR), and also the severity of diabetic retinopathy (DR).

Methods: A cross-sectional observational study was performed to retrospectively analyze UWFFA images of patients with DR. All patients underwent UWFFA and optical coherence tomography examination. Leakage index and microaneurysm (MA) count were measured using Trainable Weka Segmentation, a machine learning algorithm, and ischemic index (ISI) was measured manually. The correlation between UWFFA parameters and severity of DR was analyzed, and receiver operating characteristic curves were used to estimate their diagnostic value for DME and PDR.

Results: A total of 108 eyes from 108 patients with DR (mean age of 56.04 ± 8.85 years) were analyzed. As the severity of DR increased, the ISI and leakage index of the panretina and all subregions increased. Panretinal MA count and leakage index were significantly higher in eyes with DME than those without DME ($p = 0.044$ and 0.001, respectively). Leakage index and ISI were significantly higher in eyes with PDR than those without PDR in both panretinal and subregion-specific measurements (all $p < 0.05$). Throughout the retina and specifically in the posterior area (PoA), the leakage index had a higher diagnostic value for DME than ISI or MA count (all $p < 0.05$). The diagnostic value of MA count for PDR was lower than that of ISI and leakage index (all $p < 0.05$).

Conclusion: The ISI, leakage index, and MA count in the PoA and panretina correlated with the severity of DR, especially the posterior parameter. The leakage index was more valuable than ISI and MA count in determining the occurrence of DME. ISI and leakage index were better predictors of PDR.

Keywords: ultra-widefield fluorescein angiography (UWFFA), diabetic macular edema (DME), proliferative diabetic retinopathy (PDR), leakage index, ischemic index, microaneurysm count

INTRODUCTION

Diabetic retinopathy (DR) is one of the leading causes of vision loss and blindness and has an increasing prevalence in the working-age population worldwide from 1990 to 2020 (1). The number of patients with diabetes is expected to exceed 600 million by 2040, while DR and resulting visual impairment are becoming increasingly prevalent as people with diabetes live longer (2, 3). Diabetic macular edema (DME) and proliferative diabetic retinopathy (PDR) are severe vision-threatening endpoints in patients with DR. DR, PDR, and DME affect 34.6, 7.0, and 6.8% of patients with diabetes, respectively (3). Therefore, predicting the occurrence of DME and PDR is critical.

The pathogenesis and risk factors for DME and retinal neovascularization are complex and diverse. Fundus fluorescence angiography (FFA) is an important imaging tool for assessing the vasculopathy of DR. The range of conventional FFA is 30–55° (4, 5), and 7 Standard Field (7SF) imaging after montage has only a 75° imaging range. Ultra-widefield fluorescence angiography (UWFFA) can expand this range to about 3.2 times that of 7SF (5), achieving a 200° range in one image, allowing clinicians to better observe changes in the diabetic retinal peripheral fundus, especially in the peripheral nonperfusion area and neovascularization. UWFFA can help visualize more retinal vascular lesions in the fundus of patients with DR compared to conventional FFA (5–8).

To more accurately assess the severity of DR and its complications, a series of imaging parameters, namely, ischemic index (ISI), leakage index, microaneurysm (MA) count, retinal vascular bed area, and fractal dimension, have been established and applied to the analysis of UWFFA images (9–15). Moreover, ischemia, leakage, and MA are the most characteristic imaging changes on FFA in patients with DR. Ehlers et al. (16) first reported that the panretinal ISI, leakage index, and MA count correlate with the severity of DR and noted that the posterior leakage index and MA count correlate with the presence and severity of DME.

Different regions of the retina have different distributions of photoreceptor cells and different metabolic capacities (17). It is therefore critical to study region-specific changes in the retina with ultra-widefield (UWF) imaging. In this study, we partitioned the distribution of MA count, ISI, and leakage index in UWFFA images of patients with DR with different levels of disease severity and systematically evaluated the correlation of these parameters with DME and PDR.

METHODS

Study Participants

This is a cross-sectional observational study that retrospectively analyzed UWFFA images of patients with DR who visited the Renmin Hospital of Wuhan University from June 2016 to October 2020. This study was reviewed and approved by the Clinical Research Ethics Committee of Renmin Hospital of Wuhan University (approval number: WDRY2020-K034). Given the retrospective nature of this study, an application for an informed consent waiver for patients was submitted to and approved by the ethics committee. All the involved patients underwent slit-lamp examination, UWF fundus color photography, UWFFA, and optical coherence tomography (OCT).

Inclusion and Exclusion Criteria

Inclusion criteria were: age > 18 years; diagnosis of DR (namely, type 1 and type 2 diabetes). Exclusion criteria were: previous retinal photocoagulation and vitrectomy; antivascular endothelial growth factor (anti-VEGF) treatment within 3 months; artifacts in the UWFFA image that significantly affect the evaluation of macular edema and all parameters (such as eyelashes, eyelids, and gloves of the person who took the image); poor-quality OCT images or OCT images not centered on the macula; severe media opacity (such as cataract and vitreous hemorrhage); combined retinal vein obstruction, uveitis, and macular degeneration that may cause macular edema; optical coherence tomography image of the epiretinal membranes or vitreous macular traction and other diseases that may cause retinal thickening; the presence of tractional retinal detachment; and high myopia.

Image Acquisition

All UWF pseudocolor images and UWFFA images were obtained by Optos 200Tx or California (Optos plc, Dunfermline, UK) by the two experienced physicians. Briefly, the UWF pseudocolor images were first obtained after the pupil of patients was dilated (**Figure 1A**). After intravenous injection of 5 ml of 10% sodium fluorescein, macula-centered UWFFA images and guided eye images of the patients in the superior, inferior, nasal, and temporal directions were obtained within 0–10 min. Macula-centered images from 45 s to 1 min and 30 s (early phase) and macula-centered images from 5 to 10 min (late phase) were selected to calculate UWFFA parameters, respectively. The eyes with a wider field of view and a clearer UWFFA image were selected for analysis.

The average retinal thickness in the 1 mm range of the macula and the total retinal volume in the 1, 3, and 5 mm ranges centered on the macula were measured with RTVue XR Avanti (Optovue Inc., Fremont, CA, USA).

Image Processing

Images were processed using the public domain software Fiji (http://fiji.sc/Fiji). To speed up image processing, we first transformed the UWFFA images by bilinear interpolation from 3,900 × 3,072 pixels to a size of 1,170 × 922 pixels where the details were still distinct (18).

MA count and leakage index were obtained by Trainable Weka Segmentation, a machine learning algorithm (**Figures 1B,D**). The training features were Gaussian blur, Hessian, membrane, Sobel filters, and difference of Gaussians, and the classifier was FastRandomForest, a multithreaded version of random forest initialized with 200 trees and two random features per node. Images with distinct features were selected for training to obtain satisfactory extraction results. MA segmentation was achieved by analyzing early

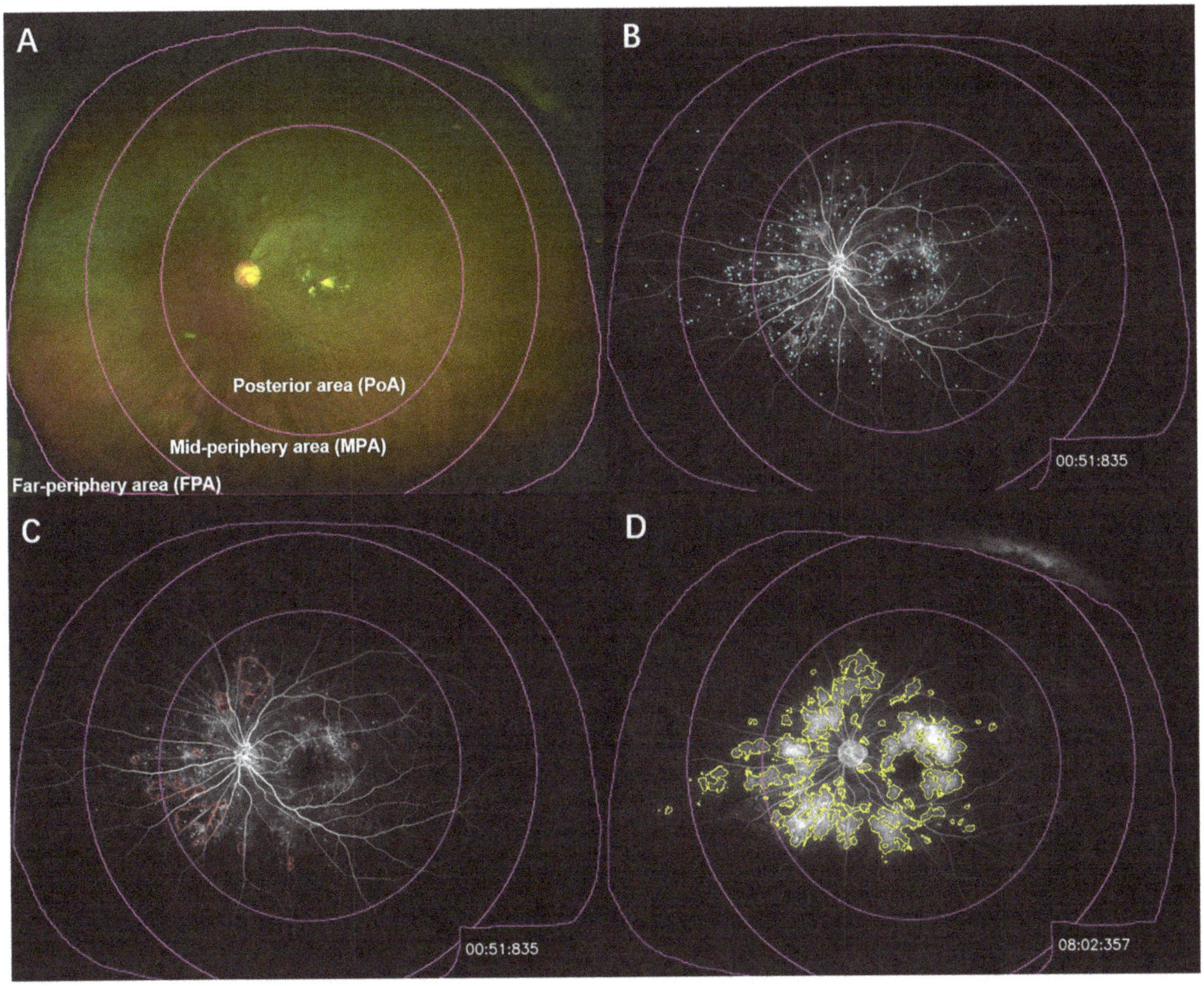

FIGURE 1 | Illustration of UWFFA partitioning and segmentation of microaneurysm, ischemia, and leakage. **(A)** The UWF pseudocolor image of patients with DR was divided into panretina, posterior area, mid-periphery area, and far-periphery area, corresponding to the subdivisions in the UWFFA images. **(B–D)** Examples of microaneurysm, ischemia, and leakage segmentation, in sequence.

UWFFA images with a trained algorithm, and MA count was obtained using the Analyze Particles tool. The leakage index was obtained by analyzing the late UWFFA images. Since the brightness and contrast of some leakage regions were relatively low, we first applied the Enhance Local Contrast tool, and then used this preprocessed image to train the algorithm and segment the leakage area. If there was no significant edema or fluorescent leakage from the optic disc, it would be manually excluded from the leakage area.

Given that nonperfusion area (NPA) is easily affected by hyperfluorescence, such as vascular filling or vascular leakage, and that peripheral background hypofluorescence is high in some patients, the segmentation of the NPA was difficult to achieve by similar automated algorithms. We, therefore, opted for a more reliable manual selection method (**Figure 1C**). By referring to the superior, inferior, nasal, and temporal UWFFA images in the middle phase, image processors delineated the NPA in the early phase.

Segmentation of ischemia, leakage, and MA was performed by a trained medical student, and the resulted segmented images were overlayed on the corresponding original images. The synthesized resultant images were reviewed by an ophthalmologist with extensive experience working with UWFFA images. For images with unsatisfactory segmentation, manual adjustment of the feature segmentation was directed by a fundus specialist. To avoid subjective factors affecting the image processing results, the retinal thickness of the patients was masked when extracting the UWFFA parameters.

The severity of DR was graded according to the Diabetic Retinopathy Disease Severity Scale using the corresponding UWF pseudocolor images (19). The DME is defined as the mean retinal thickness within 1 mm of the macula $>300\,\mu m$ or the presence of subretinal fluid within it. Leakage index is defined

TABLE 1 | Demographical and clinical characteristics of the studied eyes with diabetic retinopathy.

Characteristic	Mild NPDR (n = 11)	Moderate NPDR (n = 29)	Severe NPDR (n = 25)	PDR (n = 43)	p-value
Age, y	50.00 (46.00–65.00)	58.00 (56.00–63.50)	61.00 (56.00–64.00)	55.00 (51.00–57.00)	**0.003***
Female, n (%)	6 (54.54%)	14 (48.28%)	12 (48%)	19 (44.19%)	0.937†
Right eye, n (%)	5 (45.45%)	14 (48.28%)	15 (60%)	20 (46.51%)	0.721†
DME, n (%)	0 (0%)	5 (17.24%)	13 (52%)	18 (41.86%)	**0.003†**
CMT, μm	228.00 (210.00–253.00)	261.00 (246.00–276.45)	297.00 (268.00–510.00)	282.00 (262.00–329.00)	**<0.001***
CMV (within 1 mm), mm^3	0.18 (0.17–0.20)	0.21 (0.19–0.22)	0.23 (0.21–0.40)	0.22 (0.21–0.26)	**<0.001***
CMV (within 3 mm), mm^3	2.09(1.92–2.24)	2.29 (2.22–2.34)	2.71 (2.42–3.30)	2.50 (2.22–2.71)	**<0.001***
CMV (within 5 mm), mm^3	5.82(5.29–6.12)	6.27 (6.01–6.41)	7.51 (6.48–8.82)	7.10 (6.14–7.25)	**<0.001***
MA count (panretina), n	64.00 (8.00–93.00)	222.00 (163.67–284.00)	338.00 (295.00–390.00)	284.00 (250.00–339.00)	**<0.001***
MA count (PoA), n	41.00 (7.00–64.00)	162.00 (106.00–207.00)	257.00 (191.00–316.00)	195.00 (145.00–214.49)	**<0.001***
MA count (MPA), n	19.00 (0.00–25.00)	55.00 (32.00–88.00)	89.00 (49.00–126.00)	91.00 (62.00–105.00)	**<0.001***
MA count (FPA), n	2.00 (1.00–7.00)	11.00 (4.00–17.00)	14.00 (6.50–32.00)	17.00 (8.0–22.00)	**0.006***
ISI (panretina), %	0.00 (0.00–0.00)	0.93 (0.44–1.87)	3.47 (1.06–4.29)	4.21 (2.52–6.62)	**<0.001***
ISI (PoA), %	0.00 (0.00–0.00)	1.28 (0.79–2.63)	3.60 (1.69–9.83)	7.72 (5.48–9.77)	**<0.001***
ISI (MPA), %	0.00 (0.00–0.00)	0.53 (0.19–1.04)	1.67 (0.28–4.16)	3.35 (1.95–5.98)	**<0.001***
ISI (FPA), %	0.00 (0.00–0.00)	0.00 (0.00–0.00)	0.00 (0.00–1.58)	0.23 (0.00–1.26)	**0.004***
Leakage index (panretina), %	0.52 (0.13–1.00)	4.08 (3.00–5.84)	7.90 (3.30–9.52)	8.65 (6.71–11.01)	**<0.001***
Leakage index (PoA), %	1.60 (0.37–2.19)	9.38 (6.82–14.09)	17.19 (10.36–21.09)	20.41 (13.06–23.37)	**<0.001***
Leakage index (MPA), %	0.004 (0.00–0.24)	1.66 (0.66–2.47)	2.13 (1.12–4.35)	4.19 (2.53–5.99)	**< 0.001***
Leakage index (FPA), %	0.014 (0.00–0.38)	1.04 (0.04–1.83)	0.77 (0.01–1.99)	1.23 (0.63–2.61)	**0.006***

NPDR, nonproliferative diabetic retinopathy; PDR, proliferative diabetic retinopathy; DME, diabetic macular edema; CMT, central macular thickness; CMV, central macular volume; MA count, microaneurysm count; ISI, ischemic index; PoA, posterior area; MPA, mid-periphery area; FPA, far-periphery area.

*All quantitative parameters are expressed as median (95% CI). *p value determined by Kruskal-Wallis H test; †p-value determined by chi-squared test. Bold font indicates statistical significance.*

as the ratio of leakage area to the total area of the corresponding retina, ISI is defined as the percentage of the NPA to the total area of the corresponding retina, and MA count is defined as the total number of MAs within a certain retinal area.

To investigate the relationship between various parameters in different regions on two adverse outcomes, DME and PDR, we divided the images into three regions centered on the macula (**Figure 1A**), namely, the posterior area (PoA; 0–10 mm), the mid-periphery area (MPA; 10–15 mm), and the far-periphery area (FPA; 15 mm to the visible retinal boundary), based on the method of Silva et al. (8). Different regions were selected with the Region of Interest manager and the Specify tool.

Statistical Analysis

The normality of the data was tested by Shapiro-Wilk test and histograms. Due to the relatively small sample size, the quantitative parameters in this study were nonnormally distributed and expressed as median and 95% CI. Regional UWFFA parameters in patients with different severity levels of DR were compared using the Kruskal-Wallis H test. Correlations between UWFFA parameters and the severity of DR were analyzed using multivariate ordered logistic regression. The differences in UWFFA parameters in different regions between eyes with and without DME were determined by the Mann-Whitney U test. The discriminative capacity of the three UWFFA parameters in different regions for DME and PDR was evaluated by receiver operating characteristic (ROC) curves and the area under the ROC curve (AUC), and the optimal cut-off values were identified. Multiple linear regression analysis was used to analyze the correlation between the UWFFA parameters and central macular thickness (CMT) or central macular volume (CMV). All data processing was performed using SPSS 20.0 (version 20.0; SPSS, Chicago, IL, USA), and a p < 0.05 was considered statistically significant.

RESULTS

A total of 108 eyes from 108 patients with DR with a mean age of 56.04 ± 8.85 years were analyzed in this study, namely, 51 (47.22%) females and 54 (50%) right eyes. There were 11 eyes with mild nonproliferative diabetic retinopathy (NPDR), 29 eyes with moderate NPDR, 25 eyes with severe NPDR, and 43 eyes with PDR. A total of 36 (33.33%) eyes were diagnosed with DME. The demographic and clinical characteristics of patients with different severity levels of DR are listed in **Table 1**.

Correlation Between Panretinal and Regional UWFFA Characteristics and DR Severity

As the severity of DR increased, panretinal and subregion-specific ISI and leakage index tended to increase (**Figures 2, 3**). MA count in the NPDR group gradually increased with increasing disease severity, but it was lower in the PDR group than in the severe NPDR group. However, this difference

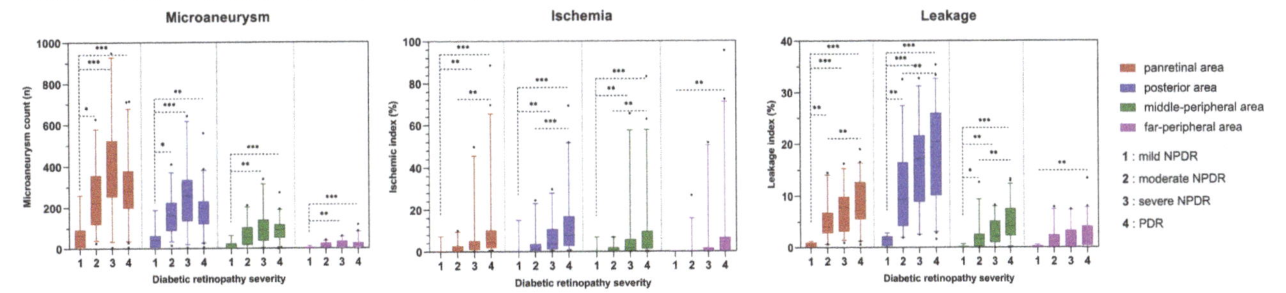

FIGURE 2 | Bar chart showing the relationship and trend between three quantitative UWFFA parameters and DR severity for panretina and each subregion. The bars are expressed as the median ± 95% CI. $^{*}p < 0.05$, $^{**}p < 0.01$, $^{***}p < 0.001$.

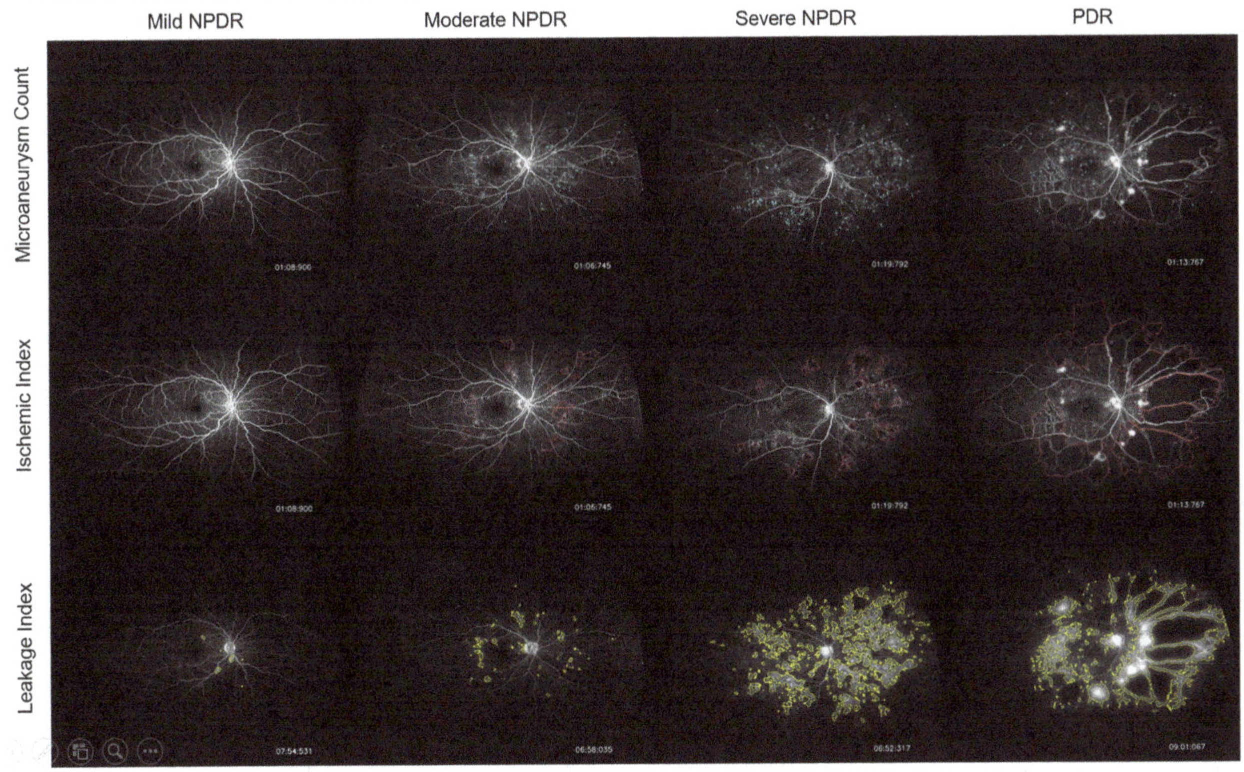

FIGURE 3 | Representative segmented images of microaneurysms, ischemia, and leakage on UWFFA images of patients with different severity of DR.

was not statistically significant (all $p > 0.05$). Meanwhile, the topographic analysis showed that all three parameters were higher in the PoA than in the MPA and FPA (all $p < 0.01$). The differences in UWFFA parameters between different DR groups with different severity levels were more pronounced in the PoA (**Figure 2**).

Multivariate ordinal logistic regression analysis showed that panretinal leakage index and ISI were associated with DR severity, while MA count was not ($p = 0.000$, 0.027, and 0.106, respectively), and posterior leakage index, ISI, and MA count were all associated with DR severity ($p = 0.026$, 0.030, and 0.002, respectively).

Comparison of UWFFA Characteristics of Eyes With and Without DME

In all the studied eyes, panretinal MA count and leakage index were significantly higher in eyes with DME than those without DME ($p = 0.044$ and 0.001, respectively). However, leakage index, ISI, and MA count in the PoA were significantly higher in eyes with DME than those without DME ($p < 0.001$, 0.022, and 0.012, respectively). Notably, there were no significant differences in any of the parameters between the two groups in the mid- and far-peripheral regions (**Table 2**).

Given that the MA count of PDR may be affected by the large NPA, and that there were many neovascularization components

TABLE 2 | Comparison of clinical characteristics between eyes with and without DME.

Characteristic	DME present ($n = 36$)	DME absent ($n = 72$)	*p*-value
Age, y	60.50 (56.00–64.00)	56.00 (55.00–58.00)	-
Female, *n* (%)	17 (47.22%)	34 (47.22)	-
Right eye, *n* (%)	18 (50%)	18 (50%)	-
CMT, μm	428.00 (397.00–502.00)	255.00 (248.51–262.00)	**<0.001***
CMV (within 1 mm), mm^3	0.34 (0.31–0.39)	0.20 (0.19–0.21)	**<0.001***
CMV (within 3 mm), mm^3	3.19 (2.90–3.48)	2.22 (2.19–2.28)	**<0.001***
CMV (within 5 mm), mm^3	8.66 (7.77–8.99)	6.11 (5.97–6.25)	**<0.001***
MA count (panretina), *n*	318.00 (262.00–356.50)	252.00 (169.00–284.00)	**0.044***
MA count (PoA), *n*	213.50 (177.00–237.00)	152.50 (114.00–191.00)	**0.012***
MA count (MPA), *n*	72.50 (61.00–105.89)	57.50 (39.00–89.00)	0.149*
MA count (FPA), *n*	12.00 (7.00–20.00)	10.50 (7.00–17.00)	0.977*
ISI (panretina), %	2.79 (1.59–4.48)	1.90 (0.99–3.53)	0.118*
ISI (PoA), %	5.10 (2.36–10.05)	2.65 (1.32–4.41)	**0.022***
ISI (MPA), %	1.69 (0.49–2.91)	1.22 (0.50–2.71)	0.590*
ISI (FPA), %	0.00 (0.00–0.24)	0.00 (0.00–0.17)	0.595*
Leakage index (panretina), %	8.90 (7.90–11.85)	4.53 (3.05–5.76)	**<0.001***
Leakage index (PoA), %	21.22 (20.20–24.78)	9.87 (7.11–11.96)	**<0.001***
Leakage index (MPA), %	3.66 (2.43–5.05)	1.65 (0.96–2.31)	**0.004***
Leakage index (FPA), %	1.42 (0.51–2.97)	0.64 (0.25–1.04)	0.077*

DME, diabetic macular edema; CMT, central macular thickness; CMV, central macular volume; MA count, microaneurysm count; ISI, ischemic index; PoA, posterior area; MPA, mid-periphery area; FPA, far-periphery area.
*All quantitative parameters are expressed as median (95% CI). *p-value determined by Mann–Whitney U-test. Bold font indicates statistical significance.*

TABLE 3 | Comparison of clinical characteristics between eyes with and without PDR.

Characteristic	PDR present ($n = 43$)	PDR absent ($n = 65$)	*p* value
Age, y	55.00 (51.00–57.00)	58.00 (56.00–61.50)	-
Female, *n* (%)	19 (44.19%)	32 (49.23%)	-
Right eye, *n* (%)	20 (46.51)	34 (52.31)	-
CMT, μm	282.00 (262.00–310.00)	266.00 (259.00–283.00)	0.361
CMV (within 1 mm), mm^3	0.22 (0.21–0.24)	0.21 (0.21–0.22)	0.350
CMV (within 3 mm), mm^3	2.50 (2.22–2.67)	2.32 (2.27–2.39)	0.770
CMV (within 5 mm), mm^3	7.07 (6.16–7.25)	6.38 (6.14–6.49)	0.516
MA count (panretina), *n*	284.00 (250.00–339.00)	260.00 (175.00–317.87)	0.222
MA count (PoA), *n*	195.00 (141.54–215.00)	168.00 (114.00–207.00)	0.609
MA count (MPA), *n*	91.00 (62.00–105.00)	55.00 (35.00–69.00)	**0.041**
MA count (FPA), *n*	17.00 (8.00–22.00)	8.00 (5.50–14.00)	0.087
ISI (panretina), %	4.21 (2.52–6.62)	1.06 (0.44–1.87)	**<0.001**
ISI (PoA), %	7.72 (5.48–10.29)	1.68 (0.94–2.69)	**<0.001**
ISI (MPA), %	3.35 (1.94–6.01)	0.48 (0.18–1.04)	**<0.001**
ISI (FPA), %	0.23 (0.00–1.26)	0.00 (0.00–0.00)	**0.006**
Leakage index (panretina), %	8.65 (6.71–11.28)	3.76 (3.06–5.62)	**<0.001**
Leakage index (PoA), %	20.41 (12.51–23.30)	9.38 (7.10–13.47)	**<0.001**
Leakage index (MPA), %	4.19 (2.63–6.6.09)	1.12 (0.66–2.17)	**<0.001**
Leakage index (FPA), %	1.23 (0.63–2.62)	0.45 (0.04–1.04)	**0.014**

PDR, proliferative diabetic retinopathy; CMT, central macular thickness; CMV, central macular volume; MA count, microaneurysm count; ISI, ischemic index; PoA, posterior area; MPA, mid-periphery area; FPA, far-periphery area.
*All quantitative parameters are expressed as median (95% CI). *p-value determined by Mann–Whitney U-test. Bold font indicates statistical significance.*

in the retinal vascular leakage, we investigated the differences in UWFFA characteristics of eyes with and without DME in NPDR and PDR groups. In patients with NPDR, the panretinal and PoA-specific leakage index, ISI, and MA count were higher in eyes with DME than those without DME (all $p < 0.05$). Multiple linear regression analysis showed that only the leakage index was associated with CMT in the panretina and PoA ($p = 0.006$ and 0.001, respectively). In patients with PDR, only panretinal, PoA-specific, and MPA-specific leakage indexes were significantly different between eyes with and without DME (all $p < 0.05$), and no significant differences were found between the other regional UWFFA parameters. Multiple linear regression analysis showed that neither panretinal nor regional UWFFA parameters were correlated with CMT (all $p > 0.05$).

Comparison of UWFFA Characteristics of Eyes With and Without PDR

The MA count in the MPA was significantly higher in eyes with PDR than those without PDR ($p = 0.041$). Leakage index and ISI were significantly higher in eyes with PDR than those without PDR, both in panretina and subregion-specific measurements (all $p < 0.05$, **Table 3**). No significant differences were found between the two groups for any other regional parameters (all $p > 0.05$).

Assessment of the Indexes Most Associated With the Two Adverse Outcomes Using ROC Curves

Since there were no significant differences in UWFFA parameters in the MPA and FPA between eyes with and without DME, we evaluated ROC curves of the three parameters in the panretina and PoA for predicting DME (**Figure 4**). For both panretinal and PoA-specific analyses, the leakage index had a higher diagnostic value for DME than ISI and MA count (all $p < 0.05$). ROC curves showed that the leakage index in the PoA had the largest AUC for the determination of DME. The cutoff value at this point was 16.704%, and its specificity and sensitivity for determining the occurrence of DME were both 75%. In addition, multiple linear regression analysis showed that among all the posterior

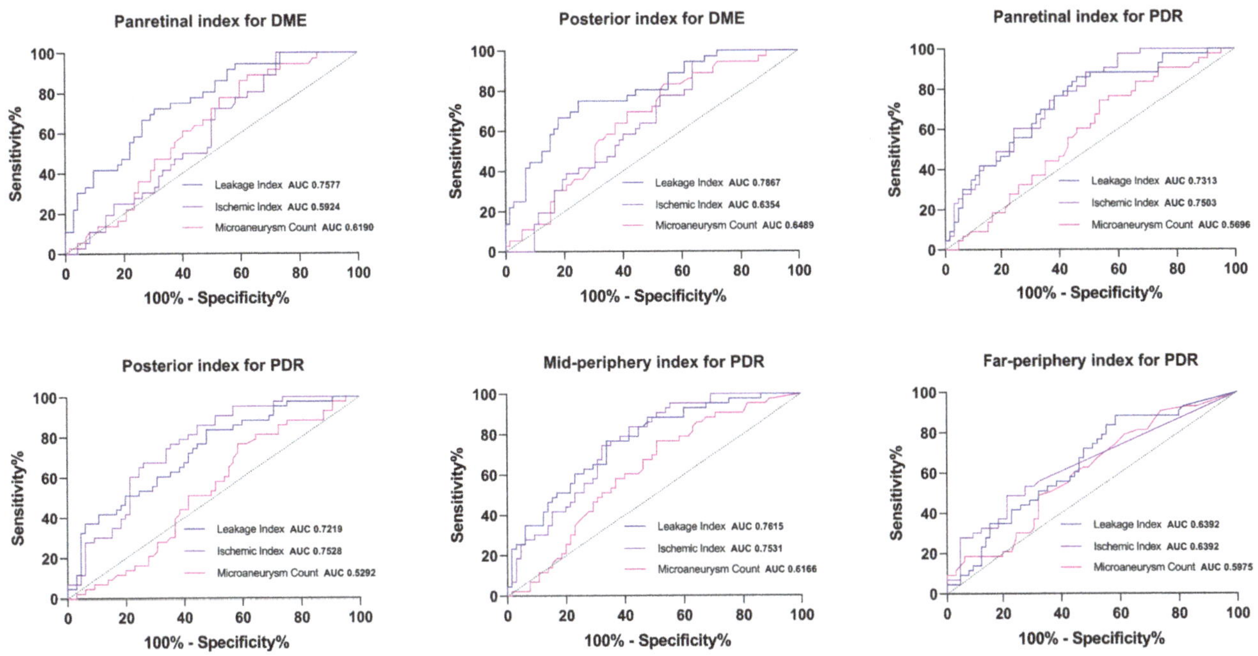

FIGURE 4 | Receiver operating characteristic curve of the regional UWFFA parameters for determining the occurrence of DME and PDR.

TABLE 4 | Optimal cut-off values and coordinates of the ROC curve for determining the presence of DME.

Characteristic	Cut-off values	Sensitivity%	Specificity%	Youden index
MA count (panretina), *n*	>153	88.89	37.50	0.2639
MA count (PoA), *n*	>129	83.33	45.83	0.2917
ISI (panretina), %	>0.34	100.00	27.78	0.2778
ISI (PoA), %	>1.01	94.44	36.11	0.3056
Leakage index (panretina), %	>6.709	72.22	69.44	0.4167
Leakage index (PoA), %	>16.704	75.00	75.00	0.5000

MA count, microaneurysm count; ISI, ischemic index; PoA, posterior area.

TABLE 5 | Optimal cut-off values and coordinates of the ROC curve for determining the presence of PDR.

Characteristic	Criterion values	Sensitivity%	Specificity%	Youden index
MA count (panretina), *n*	>222	74.42	46.15	0.2057
MA count (PoA), *n*	>119	76.74	41.54	0.1828
MA count (MPA), *n*	>50	76.74	49.23	0.2597
MA count (FPA), *n*	>5	79.07	38.46	0.1753
ISI (panretina), %	>1.058	88.37	50.77	0.3914
ISI (PoA), %	>1.7	86.05	55.38	0.4143
ISI (MPA), %	>0.64	83.72	58.46	0.4218
ISI (FPA), %	>0.325	48.84	78.46	0.2730
Leakage index (panretina), %	>4.173	86.05	53.85	0.3989
Leakage index (PoA), %	>9.393	83.72	52.31	0.3603
Leakage index (MPA), %	>2.233	76.74	66.15	0.4290
Leakage index (FPA), %	>0.044	88.37	41.54	0.2991

MA count, microaneurysm count; ISI, ischemic index; PoA, posterior area; MPA, mid-periphery area; FPA, far-periphery area.

parameters, only leakage index was significantly correlated with CMT and CMV (all $p < 0.001$), and had the highest correlation with CMV in the 5-mm range and the lowest correlation with CMV in the 1-mm range or CMT.

As for PDR, the AUC of ISI was larger than that of leakage index in both panretina and PoA-specific measurements (**Figure 4**). In the MPA, the AUC of leakage index was larger than that of ISI. Notably, the diagnostic value of MA count for PDR was lower than that of ISI and leakage index, but there was no significant difference in the diagnostic value of ISI and leakage index in any region (all $p < 0.05$, method of Delong et al., 1988). The optimal cutoff values for judging DME and PDR for different UWFFA indexes in different regions are presented in **Tables 4, 5.**

DISCUSSION

In this study, we quantified MA count, ISI, and leakage index parameters in different regions of the retina based on UWFFA images, and analyzed the correlations between these parameters and DR severity. We also evaluated the association of these parameters with DME and PDR, both of which are severe vision-threatening endpoints in patients with DR. Previous studies have demonstrated the correlation of the above three indexes with DR severity (20). Our study has validated some of their conclusions, and meanwhile provides some new findings. Although these three parameters were higher in the eyes with DME than those without DME, the leakage index was more valuable than ISI and MA count in predicting DME.

Leakage index, ISI, and MA count in the PoA were more strongly correlated with DR grade and DME occurrence than when they were measured in the panretina, and even less association was observed when they were measured in the mid- and far-periphery. ISI and leakage index, but not MA count, were powerful predictors of PDR. In addition, leakage index was better correlated with retinal volume in the 5-mm perimacular region than in the CMT or 1-mm perimacular region, suggesting that the posterior leakage index better reflects diffuse macular thickening.

Ischemia, leakage, and MA are typical fluorescein angiography features of patients with DR. The availability of UWFFA devices has enabled visualization of the peripheral retina, which was previously limited by conventional devices. Silva et al. (8) first reported that NPA and ISI on UWFFA are associated with DR severity. Ehlers et al. (12, 21) developed a semiautomatic quantitative platform for analysis of ischemia, leakage, and MA on UWFFA images, which they used to systematically evaluate the correlation of these three parameters with DR severity (20). Consistent with their results, our study showed a positive correlation between panretinal leakage index and ISI and DR severity (20). However, we found that panretinal MA count increased with increasing disease severity in the mild, moderate, and severe NPDR groups, but patients in the PDR group had lower panretinal MA count than patients with NPDR, and only MA count in the PoA was significantly correlated with DR severity. NPA in DR eyes starts in the perifoveal retina (22), and as the disease progresses, NPA may also appear in the paramacular or even peripheral retina. The extent of retinal capillary occlusion and NPA make it impossible for MAs to exist alone, and thus panretinal MA count in PDR is reduced instead. Due to the existence of significant ischemia and hypoxia in the PDR eyes, numerous MAs could still be present in the capillary perfusion areas of the PoA. The variability among the involved patients may be the reason for these different results. In addition, it is worth noting that the three parameters measured in the PoA are more meaningful than the panretinal measurements, even though more lesions may be found throughout the retina.

The mechanism of DME formation is complex and multiple factors are involved. VEGF is a potent vasopermeability factor (23), and its expression in the retina is upregulated in response to ischemia/hypoxia (24, 25). With increasing retinal vascular permeability and endothelial cell proliferation (24, 25), the breakdown of the blood-retinal barrier results in retinal edema. Previous studies showed that quantitative UWFA imaging parameters are correlated with concentrations of various aqueous cytokines, namely, VEGF and IL-6 (26). The advent of fluorescence angiography can help us observe the process of leakage of fluid from the blood vessels into tissues, and quantify the severity of leakage through fluorescence angiography images, thus facilitating our exploration of the disease.

Previous studies showed that the occurrence and severity of DME are influenced by both leakage index and MA count in the PoA (16). Our study found that only the posterior leakage index correlated with the severity of DME. Therefore, the leakage index is more important in determining the occurrence of DME than MA. Furthermore, the efficacy of the panretinal leakage index in determining DME was lower than that in the PoA, probably because posterior leakage is more likely to diffuse into the macula and contributes to the occurrence of DME than leakage in the MPA and FPA.

Retina leakage can be derived from multiple sources. Xue et al. (4) classified the causes of leakage into three types based on FFA presentation: MA-driven, peripheral ischemia, and neovascularization. We found that in patients with NPDR, MA count in PoA was significantly higher in eyes with DME than those without DME. Previous studies found a close relationship between leakage and MA (16). The leakage index has been demonstrated as the most sensitive predictor of DME. Therefore, we speculate that the presence of DME in patients with NPDR is more likely to be associated with MA-related leakage. However, in patients with PDR with reduced MA count, there were still several eyes presenting with DME because of severe leakage. Therefore, we suggest that there may be different mechanisms for the occurrence of DME in NPDR and patients with PDR and that the leaky component in patients with PDR is more likely to be of neovascular origin.

Furthermore, in NPDR eyes, the occurrence of DME was associated with ISI, but only in the PoA. The same relationship was not found in PDR eyes. In addition, no clear correlation was found between ISI and the severity of DME, in agreement with Wessel et al. (27) and Fan et al. (28).

The most important finding of this study was to explore the strongest correlations with DME and PDR from the current indexes. We found that the leakage index is optimal in the ROC curves of all three, with high accuracy in disease prediction. Based on the pathogenesis of the retinal vascular disease, MA, ischemia, or neovascularization will eventually all be accompanied by leakage in the fundus, and the leakage index may be the result of a combination of other factors. In the future, the leakage index may become an important index for assessing the severity of fundus vascular diseases.

Both leakage index and ISI are of high value for the diagnosis of PDR, and they are both superior to MA count. The occurrence of PDR can be caused by intraocular tissue hypoxia, which induces elevated levels of VEGF and other proangiogenic factors and promotes neovascularization (29). It has been reported that NPA reflects the severity of fundus hypoxia, and it may correlate with intraocular VEGF levels (5). Therefore, ISI can predict the development of neovascularization or PDR. Conversely, when neovascularization is immature and the blood-retinal barrier is highly permeable, significant leakage can be observed in fluorescence angiography images. Therefore, the leakage index is comparable to the ISI in determining PDR. Changes in these UWFFA parameters after treatment may suggest a greater significance. Babiuch et al. (30) found that patients with PDR underwent a significant reduction in leakage index on UWFFA images of panretina and all subregional areas after anti-VEGF treatment. In addition, it should not be overlooked that MA count also significantly decreased after anti-VEGF treatment (31). Leakage index and MA count may play critical roles in the assessment of treatment outcomes in patients with PDR in the future.

This study has some limitations. First, this was a retrospective observational study with small sample size. Second, peripheral image distortion is a common problem for UWF images and may affect the accuracy of image analysis. Third, only one macula-centered UWFFA image was utilized for analysis, and the complete retinal image puzzle was not acquired using the montage method. Fourth, in our clinical work, we did not set the late images at a specific point in time but within a range, which may cause some degree of variation due to the dynamic nature of fluorescence angiography.

Despite the limitations, our study complements some gaps in the current quantitative study of UWFFA in DR. We explored the in-depth relationship between each of these parameters and two adverse outcomes, PDR and DME, and found the best-evaluated parameter among several commonly used options. We also designed a quantitative method for UWFFA that can be implemented by open software, which will help improve accessibility and enrich the study of UWF images. In addition, the above limitations include common technical problems faced by current UWF image research, such as peripheral aberrations and montage. Subsequently, we expect that the development of technology will allow us to improve upon our results. In the future, studies with larger sample size and more precise timing of DR UWFFA images are needed.

In conclusion, ISI, leakage index, and MA count in the PoA and panretina were correlated with the severity of DR, especially the posterior parameter. The leakage index was more valuable than ISI and MA count in determining the occurrence of DME. ISI and leakage index were of higher value in determining PDR.

ETHICS STATEMENT

The studies involving human participants were reviewed and approved by Clinical Research Ethics Committee of Renmin Hospital of Wuhan University. Written informed consent for participation was not required for this study in accordance with the national legislation and the institutional requirements.

AUTHOR CONTRIBUTIONS

GS, XW, and CC: conception, design, and manuscript preparation. GS, XW, and JJ: image processing design. GS, XW, JJ, ZY, MF, XY, and HZ: image and data collection. HZ and CC: manuscript review and revision. All authors read and approved the final manuscript.

REFERENCES

1. Causes of blindness and vision impairment in 2020 and trends over 30 years, and prevalence of avoidable blindness in relation to VISION 2020: the Right to Sight: an analysis for the Global Burden of Disease Study. *Lancet Glob Health.* (2021) 9:e144–60. doi: 10.1016/s2214-109x(20)30489-7
2. Ogurtsova K, da Rocha Fernandes JD, Huang Y, Linnenkamp U, Guariguata L, Cho NH, et al. IDF diabetes atlas: global estimates for the prevalence of diabetes for 2015 and 2040. *Diabetes Res Clin Pract.* (2017) 128:40–50. doi: 10.1016/j.diabres.2017.03.024
3. Yau JW, Rogers SL, Kawasaki R, Lamoureux EL, Kowalski JW, Bek T, et al. Global prevalence and major risk factors of diabetic retinopathy. *Diabetes Care.* (2012) 35:556–64. doi: 10.2337/dc11-1909
4. Xue K, Yang E, Chong NV. Classification of diabetic macular oedema using ultra-widefield angiography and implications for response to anti-VEGF therapy. *Br J Ophthalmol.* (2017) 101:559–63. doi: 10.1136/bjophthalmol-2016-308704
5. Wessel MM, Aaker GD, Parlitsis G, Cho M, D'Amico DJ, Kiss S. Ultra-wide-field angiography improves the detection and classification of diabetic retinopathy. *Retina.* (2012) 32:785–91. doi: 10.1097/IAE.0b013e3182278b64
6. Silva PS, Cavallerano JD, Sun JK, Noble J, Aiello LM, Aiello LP. Nonmydriatic ultrawide field retinal imaging compared with dilated standard 7-field 35-mm photography and retinal specialist examination for evaluation of diabetic retinopathy. *Am J Ophthalmol.* (2012) 154:549–59.e2. doi: 10.1016/j.ajo.2012.03.019
7. Silva PS, Cavallerano JD, Sun JK, Soliman AZ, Aiello LM, Aiello LP. Peripheral lesions identified by mydriatic ultrawide field imaging: distribution and potential impact on diabetic retinopathy severity. *Ophthalmology.* (2013) 120:2587–95. doi: 10.1016/j.ophtha.2013.05.004
8. Silva PS, Dela Cruz AJ, Ledesma MG, van Hemert J, Radwan A, Cavallerano JD, et al. Diabetic retinopathy severity and peripheral lesions are associated with nonperfusion on ultrawide field angiography. *Ophthalmology.* (2015) 122:2465–72. doi: 10.1016/j.ophtha.2015.07.034
9. Patel RD, Messner LV, Teitelbaum B, Michel KA, Hariprasad SM. Characterization of ischemic index using ultra-widefield fluorescein angiography in patients with focal and diffuse recalcitrant diabetic macular edema. *Am J Ophthalmol.* (2013) 155:1038–44.e2. doi: 10.1016/j.ajo.2013.01.007
10. Sim DA, Keane PA, Rajendram R, Karampelas M, Selvam S, Powner MB, et al. Patterns of peripheral retinal and central macula ischemia in diabetic retinopathy as evaluated by ultra-widefield fluorescein angiography. *Am J Ophthalmol.* (2014) 158:144–53.e1. doi: 10.1016/j.ajo.2014.03.009
11. Tan CS, Chew MC, van Hemert J, Singer MA, Bell D, Sadda SR. Measuring the precise area of peripheral retinal non-perfusion using ultra-widefield imaging and its correlation with the ischaemic index. *Br J Ophthalmol.* (2016) 100:235–9. doi: 10.1136/bjophthalmol-2015-306652
12. Ehlers JP, Wang K, Vasanji A, Hu M, Srivastava SK. Automated quantitative characterisation of retinal vascular leakage and microaneurysms in ultra-widefield fluorescein angiography. *Br J Ophthalmol.* (2017) 101:696–9. doi: 10.1136/bjophthalmol-2016-310047
13. Fan W, Uji A, Nittala M, Wykoff CC, Brown D, Fleming A, et al. Retinal vascular bed area on ultra-wide field fluorescein angiography indicates the severity of diabetic retinopathy. *Br J Ophthalmol.* (2021) doi: 10.1136/bjophthalmol-2020-317488. [Epub ahead of print].
14. Fan W, Uji A, Borrelli E, Singer M, Sagong M, van Hemert J, et al. Precise measurement of retinal vascular bed area and density on ultra-wide fluorescein angiography in normal subjects. *Am J Ophthalmol.* (2018) 188:155–63. doi: 10.1016/j.ajo.2018.01.036
15. Fan W, Nittala MG, Fleming A, Robertson G, Uji A, Wykoff CC, et al. Relationship between retinal fractal dimension and nonperfusion in diabetic retinopathy on ultrawide-field fluorescein angiography. *Am J Ophthalmol.* (2020) 209:99–106. doi: 10.1016/j.ajo.2019.08.015
16. Jiang AC, Srivastava SK, Hu M, Figueiredo N, Babiuch A, Boss JD, et al. Quantitative ultra-widefield angiographic features and associations with diabetic macular edema. *Ophthalmol Retina.* (2020) 4:49–56. doi: 10.1016/j.oret.2019.08.008

17. Croft DE, Wykoff CC, van Hemert J, Verhoek M, Brown DM. Not all retina is created equal: metabolic quantification of ultra-widefield images. *Ophthalmology.* (2015) 122:2580–2. doi: 10.1016/j.ophtha.2015.05.043
18. Wang X, Sun G, Yi Z, Xu A, He L, Jiang J, et al. Leakage index on ultra-widefield fluorescence angiography in different regions of retina and its correlation with cystoid macular edema in central retinal vein occlusion eyes. *Graefes Arch Clin Exp Ophthalmol.* (2021) 259:2149–56. doi: 10.1007/s00417-021-05126-y
19. Wilkinson CP, Ferris FL, 3rd, Klein RE, Lee PP, Agardh CD, Davis M, et al. Proposed international clinical diabetic retinopathy and diabetic macular edema disease severity scales. *Ophthalmology.* (2003) 110:1677–82. doi: 10.1016/s0161-6420(03)00475-5
20. Ehlers JP, Jiang AC, Boss JD, Hu M, Figueiredo N, Babiuch A, et al. Quantitative ultra-widefield angiography and diabetic retinopathy severity: an assessment of panretinal leakage index, ischemic index and microaneurysm count. *Ophthalmology.* (2019) 126:1527–32. doi: 10.1016/j.ophtha.2019.05.034
21. Jiang A, Srivastava S, Figueiredo N, Babiuch A, Hu M, Reese J, et al. Repeatability of automated leakage quantification and microaneurysm identification utilising an analysis platform for ultra-widefield fluorescein angiography. *Br J Ophthalmol.* (2019) 104:500–3. doi: 10.1136/bjophthalmol-2019-314416
22. Kohner EM, Dollery CT. Fluorescein angiography of the fundus in diabetic retinopathy. *Br Med Bull.* (1970) 26:166–70. doi: 10.1093/oxfordjournals.bmb.a070770
23. Das A. Diabetic retinopathy: battling the global epidemic. *Invest Ophthalmol Vis Sci.* (2016) 57:6669–82. doi: 10.1167/iovs.16-21031
24. Wang W, Lo ACY. Diabetic retinopathy: pathophysiology and treatments. *Int J Mol Sci.* (2018) 19:1816. doi: 10.3390/ijms19061816
25. Gupta N, Mansoor S, Sharma A, Sapkal A, Sheth J, Falatoonzadeh P, et al. Diabetic retinopathy and VEGF. *Open Ophthalmol J.* (2013) 7:4–10. doi: 10.2174/1874364101307010004
26. Abraham JR, Wykoff CC, Arepalli S, Lunasco L, Yu HJ, Martin A, et al. Exploring the angiographic-biologic phenotype in the IMAGINE study: quantitative UWFA and cytokine expression. *Br J Ophthalmol.* (2021) doi: 10.1136/bjophthalmol-2020-318726. [Epub ahead of print].
27. Wessel MM, Nair N, Aaker GD, Ehrlich JR, D'Amico DJ, Kiss S. Peripheral retinal ischaemia, as evaluated by ultra-widefield fluorescein angiography, is associated with diabetic macular oedema. *Br J Ophthalmol.* (2012) 96:694–8. doi: 10.1136/bjophthalmol-2011-300774
28. Fan W, Wang K, Ghasemi Falavarjani K, Sagong M, Uji A, Ip M, et al. Distribution of nonperfusion area on ultra-widefield fluorescein angiography in eyes with diabetic macular edema: DAVE Study. *Am J Ophthalmol.* (2017) 180:110–6. doi: 10.1016/j.ajo.2017.05.024
29. Stitt AW, Curtis TM, Chen M, Medina RJ, McKay GJ, Jenkins A, et al. The progress in understanding and treatment of diabetic retinopathy. *Progr Retinal Eye Res.* (2016) 51:156–86. doi: 10.1016/j.preteyeres.2015.08.001
30. Babiuch AS, Wykoff CC, Srivastava SK, Talcott K, Zhou B, Hach J, et al. Retinal leakage index dynamics on ultra-widefield fluorescein angiography in eyes treated with intravitreal aflibercept for proliferative diabetic retinopathy in the recovery study. *Retina.* (2020) 40:2175–83. doi: 10.1097/iae.0000000000002727
31. Babiuch A, Wykoff CC, Hach J, Srivastava S, Talcott KE, Yu HJ, et al. Longitudinal panretinal microaneurysm dynamics on ultra-widefield fluorescein angiography in eyes treated with intravitreal aflibercept for proliferative diabetic retinopathy in the recovery study. *Br J Ophthalmol.* (2020) 105:1111–5. doi: 10.1136/bjophthalmol-2020-316952

Changes in Anterior and Posterior Corneal Elevation in Patients with Allergic Conjunctivitis

Qian Wang [1†], Fei Yu [1†], Ziqing Feng [1], Weihua Li [1], Naiyang Li [2], Xinyue Du [1], Xuan Zhao [1], Saiqun Li [1] and Jin Yuan [1*]*

[1] State Key Laboratory of Ophthalmology, Zhongshan Ophthalmic Center, Sun Yat-sen University, Guangdong Provincial Key Laboratory of Ophthalmology and Visual Science, Guangdong Provincial Clinical Research Center for Ocular Diseases, Guangzhou, China, [2] Eye Center, Zhongshan City People's Hospital, Zhongshan, China

***Correspondence:**
Saiqun Li
123213197@qq.com
Jin Yuan
yuanjincornea@126.com

† These authors have contributed equally to this work and share first authorship

Purpose: To evaluate corneal elevation changes in patients with allergic conjunctivitis (AC) and to analyze their correlations with ocular allergy signs and corneal biomechanical alterations.

Methods: Thirty patients (30 eyes) with AC and twenty normal subjects (20 eyes) were included in this prospective study. All participants underwent a complete ocular examination, including corneal tomography by Pentacam and corneal biomechanics evaluation by Corvis ST. AC patients were evaluated for their eye rubbing frequency and ocular allergic signs.

Results: The elevation at the thinnest location (TE) and the central location (CE), the elevation difference at the thinnest location (TED) and the central location (CED), and the mean value of elevation difference in the central 4 mm zoom (MED) of both the anterior and posterior corneal surface were significantly higher in the AC group than in the normal group ($p < 0.05$ for all). In AC patients, only anterior corneal elevation parameters were positively correlated with eye rubbing frequency and ocular allergy sign severity ($p < 0.05$ for all), while the tomography and biomechanical index (TBI) was positively correlated with the elevation parameters of both the anterior and posterior corneal surfaces ($p < 0.05$ for all).

Conclusion: AC patients carry an increased risk of corneal ectasia. Posterior corneal elevation parameters are sensitive and reliable predictors of keratoconus (KC) risk in AC patients.

Clinical Trial Registration: https://clinicaltrials.gov/ct2/show/NCT04299399, identifier [NCT04299399].

Keywords: allergic conjunctivitis, corneal tomography, corneal surface elevation, corneal posterior surface, corneal biomechanics

INTRODUCTION

Allergic conjunctivitis (AC) is a common ocular surface disease that affects more than 20% of the population (1). It is well established in the literature that AC is closely related to the occurrence of keratoconus (KC) (2–4). Various allergic ocular conditions, including vernal keratoconjunctivitis (VKC), atopic keratoconjunctivitis (AKC) and seasonal allergic conjunctivitis (SAC) or perennial allergic conjunctivitis (PAC), have been reported to increase the risk of developing KC (5). Although the underlying mechanisms remain unclear, increased inflammatory molecules and proteases and itch-provoked eye rubbing were thought to contribute to the development and progression of KC in AC patients (6).

AC has been found to be positively associated with early unset of KC. However, this association may still be underestimated in clinical analysis, since a considerable number of AC patients have subclinical presentation of KC (7). This subclinical population needs close monitoring for KC development. KC is characterized by progressive corneal thinning and a cone-shaped protrusion. It can be easily diagnosed in its intermediate to advanced stages, but an exact diagnosis of subclinical KC is still a major challenge because the diagnostic criteria remain to be defined (8). Several corneal topographic parameters, such as corneal elevation parameters and corneal thickness distribution indices, have been evaluated for their sensitivity to subclinical KC (9–14). Previous studies have shown that among the measured topographic parameters, including pachymetric parameters, elevation parameters and topometric parameters, anterior and posterior elevations had the greatest areas under the receiver operating characteristic curve (AUROCs) to discriminate subclinical KC from normal corneas (10, 13). KC was thought to start from the posterior surface of the cornea (15, 16). Moreover, taking into consideration that compared to the anterior corneal surface, the posterior cornea surface is less affected by corneal epithelial conditions and tear film stability, previous studies proposed posterior corneal elevations as more sensitive and reliable shape parameters for differentiating subclinical KC (15, 16).

Many studies have screened KC-like topographic and biomechanical changes in AC patients. KC-like tomography was observed in 11–20% of VKC patients (7, 17). Moreover, VKC was reported to cause a reduction in corneal biomechanics, as indicated by decreased corneal resistance factor (CRF) (18). Additionally, our previous study found alterations in the tomography and biomechanical index (TBI) in AC patients (19). In terms of posterior corneal surface changes in AC patients, studies have mainly concentrated on corneal aberrations and densitometry, and few have investigated posterior surface elevations. Barreto et al. (20) reported that VKC patients had significantly higher anterior and posterior elevations and pachymeter indices than healthy subjects. However, this study used Orbscan tomography IIz, which has been questioned by some researchers about its ability to accurately measure the posterior corneal surface. Because the Orbscan topographer works on the principle of slit scanning combined with Placido-disk technology, the posterior elevation map is derived mathematically from the Placido-disk reflection and 20 slit scans of the anterior segment (11, 14). In contrast, Pentacam uses a rotating Scheimpflug camera to capture 25 slit images and obtain a representation of the corneal shape, with which the posterior corneal elevations can be measured with high reproducibility and repeatability (21, 22).

In this study, we evaluated the corneal tomographic changes in AC patients using Pentacam, focusing on anterior and posterior surface elevation and pachymetric distribution. The correlations of these corneal tomographic changes with ocular allergic signs and corneal biomechanical changes were further analyzed. The purpose of this study was to elucidate the risk of KC development in AC patients and to identify sensitive indicators to screen high-risk patients for early intervention.

MATERIALS AND METHODS

Participants

This prospective case-control study was conducted at the Zhongshan Ophthalmic Center, Sun Yat-Sen University and was approved by the Ethics Committee of the study hospital (2020KYPJ008). This trial has been registered at ClinicalTrials.gov as trial number NCT04299399. All subjects or responsible relatives signed informed consent forms before the study.

In this study, thirty AC patients and twenty normal subjects were included. The diagnosis of AC was determined according to the presence of typical clinical manifestations, including itching, redness, conjunctival hyperemia, palpebral conjunctival papillae or Horner-Trantas dots. Only patients with a history of AC for more than 2 years were enrolled. Age-matched subjects with no remarkable medical or ocular history except for refractive error served as normal controls. The exclusion criteria were: high refractive errors (spherical equivalent >6D and/or astigmatism >2D), active ocular inflammatory diseases other than AC, previous ocular surgery or disease, systemic diseases that might lead corneal abnormalities, soft contact lens wearing within 2 weeks and rigid contact lens wearing within 1 month.

Examination Methods

Eye rubbing frequency and ocular allergy signs were evaluated in AC patients as reported in our previous study (19). Briefly, eye rubbing frequency was assessed on a scale from 1 (absent) to 5 (constant eye rubbing). Each objective ocular allergy sign (including conjunctival hyperemia, swelling, papillae, and corneal epithelial disorder) was graded on a scale from 0 (none) to 3 (severe) by the clinician.

All participants underwent a complete ophthalmic evaluation, including slit lamp examination, corneal tomography with Pentacam (Oculus, Inc., Wetzlar, Germany) and corneal biomechanics evaluation with Corneal Visualization Scheimpflug Technology (Corvis ST) (Oculus, Inc., Wetzlar, Germany). All measurements were performed by a single examiner to minimize interobserver variation.

The following Pentacam parameters were analyzed: (1) topographic parameters of the anterior and posterior corneal surface, including keratometric values [flat keratometry (K1), steep keratometry (K2), mean keratometry (Kmean), maximum keratometry (Kmax)], astigmatism and Q value; (2) Pachymetric parameters, including central and thinnest corneal thickness (CCT and TCT), pachymetric progression indices [maximum (PImax), minimum (PImin) and average (PIavg)], and Ambrosio relational thickness indices [maximum (ARTmax) minimum (ARTmin) and average (ARTavg)]. On the Belin/Ambrósio enhanced ectasia display, pachymetric progression indices (PPIs) refer to the rate of corneal thickness changes along each meridian starting from the thinnest corneal point. The maximum, minimum and average PPI are recorded. Relational thickness indices express the ratio of the TCT to each of the above three PPIs, as expressed in the following formulas: ARTavg = TCT/PIavg; ARTmin = TCT/PImin; ARTmax = TCT/PImax (16); and (3) Anterior and posterior corneal elevations, including elevations at the thinnest and central locations (TE and CE), mean elevation in the 4 mm central zone (ME), elevation differences at the thinnest and central locations (TED and CED) and in the central 4 mm zone (MED). Corneal elevations were defined as the distances between the corneal surface and the best-fit sphere (BFS) reference surfaces set at 8-mm diameter. Corneal elevation difference values were taken as the differential changes in corneal elevation values between the BFS and the enhanced BFS (with exclusion of a 3.5-mm optical zone in the thinnest portion of the cornea) obtained with Belin/Ambrósio enhanced ectasia display software. An example of the data output for corneal elevations assessment is shown in **Figure 1**. The corneal biomechanical parameters measured by Corvis ST have been presented in detail in our previous article (19). TBI was selected for analysis in this study because we previously found that only TBI showed significant differences between AC patients and normal subjects.

Statistical Analysis

To prevent bias, one eye of each participant was selected for analysis (for AC patients, the eye with more severe AC symptoms or signs was selected; for normal subjects, the eye was randomly selected). Statistical analyses were performed using SPSS software (version 25.0; SPSS, Inc., Chicago, Illinois, USA). The normality of the continuous variables was evaluated by the Kolmogorov–Smirnov test. Comparisons of continuous data between groups were performed by applying independent-sample *t*-tests. Categorical variables were compared using the χ^2 test. Correlations between the continuous and ranked data were analyzed by Spearman's correlation test. $p < 0.05$ was considered statistically significant.

RESULTS

Patient Characteristics

Twenty eyes of 20 normal subjects and thirty eyes of 30 AC patients were included in this prospective study. The demographics of the study population are shown in **Table 1**. There were no significant differences in age, sex, intraocular pressure (IOP) (measured by Corvis ST), spherical power (S), cylinder power (C) or spherical equivalent (SE) between the two groups ($p > 0.05$ for all).

Corneal Topographic Parameters

Comparisons of the main corneal topographic parameters between the normal and AC groups are shown in **Table 2**. We found no significant differences in terms of the anterior corneal surface parameters between the two groups ($p > 0.05$ for all). The astigmatism and the Q value of the posterior corneal surface were significantly higher in the AC group than in the normal group ($p = 0.02$ and $p = 0.01$, respectively). The remaining topographic parameters of the posterior surface were not significantly different between the two groups ($p > 0.05$ for all).

Corneal Pachymetric Parameters

Comparisons of the main corneal pachymetric parameters between the normal and AC groups are presented in **Table 3**. No significant difference was observed in any of the pachymetric parameters between the two groups ($p > 0.05$ for all).

Corneal Elevation Parameters

Comparisons of the corneal elevation parameters of both the anterior and posterior corneal surfaces between the normal and AC groups are shown in **Table 4**. The TE, CE, TED, CED, and MED of both the anterior and posterior corneal surfaces were significantly higher in the AC group than in the normal group ($p < 0.05$ for all).

Correlation of Corneal Elevation Parameters With Eye Rubbing Frequency and Ocular Allergy Sign Severity in AC Patients

The correlations of the corneal elevation parameters with eye rubbing frequency and ocular allergy sign severity in AC patients are presented in **Table 5**. The anterior corneal surface elevation parameters were positively related to eye rubbing frequency and the severity of ocular allergy signs, including conjunctival swelling, papillae and epithelial disorder ($p < 0.05$ for all). However, there was no correlation between the posterior corneal surface elevation parameters and eye rubbing frequency or ocular allergy sign severity ($p > 0.05$ for all).

Correlation of Corneal Elevation Parameters With the TBI in AC Patients

Table 6 shows the correlations of the corneal elevation parameters with TBI in AC patients. We found that TBI was positively correlated with TE (r = 0.608, $p < 0.001$), CE (r = 0.464, $p = 0.010$), CED (r = 0.727, $p < 0.001$), and MED (r = 0.750, $p < 0.001$) of the anterior corneal surface, as well as with TE (r = 0.563, $p = 0.001$) of the posterior corneal surface.

DISCUSSION

A close association between KC and AC has been well established in the previous literature (23–25). However, sensitive indicators for screening AC patients at high risk of developing KC are still under investigation. In our previous study, we showed that TBI could be used as an indicator of KC development risk in AC patients (19). In the current study, we found that both the anterior and posterior corneal elevation values were significantly higher in AC patients than in normal subjects and were further identified to positively correlate with the altered TBI in AC patients. Our findings provide additional evidence supporting that compared to normal subjects, AC patients have an increased risk of corneal ectasia, and corneal elevation could be used as a sensitive indicator of the risk of corneal ectasia in AC patients.

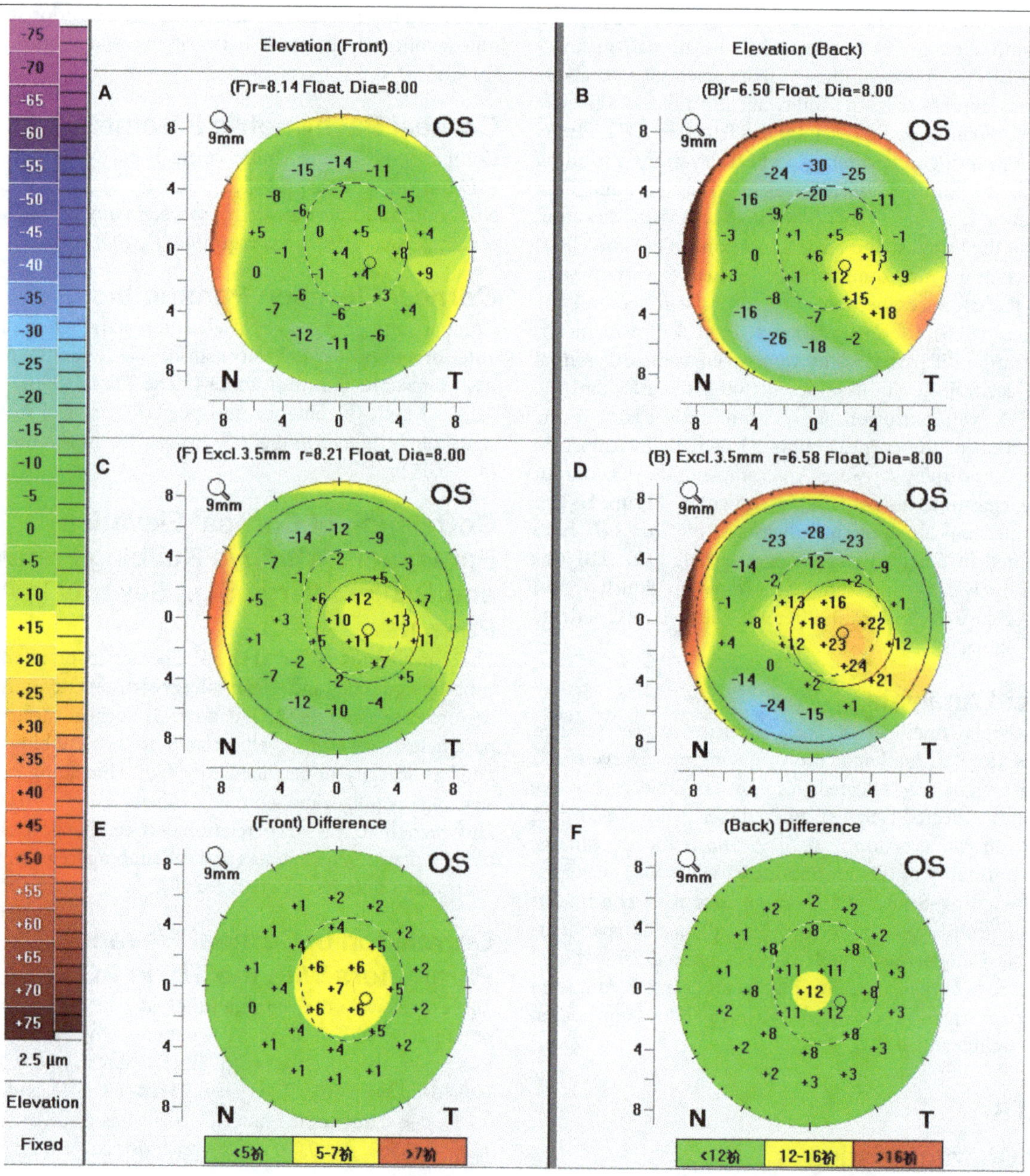

FIGURE 1 | A representative example of elevation maps in patients with allergic conjunctivitis measured by Pentacam. **(A,B)** Anterior and posterior corneal elevations correlated to the standard best-fit sphere (BFS) reference surfaces; **(C,D)** Anterior and posterior corneal elevations correlated to the enhanced BFS reference surfaces (with exclusion of a 3.5-mm optical zone in the thinnest portion of the cornea); **(E,F)** Anterior and posterior corneal elevation differences between the elevation values correlated to the standard BFS and the enhanced BFS.

The typical corneal topography characteristics in KC patients include increased corneal curvature and corneal thinning. Barreto and colleagues (20) reported a significantly greater central curvature, thinner corneal thickness and higher pachymetric index in VKC patients than in normal subjects. However, contrary to the findings by Barreto et al., our study did not find significant differences in anterior and posterior corneal surface curvature parameters or pachymetric parameters between the normal and AC groups. There are controversial findings in different studies. Similar to our results, no significant change in K1, K2 or Kmean was found in VKC patients in Ekinci's research (26). The difference in the patient characteristics might be the reason for the different results of the two studies. Barreto's study included only active VKC patients, while our study also included patients with SAC and PAC. VKC, as a more severe form of AC, was reported to have higher levels of ocular inflammatory cytokines and active proteases than SAC and PAC (27, 28),

TABLE 1 | Demographics of the normal and AC groups.

Characteristics	Normal (n = 20)	AC (n = 30)	p
Age, mean ± SD	18.75 ± 7.99	19.37 ± 10.59	0.83
Sex, male, n (%)	13 (65.0%)	20 (66.7%)	0.90
IOP (mmHg)	16.03 ± 2.40	15.90 ± 1.96	0.84
S (D)	−1.92 ± 1.91	−0.79 ± 1.55	0.14
C (D)	−0.50 ± 0.45	−0.96 ± 1.29	0.18
SE (D)	−2.22 ± 2.07	−1.28 ± 2.65	0.24

AC, allergic conjunctivitis; IOP, intraocular pressure, measured by Corvis ST; S, spherical power; C, cylinder power; SE, spherical equivalent; D, diopter; SD, standard deviation.

TABLE 2 | Comparison of corneal topographic parameters between the normal and AC groups.

Parameter	Normal Mean ± SD	AC Mean ± SD	p
Anterior corneal surface			
K1 (D)	42.41 ± 1.03	42.52 ± 1.28	0.75
K2 (D)	43.41 ± 1.05	43.87 ± 1.45	0.23
Kmean (D)	42.90 ± 1.01	43.20 ± 1.31	0.38
Kmax (D)	43.95 ± 1.13	44.46 ± 1.50	0.20
Astigmatism (D)	1.00 ± 0.54	1.34 ± 0.84	0.10
Q	−0.33 ± 0.11	−0.45 ± 0.26	0.05
Posterior corneal surface			
K1 (D)	−6.08 ± 0.16	−6.11 ± 0.21	0.59
K2 (D)	−6.40 ± 0.16	−6.5 ± 0.28	0.15
Kmean (D)	−6.23 ± 0.15	−6.29 ± 0.22	0.25
Astigmatism (D)	0.29 ± 0.12	0.38 ± 0.16	0.02*
Q	−0.26 ± 0.10	−0.34 ± 0.11	0.01*

AC, allergic conjunctivitis; K1, keratometry of the flattest meridian; K2, keratometry of the steepest meridian; Kmean, mean central keratometry; Kmax, maximum keratometry; Q, Q value; D, diopter; SD, standard deviation.
**Statistically significant (p < 0.05).*

TABLE 3 | Comparison of corneal pachymetric parameters between the normal and AC groups.

Parameter	Normal Mean ± SD	AC Mean ± SD	p
CCT (μm)	550.15 ± 21.33	554.10 ± 24.59	0.56
TCT (μm)	547.35 ± 23.45	550.43 ± 25.72	0.75
PImin	0.73 ± 0.11	0.73 ± 0.11	0.82
PImax	1.28 ± 0.10	1.36 ± 0.19	0.09
PIavg	1.03 ± 0.09	1.05 ± 0.12	0.61
ARTmin	761.30 ± 124.35	776.30 ± 150.19	0.71
ARTmax	429.55 ± 45.79	415.97 ± 72.42	0.46
ARTavg	533.65 ± 58.67	533.07 ± 80.80	0.94

AC, allergic conjunctivitis; CCT, central corneal thickness; TCT, thinnest corneal thickness; PI, pachymetric progression index; ART, Ambrosio relational thickness; min, minimum; max, maximum; avg, average; SD, standard deviation.

TABLE 4 | Comparison of corneal elevation parameters between the normal and AC groups.

Parameter	Normal Mean ± SD	AC Mean ± SD	p
Anterior corneal surface			
TE (μm)	2.80 ± 1.24	4.07 ± 2.49	0.04*
CE (μm)	2.05 ± 0.94	3.33 ± 2.45	0.03*
ME (μm)	0.12 ± 0.31	0.18 ± 0.60	0.67
TED (μm)	3.40 ± 1.10	4.67 ± 2.22	0.02*
CED (μm)	3.50 ± 1.10	4.73 ± 2.23	0.03*
MED (μm)	2.60 ± 0.79	3.64 ± 1.69	0.01*
Posterior corneal surface			
TE (μm)	5.00 ± 2.70	7.73 ± 3.23	<0.01*
CE (μm)	0.35 ± 2.06	1.90 ± 2.64	0.03*
ME (μm)	0.56 ± 0.64	0.48 ± 0.75	0.69
TED (μm)	3.90 ± 2.36	6.13 ± 2.91	0.01*
CED (μm)	4.00 ± 2.70	6.57 ± 3.08	<0.01*
MED (μm)	2.99 ± 2.01	4.95 ± 2.29	<0.01*

AC, allergic conjunctivitis; TE, elevation at the thinnest location; CE, elevation at the central location; ME, mean value of elevation in the central 4 mm zoom; ED, elevation difference; SD, standard deviation.
** Statistically significant (p < 0.05).*

which in turn could induce more severe ocular microstructure damage, indicated by a thinner corneal thickness and greater corneal curvature.

The corneal Q value is a parameter that reflects the corneal shape and represents the degree of corneal asphericity. A more negative Q value of the posterior corneal surface has been reported in early KC (15). In this study, we found greater astigmatism and a more negative Q value for the posterior corneal surface in the AC group than in the normal group. Our findings were consistent with what was reported by Dantas et al. (7). In their study, the Q value of the cornea was significantly more negative in the VKC group than in the normal group. A more negative Q value refers to a more prolate shape, with a steeper central cornea and flatter periphery. A previous study reported significant correlations between posterior elevation parameters and posterior Q values as well as posterior aberrations; hence, the authors speculated that the changes in posterior Q values and posterior corneal aberrations were attributed to alterations in corneal posterior elevation (15). Thus, we hypothesize that the more negative Q value and greater astigmatism of the corneal posterior surface in AC patients might also be induced by alterations in corneal posterior elevation.

Previous studies reported that corneal anterior and posterior elevation values were significantly higher in early KC patients than in normal subjects (10, 11, 13). Our study also found much higher corneal elevation values or elevation differences in either the anterior or posterior surface in AC patients than in normal subjects. However, whether KC-like changes in corneal elevation could predict KC development in AC patients still requires further investigation. Moreover, several studies have shown that

TABLE 5 | Correlation of altered corneal elevation parameters with eye rubbing frequency and ocular allergy sign severity in AC patients.

		Anterior corneal surface					Posterior corneal surface				
		TE	CE	TED	CED	MED	TE	CE	TED	CED	MED
Eye rubbing	r	0.251	0.414	0.424	0.452	0.462	0.277	0.023	0.247	0.226	0.211
	p	0.181	0.023*	0.020*	0.012*	0.010*	0.138	0.903	0.188	0.230	0.264
Hyperemia	r	0.011	0.082	0.099	0.109	0.077	−0.056	0.039	−0.221	−0.230	−0.256
	p	0.956	0.666	0.601	0.567	0.685	0.769	0.836	0.242	0.222	0.173
Swelling	r	0.257	0.312	0.403	0.420	0.409	0.075	0.024	−0.028	−0.075	−0.090
	p	0.170	0.093	0.027*	0.021*	0.025*	0.692	0.900	0.885	0.693	0.635
Papillae	r	0.280	0.318	0.455	0.455	0.452	0.103	0.141	0.008	−0.039	−0.024
	p	0.135	0.087	0.011*	0.011*	0.012*	0.588	0.458	0.967	0.838	0.899
Epithelial disorder	r	0.200	0.465	0.459	0.443	0.449	0.009	0.026	−0.035	−0.066	−0.070
	p	0.289	0.010*	0.011*	0.014*	0.013*	0.963	0.890	0.854	0.730	0.714

AC, allergic conjunctivitis; TE, elevation at the thinnest location; CE, elevation at the central location; TED, elevation difference at the thinnest location; CED, elevation difference at the central location; MED, mean value of elevation difference in the central 4 mm zoom.
**Statistically significant ($p < 0.05$).*

TABLE 6 | Correlation of corneal elevation parameters with TBI in AC patients.

		Anterior corneal surface					Posterior corneal surface				
		TE	CE	TED	CED	MED	TE	CE	TED	CED	MED
TBI	r	0.608	0.464	0.754	0.727	0.750	0.563	0.156	0.341	0.318	0.323
	p	<0.001*	0.010*	<0.001*	<0.001*	<0.001*	0.001*	0.412	0.065	0.087	0.081

AC, allergic conjunctivitis; TBI, tomography and biomechanical index; TE, elevation at the thinnest location; CE, elevation at the central location; CED, elevation difference at the central location; MED, mean value of elevation difference in the central 4 mm zone.
**Statistically significant ($p < 0.05$).*

posterior elevation parameters are more sensitive than anterior elevation parameters in differentiating KC from normal eyes (10, 12, 16). For example, Huseynli et al. (10) further showed that among the parameters measured by Pentacam, including corneal topographic parameters, pachymetric parameters, elevation parameters and topometric parameters, anterior and posterior elevation showed the highest AUROCs (0.935 and 0.897, respectively) to differentiate early KC patients from normal subjects. Therefore, among the parameters evaluated in their study, posterior corneal elevation changes were identified as the earliest sign of subclinical KC (15, 16). Additionally, in our study, we found that the increased elevations of both the anterior and posterior corneal surfaces were positively correlated with altered TBI, which was identified as a sensitive indicator of KC development risk in AC patients in our previous study (19). This result to a certain extent demonstrates the possibility and risk of KC occurrence in AC patients. In addition, our findings indicate that corneal elevation changes occurred earlier than the occurrence of abnormal corneal pachymetric distribution and increased corneal curvature in AC patients. Therefore, measurement of corneal elevation, especially of the posterior surface, may aid in evaluating the risk of KC development in AC patients. However, except for KC, higher corneal elevations have also been reported in other diseases such as patients with Familial Mediterranean fever (29). Even some normal subjects may have abnormal corneal elevations indicated by yellow color in the Belin/Ambrósio Enhanced Ectasia Display. Thus, it would be better to combine corneal tomography with other KC detection tools such as corneal biomechanical assessment and corneal epithelial thickness measurement to comprehensively evaluate the KC risk in AC patients.

Furthermore, we found that altered anterior corneal elevation was positively correlated with eye rubbing frequency and ocular allergy sign severity in AC patients. However, there was no significant correlation between posterior surface corneal elevation and ocular allergy sign severity. The anterior surface of the cornea could be affected by various factors. For example, AC patients often have unstable tear film and dry eye (30–33). Irregular tear films and the use of artificial tears in AC patients are factors influencing the corneal anterior surface (11, 26). Moreover, the corneal epithelial damage and thinning caused by excessive eye rubbing in AC patients could also induce increased irregularity of the anterior corneal surface. Therefore, anterior corneal elevation may not be suitable for use as an indicator of KC risk in AC patients due to its vulnerability to multiple factors, including ocular surface inflammation conditions, tear film stability and corneal epithelial defects.

Contrary to anterior corneal surface measurements, posterior corneal surface measurements were not influenced by the irregularity and allergic signs of the ocular surface. Although there was no significant correlation between altered posterior elevation and the severity of ocular allergy signs in AC patients, the alterations in posterior elevation were not necessarily independent of the inflammatory condition and the course of ocular allergy. Increased release of inflammatory cytokines, including matrix metalloproteinase (MMP)-1,−3,−7, and−13, interleukin (IL)-4,−5,−6, and−8 and tumor necrosis factor (TNF)-α and -β, induced by excessive eye rubbing in AC patients was reported to mediate pathological apoptosis of keratocytes and corneal fibroblasts, which could further induce alterations in the posterior corneal surface and corneal weakness (27, 34–36). Thus, posterior elevation parameters, which were mainly affected by corneal chronic and long-term inflammation, could be used as sensitive and stable indicators of KC risk in AC patients.

A limitation of this study is the small sample size; thus, studies with a larger sample size are needed to compare corneal tomography changes among different types of AC. Moreover, a follow-up study to explore corneal elevation changes over time is necessary.

In conclusion, compared to normal subjects, AC patients carry an increased risk of corneal ectasia, as indicated by higher corneal elevation parameters. Posterior corneal elevation parameters could be used as sensitive and stable indicators of KC risk in AC patients.

ETHICS STATEMENT

The studies involving human participants were reviewed and approved by the Ethics Committee of Zhongshan Ophthalmic Center, Sun Yat-sen University (2020KYPJ008). Written informed consent to participate in this study was provided by the participants' legal guardian/next of kin.

AUTHOR CONTRIBUTIONS

JY and SL designed and supervised the study. QW and FY analyzed and interpreted the data and prepared the manuscript. ZF, WL, NL, XD, and XZ contributed to data collection. All authors contributed to the article and approved the submitted version.

REFERENCES

1. Aydin E, Gokhale M, Azizoglu S, Suphioglu C. To see or not to see: a systematic review of the importance of human ocular surface cytokine biosignatures in ocular allergy. *Cells.* (2019) 8:620. doi: 10.3390/cells8060620
2. Ahmed AS, El-Agha MSH, Khaled MO, Shousha SM. The prevalence of keratoconus in children with allergic eye disease in an Egyptian population. *Eur J Ophthalmol.* (2020) 31:1571–76. doi: 10.1177/1120672120942691
3. Moran S, Gomez L, Zuber K, Gatinel D. A case-control study of keratoconus risk factors. *Cornea.* (2020) 39:697–701. doi: 10.1097/ICO.0000000000002283
4. Lee HK, Jung EH, Cho BJ. Epidemiological association between systemic diseases and keratoconus in a korean population: a 10-year nationwide cohort study. *Cornea.* (2020) 39:348–53. doi: 10.1097/ICO.0000000000002206
5. Sharma N, Rao K, Maharana PK, Vajpayee RB. Ocular allergy and keratoconus. *Indian J Ophthalmol.* (2013) 61:407–9. doi: 10.4103/0301-4738.116063
6. Ben-Eli H, Erdinest N, Solomon A. Pathogenesis and complications of chronic eye rubbing in ocular allergy. *Curr Opin Allergy Clin Immunol.* (2019) 19:526–34. doi: 10.1097/ACI.0000000000000571
7. Correa Dantas PE, Alves MR, Nishiwaki-Dantas MC. Topographic corneal changes in patients with vernal keratoconjunctivitis. *Arq Bras Oftalmol.* (2005) 68:593–8. doi: 10.1590/S0004-27492005000500004
8. Kataria P, Padmanabhan P, Gopalakrishnan A, Padmanaban V, Mahadik S, Ambrósio R. Accuracy of scheimpflug-derived corneal biomechanical and tomographic indices for detecting subclinical and mild keratectasia in a South Asian population. *J Cataract Refract Surg.* (2019) 45:328–36. doi: 10.1016/j.jcrs.2018.10.030
9. Golan O, Hwang ES, Lang P, Santhiago MR, Abulafia A, Touboul D, et al. Differences in posterior corneal features between normal corneas and subclinical keratoconus. *J Refract Surg.* (2018) 34:664–70. doi: 10.3928/1081597X-20180823-02
10. Huseynli S, Salgado-Borges J, Alio JL. Comparative evaluation of scheimpflug tomography parameters between thin non-keratoconic, subclinical keratoconic, and mild keratoconic corneas. *Eur J Ophthalmol.* (2018) 28:521–34. doi: 10.1177/1120672118760146
11. Mihåltz K, Kovács I, Takács Á, Nagy ZZ. Evaluation of keratometric, pachymetric, and elevation parameters of keratoconic corneas with pentacam. *Cornea.* (2009) 28:976–80. doi: 10.1097/ICO.0b013e31819e34de
12. Muftuoglu O, Ayar O, Hurmeric V, Orucoglu F, Kilic I. Comparison of multimetric D index with keratometric, pachymetric, and posterior elevation parameters in diagnosing subclinical keratoconus in fellow eyes of asymmetric keratoconus patients. *J Cataract Refract Surg.* (2015) 41:557–65. doi: 10.1016/j.jcrs.2014.05.052
13. Kamiya K, Ishii R, Shimizu K, Igarashi A. Evaluation of corneal elevation, pachymetry and keratometry in keratoconic eyes with respect to the stage of Amsler-Krumeich classification. *Br J Ophthalmol.* (2014) 98:459–63. doi: 10.1136/bjophthalmol-2013-304132
14. de Sanctis U, Loiacono C, Richiardi L, Turco D, Mutani B, Grignolo FM. Sensitivity and specificity of posterior corneal elevation measured by pentacam in discriminating keratoconus/subclinical keratoconus. *Ophthalmology.* (2008) 115:1534–9. doi: 10.1016/j.ophtha.2008.02.020
15. Elkitkat RS, Gharieb HM, Othman IS. Accuracy of the posterior corneal elevation values of pentacam HR from different reference surfaces in early ectasia diagnosis. *Int Ophthalmol.* (2021) 41:629–38. doi: 10.1007/s10792-020-01618-8
16. Muftuoglu O, Ayar O, Ozulken K, Ozyol E, Akinci A. Posterior corneal elevation and back difference corneal elevation in diagnosing forme fruste keratoconus in the fellow eyes of unilateral keratoconus patients. *J Cataract Refract Surg.* (2013) 39:1348–57. doi: 10.1016/j.jcrs.2013.03.023
17. Gautam V, Chaudhary M, Sharma AK, Shrestha GS, Rai PG. Topographic corneal changes in children with vernal keratoconjunctivitis: a report from Kathmandu, Nepal. *Contact Lens Anterior Eye.* (2015) 38:461–5. doi: 10.1016/j.clae.2015.05.013
18. Emre S, Başer E, Öztürk B, Zorlu S, Uzun Ö, Gülhan C. Corneal biochemical features of patients with vernal keratoconjunctivitis. *Graefe's Arch Clin Exp Ophthalmol.* (2013) 251:555–8. doi: 10.1007/s00417-012-2089-2

19. Wang Q, Deng Y, Li S, Du X, Zhao X, Zhang T, et al. Corneal biomechanical changes in allergic conjunctivitis. *Eye Vis.* (2021) 8:1–9. doi: 10.1186/s40662-021-00241-7
20. Barreto J, Netto MV, Santo RM, José NK, Bechara SJ. Slit-scanning topography in vernal keratoconjunctivitis. *Am J Ophthalmol.* (2007) 143:250–4. doi: 10.1016/j.ajo.2006.10.027
21. de Sanctis U, Missolungi A, Mutani B, Richiardi L, Grignolo FM. Reproducibility and repeatability of central corneal thickness measurement in keratoconus using the rotating scheimpflug camera and ultrasound pachymetry. *Am J Ophthalmol.* (2007) 144:712–718. doi: 10.1016/j.ajo.2007.07.021
22. Chen D, Lam AKC. Intrasession and intersession repeatability of the pentacam system on posterior corneal assessment in the normal human eye. *J Cataract Refract Surg.* (2007) 33:448–54. doi: 10.1016/j.jcrs.2006.11.008
23. Mazzotta C, Traversi C, Mellace P, Bagaglia SA, Zuccarini S, Mencucci R, et al. Keratoconus progression in patients with allergy and elevated surface matrix metalloproteinase 9 point-of-care test. *Eye Contact Lens.* (2018) 44:S48–S53. doi: 10.1097/ICL.0000000000000432
24. Cingu AK, Cinar Y, Turkcu FM, Sahin A, Ari S, Yuksel H, et al. Effects of vernal and allergic conjunctivitis on severity of keratoconus. *Int J Ophthalmol.* (2013) 6:370–4. doi: 10.3980/j.issn.2222-3959.2013.03.21
25. Hashemi H, Heydarian S, Hooshmand E, Saatchi M, Yekta A, Aghamirsalim M, et al. The prevalence and risk factors for keratoconus: a systematic review and meta-analysis. *Cornea.* (2020) 39:263–70. doi: 10.1097/ICO.0000000000002150
26. EKINCI DY, ALPARSLAN N, CEBECI Z, YAVUZ SARIÇAY L, DÖNMEZ GÜN R. The topographic corneal changes in patients with vernal keratoconjunctivitis. *Turkiye Klin J Ophthalmol.* (2019) 28:99–104. doi: 10.5336/ophthal.2018-63355
27. Zheng X, Yao J, Li B. Expression of TSLP and downstream molecules IL-4, IL-5, and IL-13 on the eye surface of patients with various types of allergic conjunctivitis. *J Ophthalmol.* (2016) 2016:5072781. doi: 10.1155/2016/5072781
28. Kumagai N, Yamamoto K, Fukuda K, Nakamura Y, Fujitsu Y, Nuno Y, et al. Active matrix metalloproteinases in the tear fluid of individuals with vernal keratoconjunctivitis. *J Allergy Clin Immunol.* (2002) 110:489–91. doi: 10.1067/mai.2002.126379
29. Kosekahya P, Ucgul Atilgan C, Atilgan KG, Koc M, Tekin K, Caglayan M, et al. Increased corneal ectasia risk in patients with familial mediterranean fever. *Curr Eye Res.* (2019) 44:351–5. doi: 10.1080/02713683.2018.1554150
30. Hom MM, Nguyen AL, Bielory L. Allergic conjunctivitis and dry eye syndrome. *Ann Allergy Asthma Immunol.* (2012) 108:163–6. doi: 10.1016/j.anai.2012.01.006
31. Kim M, Oh JH, Park CY, Lee SW. Dry eye disease and allergic conditions: a Korean nationwide population-based study. *Am J Rhinol Allergy.* (2016) 30:397–401. doi: 10.2500/ajra.2016.30.4361
32. Dogru M, Gunay M, Celik G, Aktas A. Evaluation of the tear film instability in children with allergic diseases. *Cutan Ocul Toxicol.* (2016) 35:49–52. doi: 10.3109/15569527.2015.1010727
33. Villani E, Rabbiolo G, Nucci P. Ocular allergy as a risk factor for dry eye in adults and children. *Curr Opin Allergy Clin Immunol.* (2018) 18:398–403. doi: 10.1097/ACI.0000000000000471
34. Leonardi A, Curnow SJ, Zhan H, Calder VL. Multiple cytokines in human tear specimens in seasonal and chronic allergic eye disease and in conjunctival fibroblast cultures. *Cl in Exp Allergy.* (2006) 36:777–84. doi: 10.1111/j.1365-2222.2006.02499.x
35. Uchio E, Ono SY, Ikezawa Z, Ohno S. Tear Levels of Interferon-γ, Interleukin (IL)−2, IL-4 and IL-5 in Patients With Vernal Keratoconjunctivitis, Atopic Keratoconjunctivitis and Allergic Conjunctivitis. *Clin Exp Allergy.* (2000) 30:103–9. doi: 10.1046/j.1365-2222.2000.00699.x
36. Leonardi A, Sathe S, Bortolotti M, Beaton A, Sack R. Cytokines, matrix metalloproteases, angiogenic and growth factors in tears of normal subjects and vernal keratoconjunctivitis patients. *Allergy Eur J Allergy Clin Immunol.* (2009) 64:710–7. doi: 10.1111/j.1398-9995.2008.01858.x

23

Evaluation of Macular and Retinal Ganglion Cell Count Estimates for Detecting and Staging Glaucoma

Yali Wu[1,2†], *Qing Cun*[2†], *Yijin Tao*[2], *Wenyan Yang*[2], *Jia Wei*[2], *Daoqing Fan*[2], *Ying Zhang*[2], *Qin Chen*[3*] *and Hua Zhong*[2*]

[1] *Department of Ophthalmology, The First Affiliated Hospital of USTC, Division of Life Sciences and Medicine, University of Science and Technology of China, Hefei, China,* [2] *The First Affiliated Hospital of Kunming Medical University, Kunming, China,* [3] *The First Affiliated Hospital of Nanjing Medical University, Nanjing, China*

***Correspondence:**
Hua Zhong
zhoculist@163.com
Qin Chen
chenkmu@163.com

† *These authors have contributed equally to this work*

Purpose: To investigate the clinical significance of macular estimated retinal ganglion cell (mRGC) and estimated retinal ganglion cell (eRGC) in the diagnosis and staging of glaucoma.

Methods: This is a cross-section study. All enrolled subjects underwent standard automated perimetry (SAP) and optical coherence tomography (OCT) examination. Swedish Interactive Threshold Algorithm (SITA)-FAST detection strategy and 24-2, 10-2 detection programs were employed in SAP assessment. The visual-field parameters and OCT parameters were calculated according to three formulas to obtain the eRGC and mRGC1 or mRGC2. The efficiency of eRGC, mRGC1, and mRGC2 estimates for the staging of glaucoma was compared. The sensitivity and specificity of each parameter for diagnosis of glaucoma were analyzed using the receiver operating characteristic (ROC) curve.

Results: A total of 119 eyes were included in the analysis. Compared with the healthy controls, eRGC, mRGC1, and mRGC2 estimates were significantly decreased in patients with glaucoma. As glaucoma progressed, eRGC, mRGC1, and mRGC2 estimates were gradually reduced. In preperimetric glaucoma, mRGC1, mRGC2, and eRGC were reduced by 13.2, 14.5, and 18%, respectively. In the mild stage of glaucoma, mRGC1, mRGC2, and eRGC were reduced by 28, 34, and 38%, respectively. In the advanced stage of glaucoma, mRGC1, mRGC2, and eRGC were reduced by 81, 85, and 92% respectively. The proportion of retinal ganglion cell (RGC) loss in the macula was close to that outside the macula. The specificity at 95% gave a sensitivity of 95.51, 86.52, and 87.64% for eRGC, mRGC1, and mRGC2, respectively. The sensitivity of structural parameters macular ganglion cell complex thickness and retinal nerve fiber layer (RNFL) were 98.88 and 95.51%, respectively. The sensitivity of functional parameters mean deviation (24-2) and visual field index (VFI) were 80.90 and 73.03%, respectively. The area under ROC curve of mRGC1, mRGC2, and eRGC were 0.982, 0.972, and 0.995 ($P < 0.0001$), respectively.

Conclusion: Estimated retinal ganglion cell, mRGC1, and mRGC2 provide value to the staging of glaucoma and better diagnostic performance. Macular RGC estimatesthat integration of both structural and functional damages in macular may serve as a sensitive indicator for assessing macular damage in glaucoma and are of importance for the diagnosis and progression management of glaucoma.

Keywords: glaucoma, estimated retinal ganglion cell, standard automated perimetry, retinal nerve fiber layer, ganglion cell complex

INTRODUCTION

A glaucoma is a group of progressive optic neuropathies characterized by thinning of the retinal nerve fiber layer (RNFL) and cupping of the optic disc (1). Such structural changes are usually accompanied by functional impairments, which may eventually lead to irreversible vision loss. Both the characteristic structural and functional changes are related to pathological loss of retinal ganglion cell (RGC) somas and axons (2). Clinical measurements of structural and functional damage in glaucoma are currently using standard automated perimetry (SAP) and optical coherence tomography (OCT), respectively, for diagnosis and staging of disease. However, these measurements of structural and functional changes are variable and inconsistently related to one another in many cases. For instance, studies have shown that visual field changes precede neural structural loss in mild stages of diseases (3–11); on the contrary, evidence is found that visual field changes are only detected when damages to the nerve fiber layer reach 40% or more (6, 7, 12, 13). Such common inconsistency between structural and functional measurements is largely considered attributed to different measurement scales and computational methods. Therefore, single structural or functional measures are not enough to identify and monitor progressive glaucomatous damage.

Harwerth et al. demonstrated that structural and functional tests are in agreement as long as one uses appropriate measurement scales for neural and sensitivity losses and takes the effect of aging and eccentricity into account on estimates of neural losses. Consecutive studies have found that the estimates of RGC losses from visual field detection using perimetry closely fit that from RNFL detection using OCT (14). In addition, ganglion cell complex (GCC) thickness had been recognized as an important indicator for glaucoma. Based on the original RGC estimation model proposed by Harwerth et al. (14, 15) and Medeiros et al. (16, 17), we incorporated the macular RGC estimation model (18) and made appropriate adaptations. The structural evaluation was modified and peripapillary RNFL thickness measurements were replaced by macular structural parameter GCC. SAP program 24-2 (6° interval) was changed to program 10-2 (2° interval). We sought to integrate macular structural and functional parameters to obtain macular estimated retinal ganglion cell (mRGC) and to determine whether these parameters are superior to structural or functional analysis individually in the discrimination of glaucomatous from healthy eyes and its performance in staging the disease.

METHOD

Study Design and Participants

This was an observational, cross-sectional study. The study has been approved by the Ethics Committee of the First Affiliated Hospital of Kunming Medical University and was implemented following the Declaration of Helsinki. All participants gave written informed consent before the study. All patients underwent a detailed and comprehensive medical history and ophthalmologic examinations, namely, ophthalmic routine slit-lamp examination, diopter examination, anterior chamber angle, and fundus photography, A-scan measures central corneal thickness and axial length, Goldmann intraocular pressure (IOP), and average RNFL thickness, and visual field examination. A total of 89 eyes of patients diagnosed with primary open-angle glaucoma (POAG) in the First Affiliated Hospital of Kunming Medical University from February 2015 to February 2017 were included, according to the Advanced Glaucoma Intervention Study (AGIS) visual field scoring system, 20 eyes with preperimetric glaucoma, 20 eyes with the mild stage of disease (1–5 points), 20 eyes with the moderate stage (6–12 points), and 29 eyes with the severe stage (13–20 points). The normal control group includes 30 eyes of healthy examined subjects at the same period. Inclusion criteria were: the best-corrected visual acuity was not less than 20/40, spherical refraction ranged from -5 to $+5$ D, cylinder correction ranged from -3 to $+3$ D, and subjects were excluded if they presented with nonglaucomatous visual field defective diseases, such as optic neuritis, history of ocular trauma, macular lesions, or intraocular surgery.

Visual Field Testing

All subjects were examined with the Humphrey Visual Field Analyzer II (Carl Zeiss Meditec, Dublin, CA, USA) using Swedish Interactive Threshold Algorithm (SITA)-FAST 24-2 and 10-2 programs. Each visual field test was performed by the same physician. Visual fields with a solid fixation loss rate of $<20\%$, a false-negative rate of $<33\%$, and a false-positive rate of $<15\%$ were considered reliable results. The visual field that the false-negative rate was higher than 33% but indicative of severe disease progression (mean deviation (MD) value below -12 dB) was also considered for the calculation. Repeated visual field examinations were required if eyelid masking, fatigue, incorrect fixation, or learning effects were present.

Optical Coherence Tomography

Subjects underwent optic nerve head (ONH) scanning program for ONH examination and GCC program for macula using the ultrahigh speed 70 kHz Fourier domain OCT system (RTVue XR Avanti, Optovue, Inc., Fremont, CA, USA). Peripapillary RNFL and GCC thickness probability maps with eight partitions were obtained by measuring the RNFL thickness of the optic disc and the macular GCC thickness. High-quality images with signal intensity index >50 without motion and vitreous floaters were considered for analysis. OCT testing and visual field testing were performed on the same day.

Integrated Structure-Function Estimate of RGC Counts

Harwerth et al. (19) proposed an empirical formula for estimating the counts of corresponding RGCs based on experimental studies on rhesus monkeys, namely, SAPrgcs from the visual field (Humphrey 24-2) detection as function measurements and OCTrgc obtained OCT detection as peripapillary structure measurements. The experimental model was translated to clinical perimetry in humans and has been validated in glaucoma and normal IOP glaucoma (5, 14, 20). Considering the effects of aging on axonal degeneration and varying severity of the disease, factors such as age and MD have been adjusted in OCTrgc. The use of this model would translate region-specific visual field sensitivity into estimate RGC for the corresponding regions.

$$m = [0.054(ec \times 1.32)] + 0.9$$
$$b = [-1.5(ec \times 1.32)] - 14.8$$
$$gc = \{[(s-1) - b]/m\} + 4.7$$
$$SAPrgc = \sum 10\hat{}(gc \times 0.1)$$
$$d = (-0.007 \times \text{age}) + 1.4$$
$$c = (-0.26 \times MD) + 0.12$$
$$a = \text{average RNFL thickness} \times 10{,}870 \times \text{d}$$
$$OCTrgc = 10\hat{}\{[\log(a) \times 10 - c] \times 0.1\}$$

In the above formulas, *ec* is the retinal eccentricity, which refers to the distance from the central fixation to a certain point on the retina. Based on the results, the values of *ec* were taken separately as 4.2 (3 × 3 deg), 12.8 (9 × 9 deg), 21.2 (15 × 15 deg), and 24 (nasal side of the visual field 21 × 3 deg and 27 × 3 deg). *m* and *b* represent the slope and intercept of the linear relationship relating ganglion cell count and visual field sensitivity at a given *ec* value. *s* refers to visual acuity at a certain locus of the visual field in dB. *d* refers to the axonal density (axons/μm^2). *c* is highly related to the severity of the disease and is used to correct the ratio of axonal to nonaxonal cell composition of RGC cells in the model.

Considering that the mild manifestation of glaucoma derived mainly from RNFL damage while the severe stage reveals a more variable MD damage in the visual field, Medeiros et al. (15–17) performed a weighted integration by which the model relates structure to function.

$$Estimate\ RGC\ count = (1 + MD/30) \times OCTrgc + (-MD/30) \times SAPrgc$$

The Original Model for an Estimate of Macular Ganglion Cell Count

Hood et al. found that mild glaucoma damages were detected in the macula (21, 22). Based on the previous model for eRGC estimation, Medeiros et al. (18) have modified the visual function test. The scattered loci in the Humphrey 24-2 SAP were changed to focused 16 loci of the retinal sensitivity within 10° of the macular fixation areas.

$$m = [0.054(ec \times 1.32)] + 0.9$$
$$b = [-1.5(ec \times 1.32)] - 14.8$$
$$gc = \{[(s-1) - b]/m\} + 4.7$$
$$macular\ SAPrgc = \sum 10\hat{}(gc \times 0.1)$$
$$d = (-0.007 \times age) + 1.4$$
$$c = (-0.26 \times TD) + 0.12$$
$$a = average\ temporal\ RNFL\ thickness \times 0.51 \times 10{,}870 \times d$$
$$macular\ OCTrgc = 10\hat{}\{[\log(a) \times 10 - c] \times 0.1\}$$

In the above formulas, *ec* was denoted as 4.2 (3 × 3 deg), 9.5 (3 × 9 deg and 9 × 3 deg), and 12.8 (9 × 9 deg). TD is the mean value of retinal sensitivity at 16 loci corresponding to 10° of the center of total deviation using 24-2 SAP. Corresponding estimated RGC count, namely, the macular *SAPrgc* was obtained by applying the value of each point detected by SAP to the above formula. Similarly, structural parameters were changed to mean RNFL of the temporal, superior, and inferior temporal regions of the optic disc corresponding to the macula.

The aforementioned formulas gave the OCT measurements in the macula, namely, *macular OCTrgc*. The formulas were weighted and integrated according to the previous description by Medeiros et al. and the obtained RGC remained both structural and functional components.

$$mRGC2 = (1 + MD/30) \times mOCTrgc + (-MD/30) \times mSAPrgc$$

A New Model for RGC Estimation in the Macula

Three innermost layers of the retina are preferentially involved when there is glaucomatous damage in the macular: the nerve fiber layer, the ganglion cell layer, and the inner plexiform layer. These three layers contain ganglion cell axons, ganglion cell body, and ganglion cell dendrites, which are collectively called the GCC. The latest frequency-domain OCT uses Fourier technology and broadband light source technology to acquire and process data, which has higher resolution, sensitivity, and faster scanning speed than time-domain OCT, and can acquire and analyze the structural images and data information of GCC

TABLE 1 | Demographic and clinical characteristics of healthy eyes and primary open-angle glaucoma (POAG) eyes in different stages.

Variables	Healthy (n = 30)	Glaucoma				P value
		PPG (n = 20)	Mild (n = 20)	Moderate (n = 20)	Severe (n = 29)	
Age (years)	48.2 ± 12.6	46.4 ± 10.2	48.1 ± 15.2	50.5 ± 18.5	48.9 ± 14.1	0.921
VFI(%)	98.2 ± 1.9	97.2 ± 2.4	90.2 ± 4.9	65.6 ± 9.3	24.0 ± 17.4	0.000
MD24-2(dB)	−1.54 ± 0.97	−2.59 ± 1.26	−4.82 ± 2.11	−14.85 ± 3.44	− 26.73 ± 4.41	0.000
MD10-2(dB)	−0.37 ± 0.81	−0.63 ± 1.40	− 3.78 ± 2.48	−9.57 ± 4.30	− 21.37 ± 8.29	0.000
GCC(um)	105.95 ± 4.83	92.38 ± 4.10	84.04 ± 8.98	71.23 ± 7.63	61.40 ± 6.37	0.000
RNFL(um)	110.37 ± 4.90	95.65 ± 6.34	87 ± 9.40	72.60 ± 10.94	58.76 ± 11.93	0.000
mRGC1	11,739,81 ± 77,580	10,189,84 ± 60156	8,487,95 ± 110,610	6,428,02 ± 157,538	2,272,90 ± 42,206	0.000
mRGC2	6,195,39 ± 58,775	5,293,83 ± 37,422	4,087,60 ± 67,796	2,322,21 ± 56,410	921,18 ± 80978	0.000
eRGC	11,021,08 ± 72,669	8,939,76 ± 87,103	6,809,84 ± 118,903	2,897,88 ± 96,051	822,68 ± 72,653	0.000

eRGC, estimated retinal ganglion cell; mRGC, macular estimated retinal ganglion cell; GCC, ganglion cell complex; MD, mean deviation; POAG, primary open-angle glaucoma; PPG, preperimetric glaucoma; RNFL, retinal nerve fiber layer; VFI, visual field index.

in the macula in a short time. The estimation model built by Harwerth and Medeiros was adopted in the modified macular structure-function model. SAP test was changed to Humphrey 10-2 program which focuses on 16 loci within 10° of the macula (2° interval). *ec* was taken as 1.4 (1 × 1 deg), 4.2 (3 × 3 deg), 7.0 (5 × 5 deg), and 8.6 (7 × 5 deg). Macular SAPrgc, corresponding to the estimated RGC count was obtained by applying the value of each point detected by SAP to the formula.

$$m = [0.054(ec \times 1.32)] + 0.9$$
$$b = [-1.5(ec \times 1.32)] - 14.8$$
$$gc = \{[(s-1) - b]/m\} + 4.7$$
$$macular\ SAPrgc = \sum 10\hat{}(gc \times 0.1)$$

Ganglion cell complex thickness of the macula was taken as the structural parameter. MD is the value used for the center of the visual field in Humphrey SAP 10-2 program (interval 2°). Macular OCTrgc was obtained by the OCT measurements of the macula for RGC estimates.

$$d = (-0.007 \times age) + 1.4$$
$$c = (-0.26 \times TD) + 0.12$$
$$a = average\ macular\ GCC\ thickness \times 10,870 \times d$$
$$macular\ OCTrgc = 10\hat{}\{[\log(a) \times 10 - c] \times 0.1\}$$

The formula for modified macular SAPrgc is the same used in the above model for RGCs estimate.

$$mRGC1 = (1 + MD/30) \times mOCTrgc + (-MD/30) \times mSAPrgc$$

Statistical Analysis

Continuous variables were checked to meet the normality conditions of the Shapiro-Wilk test. ANOVA test and the least significant difference *post-hoc* test with Bonferroni adjustment were used for intergroup comparisons for normally distributed variables. Dichotomic variables were analyzed using the χ^2 test or the Fisher's exact test. Receiver operating characteristic (ROC) curve analyses were used to assess the diagnostic accuracy of eRGC, mRGC1, and mRGC2. The area under the ROC curve (AUC), sensitivity, specificity were calculated to assess the performance of the prediction model. Yorden's index, defined as the sensitivity + specificity − 1, was used to determine the optimal cut-off values to maximize diagnostic efficiency. Statistical significance was set at $P \leq 0.05$. By setting the alpha to 0.05 to declare the slope of RGC loss as statistically significant, we were able to maintain a specificity of 95%, as demonstrated in the previous study that estimated rates of RGC loss obtained from SAP and OCT (16). At 95% specificity, approximately six of the 119 eyes would be expected to show significant slopes just by chance. The SPSS program package version 21.0 (Statistic Package for the Social Science, Inc., Chicago, IL, USA) was used for statistical analysis.

RESULTS

Comparison of the Demographic and Clinical Characteristics of Healthy Eyes and POAG Eyes in Different Stages

A total of 89 eyes with POAG meeting the diagnostic criteria were enrolled. Healthy control included 30 eyes of healthy examined subjects. According to the AGIS scoring system, POAG eyes were divided using Humphrey SAP 24-2 program, namely, 20 eyes with preperimetric glaucoma, 20 eyes with the mild stage of glaucoma, 20 eyes with moderate stage, and 29 eyes with advanced stage. The demographic and clinical characteristics of subjects among the groups were shown in **Table 1**. The glaucomatous eyes have significantly worse visual field index (VFI), MD (24-4 and 10-2), GCC, RNFL, eRGC, mRGC2, and mRGC1 than healthy eyes ($P < 0.001$).

Comparison of the Three Estimated Values for Each Group

Compared with normal individuals (**Figure 1**), eRGC, mRGC1, and mRGC2 obtained from the three models decreased markedly in glaucoma, and as glaucoma progressed, RGC estimates reduced gradually from mild to severe stage.

Compared with the estimated RGCs in healthy eyes, preperimetric glaucomatous eyes had mRGC1 reduced to 13.2%, mRGC2 reduced to 14.5%, and eRGC reduced to 18%. Glaucomatous eyes with mild stages had mRGC1 reduced to 28%, mRGC2 reduced to 34%, and eRGC reduced to 38%. In the severe stage, the reduction proportion for mRGC1, mRGC2, and eRGC was 81, 85, and 92%, respectively, indicating that mRGC1 has a good staging performance and may serve as a candidate model for estimating RGC counts in the macula.

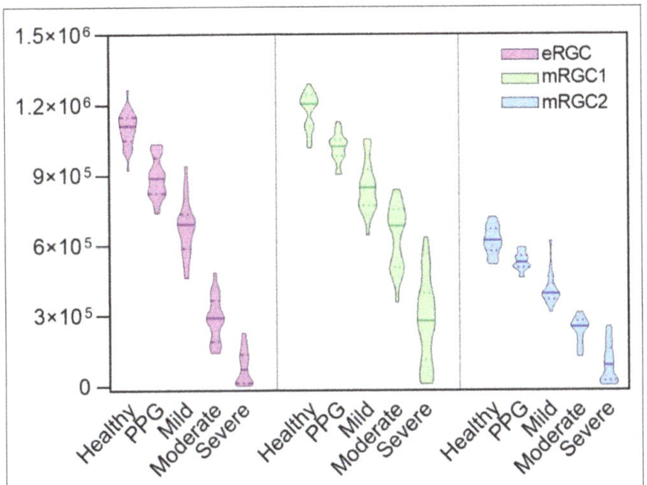

FIGURE 1 | Violin plots illustrating that estimated retinal ganglion cell (eRGC), macular estimated retinal ganglion cell (mRGC1), and mRGC2 were obtained from the three models at five stages. It showed that eRGC, mRGC1, and mRGC2 decreased markedly from preperimetric glaucoma (PPG) to severe stage of glaucoma ($P < 0.05$).

Diagnostic Efficacy and Sensitivity Analysis of eRGC, mRGC1, and mRGC2 and Related Structural/Functional Parameters

To analyze the capability of eRGC, mRGC1, and mRGC2 and also structural parameters (GCC and RNFL) and functional parameters (VFI and MD24-2) in differentiating between POAG and healthy eyes, ROC curves were conducted. The results showed that the AUCs of all parameters were above 0.9. As shown in **Figure 2**, AUC of eRGC, mRGC1, and mRGC2 was 0.992 (95% CI, 0.954~1), 0.982 (95% CI, 0.939~0.998), and 0.972 (95% CI, 0.924~0.994), respectively. The AUC of structural parameter GCC was 0.995 (95% CI, 0.960~1) and the AUC of peripapillary RNFL was 0.992 (95% CI, 0.954~1). The AUCs for the functional parameters VFI and MD (24-2) were 0.906 (95% CI, 0.839–0.952) and 0.927 (95% CI, 0.865–0.967), respectively. All these indicators offered relatively good predictive performances to distinguish glaucoma from a healthy population.

For a 95% specificity as shown in **Table 2**, eRGC had a sensitivity of 95.51%, with a relatively low sensitivity of 86.52 and 87.64% for mRGC1 and mRGC2, respectively. The sensitivity of structural parameters GCC and RNFL were 98.88 and 95.51%, respectively, while the sensitivity of the functional parameter MD24-2 is 80.90%, the VFI sensitivity is 73.03%, much lower than the sensitivity of mRGC1 and mRGC2.

DISCUSSION

Previous studies have built a model that combines structure and function measures to estimate RGC losses and validated it in both experimental studies and human glaucoma (5, 14, 19). Along with this, the involvement of the macula has been evidenced in mild glaucomatous damage (21). However, the

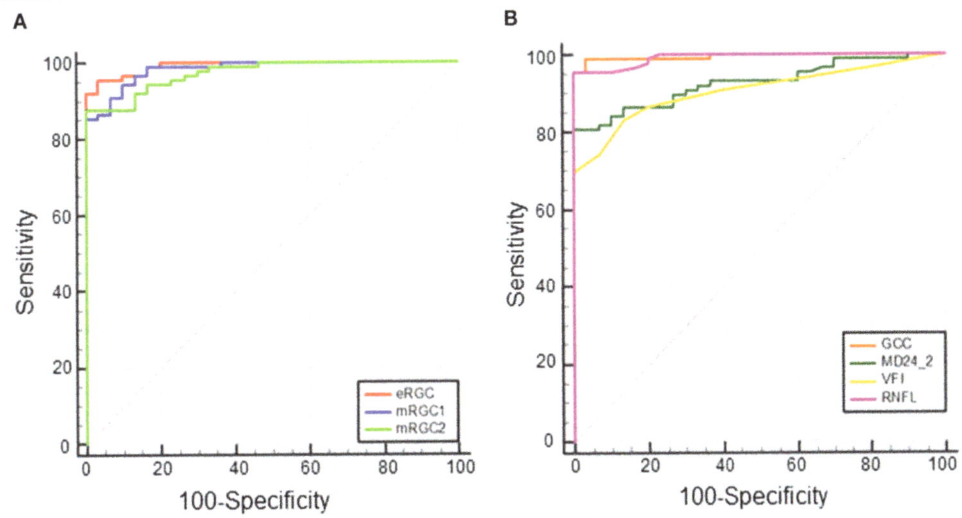

FIGURE 2 | Receiver operating characteristic (ROC) curve of total eRGC, mRGC1, and mRGC2 and structural/functional parameters in POAG, **(A)** Area under the ROC curve (AUC) of eRGC, mRGC1, and mRGC2 was 0.992 (95% CI, 0.954~1.000), 0.982 (95% CI, 0.939~0.998), 0.972 (95% CI, 0.924~0.994), respectively, and **(B)** AUC of ganglion cell complex (GCC), retinal nerve fiber layer (RNFL), visual field index (VFI), and MD (24-2) was 0.995 (95% CI, 0.960~1.000), 0.992 (95% CI, 0.954~1.000), 0.906 (95% CI, 0.839–0.952), and 0.927 (95% CI, 0.865–0.967), respectively.

TABLE 2 | Diagnostic efficacy and sensitivity analysis of eRGC, mRGC1, and mRGC2 and related structural/functional parameters.

Variables	Sensitivity at 95% specificity	AUC (95% CI)	Yorden index	*P* value
eRGC	95.51%(87.64~100.00%)	0.992(0.954~1.000)	0.9217	<0.0001
mRGC1	86.52%(74.16~94.38%)	0.982(0.939~0.998)	0.8539	<0.0001
mRGC2	87.64%(78.65~93.26%)	0.972(0.924~0.994)	0.8764	<0.0001
GCC(um)	98.88%(91.01~100.00%)	0.995(0.960~1.000)	0.9554	<0.0001
RNFL(um)	95.51%(88.76~98.88%)	0.992(0.954~1.000)	0.9551	<0.0001
MD24-2(dB)	80.90%(69.66~87.64%)	0.927(0.865~0.967)	0.8090	<0.0001
VFI(%)	73.03%(56.68~83.15%)	0.906(0.839~0.952)	0.6981	<0.0001

eRGC, estimated retinal ganglion cell; GCC, ganglion cell complex; mRGC, macular estimated retinal ganglion cell; RNFL, retinal nerve fiber layer; MD, mean deviation; VFI, visual field index.

current assessment of structural damage in glaucoma is mainly based on damages to the optic disc and peripapillary RNFL, few studies have investigated the clinical significance of macular damage for diagnosis and staging in glaucoma. The original model for macular RGC estimation structurally applied the temporal RNFL thickness of the optic disc and functionally applied 16 central points of the 24-2 SAP test corresponding to the central 10° to assess macular RGC loss. However, there are two limitations in this model: the first is that the temporal RNFL of the optic disc does not reflect the real situation of ganglion cell damage in the macula. Second, approximately 50% of RGCs are located within 16° of the central macula, an area that accounts for only 7.3% of the total retinal area. In the SAP test 24-2 program, only 12 (22%) of the 54 loci (6° interval) were located in this region, so mild glaucomatous visual field defects may be missed and also a large difference in the real number of residual RGCs in the macula was observed. Therefore, in this study, we made adjustments to the original model and sought to propose a novel improved macular RGC estimation model with the combination of both structural and functional measurements. The structural parameter for temporal peripapillary RNFL thickness measurement was changed to the macular structural parameter GCC thickness. The SAP testing program and location were changed from 24-2 with a large range (interval 6°) to 10-2, focusing on visual sensitivity that has 16 loci within 10° of the macular fixation points (interval 2°).

Table 1 and **Figure 1** showed that eRGC, mRGC1, and mRGC2 were significantly higher in normal subjects than in patients with glaucoma and that the eRGC decreased gradually in patients with glaucoma as the disease progressed, with statistically significant differences between all groups. eRGC, mRGC1, and mRGC2 provided good performance in discriminating glaucomatous from healthy eyes, and different degrees of severity or progression. Compared with the normal controls, mRGC1, mRGC2, and eRGC were reduced by 13.2, 14.5, and 18%, respectively, in preperimetric glaucoma. In mild glaucoma, mRGC1, mRGC2, and eRGC were reduced by 28, 34, and 38%, respectively. In the advanced disease, mRGC1, mRGC2, and eRGC were reduced by 81, 85, and 92%, respectively. The proportion of RGC loss in the macula was close to the proportion outside the macula in different stages of POAG, indicating that the macular ganglion cell damage started at early stages, and as the disease progresses, parallel damages would be observed both in the macula and outside the macula. In the preperimetric stage, there was already about 13.2% (14.5% for mRGC2 estimation) RGC loss in the macula and the decline of MD in SAP 10-2 was 0.63 dB, 0.3 dB lower than normal controls; however, in the progression stage, there was a considerate loss of macular and eRGC estimations, and the MD declined significantly, suggesting that SAP was not sensitive in the detection of mild glaucoma. While the macular had the highest RGC density, thus in the early stage of disease, a significant reduction of mRGC1 and mRGC2 could be observed, which is helpful in the early diagnosis.

Several studies have revealed that RGC estimates that integrate structural and functional parameters have higher diagnostic efficacy for glaucoma than structural or functional parameters applied alone. Medeiros et al. (23) found that RGC estimates were superior to mean RNFL thickness in distinguishing glaucomatous from healthy eyes (AUCs 0.95 and 0.88, respectively). Our data demonstrated that the AUCs of mRGC1, mRGC2, and eRGC in the three RGC estimation models of POAG were 0.982 (95% CI, 0.939–0.998), 0.972 (95% CI, 0.924–0.994), and 0.992 (95% CI, 0.954–1.000), respectively, which were higher than those of the separate functional AUC 0.906 (95% CI, 0.839~0.952) and 0.927 (95% CI, 0.865~0.967) for VFI and MD (24-2). At 95% specificity, eRGC had a sensitivity of 95.51%, and the sensitivity of mRGC1 and mRGC2 estimates were relatively low, with 86.52 and 87.64% respectively. The macular region analyzed in the macular structure-function model may contain only about 50% of RGCs, while the RNFL in the conventional optic disc-visual field model contains axons of ganglion cells in a wide area of the retina and can detect glaucomatous damage in more locations outside the macula, resulting in higher diagnostic efficacy for eRGC. For a 95% specificity, the structural parameter GCC was 98.88%, significantly higher than the functional parameters MD (24-2) with a sensitivity of 80.90% and VFI with a sensitivity of 73.03%. In addition, because the macular region is less affected by blood vessels during OCT imaging, thus making GCC is an ideal tool for glaucoma detection.

It is also worth noting that there are some limitations to this study. The number of RGCs is based on models and formulas from SAP and OCT data, not directly derived from histologic data. Although the formula has been validated in animals and glaucoma populations, there are still some deviations from the real RGCs number. Furthermore, differences in detection equipment and individual variability in disc-macula structures should also be taken into account, which may indirectly or directly affect the accuracy of macular RGCs count estimation. Another limitation is that the macular estimated RGC count could be affected by macular diseases. The macular examination is, therefore, required to exclude any macular affection. Future prospective studies are needed to further validate our macular structure-function model for estimating the number of macular RGCs.

In conclusion, this study performed a comparative analysis for three RGC estimation models. Our results showed that mRGC1, mRGC2, and eRGC all provided good performances in the severity grading of glaucoma. No significant differences were observed in diagnostic efficacy between the new modified macular structure-function models mRGC1 and eRGC. Meanwhile, the results of GCC were more stable with fewer individual differences. Thus, our model combining structure and function is expected to be a new strategy for the evaluation of glaucomatous damage in the macula and has significant clinical implications regarding the diagnosis and early detection of glaucoma progression.

ETHICS STATEMENT

The studies involving human participants were reviewed and approved by the Ethics Committee of The First Affiliated Hospital of Kunming Medical University. The patients/participants provided their written informed consent to participate in this study.

AUTHOR CONTRIBUTIONS

YW, HZ, and QC designed the study and wrote the manuscript. YW, QC, YT, WY, JW, and DF collected data of the patients and performed various clinical examinations. YW, YZ, and QC analyzed the data. HZ gained the fund and supervised the process. All the authors approved the final version of the article.

ACKNOWLEDGMENTS

We would thank all the participants and staff for their valuable contributions to this research.

REFERENCES

1. Weinreb RN, Leung CK, Crowston JG, Medeiros FA, Friedman DS, Wiggs JL, et al. Primary open-angle glaucoma. *Nat Rev Dis Primers.* (2016) 2:16067. doi: 10.1038/nrdp.2016.67
2. Weinreb RN, Aung T, Medeiros FA. The pathophysiology and treatment of glaucoma: a review. *JAMA.* (2014) 311:1901–11. doi: 10.1001/jama.2014.3192
3. Medeiros FA, Alencar LM, Zangwill LM, Bowd C, Sample PA, Weinreb RN. Prediction of functional loss in glaucoma from progressive optic disc damage. *Arch Ophthalmol.* (2009) 127:1250–6. doi: 10.1001/archophthalmol.2009.276
4. Hood DC, Kardon RH. A framework for comparing structural and functional measures of glaucomatous damage. *Prog Retin Eye Res.* (2007) 26:688–710. doi: 10.1016/j.preteyeres.2007.08.001
5. Harwerth RS, Carter-Dawson L, Smith EL. 3rd, Barnes G, Holt WF, Crawford ML. Neural losses correlated with visual losses in clinical perimetry. *Invest Ophthalmol Vis Sci.* (2004) 45:3152–60. doi: 10.1167/iovs.04-0227
6. Kass MA, Heuer DK, Higginbotham EJ, Johnson CA, Keltner JL, Miller JP, et al. The Ocular Hypertension Treatment Study: a randomized trial determines that topical ocular hypotensive medication delays or prevents the onset of primary open-angle glaucoma. *Arch Ophthalmol.* (2002) 120:701–13. doi: 10.1001/archopht.120.6.701
7. Miglior S, Zeyen T, Pfeiffer N, Cunha-Vaz J, Torri V, Adamsons I, et al. Results of the European glaucoma prevention study. *Ophthalmology.* (2005) 112:366–75. doi: 10.1016/j.ophtha.2004.11.030
8. Wollstein G, Schuman JS, Price LL, Aydin A, Stark PC, Hertzmark E, et al. Optical coherence tomography longitudinal evaluation of retinal nerve fiber layer thickness in glaucoma. *Arch Ophthalmol.* (2005) 123:464–70. doi: 10.1001/archopht.123.4.464
9. Strouthidis NG, Scott A, Peter NM, Garway-Heath DF. Optic disc and visual field progression in ocular hypertensive subjects: detection rates, specificity, and agreement. *Invest Ophthalmol Vis Sci.* (2006) 47:2904–10. doi: 10.1167/iovs.05-1584
10. Medeiros FA, Alencar LM, Zangwill LM, Sample PA, Weinreb RN. The Relationship between intraocular pressure and progressive retinal nerve fiber layer loss in glaucoma. *Ophthalmology.* (2009) 116:1125–33. doi: 10.1016/j.ophtha.2008.12.062
11. Leung CK, Cheung CY, Weinreb RN, Qiu K, Liu S, Li H, et al. Evaluation of retinal nerve fiber layer progression in glaucoma: a study on optical coherence tomography guided progression analysis. *Invest Ophthalmol Vis Sci.* (2010) 51:217–22. doi: 10.1167/iovs.09-3468
12. Artes PH, Chauhan BC. Longitudinal changes in the visual field and optic disc in glaucoma. *Prog Retin Eye Res.* (2005) 24:333–54. doi: 10.1016/j.preteyeres.2004.10.002
13. Schulzer M. Errors in the diagnosis of visual field progression in normal-tension glaucoma. *Ophthalmology.* (1994) 101:1589–94.
14. Harwerth RS, Wheat JL, Fredette MJ, Anderson DR. Linking structure and function in glaucoma. *Prog Retin Eye Res.* (2010) 29:249–71. doi: 10.1016/j.preteyeres.2010.02.001
15. Medeiros FA, Lisboa R, Weinreb RN, Girkin CA, Liebmann JM, Zangwill LM. A combined index of structure and function for staging glaucomatous damage. *Arch Ophthalmol.* (2012) 130:1107–16. doi: 10.1001/archophthalmol.2012.827
16. Medeiros FA, Zangwill LM, Anderson DR, Liebmann JM, Girkin CA, Harwerth RS, et al. Estimating the rate of retinal ganglion cell loss in glaucoma. *Am J Ophthalmol.* (2012) 154:814–24 e811. doi: 10.1016/j.ajo.2012.04.022
17. Medeiros FA, Zangwill LM, Bowd C, Mansouri K, Weinreb RN. The structure and function relationship in glaucoma: implications for detection of progression and measurement of rates of change. *Invest Ophthalmol Vis Sci.* (2012) 53:6939–46. doi: 10.1167/iovs.12-10345

18. Zhang C, Tatham AJ, Weinreb RN, Zangwill LM, Yang Z, Zhang JZ, et al. Relationship between ganglion cell layer thickness and estimated retinal ganglion cell counts in the glaucomatous macula. *Ophthalmology.* (2014) 121:2371–9. doi: 10.1016/j.ophtha.2014.06.047
19. Harwerth RS, Vilupuru AS, Rangaswamy NV, Smith EL, 3rd. The relationship between nerve fiber layer and perimetry measurements. *Invest Ophthalmol Vis Sci.* (2007) 48:763–73. doi: 10.1167/iovs.06-0688
20. Chauhan BC, Blanchard JW, Hamilton DC, LeBlanc RP. Technique for detecting serial topographic changes in the optic disc and peripapillary retina using scanning laser tomography. *Invest Ophthalmol Vis Sci.* (2000) 41:775–82.
21. Hood DC, Raza AS, de Moraes CG, Liebmann JM, Ritch R. Glaucomatous damage of the macula. *Prog Retin Eye Res.* (2013) 32:1–21. doi: 10.1016/j.preteyeres.2012.08.003
22. Hood DC, Raza AS, de Moraes CG, Odel JG, Greenstein VC, Liebmann JM, et al. Initial arcuate defects within the central 10 degrees in glaucoma. *Invest Ophthalmol Vis Sci.* (2011) 52:940–6. doi: 10.1167/iovs.10-5803
23. Medeiros FA, Lisboa R, Weinreb RN, Liebmann JM, Girkin C, Zangwill LM. Retinal ganglion cell count estimates associated with early development of visual field defects in glaucoma. *Ophthalmology.* (2013) 120:736–44. doi: 10.1016/j.ophtha.2012.09.039

24

Low-Reflectivity Drusen with Overlying RPE Damage Revealed by Spectral-Domain OCT: Hint for the Development of Age-Related Macular Degeneration

Shasha Yang[1], Zongyin Gao[1], Haijiang Qiu[1], Chengguo Zuo[2], Lan Mi[2], Hui Xiao[2] and Xing Liu[2]*

[1] Department of Ophthalmology, Guangzhou First People's Hospital, School of Medicine, South China University of Technology, Guangzhou, China, [2] State Key Laboratory of Ophthalmology, Zhongshan Ophthalmic Center, Sun Yat-sen University, Guangzhou, China

***Correspondence:**
Xing Liu
liuxing@mail.sysu.edu.cn

Purpose: To observe the relationship between the characteristic changes in the drusen morphology revealed by the spectral-domain optical coherence tomography (SD-OCT) and the progression of age-related macular degeneration (AMD).

Methods: A total of 380 drusen in 45 eyes in 35 patients with the intermediate drusen were longitudinally followed up every 6 months by SD-OCT for a period of 24 months. The drusen were divided into the dynamic group and stable group according to the following parameters: number, volume, concurrent retinal pigment epithelium (RPE)/ellipsoid zone (EZ) damage, and the development of advanced AMD. The morphological characteristics of the progressive or stable drusen were further analyzed. Odds ratios (ORs) and the risk for the drusen progression were calculated.

Results: The level of interobserver and intraobserver agreement for each drusen tomographic morphological parameters ranged from 82.7 to 90%. At the end of an average follow-up of 15.92 $\pm$ 6.99 months, six patients developed choroidal neovascularization and no patients developed geographic atrophy. Finally, 139 drusen changed and 241 drusen remained stable. The drusen with low reflectivity ($p < 0.001$; OR: 5.26; 95% CI: 2.24–12.36), non-homogeneity without a core ($p < 0.001$; OR: 4.31; 95% CI: 2.08–8.92), RPE damage ($p < 0.001$; OR: 28.12; 95% CI: 9.43–83.85), and the EZ damage ($p < 0.001$; OR: 14.01; 95% CI: 5.28–37.18) were significantly associated with active change; the drusen with low reflectivity ($p = 0.01$; OR: 2.95; 95% CI: 1.29–6.75) and decreased overlying RPE reflectivity ($p < 0.001$; OR: 21.67; 95% CI: 9.20–51.02) were the independent predictors for progression. The drusen with high reflectivity were significantly associated with stabilization ($p = 0.03$; OR: 0.17; 95% CI: 0.04–0.84).

Conclusion: Spectral-domain optical coherence tomography is an optimized, accurate, and efficient method to follow-up the drusen. The intermediate non-exudative AMD prognosis of the patient was most strongly correlated with the drusen reflectivity and disruption of the overlying RPE layer. The drusen with low reflectivity and overlying RPE damage were more likely to progress and required frequent follow-up.

Keywords: drusen, age-related macular degeneration (AMD), optical coherence tomography, character, predictor

INTRODUCTION

Age-related macular degeneration (AMD) is the leading cause of vision loss among people over 60 years of age in the developed countries (1). With vision loss, the life of a person with AMD becomes inconvenient and elderly people with AMD have a higher risk of depression and anxiety than unaffected elderly people (2). Because there are no vision-restoring therapies, the individuals with intermediate AMD are just as anxious about losing vision as the individuals who are actually blind (3). Thus, it is crucial to find the predictors of intermediate AMD progression, which is only slightly understood at present.

Macular drusen are the characteristic lesions of intermediate AMD (4). Therefore, the size and number of the drusen are used for AMD staging and for predicting the likelihood of the disease progression and vision loss. Color fundus photographs are commonly used to evaluate the morphology of the drusen over time (5–10). However, the color images do not provide detailed information about the changing internal morphology of the drusen (11). There is usually a long process before the drusen progress to advanced AMD. Historically, based on the color photographs, the large drusen and pigmentary changes have been identified as the risk factors for progression (7). However, these factors do not provide enough information to allow a clear understanding of the course of the disease to be achieved. The introduction of spectral-domain optical coherence tomography (SD-OCT) has enabled the investigation of the ultrastructural morphological characteristics of the drusen *in vivo* and the distinction of subclasses of the drusen types (12–15). SD-OCT can provide important information, which will facilitate further understanding of the disease pathogenesis, identification of the potential risk factors for progression to advanced AMD (16), and the development of early interventions before disease progression to the advanced stages.

METHODS

Patients

We enrolled 35 patients with binocular AMD and eventually excluded eyes with choroidal neovascularization (CNV) or geographic atrophy (GA) at baseline. The mean age of the patients was 69.94 ± 7.30 years, ranging from 55 to 81 years. We defined early AMD as the presence of at least one drusen on any of the B-scan (6 × 6 mm) centered on the fovea on OCT (12). This study was approved by the Human Ethics Committee of Zhongshan Ophthalmic Center and informed consent was obtained from all the participants in accordance with the Declaration of Helsinki.

The study participants had to be able to fix their eyes for at least 1 min to allow adequate SD-OCT scanning. At the beginning of the follow-up period, the eligibility criteria were as follows: (1) age between 50 and 85 years; (2) bilateral large drusen (125 μm) or large drusen in one eye and advanced AMD in the fellow eye (17); (3) the drusen within 3,000 μm of the foveola; and (4) no signs of any other retinopathy or advanced AMD in the study eye. The exclusion criteria were as follows: (1) bilateral late-stage AMD, including a large area (>1,500 μm) of central GA or CNV; (2) significant opacity of the cornea or media; (3) amblyopia; (4) retinal abnormalities other than AMD; (5); diabetes; (6) uncontrolled hypertension (systolic blood pressure > 150 mm Hg and diastolic blood pressure > 90 mm Hg); (7) neurological or systemic disease that could compromise vision; (8) use of medication known to affect the retina (e.g., hydroxychloroquine); (9) use of antioxidant agent one month prior to study entry and during the period of follow-up; and (10) physical and/or mental impairment or inability to sign a consent form. None of the participants had a history of high myopia, ocular trauma, or ocular surgery.

Image Acquisition

All the study participants were examined five times during a six month interval within a follow-up period of 24 months. At each visit, visual acuity was recorded with the Early Treatment Diabetic Retinopathy Study (ETDRS) charts. SD-OCT images were obtained with a Spectralis^{TM} OCT system (Heidelberg Engineering, Germany) after pupil dilation with 0.5% tropicamide and 5% phenylephrine. A standardized SD-OCT scan (λ = 870 nm; 40,000 A-scans/s; 38 B-scans) was performed in each study eye with a transverse resolution of 6 μm and an axial resolution of 5 μm. Because of the independent pairs of the scanning mirrors, the eye movements were automatically corrected by the in-system "eye tracking" device, which enabled the identification of the same scanning location during the follow-up visits. To increase the image quality, the automatic real-time analysis scanning of the same location was performed and the images were averaged to reduce the signal-to-noise ratio. The automatic real-time averaging settings were 7 and the scan quality was 23–36 dB (15, 18).

Spectral Domain-Optical CT Classification of the Drusen Ultrastructure

The images were always evaluated as white-on-black in the HEYEX software. In high-speed mode, the vertical presentation of the OCT scan was magnified twice (19). The graded and analyzed morphological characteristics of the drusen included shape, internal reflectivity, homogeneity, and status of the retinal pigment epithelium (RPE) or ellipsoid zone (EZ) layer above the drusen (20–23). The shape of the drusen was classified as domed, saw-toothed, pointed, or cuticular. The internal reflectivity of the drusen was graded as a low, medium, or high compared with the reflectivity of the adjacent RPE layer on the same scan. Homogeneity was evaluated and classified as follows: non-homogeneous without a core (a distinct focus of hyperreflectivity inside the drusen), non-homogeneous with a central core, or homogeneous (relatively uniform internal reflectivity). The status of the RPE layer and EZ layer above the drusen was determined to be intact/present or disrupted/absent.

The SD-OCT characteristics of the drusen were analyzed by two trained independent graders (SSY and LM) and a senior grader (XL) decided in the case of a discrepancy. Interobserver reliability was determined for each parameter by calculating Cohen's kappa coefficient.

Image Analysis

The SD-OCT characteristics of the drusen were graded and analyzed every six months. The drusen were divided into the dynamic group and the stable group according to the follow-up results.

(1) Dynamic group: An increase or decrease in the number or volume of the drusen over time, the appearance or expansion of RPE damage, the appearance or expansion of the EZ damage scope, or progression into CNV or GA.

(2) Stable group: After 24 months of follow-up, no obvious changes in the number or volume of the drusen, no increase in the RPE or EZ damage, and no development of CNV or GA.

Statistical Analysis

Statistical analysis was performed by using SPSS Statistical Software version 20 (Chicago, Illinois, USA). The prevalence of each basic morphological pattern was calculated and analyzed with descriptive statistics. The chi-squared test was used for the analysis of the categorical data. Enumeration data were analyzed by t-test. The strength of the association of the different drusen characteristics between the dynamic drusen group and the stable drusen group is shown as the odds ratio (OR) with 95% CI. For all the tests, a $p < 0.05$ was considered statistically significant.

RESULTS

A total of 380 drusen were observed in 45 eyes of 35 patients. The mean age of the patients was 69.94 ± 7.30 years, ranging from 55 to 81 years; 8 patients were women and 27 patients were men. The mean follow-up period was 15.92 ± 6.99 months (range: 3–27 months). At the end of the follow-up period, 139 drusen had changed and 241 drusen had remained stable. During the follow-up period, the number of the drusen increased in 13 eyes and decreased in 2 eyes; the volume of the drusen increased in 18 eyes and decreased in 3 eyes; the range of RPE damage increased in 21 eyes; and the range of the EZ damage increased in 20 eyes. There were no cases of a decrease in the range of the RPE or EZ damage. In addition, there were six cases (six eyes) of CNV development and no cases of GA development. **Table 1** shows the shape, internal reflectivity, homogeneity, RPE status, and EZ integrity in the dynamic and stable drusen groups.

At the end of the follow-up period, the drusen in approximately 60% (21/35) of eyes and 62.2% (28/45) of eyes had changed. Among them, there were six cases (six eyes) of neovascular AMD development. All the eyes had the drusen with RPE damage and five eyes had the drusen with the EZ damage. In the six development eyes of neovascular AMD, we noticed an interesting phenomenon: there were no changes in the drusen shape or homogeneity on SD-OCT, but in three cases, the medium-reflectivity drusen converted to the low-reflectivity drusen (**Figures 1, 2**). These may be due to the internal reflectivity change of the drusen or due to the greater thickness and shadowing of the hemorrhagic change on the appearance of the underlying drusen.

Univariate analysis showed that the low-reflectivity drusen (OR: 5.26, $p < 0.001$), the non-homogeneous drusen without a core (OR: 4.31, $p < 0.001$), the drusen with RPE damage (OR: 28.12, $p < 0.001$), and the drusen with the EZ damage (OR: 14.01, $p < 0.001$) were associated with progression. Furthermore, multivariate analysis [generalized estimating equation (GEE) model] showed that the low-reflectivity drusen and the drusen

TABLE 1 | Summary of the drusen basic morphological parameters seen in the drusen dynamic group and the drusen stable group.

		Dynamic drusen		Stable drusen	
		No.	%	No.	%
Shape					
Dome	244	112	45.9	132	54.1
Saw-toothed	66	14	21.2	52	78.8
Pointed	47	13	27.7	34	72.3
Cuticular	23	0	0	23	100
Reflectivity					
Low	91	70	76.9	21	23.1
Medium	202	65	32.2	137	67.8
High	87	4	4.6	83	95.4
Homogeneity					
Homogeneous	290	71	24.5	219	75.5
Nonhomogeneous with a core	7	3	42.9	4	57.1
Nonhomogeneous without a core	83	65	78.3	18	21.7
RPE damage					
Present	129	114	88.4	15	11.6
Absent	251	25	10.0	226	90.0
EZ damage					
Present	77	74	96.1	3	3.9
Absent	303	65	21.5	238	78.5

RPE, retinal pigment epithelium; EZ, ellipsoid zone.

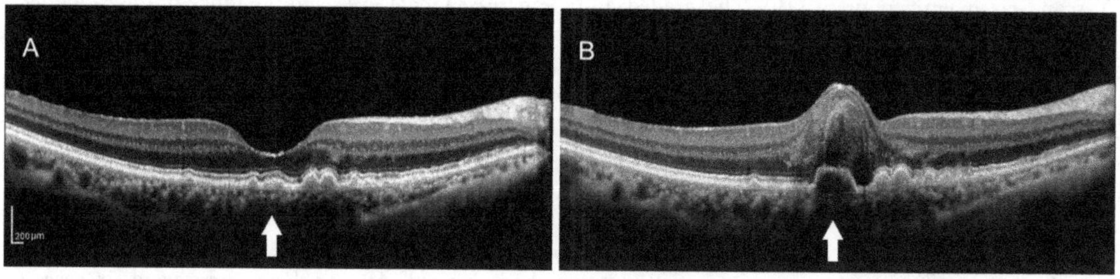

FIGURE 1 | (A) Spectral-domain optical coherence tomography (SD-OCT) image of a 64-year-old female dry patient with age-related macular degeneration (AMD) showing the medium-reflectivity drusen without the retinal pigment epithelium (RPE) or ellipsoid zone (EZ) damage at the fovea. **(B)** SD-OCT image of the same patient 1.5 years later, demonstrating the notable changes in the fovea, including retinal neuroepithelial hemorrhagic detachment with the local RPE and EZ disruption, which were associated with choroidal neovascularization (CNV). Note that the detected drusen (white arrow) developed into the low-reflectivity fusion drusen corresponding to the presence of the above changes.

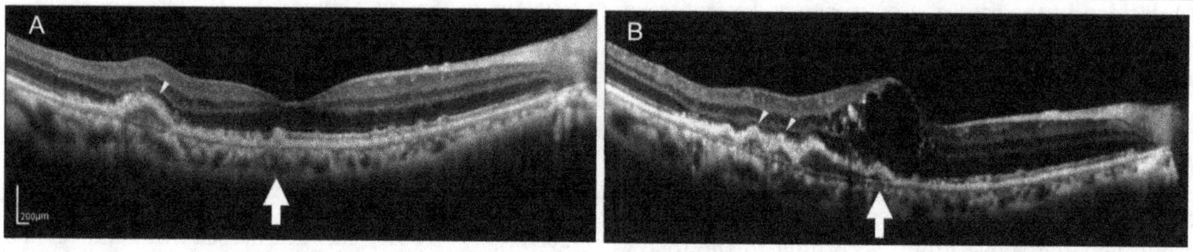

FIGURE 2 | (A) SD-OCT image of a 75-year-old male dry AMD patient showing the multiple, medium-reflectivity drusen with the extensive RPE and EZ damage surrounding the fovea. **(B)** SD-OCT image of the same patient 1 year later, demonstrating retinal neuroepithelial serous detachment with the additional and expanded drusen in his right macula. Note that the detected drusen (yellow arrowheads and white arrow) developed into the low-reflectivity confluent drusen corresponding to the presence of the above changes. Note that some drusen (white arrow) showed low reflectivity under the hemorrhagic shadow, whereas others appearing hyporeflective (yellow arrowheads) that were not covered by the hemorrhagic shadow.

with RPE damage were independent predictors for progression with OR values of 2.95 and 21.67, while the high-reflectivity drusen were less likely to progress with an OR value of only 0.17 (**Table 2**).

The interobserver and intraobserver agreement of the drusen grading data is shown in **Table 3**. In summary, the interobserver agreement was highest for reflectivity (95.2%) followed by shape (93.8%), presence of RPE damage (91.5%), presence of the EZ damage (89.7%), and homogeneity (83.4%). The intraobserver agreement was similar in the two groups. Observer 1 had a slightly higher intraobserver agreement compared to observer 2.

DISCUSSION

Drusen are an important quantifier of AMD severity. Drusen contain a great diversity of the compounds that appear to influence the complex pathogenesis of AMD (24, 25). Different clinical subtypes of the drusen have been described in AMD. Large (≥125 μm, width of a large vein at the disk margin) drusen with a soft, fuzzy boundary and pigmentary abnormalities are the well-recognized predictors for the progression to advanced AMD (26). However, these predictors are mainly based on the color fundus photography findings. However, the changes taking place within these high-risk drusen are unknown.

Recent developments in retinal imaging, especially with the introduction of high-resolution SD-OCT, have expanded the understanding of the complex ultrastructure of the drusen. Based on the SD-OCT morphological characteristics, 17 distinct subclasses of the drusen types were described by Khanifar et al. (20, 21). Approximately, 50% of the soft-indistinct drusen on color photography have a different appearance on SD-OCT (16, 27–29). We propose that investigating changes in the appearance of the various characteristics within the drusen *via* SD-OCT may contribute to a better understanding of the genotype, severity of disease, and risk of progression in AMD. They are consistent with that SD-OCT can provide more information about the risk factors for progression based on color photography described by Khanifar et al. (21). In this study, we used longitudinal SD-OCT photography to investigate the dynamic process of the drusen development to provide a clinically useful judgment regarding the risk of progression to vision-threatening AMD in the patients with the drusen. Drusen with low reflectivity and an overlying RPE or the EZ layer with decreased reflectivity were more likely to progress, whereas the high-reflectivity drusen were more likely to remain stable (**Figures 3, 4**).

There was considerable interobserver and intraobserver agreement in the grading of the drusen according to the morphological parameters on SD-OCT compared with the grading of the drusen according to the findings on color

TABLE 2 | The generalized estimating equation (GEE) model analysis of the drusen progression factors.

Influencing factors	Univariate analysis		Multivariate analysis	
	OR (95% CI)	***P***	**OR (95% CI)**	***P***
Age (per year)	1.06 (1.00–1.12)	0.066	–	–
Gender (Male vs. Female)	1.99 (0.84–4.74)	0.120	–	–
Reflectivity (Low vs. Medium)	5.26 (2.24–12.36)	< 0.001	2.95 (1.29–6.75)	0.010
Reflectivity (High vs. Medium)	0.48 (0.21–1.07)	0.074	0.17 (0.04–0.84)	0.030
Homogeneity (Nonhomogeneous with a core vs. Homogeneous)	2.52 (0.48–13.23)	0.275	–	–
Homogeneity (Nonhomogeneous without a core vs. Homogeneous)	4.31 (2.08–8.92)	< 0.001	–	–
RPE damage (Present vs. Absent)	28.12 (9.43–83.85)	< 0.001	21.67 (9.20–51.02)	< 0.001
EZ damage (Present vs. Absent)	14.01 (5.28–37.18)	< 0.001	2.72 (0.91–8.14)	0.074

RPE, retinal pigment epithelium; EZ, ellipsoid zone.

TABLE 3 | Interobserver and intraobserver agreement in the drusen grading of the morphological parameters.

Agreement	Shape		Reflectivity		Homogeneity		RPE damage		EZ damage	
Interobserver	93.8		95.2		83.4		91.5		89.7	
	Obs1	Obs2	Obs1	Obs2	Obs1	Obs2	Obs1	Obs2	Obs1	Obs2
Intraobserver	94.1	92.0	94.8	91.6	88.9	82.7	94.4	91.2	90.1	87.3

Obs1, observer 1; Obs2, observer 2.

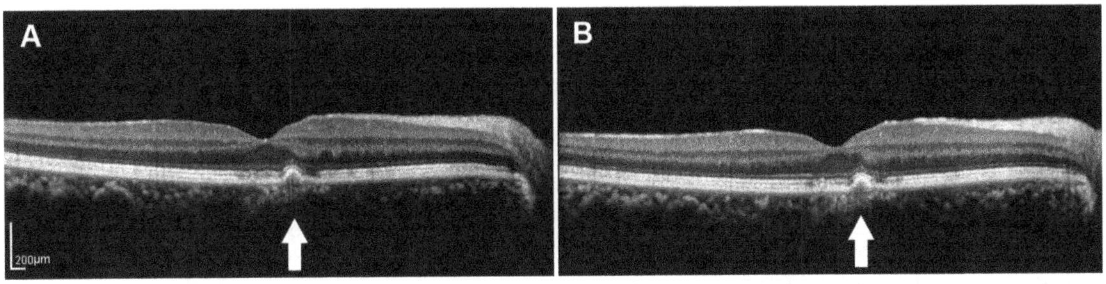

FIGURE 3 | (A) SD-OCT image of a 65-year-old male dry AMD patient showing the medium-reflectivity drusen without the RPE damage and the EZ is focally thinned at the fovea. **(B)** SD-OCT image of the same patient 1.5 years later, demonstrating the changes in neither the number nor the volume of the drusen. White arrows showed the drusen remained stable during the follow-up.

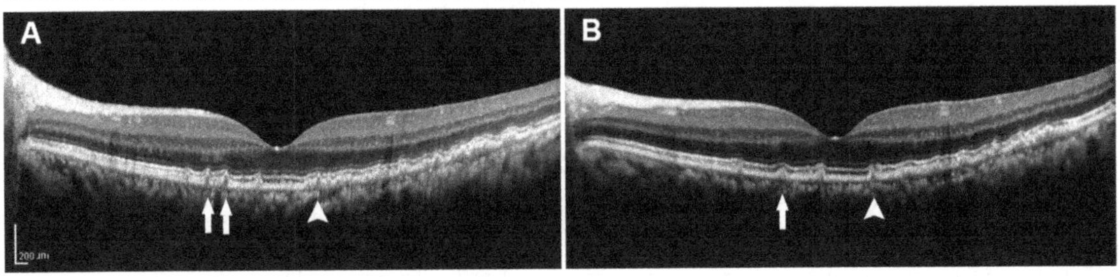

FIGURE 4 | (A) SD-OCT image of a 57-year-old female dry AMD patient showing the cuticular drusen without the RPE or the EZ damage around the fovea. **(B)** SD-OCT image of the same patient 2 years later, demonstrating a decrease in the number (arrow) and volume (arrowhead) of the drusen. SD-OCT, spectral domain-optical coherence tomography; AMD, age-related macular degeneration; RPE, retinal pigment epithelium; EZ, ellipsoid zone.

photography. In the Wisconsin age-related maculopathy grading system, the interobserver agreement for the type of the drusen was 70.6% and the intraobserver agreement for the type of the drusen was 62.5% (30). The Age-Related Eye Disease Study (AREDS) research group found that the reproducibility of the type of the drusen ranges from 59.0 to 77.5% (exact agreement) (31). In this study, there were only two readers and they were from the same center and the reading standards were unified before reading; thus, our interobserver agreement was different from that reported by the Classification of Atrophy Meetings (CAM) group (32) (by 12 readers from 6 reading centers). In this study, the level of interobserver and intraobserver agreement for each morphological parameter was generally more than 90% for the drusen reflectivity, shape, and RPE damage, while the drusen homogeneity and the EZ damage showed the lowest agreement at 82.7%.

In this study, out of the 380 drusen, approximately one-third (139/380) were the dynamic drusen and two-thirds (241/380) were the stable drusen. Univariate analysis regarding the differences in the SD-OCT morphological characteristics between the dynamic and stable drusen showed that the low-reflectivity drusen, the non-homogeneous drusen without a core, the drusen with RPE damage, and the drusen with the EZ damage were more likely to be the dynamic drusen ($p < 0.001$).

Further multivariate analysis showed that the low-reflectivity drusen and the drusen with RPE damage were the independent predictors for AMD progression. In particular, the progressive OR of the low-reflectivity drusen was 2.95, while the high-reflectivity drusen was only 0.17 indicating that the low-reflectivity drusen were most likely to progress into advanced AMD and the high-reflectivity drusen were most likely to remain stable. These findings are consistent that the transition to a low internal reflectivity in the drusen is a dangerous signal of a transition toward CNV.

We found that all the six patients with the drusen with RPE damage eventually developed neovascular AMD including five patients with the drusen with the EZ damage. Multivariate analysis also showed that the progressive OR of the drusen with RPE damage over the drusen without RPE damage was 21.67. This is consistent with the traditional concept that RPE impairment significantly contributes to AMD (33–35). Ellipsoid corresponds to the outer part of the cone photoreceptor of the inner segments that are packed with the mitochondria and shows a continuous, high-reflection signal layer located over the RPE layer on SD-OCT (34, 36). The integrity of the EZ is an important indicator of the structural integrity of the photoreceptor. Disruption of the EZ caused by the various fundus diseases has been proven to be obviously correlated with abnormal photoreceptor function (37–39). Since the apical side of the RPE cells is in intimate contact with the outer segments of the photoreceptor and the drusen with RPE damage were independent predictors for AMD progression, drusen with the overlying EZ disruption ought to be a reasonable predictor for AMD progression. However, the p-value of this factor slightly exceeded 0.05 in the GEE analysis. However, the result could be different if more eyes were included in this study. We did not observe a decrease in the range of the RPE or EZ damage in any case suggesting that the RPE or EZ damage might be irreversible.

Sarks (40) studied the drusen by using panoramic electron microscopy and proved that the clinical drusen phenotypes differed in ultrastructure and, thus, in composition. He found that the amorphous substance in the small hard drusen was dense. When the small hard drusen grew larger than approximately 63 µm in size, the amorphous content became less compact. When the drusen reached confluence, the content of the drusen broke down and the particles of the amorphous material were of a smaller size. Histologically, the confluent soft drusen contain granular material apparently derived from the breakdown of the small hard drusen. When the globules break down further to very finely granular material, the drusen appeared empty or very finely granular on electron microscopy. On the other hand, Sarks (40) also noted that as the content breakdown, the drusen tended to lose both the sharp boundary and the nodular surface elevation, whereas the RPE over the broken-down drusen seemed to disappear, the photoreceptors appeared stunted, and there was a loss of overlying photoreceptor nuclei. Curcio proposed that the soft drusen/basal linear deposits (BLinDs) and subretinal drusenoid deposits (SDDs) confer the risk for end-stage atrophy and neovascularization. The life cycle of the soft drusen includes growth, anterior migration of RPE atop drusen, collapse, and atrophy (41, 42).

Lipid particles accumulate between the RPE and Bruch's membrane and form the drusen (43, 44). Due to the age-related changes, apoB100 lipoprotein accumulates in Bruch's membrane. Furthermore, the RPE synthesizes and secretes very-low-density lipoprotein (VLDL) and low-density lipoprotein (LDL) (45). Failure of the choriocapillaris–Bruch's membrane complex to clear the normal RPE secretions to plasma can lead to the accumulation of the drusen (40, 41, 45, 46). Differences in the lipid particle composition are most likely to result in the differences in internal reflectivity and the changes in the lipid particle composition within the drusen may be a sign of a poor prognosis for the drusen.

Vande Ven et al. (47) studied 19 eyes of 10 patients with the basal laminar drusen by using SD-OCT and found that the small hard drusen were subjected to the constant changes in volume during four months of follow-up. Small hard drusen with decreased reflectivity of the overlying RPE or photoreceptor layer were more likely to show volume regression, whereas the pointed, small hard drusen were more likely to show volume progression. The term basal laminar drusen has been superseded by the cuticular drusen (23). Balaratnasingam et al. (23) considered that the ultrastructural characteristics of the cuticular drusen appear similar to those of the hard drusen; however, their life cycle and macular complications are more comparable to those of the soft drusen. With more than five years of follow-up, the neovascularization and GA occurred at a frequency of 12.5 and 25% cuticular drusen eyes, respectively. In this study, the shape of the drusen was unrelated to the notable changes in SD-OCT in the subjects, which may be due to the relatively small sample size and a short follow-up period.

The limitations of this study include the consideration of SDDs accumulating in a different layer of the outer retina, appearing differently in the terms of retinal topography, and having a different pathological basis and pathogenicity than the drusen; therefore, the SDDs were not included in this study. As the focus of this article is on the relationship between the internal SD-OCT characteristics of the drusen and the prognosis of AMD, the hyperreflective foci above the drusen were not involved in the analysis. The other limitation of this study is that because the follow-up interval was up to six months, the study missed capturing the moment when the reflectivity of the drusen changed before the transformation into the neovascular lesions. Therefore, these results need to be confirmed in a clinical cohort study with larger sample size and a longer follow-up period with shorter follow-up intervals.

This study demonstrated the differences between the drusen that were stable and those that were dynamic, even with the relatively small sample size. To the best of our knowledge, this is the first prospective cohort study on the drusen in Chinese people.

In conclusion, the findings of this study suggest that the prognosis of the drusen is most strongly correlated with the reflectivity of the drusen and disruption of the overlying RPE layer. For the patients with the drusen of low inner reflectivity and concurrently decreased reflectivity of the overlying RPE and EZ layers on SD-OCT, an increased follow-up frequency is strongly recommended to avoid missing the opportunity of optimum treatment.

ETHICS STATEMENT

The studies involving human participants were reviewed and approved by the Human Ethics Committee of Zhongshan Ophthalmic Center. The patients/participants provided their written informed consent to participate in this study. Written informed consent was obtained from the individual(s) for the publication of any potentially identifiable images or data included in this article.

AUTHOR CONTRIBUTIONS

SY: study design, acquisition of data, analysis and interpretation of data, and drafting of the manuscript. XL: study design, analysis and interpretation of data, drafting of the manuscript, and critical revision. HX: analysis and interpretation of data. LM: acquisition of data and analysis and interpretation of data. HQ: recruiting patients and analysis and interpretation of data. ZG: study design, recruiting patients, and analysis and interpretation of data. CZ: drafting of the manuscript and critical revision. All authors contributed to the article and approved the submitted version.

REFERENCES

1. Congdon N, O'Colmain B, Klaver CC, Klein R, Muñoz B, Friedman DS, et al. Causes and prevalence of visual impairment among adults in the United States. *Arch Ophthalmol.* (2004) 122:477–85. doi: 10.1001/archopht.122.4.477
2. Augustin A, Sahel JA, Bandello F, Dardennes R, Maurel F, Negrini C, et al. Anxiety and depression prevalence rates in age-related macular degeneration. *Invest Ophthalmol Vis Sci.* (2007) 48:1498–503. doi: 10.1167/iovs.06-0761
3. Berman K, Brodaty H. Psychosocial effects of age-related macular degeneration. *Int Psychogeriatr.* (2006) 18:415–28. doi: 10.1017/S1041610205002905
4. Klein R, Klein BE, Tomany SC, Meuer SM, Huang GH. Ten-year incidence and progression of age-related maculopathy: The Beaver Dam eye study. *Ophthalmology.* (2002) 109:1767–79. doi: 10.1016/S0161-6420(02)01146-6
5. Bressler NM, Munoz B, Maguire MG, Vitale SE, Schein OD, Taylor HR, et al. Five-year incidence and disappearance of drusen and retinal pigment epithelial abnormalities. *Arch Ophthalmol.* (1995) 113:301–8. doi: 10.1001/archopht.1995.01100030055022
6. Zhang Y, Wang X, Godara P, Zhang T, Clark ME, Witherspoon CD, et al. Dynamism of dot subretinal drusenoid deposits in age-related macular degeneration demonstrated with adaptive optics imaging. *Retina.* (2018) 38:29–38. doi: 10.1097/IAE.0000000000001504
7. Tan AC, Pilgrim M, Fearn S, Bertazzo S, Tsolaki E, Morrell A, et al. Calcified nodules in retinal drusen are associated with disease progression with age-related macular degeneration. *Sci Transl Med.* (2018) 10:466–77. doi: 10.1126/scitranslmed.aat4544
8. Jaffe GJ, Chakravarthy U, Freund KB, Guymer RH, Holz FG, Liakopoulos S, et al. Imaging features associated with progression to geographic atrophy in age-related macular degeneration: CAM Report 5. *Ophthalmology.* (2020) 5:855–67. doi: 10.1016/j.oret.2020.12.009
9. Chen L, Messinger JD, Sloan KR, Wong J, Roorda A, Duncan JL, et al. Abundance and multimodal visibility of soft drusen in early age-related macular degeneration: a clinicopathologic correlation. *Retina.* (2020) 40:1644–8. doi: 10.1097/IAE.0000000000002893
10. Chen L, Messinger JD, Ferrara D, Freund KB, Curcio CA. Fundus autofluorescence in neovascular age-related macular degeneration, a clinicopathologic correlation relevant to macular atrophy. *Ophthalmology.* (2021). doi: 10.1016/j.oret.2021.01.012
11. Smith RT, Sohrab MA, Pumariega N, Chen Y, Chen J, Lee N, et al. Dynamic soft drusen remodelling in age-related macular degeneration. *Br J Ophthalmol.* (2010) 94:1618–23. doi: 10.1136/bjo.2009.166843
12. Lei J, Balasubramanian S, Abdelfattah NS, Nittala M, Sadda SR. Proposal of a simple optical coherence tomography-based scoring system for progression of age related macular degeneration. *Graefes Arch Clin Exp Ophthalmol.* (2017) 255:1551–8. doi: 10.1007/s00417-017-3693-y
13. Curcio CA, Zanzottera EC, Ach T, Balaratnasingam C, Freund KB. Activated retinal pigment epithelium, an optical coherence tomography biomarker for progression in age-related macular degeneration. *Invest Ophthalmol Vis Sci.* (2017) 58:BIO211-BIO226.
14. Oishi A, Thiele S, Nadal J, Oishi M, Fleckenstein M, Schmid M, et al. Prevalence, natural course, and prognostic role of refractile drusen in age-related macular degeneration. *Invest Ophthalmol Vis Sci.* (2017) 58:2198–206. doi: 10.1167/iovs.16-20781
15. Dolz-Marco R, Balaratnasingam C, Messinger JD, Li M, Ferrara D, Freund KB, et al. The border of macular atrophy in age-related macular degeneration: a clinicopathologic correlation. *Am J Ophthalmol.* (2018) 193:166–77. doi: 10.1016/j.ajo.2018.06.020
16. Jain N, Farsiu S, Khanifar AA, Bearelly S, Smith RT, Izatt JA, et al. Quantitative comparison of drusen segmented on SD-OCT versus drusen delineated on color fundus photographs. *Invest Ophthalmol Vis Sci.* (2010) 51:4875–83. doi: 10.1167/iovs.09-4962

17. Leuschen JN, Schuman SG, Winter KP, McCall MN, Wong WT, Chew EY, et al. Spectral-domain optical coherence tomography characteristics of intermediate age-related macular degeneration. *Ophthalmology.* (2013) 120:140–50. doi: 10.1016/j.ophtha.2012.07.004
18. Li M, Dolz-Marco R, Huisingh C, Messinger JD, Feist RM, Ferrara D, et al. Clinicopathologic correlation of geographic atrophy secondary to age-related macular degeneration. *Retina.* (2019) 39:802–16. doi: 10.1097/IAE.0000000000002461
19. Fleckenstein M, Charbel Issa P, Helb HM, Schmitz-Valckenberg S, Finger RP, Scholl HP, et al. High-resolution spectral domain-OCT imaging in geographic atrophy associated with age-related macular degeneration. *Invest Ophthalmol Vis Sci.* (2008) 49:4137–44. doi: 10.1167/iovs.08-1967
20. Gregori G, Wang F, Rosenfeld PJ, Yehoshua Z, Gregori NZ, Lujan BJ, et al. Spectral domain optical coherence tomography imaging of drusen in nonexudative age-related macular degeneration. *Ophthalmology.* (2011) 118:1373–9. doi: 10.1016/j.ophtha.2010.11.013
21. Khanifar AA, Koreishi AF, Izatt JA, Toth CA. Drusen ultrastructure imaging with spectral domain optical coherence tomography in age-related macular degeneration. *Ophthalmology.* (2008) 115:1883–90. doi: 10.1016/j.ophtha.2008.04.041
22. Staurenghi G, Sadda S, Chakravarthy U, Spaide RF. Proposed lexicon for anatomic landmarks in normal posterior segment spectral-domain optical coherence tomography: the IN*OCT consensus. *Ophthalmology.* (2014) 121:1572–8. doi: 10.1016/j.ophtha.2014.02.023
23. Balaratnasingam C, Cherepanoff S, Dolz-Marco R, Killingsworth M, Chen F, Mendis KR, et al. Cuticular drusen: clinical phenotypes and natural course defined using multimodal imaging. *Ophthalmology.* (2018) 125:100–18. doi: 10.1016/j.ophtha.2017.08.033
24. Ennis S, Gibson J, Cree AJ, Collins A, Lotery AJ. Support for the involvement of complement factor I in age-related macular degeneration. *Eur J Hum Genet.* (2010) 18:15–6. doi: 10.1038/ejhg.2009.113
25. Klein RJ, Zeiss C, Chew EY, Tsai JY, Sackler RS, Haynes C. Complement factor H polymorphism in age-related macular degeneration. *Science.* (2005) 308:385–9. doi: 10.1126/science.1109557
26. Ferris FL, Davis MD, Clemons TE, Lee LY, Chew EY. A simplified severity scale for age-related macular degeneration: AREDS Report No 18. *Arch Ophthalmol.* (2005) 123:1570–74. doi: 10.1001/archopht.123.11.1570
27. Folgar FA, Yuan EL, Sevilla MB, Chiu SJ, Farsiu S, Chew EY, et al. Drusen volume and retinal pigment epithelium abnormal thinning volume predict 2-year progression of age-related macular degeneration. *Ophthalmology.* (2016) 123:39–50 e31. doi: 10.1016/j.ophtha.2015.09.016
28. Veerappan M, El-Hage-Sleiman AM, Tai V, Chiu SJ, Winter KP, Stinnett SS, et al. Optical coherence tomography reflective drusen substructures predict progression to geographic atrophy in age-related macular degeneration. *Ophthalmology.* (2016) 123:2554–70. doi: 10.1016/j.ophtha.2016.08.047
29. Sleiman K, Veerappan M, Winter KP, McCall MN, Yiu G, Farsiu S, et al. Optical coherence tomography predictors of risk for progression to non-neovascular atrophic age-related macular degeneration. *Ophthalmology.* (2017) 124:1764–77. doi: 10.1016/j.ophtha.2017.06.032
30. Klein R, Davis MD, Magli YL, Segal P, Klein BE, Hubbard L. The wisconsin age-related maculopathy grading system. *Ophthalmology.* (1991) 98:1128–34. doi: 10.1016/S0161-6420(91)32186-9
31. Age-Related Eye Disease Study Research, Group. (2001). The Age-Related Eye Disease Study system for classifying age-related macular degeneration from stereoscopic color fundus photographs: the Age-Related Eye Disease Study report number 6. *Am J Ophthalmol.* 132:668–81. doi: 10.1016/S0002-9394(01)01218-1
32. Wu Z, Pfau M, Blodi BA, Holz FG, Jaffe GJ, Liakopoulos S, et al. Optical coherence tomography signs of early atrophy in age-related macular degeneration: inter-reader agreement: CAM Report 6. *Ophthalmol.* (2021) doi: 10.1016/j.oret.2021.03.008
33. Yang P, Tyrrell J, Han I, Jaffe GJ. Expression and modulation of RPE cell membrane complement regulatory proteins. *Invest Ophthalmol Vis Sci.* (2009) 50:3473–81. doi: 10.1167/iovs.08-3202
34. Seddon JM, McLeod DS, Bhutto IA, Villalonga MB, Silver RE, Wenick AS, et al. Histopathological insights into choroidal vascular loss in clinically documented cases of age-related macular degeneration. *JAMA Ophthalmol.* (2016) 134:1272–80. doi: 10.1001/jamaophthalmol.2016.3519
35. Schlanitz F, Baumann B, Sacu S, Baumann L, Pircher M, Hitzenberger CK, et al. Impact of drusen and drusenoid retinal pigment epithelium elevation size and structure on the integrity of the retinal pigment epithelium layer. *Br J Ophthalmol.* (2019) 103:227–232. doi: 10.1136/bjophthalmol-2017-311782
36. Suh MH, Seo JM, Park KH, Yu HG. Associations between macular findings by optical coherence tomography and visual outcomes after epiretinal membrane removal. *Am J Ophthalmol.* (2009) 147:473–480. doi: 10.1016/j.ajo.2008.09.020
37. Scarinci F, Jampol LM, Linsenmeier RA, Fawzi AA. Association of diabetic macular nonperfusion with outer retinal disruption on optical coherence tomography. *JAMA Ophthalmol.* (2015) 133:1036–44. doi: 10.1001/jamaophthalmol.2015.2183
38. Oishi A, Shimozono M, Mandal M, Hata M, Nishida A, Kurimoto Y. Recovery of photoreceptor outer segments after anti- VEGF therapy for age-related macular degeneration. *Graefes Arch Clin Exp Ophthalmol.* (2013) 251:435–40. doi: 10.1007/s00417-012-2034-4
39. Spaide R, Curcio CA. Anatomic correlates to the bands seen in the outer retina by optical coherence tomography: literature review and model. *Retina.* (2011) 31:1609–19. doi: 10.1097/IAE.0b013e3182247535
40. JP, Sarks SH, Killingsworth MC. Evolution of soft drusen in age-related macular degeneration. *Eye.* (1994) 8:269–83. doi: 10.1038/eye.1994.57
41. Curcio CA. Soft drusen in age-related macular degeneration: biology and targeting, via the Oil Spill Strategy. *Invest Ophthalmol Vis Sci.* (2018) 59:AMD160-AMD181. doi: 10.1167/iovs.18-24882
42. Mullins RF, Khanna A, Schoo DP, Tucker BA, Sohn EH, Drack AV, et al. Is age-related macular degeneration a microvascular disease? *Adv Exp Med Biol.* (2014) 801:283–9. doi: 10.1007/978-1-4614-3209-8_36
43. An E, Lu X, Flippin J, Devaney JM, Halligan B, Hoffman EP, et al. Secreted proteome profiling in human RPE cell cultures derived from donors with age related macular degeneration and age matched healthy donors. *J Proteome Res.* (2006) 5:2599–610. doi: 10.1021/pr060121j
44. Curcio CA. Antecedents of Soft Drusen, the Specific Deposits of Age-Related Macular Degeneration, in the Biology of Human Macula. *Invest Ophthalmol Vis Sci.* (2018) 59:AMD182–194. doi: 10.1167/iovs.18-24883
45. Curcio CA, Johnson M, Huang JD, Rudolf M. Apolipoprotein B-containing lipoproteins in retinal aging and age-related macular degeneration. *J Lipid Res.* (2010) 51:451–67. doi: 10.1194/jlr.R002238
46. Pilgrim MG, Lengyel I, Lanzirotti A, Newville M, Fearn S, Emri E, et al. Sub-retinal pigment epithelial deposition of drusen components including hydroxyapatite in a primary cell culture model. *Invest Ophthalmol Vis Sci.* (2017) 58:708–19. doi: 10.1167/iovs.16-21060
47. van de Ven JP, Boon CJ, Smailhodzic D, Lechanteur YT, den Hollander AI, Hoyng CB, et al. Short-term changes of Basal laminar drusen on spectral-domain optical coherence tomography. *Am J Ophthalmol.* (2012) 154(3):560–567. doi: 10.1016/j.ajo.2012.03.012

25

Diagnosability of Keratoconus Using Deep Learning with Placido Disk-Based Corneal Topography

Kazutaka Kamiya[1], Yuji Ayatsuka[2], Yudai Kato[2], Nobuyuki Shoji[3], Yosai Mori[4] and Kazunori Miyata[4]*

[1] Visual Physiology, School of Allied Health Sciences, Kitasato University, Kanagawa, Japan, [2] Cresco Ltd., Tokyo, Japan, [3] Department of Ophthalmology, School of Medicine, Kitasato University, Kanagawa, Japan, [4] Department of Ophthalmology, Miyata Eye Hospital, Miyazaki, Japan

***Correspondence:**
Kazutaka Kamiya
kamiyak-tky@umin.ac.jp*

Purpose: Placido disk-based corneal topography is still most commonly used in daily practice. This study was aimed to evaluate the diagnosability of keratoconus using deep learning of a color-coded map with Placido disk-based corneal topography.

Methods: We retrospectively examined 179 keratoconic eyes [Grade 1 (54 eyes), 2 (52 eyes), 3 (23 eyes), and 4 (50 eyes), according to the Amsler-Krumeich classification], and 170 age-matched healthy eyes, with good quality images of corneal topography measured with a Placido disk corneal topographer (TMS-4^{TM}, Tomey). Using deep learning of a color-coded map, we evaluated the diagnostic accuracy, sensitivity, and specificity, for keratoconus screening and staging tests, in these eyes.

Results: Deep learning of color-coded maps exhibited an accuracy of 0.966 (sensitivity 0.988, specificity 0.944) in discriminating keratoconus from normal eyes. It also exhibited an accuracy of 0.785 (0.911 for Grade 1, 0.868 for Grade 2, 0.920 for Grade 3, and 0.905 for Grade 4) in classifying the stage. The area under the curve value was 0.997, 0.955, 0.899, 0.888, and 0.943 as Grade 0 (normal) to 4 grading tests, respectively.

Conclusions: Deep learning using color-coded maps with conventional corneal topography effectively distinguishes between keratoconus and normal eyes and classifies the grade of the disease, indicating that this will become an aid for enhancing the diagnosis and staging ability of keratoconus in a clinical setting.

Keywords: deep learning, keratoconus, diagnosis, accuracy, corneal topography

INTRODUCTION

Keratoconus has been widely recognized as a progressive disease characterized by anterior bulging and local thinning of the cornea. Based on the fact that keratoconic patients tend to have high myopic astigmatism, the percentage of such patients among all candidates for corneal refractive surgery has shown to be relatively high. Therefore, it is clinically essential to effectively exclude keratoconus among refractive surgery candidates to prevent the post-operative occurrence of iatrogenic keratectasia.

In previous studies, simple multi-layer neural networks, support vector machines, or decision trees were applied to machine learning for keratoconus detection. We assume that the use of a convolutional neural network has advantages over other machine learning methods, since a convolutional neural network can directly extract the morphological characteristics from the obtained images without preliminary learning, and subsequently provide a higher classification precision, especially in the field of image recognition.

We previously reported that deep learning using multiple color-coded maps obtained from the anterior segment optical coherence tomography (OCT) was effective not only for the screening of keratoconus, but also for the grade classification (1). Placido disk-based corneal topography provides a high sensitivity and specificity to discriminate keratoconus from normal eyes, and is still widely used especially at private eye clinics in a clinical setting. Although corneal topography only examines the anterior corneal surface, it is still most commonly used in daily practice. However, deep learning technique has so far not been fully elucidated for keratoconus detection using Placido disk-based corneal topography. Moreover, this technique has not been applied for the keratoconus staging capability using corneal topography. It may be clinically meaningful not only as a pre-operative screening test of refractive surgery candidates, but also as a staging test for understanding the severity of the disease, especially in consideration of high prevalence of such devices. The goal of the present study is to evaluate the diagnostic capability of deep learning using conventional corneal topography, in terms of the disease screening and the stage classification.

METHODS

Study Population

We registered the study protocol with the University Hospital Medical Information Network Clinical Trial Registry (000040128). A total of 349 eyes with good quality images of corneal topography measured with a Placido disk corneal topographer (TMS-4^{TM}, Tomey, Aichi, Japan) were included in this case series. Multiple corneal specialists diagnosed keratoconus with distinctive features (e.g., corneal color-coded map with asymmetric bow-tie pattern with or without skewed axes), and at least one keratoconus sign (e.g., stromal thinning, conical bulging, Fleischer ring, Vogt striae, or apical scar) (2). We utilized the Amsler-Krumeich classification to evaluate the grade of the disease [Grade 1 (54 eyes), 2 (52 eyes), 3 (23 eyes), and 4 (50 eyes)] (3). As a control group we examined 170 eyes in subjects with normal ocular findings applying for a contact lens fitting or for a refractive surgery consultation, who had a refractive error of <6 diopters (D) as well as astigmatism of <3 D. We asked the patients who wore rigid and soft contact lenses to stop wearing them for 3 and 2 weeks, respectively. This review was approved by the Institutional Review Board of Miyata Eye Hospital (CS-315), and followed the tenets of the Declaration of Helsinki. The Institutional Review Board waived the requirement for informed consent for this retrospective study.

Placido Disk-Based Corneal Topography

We performed corneal topography using a Placido disk-based corneal topographer (TMS-4^{TM}, Tomey Corporation, Nagoya, Japan). Patients were asked to blink just before starting measurements. We obtained an absolute topography map (9.0–101.5 diopter (D), 5 D step), in accordance with the manufacturer's instructions, because this scale is widely used in daily practice. We acquired at least three topographic images with this corneal topographer. We manually excluded poor-quality data (e.g., blinking artifacts, or poor detections of topographic images), and selected one topographic map with a high image quality.

Deep Learning

Detailed methods for deep learning were described previously (1). In brief, we exported the data of a single image by taking a screenshot, and stored it in a lossless compression format such as PNG. We excluded the color-scaled bar for this image analysis. We made one classifier for the Placido disk-based color-coded map. We utilized an open source deep learning platform (PyTorch) for deep learning with a VGG-16 network model. This model has been pre-trained by 3,390 color-coded map images that were composed of anterior and posterior elevation, anterior and posterior curvature, total refractive power, and pachymetry maps obtained with an anterior segment OCT (CASIA2^{TM}, Tomey Corporation, Nagoya, Japan) (1). Each input image without the color-scaled bar was resized to 224-by-224 pixels without deformation. The output (one value of 0–4) can be mapped to the grades (including normal eyes). "Normal" is represented as "0," and grades 1, 2, 3, and 4 are denoted as "1," "2," "3," and "4" in teaching data. Each network classifies an image into 0–4. The output value of neural network for an image is a real number, so that we aligned it to the nearest integer value to interpret. For example, if the output value is "2.67," it is interpreted as "3" (classified as Grade 3). A total of 349 eyes were split into seven groups (49 or 50 eyes in each group) based on our preliminary evaluation. We applied 7-fold cross-validation with validation and test set to increase the reliability of the accuracy outcomes of the classifier. For each fold, five of seven sets were used for training and one of the remaining two sets was used for validation, finally the model was tested with the remaining one set after the training finished (training set: validation set: test set = 5:1:1). We calculated the sensitivity, the specificity, and the accuracy as follows: sensitivity = true positive / (true positive + false negative), specificity = true negative/(true negative + false positive), and accuracy = (true positive + true negative)/(true positive + false positive + true negative + false negative). We also calculated the receiver operating characteristic curve and the area under the curve (AUC) as the area under the cumulative distribution function of the sensitivity on the y-axis vs. the cumulative distribution function of (1-specificity) on the x-axis, using a statistical software (Bellcurve for Excel, Social Survey Research Information Co, Ltd., Tokyo, Japan).

RESULTS

Table 1 shows the patient demographics of the study population. **Figure 1** shows a representative color-coded map measured with the Placido disk-based corneal topography. **Table 2** shows the output data of deep learning of single color-coded maps

TABLE 1 | The demographics of the study population according to the Amsler-Krumeich classification.

Characteristic	Control	Grade 1	Grade 2	Grade 3	Grade 4
Age (years)	36.9 ± 12.5	34.1 ± 18.0	35.4 ± 14.1	35.4 ± 15.0	39.4 ± 14.6
LogMAR UCVA	0.76 ± 0.66	0.48 ± 0.55	0.94 ± 0.60	0.91 ± 0.56	1.27 ± 0.58
LogMAR BSCVA	−0.17 ± 0.04	−0.03 ± 0.12	0.15 ± 0.32	0.23 ± 0.32	0.46 ± 0.38
Manifest sphere (D)	−3.07 ± 3.44	−2.32 ± 3.52	−4.74 ± 4.63	−4.23 ± 3.99	−4.67 ± 5.43
Manifest cylinder (D)	−0.67 ± 0.73	−2.10 ± 1.77	−3.40 ± 1.86	−3.24 ± 1.55	−2.68 ± 2.61
Flat keratomtry (D)	43.1 ± 1.2	43.2 ± 1.7	46.2 ± 3.0	49.8 ± 4.7	52.6 ± 4.6
Steep keratometry (D)	44.6 ± 1.5	46.3 ± 2.1	51.0 ± 3.8	55.7 ± 5.0	58.8 ± 6.4

LogMAR, logarithm of the minimal angle of resolution; UCVA, uncorrected visual acuity; BSCVA, best spectacle corrected visual acuity; D, diopter.

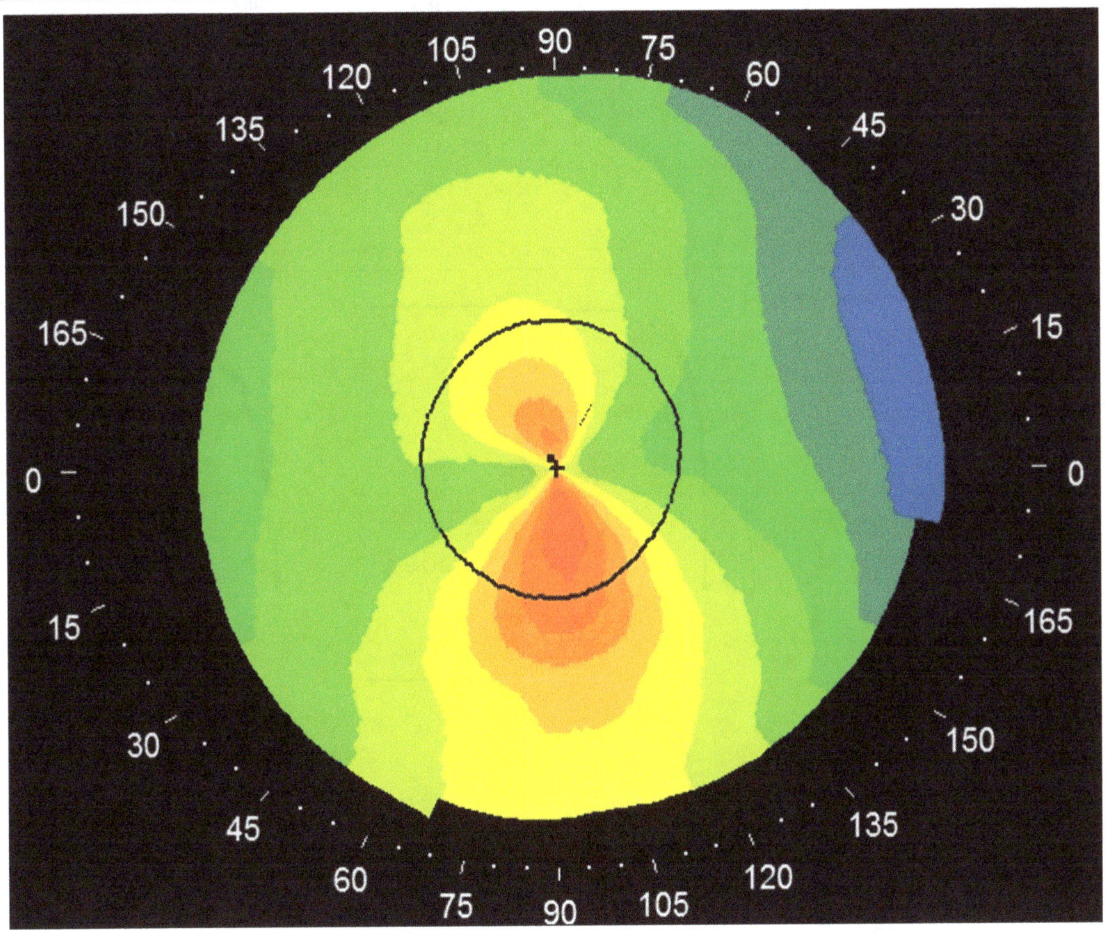

FIGURE 1 | A representative image of a single color-coded map (absolute axial map) by the Placido disk-based corneal topography. A color-scale bar was eliminated for deep learning.

with corneal topography in terms of the grade classification for test data sets. **Table 3** shows the sensitivity, the specificity, and the accuracy of deep learning of a single color-coded map with corneal topography in the grade classification according to the Amsler-Krumeich classification. Deep learning of the color-coded map exhibited an accuracy of 0.966 (sensitivity 0.988, specificity 0.944), in discriminating keratoconus from normal cornea. It also exhibited an overall accuracy of 0.785 (sensitivity 0.611, specificity 0.966 for Grade 1, sensitivity 0.615, specificity 0.912 for Grade 2, sensitivity 0.281, specificity 0.957 for Grade 3, and sensitivity 0.640, specificity 0.950 for Grade 4) in classifying the stage of the disease. **Figure 2** shows the receiver operating characteristic curves of classifying normal and Grade 1 to 4 keratoconic eyes, and the AUC value was 0.997, 0.955, 0.899, 0.888, and 0.943 as Grade 0 (normal) to 4 grading tests, respectively.

TABLE 2 | The output data for test sets of deep learning in the grade classification according to the Amsler-Krumeich classification.

	Output of Convolutional Neural Network					
Actual Category	**Normal**	**G1**	**G2**	**G3**	**G4**	**Total**
Normal	168	2	0	0	0	170
G1	9	33	11	0	1	54
G2	0	6	32	8	6	52
G3	0	1	5	9	8	23
G4	1	1	10	6	32	50

TABLE 3 | The sensitivity, the specificity, and the accuracy of deep learning in the grade classification according to the Amsler-Krumeich classification.

Category	True positive	True negative	False negative	False positive	Sensitivity	Specificity	Accuracy
Normal	168	169	2	10	0.988	0.944	0.966
G1	33	285	21	10	0.611	0.966	0.911
G2	32	271	20	26	0.615	0.912	0.868
G3	9	312	14	14	0.281	0.957	0.920
G4	32	284	18	15	0.640	0.950	0.905
Total							0.785

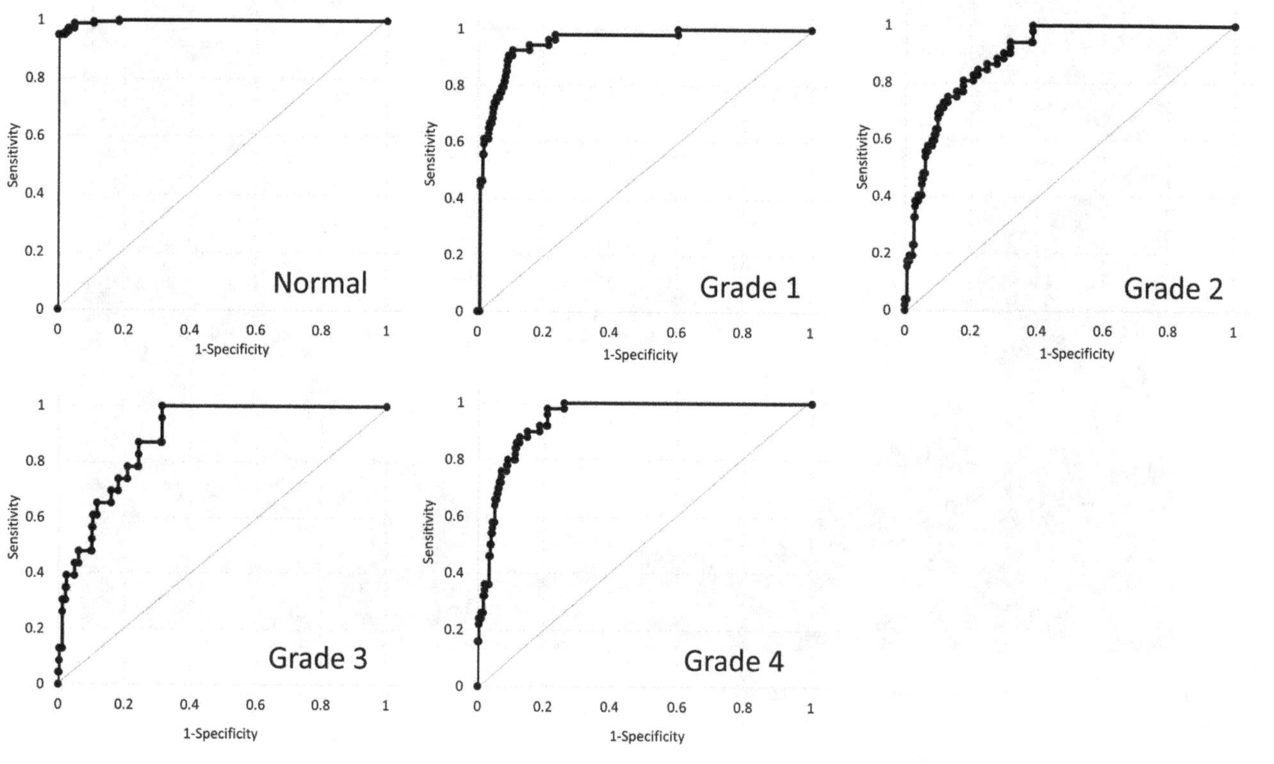

FIGURE 2 | Receiver operating characteristic curves of classifying normal and Grade 1 to 4 keratoconic eyes using deep learning.

DISCUSSION

In the current study, our findings demonstrated that deep learning of a single color-coded map with a corneal topographer will be beneficial not only for the disease screening, but also for the stage classification. To our knowledge, this is the first study to investigate both the diagnostic and disease staging capability of deep learning of a single image with conventional Placido disk-based corneal topography. In terms of simple keratoconus detection, Kuo et al. compared deep learning algorithms to detect keratoconus on the basis of corneal topography, showing that the accuracy was 0.931, 0.931, and 0.958, when using the

VGG16, InceptionV3, ResNet152 models, respectively. However, this study was not age-matched with a significant difference in age between the groups, and the numbers of the subjects (94 and 84) were still limited in the keratoconus and control groups, respectively (4). Since it is still difficult to differentiate keratoconus from normal cornea in daily practice, when using only slit-lamp examination, we assume that it will become an aid as a screening and staging test for keratoconus, especially in consideration of the higher prevalence of corneal topography in a clinical setting.

So far many studies on keratoconus detection have been conducted using machine learning methods. However, most studies have just utilized topographic or tomographic numeric indices that can grasp the overall corneal shape, but this hides the spatial gradients and distributions of the corneal curvature. In recent years, several studies on keratoconus detection using deep learning have been reported (1, 5–9). Dos Santos et al. stated that a custom neural network architecture could segment both healthy and keratoconus images with high accuracy (5). Abdelmotaal et al. demonstrated, using color-coded Scheimpflug images, that a convolutional neural network classified four map-selectable display images with average accuracies of 0.983 and 0.958 for the training and test sets, respectively (7). Elsawy et al. developed the multi-disease deep learning diagnostic algorithm providing an F1 score >0.90 for keratoconus detection using the As-OCT images (8). Feng et al. proposed an end-to-end deep learning approach utilizing raw data obtained by the Pentacam system for keratoconus and subclinical keratoconus detection (9). Chen et al. also showed that convolutional neural network provides excellent performance for keratoconus detection and grading classification using the axial map, anterior and posterior elevation map, and pachymetry maps obtained by the Scheimpflug camera (10). We assume that the use of a color-coded map has advantages over that of numeric values for machine learning, because it can bring us a larger amount of anterior corneal curvature information than these numeric values. These findings were in agreement with our current findings using corneal topography. Our study is somewhat different from their study in that we assessed the stage-classification capability of the disease, which is clinically meaningful to determine the surgical indication, as well as to predict the visual prognosis of such keratoconic patients, and that adopt a cross-validation with validation and test set to increase the reliability of the accuracy outcomes of the classifier.

In the current study, the overall accuracy using a single map with Placido disk-based corneal topography was slightly lower than that using multiple maps with the OCT, in terms of the keratoconus screening (vs. 0.991) and the keratoconus staging (vs. 0.874) (1). Moreover, even when we compared the same single absolute map of anterior corneal curvature between the two instruments, the accuracy using the corneal topography was slightly lower than that using the OCT (vs. 0.976). We previously reported, using the rotating Scheimpflug tomography, that the cases of lower staging had a larger area under the receiver operating characteristic curve in the posterior elevation differences than in the anterior elevation differences (11), and that the accuracy of various elevation, pachymetry, and keratometry indices was overall high, but that posterior and anterior elevation differences were the most effective parameters for the diagnosis of keratoconus (12). These findings highlight the importance of the corneal posterior information as a diagnostic ability using the corneal tomographer. Based on our current and previous findings, we can detect keratoconus only using the Placido-based corneal topography in almost all eyes, but the use of OCT-based or Scheimpflug-based corneal tomography is still recommended to further improve the diagnostic accuracy, especially for the early diagnosis of keratoconus.

Our limitations to this study are as follows: Firstly, we only used normal corneas as a control group, and that we did not include other corneal disorders, such as forme fruste keratoconus, subclinical keratoconus, or post-keratoplasty eyes. Accordingly, we cannot refute the possibility that the disease category and the inclusion criteria might influence the diagnosability of keratoconus. Secondly, we did not totally eliminate the effect of rigid or soft contact lenses on corneal topographic measurements. Although we asked the patients to stop wearing rigid gas permeable lenses and soft contact lenses for 3 and 2 weeks, respectively, before this evaluation, it is clinically difficult for such patients to stop wearing contact lenses for a long period of time, in consideration of their daily life activities. Thirdly, it is still difficult to accurately diagnose keratoconus by ophthalmologists, and its diagnosis can be influenced not only by the definition but also by the severity of the disease. We still need to have ophthalmologists read the same dataset and compare the performance of this model with the ophthalmologists' readings. Fourthly, we used healthy eyes with astigmatism of <3 D as a control group, in accordance with previous studies on keratoconus detection. Therefore, we did not guarantee that healthy eyes with a large amount of astigmatism could be classified as normal eyes using this network. A further research in another population is still necessary to clarify this point.

CONCLUSIONS

In summary, our findings may support the view that deep learning of a single color-coded map with a conventional corneal topographer is clinically helpful not only for keratoconus screening, but also for stage classification. We assume that it will also become an aid for keratoconus detection using a conventional topography in daily practice. We await a further external validation using another study population to confirm the authenticity of our results.

ETHICS STATEMENT

The studies involving human participants were reviewed and approved by Institutional Review Board of Miyata Eye Hospital (CS-315). Written informed consent from the participants' legal guardian/next of kin was not required to participate in this study in accordance with the national legislation and the institutional requirements.

AUTHOR CONTRIBUTIONS

KK, NS, and KM were involved in the design and conducted the study. KK, YA, YK, and YM were involved in collection, management, analysis, and interpretation of data. KK, YA, YK, NS, YM, and KM were involved in preparation, review, and final approval of the manuscript. All authors contributed to the article and approved the submitted version.

REFERENCES

1. Kamiya K, Ayatsuka Y, Kato Y, Fujimura F, Takahashi M, Shoji N, et al. Keratoconus detection using deep learning of colour-coded maps with anterior segment optical coherence tomography: a diagnostic accuracy study. *BMJ Open.* (2019) 9:e031313. doi: 10.1136/bmjopen-2019-031313
2. Rabinowitz YS. Keratoconus. *Surv Ophthalmol.* (1998) 42:297–319. doi: 10.1016/S0039-6257(97)00119-7
3. Krumeich JH, Kezirian GM. Circular keratotomy to reduce astigmatism and improve vision in stage I and II keratoconus. *J Refract Surg.* (2009) 25:357–65. doi: 10.3928/1081597X-20090401-07
4. Kuo BI, Chang WY, Liao TS, Liu FY, Liu HY, Chu HS, et al. Keratoconus screening based on deep learning approach of corneal topography. *Transl Vis Sci Technol.* (2020) 9:53. doi: 10.1167/tvst.9.2.53
5. Dos Santos VA, Schmetterer L, Stegmann H, Pfister M, Messner A, Schmidinger G, et al. CorneaNet: fast segmentation of cornea OCT scans of healthy and keratoconic eyes using deep learning. *Biomed Opt Express.* (2019) 10:622–41. doi: 10.1364/BOE.10.000622
6. Xie Y, Zhao L, Yang X, Wu X, Yang Y, Huang X, et al. Screening candidates for refractive surgery with corneal tomographic-based deep learning. *JAMA Ophthalmol.* (2020) 138:519–26. doi: 10.1001/jamaophthalmol.2020.0507
7. Abdelmotaal H, Mostafa MM, Mostafa ANR, Mohamed AA, Abdelazeem K. Classification of color-coded scheimpflug camera corneal tomography images using deep learning. *Transl Vis Sci Technol.* (2020) 9:30. doi: 10.1167/tvst.9.13.30
8. Elsawy A, Eleiwa T, Chase C, Ozcan E, Tolba M, Feuer W, et al. Multidisease deep learning neural network for the diagnosis of corneal diseases. *Am J Ophthalmol.* (2021) 226:252–61. doi: 10.1016/j.ajo.2021.01.018
9. Feng R, Xu Z, Zheng X, Hu H, Jin X, Chen DZ, et al. KerNet: a novel deep learning approach for keratoconus and sub-clinical keratoconus detection based on raw data of the pentacam system. *IEEE J Biomed Health Inform.* (2021). doi: 10.1109/JBHI.2021.3079430. [Epub ahead of print].
10. Chen X, Zhao J, Iselin KC, Borroni D, Romano D, Gokul A, et al. Keratoconus detection of changes using deep learning of colour-coded maps. *BMJ Open Ophthalmol.* (2021) 6:e000824. doi: 10.1136/bmjophth-2021-000824
11. Ishii R, Kamiya K, Igarashi A, Shimizu K, Utsumi Y, Kumanomido T. Correlation of corneal elevation with severity of keratoconus by means of anterior and posterior topographic analysis. *Cornea.* (2012) 31:253–8. doi: 10.1097/ICO.0B013E31823D1EE0
12. Kamiya K, Ishii R, Shimizu K, Igarashi A. Evaluation of corneal elevation, pachymetry and keratometry in keratoconic eyes with respect to the stage of Amsler-Krumeich classification. *Br J Ophthalmol.* (2014) 98:459–63. doi: 10.1136/bjophthalmol-2013-304132

26

Clinical and Multi-Mode Imaging Features of Eyes with Peripapillary Hyperreflective Ovoid Mass-Like Structures

Xiao Xie[1,2,3,4], *Tingting Liu*[2,3,4,5*], *Wenqi Wang*[1,2,3,4], *Ge Tian*[2,3,4,5], *Jinyan Wang*[2,3,4,5], *Jitian Guan*[2,3,4,5], *Meng Chen*[6], *Xunchang Wang*[2,3,4,5] and *Qingjun Zhou*[3,4,5,7]

[1] *The First Clinical Medical College of Shandong University of Traditional Chinese Medicine, Jinan, China,* [2] *Eye Hospital of Shandong First Medical University (Shandong Eye Hospital), Jinan, China,* [3] *State Key Laboratory Cultivation Base, Shandong Provincial Key Laboratory of Ophthalmology, Shandong Eye Institute, Qingdao, China,* [4] *Shandong First Medical University and Shandong Academy of Medical Sciences, Qingdao, China,* [5] *School of Ophthalmology, Shandong First Medical University, Jinan, China,* [6] *Zaozhuang Shizhong District People's Hospital, Zaozhuang, China,* [7] *Qingdao Eye Hospital of Shandong First Medical University, Qingdao, China*

***Correspondence:**
Tingting Liu
tingtingliu@vip.sina.com

Purpose: To observe and analyze the clinical and multi-mode imaging features of eyes with PHOMS, and to introduce two cases of PHOMS which underwent multi-mode imaging.

Methods: Retrospective clinical observational study. A total of 26 patients (37 eyes) with hyperreflective structures surrounded by hyporeflective edges around the optic discs who were examined and diagnosed at Shandong Eye Hospital between January 2019 and June 2021 were included in the study. Among these patients, 12 were male and 14 were female. Fifteen were monocular. The average age was 39 years. All patients underwent the following examinations: Best-corrected visual acuity (BCVA), intraocular pressure examinations, slit-lamp anterior segment examinations, indirect ophthalmoscopy, visual field examinations, fundus color photography, fundus autofluorescence (FAF), optical coherence tomography (OCT), and optical coherence tomography angiography (OCTA). Some of the patients were examined with fundus fluorescein angiography (FFA). Clinical data and imaging characteristics from the OCT, OCTA, and FFA were analyzed retrospectively.

Results: We found the hyperreflective structures surrounded by hyporeflective edges around the optic discs in 37 eyes. EDI-OCT results revealed hyperreflective structures surrounded by hyporeflective edges around the optic discs in all eyes. Typical hyperreflexia lesions occurred around the optic disc, located subretinally and above Bruch's membrane. OCTA revealed that the highly reflective perioptic material also had vascular structures.

Conclusion: EDI-OCT of PHOMS showed hyperreflective structures surrounded by hyporeflective edges around all of the optic discs. Infra-red photography showed temporal hyperreflexia. These characteristics can be seen in a variety of diseases and may be a relatively common feature revealed by EDI-OCT scanning. These characteristics may also be seen in elderly patients as well as children. PHOMS may be found in optic disc drusen (ODD), tilted disc syndrome (TDS), optic neuritis, ischemic optic neuropathy, and in white dot syndromes. Few patients may be developed into macular neovascularization (MNV). In order to improve the accuracy and robustness of the conclusions and provide better clinical guidance, we need to conduct more comprehensive research in the subsequent clinical work.

Keywords: peripapillary hyperreflective ovoid mass-like structures, optic disc drusen, optic disc edema, optical coherence tomography, regional blood flow imaging, multi-mode imaging features

INTRODUCTION

Peripapillary hyperreflective ovoid mass-like structures (PHOMS) are new imaging feature that have recently been revealed by EDI-OCT. In previously published literature, PHOMS was often diagnosed as buried optic disc drusen (ODD). It is also easily confused with optic disc edema (ODE) (1–7). In 2018, the term "PHOMS" was proposed by the Optic Disc Drusen Studies (ODDS) consortium to characterize the hyperreflective ovoid mass-like structures found on OCT images in the areas around the optic disc (8). The pathogenesis of PHOMS is not clear. Most researchers think it is a herniation of nerve fibers or axoplasmic stasis, or is related to congestion in the prelaminar optic nerve head (9, 10). Understandings of PHOMS have improved because of the application of optical coherence tomography (OCT), enhanced depth imaging optical coherence tomography (EDI-OCT) and optical coherence tomography angiography (OCTA). We recommend adopting this refined definition (11). Although there have been some reports about this disease, there are few studies about the clinical features of PHOMS that are based on multi-modal imaging. Here, we retrospectively analyzed the clinical manifestations and multi-modal imaging features of eyes with PHOMS. The OCT finding was investigated in a larger, more definitive, series of patients and termed PHOMS, and we found that PHOMS existed in some optic nerve diseases. This may indicate that PHOMS are novel and not well-characterized OCT findings occurring in several disorders of the optic nerve. We expect to provide more evidence for the clinical diagnosis and treatment of the disease.

METHODS

This was a retrospective clinical observational study. The study was approved by the Institutional Ethics Committee of Shandong eye hospital (approval No. 2019-G-012) on March 12, 2019. All experimental procedures were conducted in accordance with the Declaration of Helsinki (World Medical Association, as amended 2013) and the Health Insurance Portability and Accountability Act. All of the patients in this study agreed to provide identification information that was relevant to their pathology, and signed informed consent as required. A total of 26 patients (37 eyes) with PHOMS who were examined and diagnosed at Shandong Eye Hospital between January 2019 and June 2021 were included in the study. Among these patients, 12 were male and 14 were female. Fifteen were monocular. The average age was 39 years. The time from symptom onset to treatment ranged from 1 to 45 days, with an average time of 11 days. All patients complained of vision loss.

Inclusion Criteria

(1) The rim of the optic disc was blurred and bleeding could be seen in fundus color photography; (2) EDI-OCT revealed a hyperreflective structure surrounded by a hyporeflective edge around the optic disc.

Exclusion Criteria

(1) The ocular fundus was affected by severe refractive stroma opacity; (2) After repeated measurements, it was still not possible to obtain images that meet the analysis requirements.

All patients underwent the following examinations: Best-corrected visual acuity (BCVA) [with the international standard chart of vision and the minimum resolution logarithmic (LogMAR) vision chart], intraocular pressure examinations, slit-lamp examinations, indirect ophthalmoscopy, visual field examinations, fundus color photography, fundus autofluorescence (FAF), optical coherence tomography (OCT), and optical coherence tomography angiography (OCTA). Some of the patients were examined with fundus fluorescein angiography (FFA). We retrospectively analyzed the patients' clinical data OCT, OCTA, and FFA imaging characteristics.

OCT, OCTA, and FFA

We selected Heidelberg Spectralis HRA+OCT (Heidelberg Engineering, Heidelberg, Germany) for these examinations. The IR mode was used to track the subjects' optic discs, followed by the appropriate mode was used to obtain the structural images or retinal blood flow of the optic discs. When patients underwent FFA examinations, their skin tests were negative, and 3 ml of 20% fluorescein sodium was quickly injected into the middle elbow vein within a 5 s window.

Each patients' examinations were performed by the same doctor on the same day. If the position and quality of the image were not satisfactory, or if there were too many motion artifacts, the images were recorded again. The resulting images were reviewed by two other ophthalmologists with professional training. When there was a discrepancy between the ophthalmologists, a third ophthalmologist reviewed the scans so they could all reach a consensus. After the diagnosis, the primary disease treatment principle carried through intervention treatment, and patients received regular follow-up care.

TABLE 1 | Basic patient characteristics.

Number	Sex	Age	Eye	BCVA* (LogMAR)	PHOMS*	
					Width (μm)	Height (μm)
1	Male	54	OD	0.1	1427	504
2	Male	41	OS	1.0	619	312
3	Male	55	OD	0.7	678	402
			OS	0.4	602	377
4	Male	45	OD	0.3	560	386
			OS	0.1	745	333
5	Male	48	OD	0.2	729	225
6	Male	20	OD	0.3	555	454
			OS	0.3	757	640
7	Male	67	OD	0.2	898	547
8	Male	33	OD	0.8	485	321
			OS	0.9	530	517
9	Male	55	OD	1.0	685	503
			OS	0.9	342	279
10	Male	48	OD	0.1	845	306
			OS	0.1	793	452
11	Male	55	OD	1.0	347	247
			OS	0	309	256
12	Male	66	OS	0.2	855	404
13	Female	9	OD	0	2285	798
			OS	0.5	1604	839
14	Female	13	OS	0.9	424	427
15	Female	61	OD	0.7	464	219
			OS	1.0	598	301
16	Female	14	OD	1.0	625	286
			OS	0.9	596	372
17	Female	14	OD	0.3	766	392
18	Female	36	OS	1.0	556	243
19	Female	44	OD	0.9	722	365
20	Female	9	OS	0.7	952	490
21	Female	24	OS	1.0	492	413
22	Female	18	OD	1.0	512	595
23	Female	64	OS	0.4	693	378
24	Female	54	OD	1.0	506	319
25	Female	29	OD	0	471	194
			OS	0	875	422
26	Female	29	OD	0.6	780	256

**BCVA, best-corrected visual acuity; PHOMS, peripapillary hyperreflective ovoid mass-like structures; OD, oculus dexter; OS, oculus sinister.*

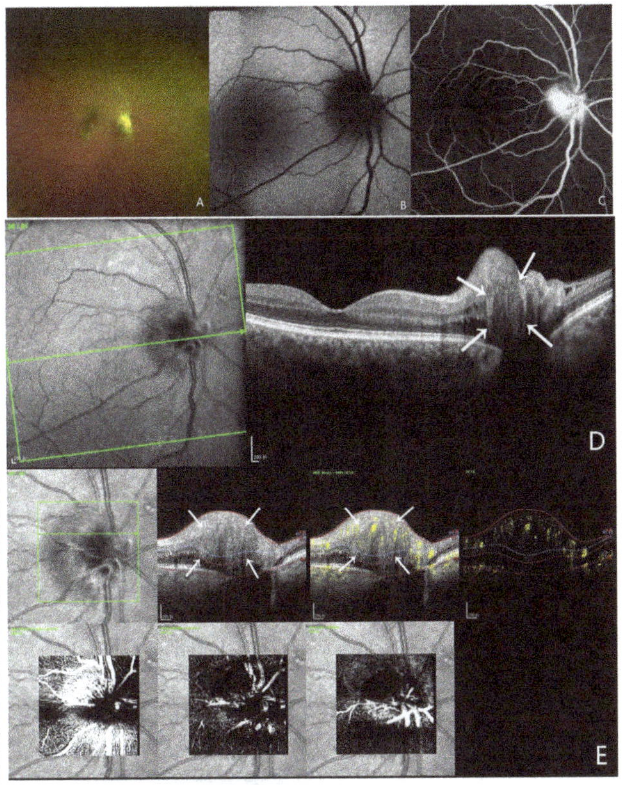

FIGURE 1 | Multi-modal image data of case 1. **(A)** Color fundus photography showed blurred boundaries and bleeding of the optic disc. **(B)** This case did not show autofluorescence. **(C)** FFA shows a hyperreflective optic disc with poorly defined boundaries. **(D)** OCT confirmed the presence of PHOMS, which is a hyperreflective ovoid mass-like structure surrounded by a hyporeflective edge around the optic disc. **(E)** OCTA showed a vascular complex, and there was a strong blood flow signal within this hyperreflective lesion.

RESULTS

Basic Characteristics of Patients

We found the hyperreflective structures surrounded by hyporeflective edges around the optic discs in 26 patients (37 eyes). As shown in **Table 1**, Among these patients, 12 were male and 14 were female. Fifteen were monocular. The average age was 38.65 ± 18.76 (Mean ± SD) years. The average BCVA was 0.55 ± 0.38 (Mean ± SD). PHOMS was present in patients diagnosed with a variety of diseases, including optic disc drusen (nine eyes), tilted disc syndrome (two eyes), optic neuritis (11 eyes), ischemic optic neuropathy (12 eyes), white dot syndromes (two eyes) and macular neovascularization (one eye). PHOMS widths ranged from 309 μm to 2285 μm (Mean ± SD: 721.14 ± 365.11), and their heights ranged from 194 μm to 839 μm (Mean ± SD: 399.30 ± 145.98).

Cases Sharing

Below, we have selected two cases with different characteristics to introduce PHOMS in detail.

Case 1

A 54-year-old man came to our department complaining of reduced visual acuity in the right eye. LogMAR BCVA was 0.1 for right eye. Intraocular pressure and slit-lamp anterior segment examinations were normal. The initial diagnosis was ischemic optic neuropathy in the right eye (**Figure 1**).

Case 2

A 9-year-old girl was brought to our department by her mother complaining of reduced visual acuity in the left eye. LogMAR BCVA examination was 0 for the right eye and 0.5 for the

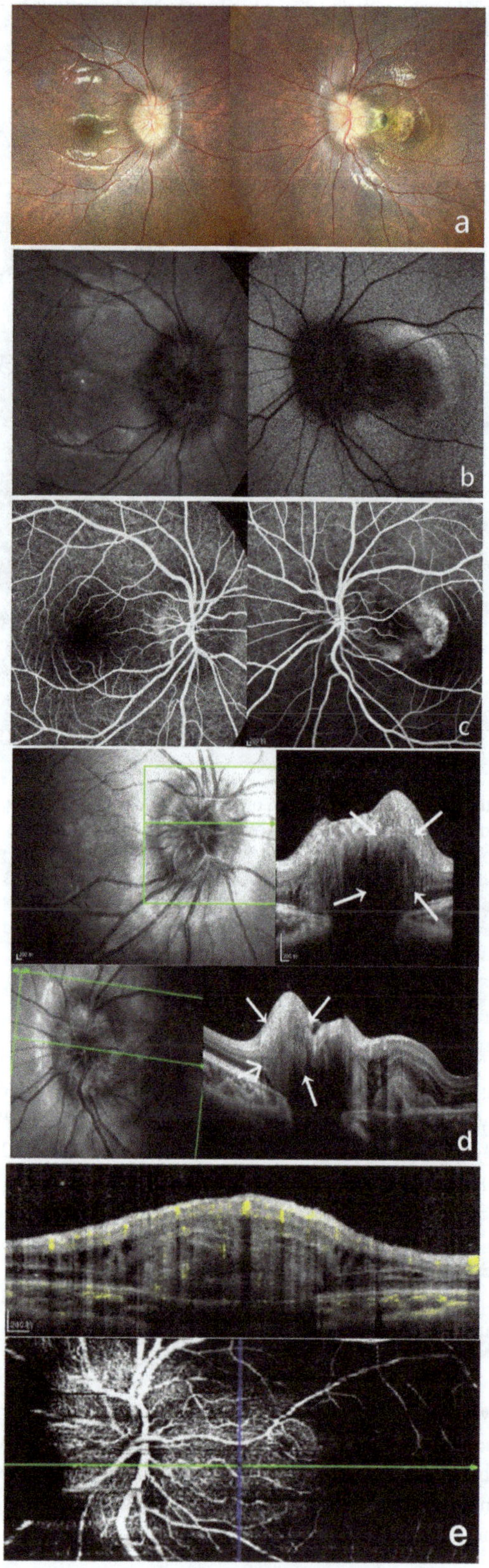

FIGURE 2 | Multi-modal image data of case 2. **(a)** Color fundus photography showed unclear optic disc boundaries, as well as are fibrosis and serous detachment of the retina in macular area. **(b)** This case did not show

(Continued)

FIGURE 2 | autofluorescence. **(c)** FFA shows a hyperreflective optic disc with poorly defined boundaries. **(d)** OCT shows a hyperreflective ovoid mass-like structure surrounded by a hyporeflective edge around the optic disc. **(e)** OCTA shows blood flow within this hyperreflective lesion.

left eye. Intraocular pressure and slit-lamp anterior segment examinations were normal. The initial diagnosis was binocular optic disc drusen (**Figure 2**).

DISCUSSION

In previous studies, PHOMS was found in cases of optic disc drusen (ODD), optic disc edema (ODE), pseudo-optic disc edema, tilted disc syndrome (TDS), and optic neuritis, as well as other diseases (8, 12–15). We found that PHOMS was also present in ischemic optic neuropathy and white dot syndromes. Further, some patients may be developed into macular neovascularization (MNV). Of the 26 patients (37 eyes) that we included in this study, 12 were male and 14 were female. The average age was 38.65 ± 18.76 (Mean ± SD) years. The average BCVA was 0.55 ± 0.38 (Mean ± SD). The average BCVA of patients under 50 years old was 0.54 ± 0.38 (Mean ± SD) and that of patients over 50 years old was 0.58 ± 0.37 (Mean ± SD). There was no significant difference, and there seemed to be no correlation between age and BCVA. Among them, including optic disc drusen (nine eyes), tilted disc syndrome (two eyes), optic neuritis (11 eyes), ischemic optic neuropathy (12 eyes), white dot syndromes (two eyes) and macular neovascularization (one eye). PHOMS widths ranged from 309 μm to 2285 μm (Mean ± SD: 721.14 ± 365.11). In females patients, there is only a 9-year-old girl whose PHOMS widths are larger. At the same time, there is also a 54-year-old man whose PHOMS width is larger. We think this was caused by individual differences. Excluding these two patients, the average PHOMS width of male patients was 629.67 ± 174.52 μm (Mean ± SD) and that of female patients was 627 ± 151.72 μm (Mean ± SD). There was no significant difference. Their heights ranged from 194 μm to 839 μm (Mean ± SD: 399.30 ± 145.98). We also found that PHOMS tended to be located outside and around the optic disc. PHOMS is defined as a hyperreflective ovoid mass-like structure with a hyperreflective interior without sharp outer edges or a hyporeflective core. PHOMS can typically not be found using fluorescence methods, and is not visible on B-scan ultrasonography despite its superficial location (16). It can also be seen in patients without apparent optic disc edema or poorly demarcated optic discs. During our follow-up, we found that PHOMS did not disappear. These findings are roughly the same as what has been previously reported in the literature (8, 9, 11, 17).

Early definitions of PHOMS were made with the context that they often occur alongside optic disc drusen (ODD) (18). With the development of multi-modal imaging, however, it appears that there are several features of PHOMS that are distinct from ODD, even though some symptoms overlap (8, 12, 13, 19–21). PHOMS does tend to be more common in patients with ODD. However, 26% of patients without ODD but with disc edema from NODD-AION had PHOMS (22). PHOMS do not correspond to clinically visible ODD. The same OCT findings can also be seen in patients without ODD (16).

In addition, PHOMS should be differentiated from true optic disc edema. Optic disc edema is caused by increased intracranial pressure or optic neuritis, and can be a serious threat to vision and life (3, 23). PHOMS may be caused by some degree of optic disc congestion or axonal stasis (17). Under certain circumstances, it is necessary to examine the patient's intracranial pressure at the time of initial diagnosis, and to examine the cause of intracranial pressure, using methods such as neuroimaging and lumbar punctures. In addition, OCT features of normal vessels are similar to those of vessels with PHOMS. However, the retina's vascular structures are located on the surface of the optic disc, and PHOMS structures are located subretinally and above Bruch's membrane (14). PHOMS were also observed in patients with myopic tilted discs, which is not related to papilledema nor ODD. It is now suggested, PHOMS are non-specific OCT findings of axonal distension and crowding that can be seen in acquired and dysplastic anomalies of the ONH (16). PHOMS is a new clinical feature found on the EDI-OCT in recent years. Multi-mode imaging has been proved to be a better way to identify PHOMS. EDI-OCT is the most sensitive and specific technique to identify PHOMS and thus serves as the mainstay of diagnosis.

Later with the advent of OCTA, we also found vascular complexes in PHOMS using OCTA. The OCTA revealed significant blood flow signals in these hyperreflective lesions, which may indicate there are vascular structures within them. This phenomenon has been described in several previous studies based on OCTA findings (8, 12, 13, 15), but PHOMS is a new clinical feature that has been demonstrated using EDI-OCT in recent years. Multi-modal imaging, especially OCTA, may be a better way to identify PHOMS.

Most researchers think PHOMS is caused by herniation of nerve fibers or axoplasmic stasis, or by prelaminar optic nerve head. Some histopathological evidence suggests that PHOMS is related to lateral bulges of nerve fibers in the retina. It might bring deeper vessels deputed at the irroration of the optic nerve into the retina. It may even lead to increased levels of vascular endothelial growth factor (VEGF) and the development of neovessels (8–10, 24), which could then lead to secondary CNV. Studies by Shinohara and Pichi et al. (based on OCT images) showed that the PHOMS protrudes from the upper edges of Bruch's membrane and choroid, and courses toward. This may help pinpoint PHOMS locations (12, 13). In recent years, OCTA technology has been able to better display fundus blood flow lesions, thus expanding the evaluation of deeper vascular layers (25). However the exact mechanisms that lead to the formation of PHOMS remain unknown, and more study is needed.

There are some limitations of our study. Patients' clinical features were not collected completely due to unfamiliarity with PHOMS features. This study is also limited to morphological analysis of PHOMS, and the exact pathophysiology remains unknown. In addition, due to the difficulty of following up on some patients, sufficient longitudinal data were not always collected. As a result, we have not carried out a comprehensive longitudinal discussion in this respect. Our study also had a small case number. We also did not look at the correlation between PHOMS and visual field defects. Although we have collected the quantitative measurement of PHOMS, certain clinical characteristics of PHOMS, and the pathogenesis of the disease, need further analysis. This could look like studying in whether PHOMS can be used to predict visual outcomes in neuro-ophthalmic disease, whether PHOMS size is associated with other measurements of optic disc edema, whether early discovery of PHOMS by OCT could be used to predict papilledema recurrence, and whether the size or location of a PHOMS could predict visual field (15). In order to improve the accuracy and robustness of the conclusions and provide better clinical guidance, we need to conduct more comprehensive research in the subsequent clinical work.

CONCLUSION

EDI-OCT is the most sensitive and specific technique to identify PHOMS and thus serves as the mainstay of diagnosis. EDI-OCT of PHOMS showed hyperreflective structures surrounded by hyporeflective edges around the optic discs. These characteristics may be unique features revealed by EDI-OCT and can be found in a variety of optic nerve diseases. Later with the advent of OCTA, we found that it may be developed into CNV. Future larger longitudinal studies may reveal the exact mechanisms leading to the OCT finding.

ETHICS STATEMENT

The study was approved by the Institutional Ethics Committee of Shandong Eye Hospital (approval No. 2019-G-012) on March 12, 2019. Written informed consent to participate in this study was provided by the participants' legal guardian/next of kin. Written informed consent was obtained from the individual(s), and minor(s)' legal guardian/next of kin, for the publication of any potentially identifiable images or data included in this article.

AUTHOR CONTRIBUTIONS

TL and XX designed research, conducted clinical examination, and drafted and revised the manuscript.

WW, GT, JW, JG, MC, XW, and QZ generated the figures and tables and organized the data and tables. All authors contributed to the article and approved the submitted version.

REFERENCES

1. Lee KM, Woo SJ, Hwang JM. Morphologic characteristics of optic nerve head drusen on spectral-domain optical coherence tomography. *Am J Ophthalmol.* (2013) 155:1139–47.e1. doi: 10.1016/j.ajo.2013.01.024
2. Bassi ST, Mohana KP. Optical coherence tomography in papilledema and pseudopapilledema with and without optic nerve head drusen. *Indian J Ophthalmol.* (2014) 62:1146–51. doi: 10.4103/0301-4738.149136
3. Lee KM, Woo SJ, Hwang JM. Differentiation of optic nerve head drusen and optic disc edema with spectral-domain optical coherence tomography. *Ophthalmology.* (2011) 118:971–7. doi: 10.1016/j.ophtha.2010.09.006
4. Gili P, Flores-Rodríguez P, Yangüela J, Orduña-Azcona J, Martín-Ríos MD. Sensitivity and specificity of monochromatic photography of the ocular fundus in differentiating optic nerve head drusen and optic disc oedema: optic disc drusen and oedema. *Graefes Arch Clin Exp Ophthalmol.* (2013) 251:923–8. doi: 10.1007/s00417-012-2223-1
5. Lee KM, Woo SJ, Hwang JM. Factors associated with visual field defects of optic disc drusen. *PLoS ONE.* (2018) 13:e0196001. doi: 10.1371/journal.pone.0196001
6. Friedman AH, Beckerman B, Gold DH, Walsh JB, Gartner S. Drusen of the optic disc. *Surv Ophthalmol.* (1977) 21:373–90. doi: 10.1016/0039-6257(77)90041-8
7. Tso MO. Pathology and pathogenesis of drusen of the optic nervehead. *Ophthalmology.* (1981) 88:1066–80. doi: 10.1016/S0161-6420(81)80038-3
8. Malmqvist L, Bursztyn L, Costello F, et al. The Optic Disc Drusen Studies Consortium Recommendations for Diagnosis of Optic Disc Drusen Using Optical Coherence Tomography. *J Neuroophthalmol.* (2018) 38:299–307. doi: 10.1097/WNO.0000000000000585
9. Borrelli E, Barboni P, Battista M, Digre K, Fraser JA, Fraser C, et al. Peripapillary hyperreflective ovoid mass-like structures (PHOMS): OCTA may reveal new findings. *Eye (Lond).* (2021) 35:528–31. doi: 10.1038/s41433-020-0890-4
10. Lyu IJ, Park KA, Oh SY. Association between myopia and peripapillary hyperreflective ovoid mass-like structures in children. *Sci Rep.* (2020) 10:2238. doi: 10.1038/s41598-020-58829-3
11. Wang DD, Leong JCY, Gale J, Wells AP. Multimodal imaging of buried optic nerve head drusen. *Eye (Lond).* (2018) 32:1145–6. doi: 10.1038/s41433-017-0009-8
12. Shinohara K, Moriyama M, Shimada N, Nagaoka N, Ishibashi T, Tokoro T, et al. Analyses of shape of eyes and structure of optic nerves in eyes with tilted disc syndrome by swept-source optical coherence tomography and three-dimensional magnetic resonance imaging. *Eye (Lond).* (2013) 27:1233–42. doi: 10.1038/eye.2013.202
13. Pichi F, Romano S, Villani E, Lembo A, Gilardoni F, Morara M, et al. Spectral-domain optical coherence tomography findings in pediatric tilted disc syndrome. *Graefes Arch Clin Exp Ophthalmol.* (2014) 252:1661–7. doi: 10.1007/s00417-014-2701-8
14. Mezad-Koursh D, Klein A, Rosenblatt A, Teper Roth S, Neudorfer M, Loewenstein A, et al. Peripapillary hyperreflective ovoid mass-like structures-a novel entity as frequent cause of pseudopapilloedema in children. *Eye (Lond).* (2021) 35:1228–34. doi: 10.1038/s41433-020-1067-x
15. Fraser JA, Sibony PA, Petzold A, Thaung C, Hamann S. ODDS consortium. Peripapillary Hyper-reflective Ovoid Mass-like Structure (PHOMS): an optical coherence tomography marker of axoplasmic stasis in the optic nerve head. *J Neuroophthalmol.* (2021) 41:431–41. doi: 10.1097/WNO.0000000000001203
16. Ahn YJ, Park YY, Shin SY. Peripapillary hyperreflective ovoid mass-like structures (PHOMS) in children. *Eye (Lond).* (2021). [Epub ahead of print]. doi: 10.1038/s41433-021-01461-w
17. Wibroe EA, Malmqvist L, Hamann S. OCT based interpretation of the optic nerve head anatomy and prevalence of optic disc drusen in patients with Idiopathic Intracranial Hypertension (IIH). *Life (Basel).* (2021) 11:584. doi: 10.3390/life11060584
18. Petzold A, Biousse V, Bursztyn L, Costello F, Crum A, Digre K, et al. Multirater Validation of peripapillary hyperreflective ovoid mass-like structures (PHOMS). *Neuroophthalmology.* (2020) 44:413–4. doi: 10.1080/01658107.2020.1760891
19. Malmqvist L, Bursztyn L, Costello F, Digre K, Fraser JA, Fraser C, et al. Peripapillary hyperreflective ovoid mass-like structures: is it optic disc drusen or not?: Response. *J Neuroophthalmol.* (2018) 38:568–70. doi: 10.1097/WNO.0000000000000674
20. Teixeira FJ, Marques RE, Mano SS, Couceiro R, Pinto F. Optic disc drusen in children: morphologic features using EDI-OCT. *Eye (Lond).* (2020) 34:1577–84. doi: 10.1038/s41433-019-0694-6
21. Yan Y, Ludwig CA, Liao YJ. Multimodal imaging features of optic disc drusen. *Am J Ophthalmol.* (2021) 225:18–26. doi: 10.1016/j.ajo.2020.12.023
22. Hamann S, Malmqvist L, Wegener M, Fard MA, Biousse V, Bursztyn L, et al. Young adults with anterior ischemic optic neuropathy: a multicenter optic disc drusen study. *Am J Ophthalmol.* (2020) 217:174–81. doi: 10.1016/j.ajo.2020.03.052
23. Chen JJ, Bhatti MT. Papilledema. *Int Ophthalmol Clin.* (2019) 59:3–22. doi: 10.1097/IIO.0000000000000274
24. Petzold A, Coric D, Balk LJ, Hamann S, Uitdehaag BMJ, Denniston AK, et al. Longitudinal development of peripapillary hyper-reflective ovoid masslike structures suggests a novel pathological pathway in multiple sclerosis. *Ann Neurol.* (2020) 88:309–19. doi: 10.1002/ana.25782
25. Borrelli E, Sadda SR, Uji A, Querques G. Pearls and pitfalls of optical coherence tomography angiography imaging: a review. *Ophthalmol Ther.* (2019) 8:215–26. doi: 10.1007/s40123-019-0178-6

27

Ocular Biometry of Primary Angle-Closure Disease in Younger Patients

Shufen Lin[1†], *Chengguo Zuo*[1†], *Yuan Liu*[1], *Hui Xiao*[1], *Lei Fang*[1], *Yihua Su*[1,2], *Liming Chen*[1], *Mingkai Lin*[1], *Yunlan Ling*[1] *and Xing Liu*[1*]

[1] *State Key Laboratory of Ophthalmology, Zhongshan Ophthalmic Center, Sun Yat-sen University, Guangzhou, China,* [2] *The First Affiliated Hospital, Sun Yat-sen University, Guangzhou, China*

Correspondence:
Xing Liu
liuxing@mail.sysu.edu.cn

† *These authors have contributed equally to this work and share first authorship*

Background: The purpose of this study was to analyze the ocular biometric parameters of primary angle-closure disease (PACD) in younger patients and compare them with those of elderly patients.

Methods: This clinic-based, cross-sectional study included 154 eyes of 154 patients with PACD, consisting of 77 eyes of patients aged 40 years or younger and 77 eyes of patients older than 40. The PACD case definition was compatible with the ISGEO definition. Anterior segment parameters were measured by ultrasound biomicroscopy, axial length (AL) and lens thickness (LT) were measured by A-scan ultrasonography measurements, and the thickness of the retina and choroid were measured by optical coherence tomography. The differences in ocular biometric parameters between different age groups were compared by independent sample *t*-tests or Mann-Whitney *U* tests, and the correlation between the parameters and age was analyzed.

Results: Compared to older PACD patients, the lens vault(LV),LV/LT and subfoveal choroidal thickness (SFCT) of younger patients were larger, while the peripheral and mean iris thickness (IT), trabecular-ciliary angle (TCA), ciliary body thickness (CBT), AL and LT were smaller (all $P < 0.01$). There was no significant difference in anterior chamber depth, anterior chamber width, pupil diameter, angle opening distance at 500 μm from the scleral spur, anterior chamber angle and iris convexity between the two groups (all $P > 0.05$). AL, LT, IT, TCA and CBT were positively associated with age (all $P < 0.001$), while LV and SFCT were negatively associated with age ($P = 0.027$ and $P < 0.001$, respectively).

Conclusions: Compared with elderly patients, younger PACD patients had more anteriorly positioned lenses, thinner and more anteriorly rotated ciliary bodies, thicker choroids, and shorter axial length. These characteristics might be important anatomical bases for the earlier onset of PACD and the higher risk of malignant glaucoma after filtering surgery.

Keywords: ocular biometric parameter, primary angle-closure disease, younger patients, ultrasound biomicroscopy, anterior segment

INTRODUCTION

Primary angle-closure disease (PACD) is a group of diseases that mainly affect Asian populations (1–3). It is commonly a disease of older persons and is rare in younger individuals (4–6). Ritch et al. (5) defined "young" as "40 years old or younger" for the first time. Previous studies have found that younger PACD patients had a higher risk of malignant glaucoma after trabeculectomy (7, 8), suggesting that the ocular biometric structure of younger patients might be different from that of older patients. However, most of the current studies on the ocular biometric parameters of PACD have focused on elderly patients (9–16). The characteristics of the ocular biometric structure of younger PACD patients and their differences with those of older patients remain unknown.

In this study, PACD patients were divided into a ≤40-year-old group and a >40-year-old group. The ocular biometric parameters of the anterior chamber, anterior chamber angle, iris, ciliary body, retina, choroid, axial length, and lens thickness were measured by ultrasound biomicroscopy (UBM), optical coherence tomography (OCT), and A-scan ultrasonography measurements. We quantitatively analyzed the ocular biometric parameters of younger PACD patients, and compared them with those of elderly patients.

METHODS

Study Design and Subjects

This retrospective cross-sectional study included patients who were initially diagnosed with PACD by the same glaucoma specialist (XL) between January 2012 and December 2019 in Zhongshan Ophthalmic Center. PACD patients aged 40 or younger were continuously included, while patients >40 years old were randomly selected during the same period. This investigation adhered to the tenets of the Declaration of Helsinki and was approved by the human research ethics committee of Zhongshan Ophthalmic Center of Sun Yat-sen University in Guangzhou (2021KYPJ003).

PACD was diagnosed based on the criteria of International Society of Geographical and Epidemiological Ophthalmology (ISGEO), including primary angle-closure suspect (PACS), primary angle-closure (PAC), and primary angle-closure glaucoma (PACG) (17). PACS was defined as an eye with iridotrabecular contact (ITC) for at least 180 degrees on indentation gonioscopy in the primary position (without peripheral synechiae), with normal intraocular pressure (IOP) and no optic nerve damage. PAC was defined as an eye with ITC for at least 180 degrees on indentation gonioscopy in the primary position, with peripheral anterior synechiae, with or without elevated IOP, and without glaucomatous optic neuropathy. PACG was defined as PAC together with chronically elevated IOP and evidence of glaucomatous optic changes (defined as a vertical cup-to-disc ratio [CDR] > 0.7 and/or CDR asymmetry > 0.2), and with glaucoma hemifield test outside normal limits (17). The right eye in each subject was selected for analysis if both eyes met the inclusion criteria. Patients with blurred UBM images, secondary factors that can cause angle-closure glaucoma, a history of laser therapy or incisional surgery or eye trauma, a history of acute angle-closure crisis, or a rigid pupil or a change in the pupil shape after long-term use of miotics were excluded.

Ocular Biometric Measurements

All patients received a comprehensive ocular examination. The best-corrected visual acuity (BCVA) measured with the Snellen chart and converted into a logMAR equivalent. IOP was measured with a Goldmann applanation tonometer. Anterior segments were examined with slit-lamp microscopy, and ocular fundus were examined with a 90 diopter (D) preset lens in a natural pupil state. Anterior chamber angle was analyzed in the dark with Goldmann gonioscopy by the same glaucoma specialist (XL). Axial length (AL) and lens thickness (LT) were measured with A-scan ultrasonography measurements (model US-1800, Nidek), while visual field was measured with Humphrey perimetry (Carl Zeiss Meditec, Dublin). The mean retinal nerve fiber layer thickness (mRNFLT), foveal retinal thickness (FRT), and subfoveal choroidal thickness (SFCT) were measured with optical coherence tomography (OCT; Heidelberg Engineering, Heidelberg, Germany).

Ultrasound Biomicroscopy (UBM)

The standardized protocol for obtaining UBM images has been reported previously (18, 19). The UBM (model SW-3200L; Tianjin Sower Electronic Technology Co., Ltd., Tianjin, China) examination was performed on the patients by a skilled physician (LC) at the initial consultation. Patients were examined under dark lighting conditions (illumination 60–70 lux) in a supine position. Each eye was assessed with central and 360 degree radiation of the anterior segment. Radial scans were performed at the 12, 3, 6, and 9 o'clock positions centered over the limbus. The images that clearly showed the scleral spur, corneal epithelium/endothelial, iris pigment epithelium, and lens anterior capsule were saved for analysis.

The UBM parameters of the anterior segment measured in the current study were as follows. Average values of the four quadrants were obtained for all parameters except for anterior chamber depth (ACD) (**Figure 1**).

1) ACD is the distance from the corneal endothelium to the anterior surface of the lens centered over the pupil (18).
2) The anterior chamber width (ACW) is the horizontal scleral spur-to-spur distance (19).
3) The lens vault (LV) is the perpendicular distance between the anterior surface of lens and the horizontal line joining the two scleral spurs (ACW) (10).
4) The angle opening distance at 500 μm from the scleral spur (AOD500) is the distance between the posterior corneal surface and the anterior iris measured on a line perpendicular to the plain of the trabecular meshwork at 500μm from the scleral spur (18).
5) The anterior chamber angle (ACA) is the angle between the posterior corneal surface and the anterior surface of the iris with the scleral spur as the apex (18).
6) Iris convexity (IC) is the distance from the greatest convexity point on the posterior surface of the iris to the line joining the pupillary margin and the iris root (20).

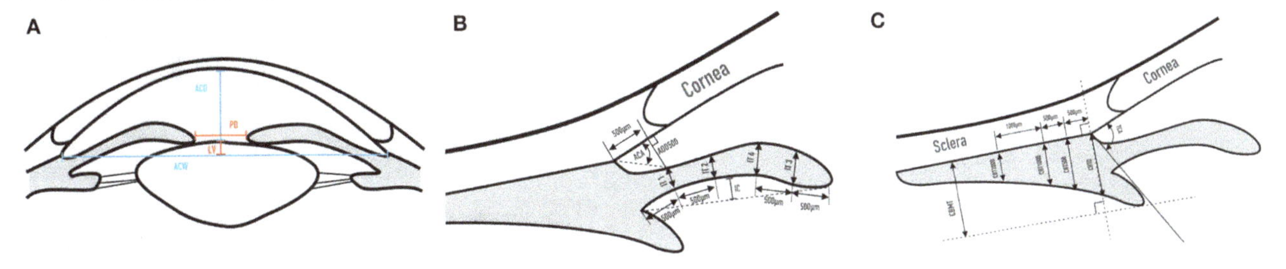

FIGURE 1 | UBM measurement parameters of the anterior segment. **(A)** ACD, ACW, LV, PD; **(B)** AOD500, ACA, IT1, IT2, IT3, IT4, IC; **(C)** TCA, CBT0, CBT500, CBT1000, CBT2000, CBMT.

7) Five parameters of iris thickness (IT) were measured. IT1 is the thickness of the iris at a distance of 500 μm from the root of the iris; IT2 is the thickness of the iris at 1,000 μm from the root of the iris; IT3 is the thickness of the iris at 500 μm from the pupillary margin; IT4 is the thickness of the iris at 1,000 μm from the pupillary margin; and the mean iris thickness (MIT) is the average value of IT1, IT2, IT3, and IT4 (21).
8) The trabecular-ciliary process angle (TCA) is the angle between the most anterior surface of the ciliary body and the posterior corneal surface with the scleral spur as the apex (18).
9) The ciliary body thickness at the point of the scleral spur (CBT0) is the distance between the inner surface of the ciliary body and the inner surface of the scleral at the point of the scleral spur; CBT500, CBT1000, and CBT2000 are ciliary body thickness at 500, 1,000, 2,000 μm from the scleral spur; Ciliary body max thickness (CBMT) is the distance from the most inner point of the ciliary body perpendicular to the inner surface of the sclera or its extended line (18).

All UBM parameters were measured by the same trained physician (SL) who was blinded to the clinical data of the subjects. After an interval of more than 2 weeks, 15 pictures were randomly selected by the same doctor for repeated measurements. The data were evaluated with an intraclass correlation coefficient (ICC) for intraobserver reproducibility (22).

Statistical Analyses

Statistical analyses were conducted using the statistic package social science version 22.0 (SPSS, Inc., Chicago, IL). The Shapiro-Wilk *W* test was applied for a normality test of the examined parameters. According to the distribution of the data, the differences in parameters between the ≤40-year-old group and >40-year-old group were compared using the independent *t*-test or the Mann-Whitney *U* test. The chi-square test was implemented for the qualitative variables. Spearman's rank correlation was used to analyze the correlation between age and ocular biological parameters. The intraclass correlation coefficient (ICC) was applied to evaluate the intraobserver reproducibility. $P < 0.05$ was considered statistically significant.

TABLE 1 | Basic clinical data of PACD of different age groups.

Parameters	≤40 years old	>40 years old	$t/Z/\chi^2$	*P*
Eyes	77	77		
Age, years	34.0 (29.0 to 37.5)	58.0 (45.0 to 63.5)	−10.717	**<0.001**‡
Male/female	14/63	22/55	2.320	0.128*
PACS/PAC/PACG	9/24/44	4/29/44	2.395	0.302*
BCVA (LogMAR)	0 (0 to 0.3)	0.1 (0 to 0.2)	−0.911	0.362‡
IOP (mmHg)	31.06 ± 13.35	29.14 ± 12.26	0.929	0.354†
PAS (degrees)	240.0 (153.0 to 330.0)	180.0 (130.0 to 270.0)	−1.501	0.133‡
CDR	0.7 (0.3 to 0.9)	0.6 (0.4 to 0.8)	−0.839	0.401‡
MD (dB)	−11.13 (−27.49 to −2.42)	−16.24 (−21.47 to −3.28)	−0.732	0.464‡
AL (mm)	21.63 ± 0.78	22.31 ± 0.81	−5.231	**<0.001**†
LT (mm)	4.68 (4.39 to 4.92)	5.10 (4.84 to 5.37)	−5.622	**<0.001**‡
RNFLT (μm)	73.0 (48.0 to 110.3)	86.0 (53.3 to 106.8)	−0.319	0.749‡
FRT (μm)	181.8 (170.6 to 194.0)	188.0 (175.0 to 200.4)	−5.781	0.241‡
SFCT (μm)	423.0 (341.0 to 512.0)	291.0 (231.0 to 392.3)	−5.273	**<0.001**‡

(mean ± SD) or (median, IQR).
IQR = interquartile range, shown as (25%, 75%).
† Independent-Samples t- test.
‡ Mann-Whitney U test.
**Chi-square test.*
P-values with statistical significance (<0.05) are highlighted in bold.

RESULTS

Demographic Data and Basic Characteristics of the Study Subjects

In this study, 1,157 patients with PACD were screened, of which 109 cases were ≤40 years old. After excluding patients with a history of acute angle-closure attack ($N = 15$), low-quality UBM images ($N = 5$), and history of miotic use ($N = 12$), 77 eyes of 77 younger patients were included. Seventy-seven eyes of 77 PACD patients older than 40 were randomly selected during the same period. Except for age ($P < 0.001$), there was no significant

TABLE 2 | Parameters of anterior segment of different age groups.

Parameters	≤40 years old	>40 years old	t/z	P
ACD (mm)	1.99 ± 0.36	1.96 ± 0.23	0.688	0.492†
ACW (mm)	12.01 ± 0.69	11.90 ± 0.56	0.953	0.343†
PD (mm)	3.97 ± 1.14	3.85 ± 0.88	0.725	0.470†
LV (mm)	1.21 ± 0.22	1.10 ± 0.22	2.811	**0.006†**
AOD500 (mm)	0.016 (0∼0.034)	0.020 (0.006∼0.040)	−1.955	0.051‡
ACA (degree)	1.75(0∼3.93)	2.28(0.64∼4.59)	−1.955	0.051‡
IT1 (mm)	0.37 ± 0.08	0.42 ± 0.08	−4.032	**<0.001†**
IT2 (mm)	0.43 ± 0.08	0.47 ± 0.08	−2.977	**0.003†**
IT3 (mm)	0.50 ± 0.12	0.51 ± 0.10	−0.683	0.496†
IT4 (mm)	0.59(0.49∼0.62)	0.58(0.54∼0.63)	−0.314	0.754‡
MIT (mm)	0.47 ± 0.07	0.50 ± 0.06	−2.663	**0.009†**
IC (mm)	0.16(0.11∼0.23)	0.18(0.12∼0.27)	−1.606	0.108‡
TCA (degree)	47.40 ± 13.25	53.03 ± 12.17	−2.735	0.007†
CBT0 (mm)	0.82 ± 0.13	0.90 ± 0.12	−3.692	**<0.001†**
CBT500 (mm)	0.77(0.71∼0.82)	0.83(0.75∼0.93)	−2.963	**0.003‡**
CBT1000 (mm)	0.59 ± 0.11	0.66 ± 0.12	−3.917	**<0.001†**
CBT2000 (mm)	0.30 ± 0.05	0.35 ± 0.06	−4.626	**<0.001†**
CBMT (mm)	0.96 ± 0.11	1.00 ± 0.11	−2.630	**0.009†**
LV/LT	0.26 ± 0.05	0.21 ± 0.04	5.822	**<0.001†**

(mean ± SD) or (median, IQR).
IQR = interquartile range, shown as (25%, 75%).
†Independent-Samples t-test.
‡Mann-Whitney U test.
P-values with statistical significance (<0.05) are highlighted in bold.

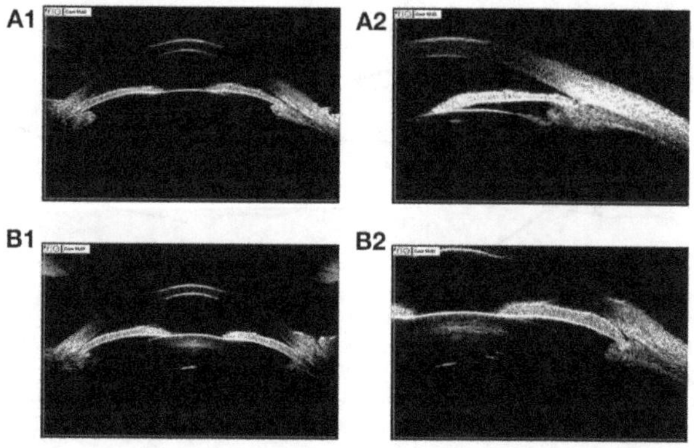

FIGURE 2 | (A1,A2) UBM images of a 36-year-old female PACG patient. ACD 1.93 mm, ACW 10.77 mm, LV 0.869 mm, PD 2.17 mm, AOD 0.02 mm, ACA 2.1°, IT1 0.352 mm, IT2 0.338 mm, IT3 0. 459 mm, IT4 0.460 mm, MIT 0.402 mm, IC 0.215 mm, TCA 41.0°, CBT0 0.981 mm, CBT500 0.856 mm, CBT1000 0.710 mm, CBT2000 0.460 mm, CBMT 1.046 mm; **(B1,B2)** UBM images of a 68-year-old female PACG patient. ACD 2.00 mm, ACW 11.47 mm, LV 0.915 mm, PD 2.84 mm, AOD 0.02 mm, ACA 2.5°, IT1 0.392 mm, IT2 0.442 mm, IT3 0. 500 mm, IT4 0.554 mm, MIT 0.472mm, IC 0.293 mm, TCA 62.1°, CBT0 0.906 mm, CBT500 0.911 mm, CBT1000 0.674 mm, CBT2000 0.446 mm, CBMT 1.082 mm.

difference in sex or diagnosis between these two groups ($P > 0.05$) (**Table 1**). The basic ocular characteristics of various age groups measured by OCT and A-scan ultrasonography measurements are summarized in **Table 1**. Compared to patients older than 40, younger patients had shorter axial lengths, thinner lenses and thicker SFCTs (all $P < 0.001$).

Parameters of Anterior Chamber, Iris, and Ciliary Body

The comparisons of anterior segment biometric measurements detected by UBM between younger and elderly PACD patients are shown in **Table 2**. Compared to elderly patients, patients aged 40 or younger had thinner MIT and peripheral iris thickness (IT1, IT2) ($P < 0.01$), relatively anterior positioned lenses (LV, LV/LT were larger) ($P < 0.01$), more anteriorly rotated ciliary bodies (TCA was smaller) ($P = 0.007$), and thinner ciliary bodies (CBT0,CBT500, CBT1000,CBT2000, CBMT) ($P < 0.01$) (**Table 2, Figure 2**).

Correlation Analysis Between Ocular Biometric Parameters and Age

The current study found that ocular biological parameters including AL, LT, SFCT, LV, IT1, IT2, MIT, TCA, CBT0, CBT500, CBT1000, CBT2000, and CBMT were significantly different between different age groups. The correlation between these parameters and age was analyzed. The result indicated that AL, LT, IT1, IT2, MIT, TCA, CBT0, CBT500, CBT1000, CBT2000, and CBMT were positively associated with age ($r = 0.501, 0.630, 0.352, 0.268, 0.244, 0.272, 0.357, 0.340, 0.427, 0.391, 0.290$, all $P < 0.001$), while LV and SFCT were negatively associated with age ($r = -0.208, P = 0.027$; $r = -0.636, P < 0.001$) (**Figure 3**).

Reproducibility Analysis of UBM Parameters

The UBM images of 15 eyes were randomly selected to analyze the repeatability of the UBM parameter measurement (**Table 3**), except that the ICC value of CBT2000 was 0.526. All the other parameters verified excellent reproducibility with ICCs (ICC 0.778–0.996).

DISCUSSION

This study measured the ocular biometric parameters of PACD in younger patients, and compared them with those of older patients. We found that compared with older patients, younger patients had more anteriorly positioned lenses, thinner and more anteriorly rotated ciliary bodies, thicker choroids, and shorter axial lengths. The anatomical characteristics of younger patients might play an important role in the early onset of PACD.

There were obvious differences in anterior anatomical structure between PACD patients and normal people, including short axial length, shallow anterior chamber, narrow angle, and thicker and relatively anteriorly positioned lenses (10–13). However, previous studies that investigated the biological characteristics of PACD mainly focused on older patients. Few systematic study has reported the ocular biometric parameters of young PACD patients or their differences with those of elderly patients.

In this study, we found that the LT of young patients was thicker than that of normal populations of the same age group (3.95 ± 0.30 mm) (23), and the LV was larger than that of normal

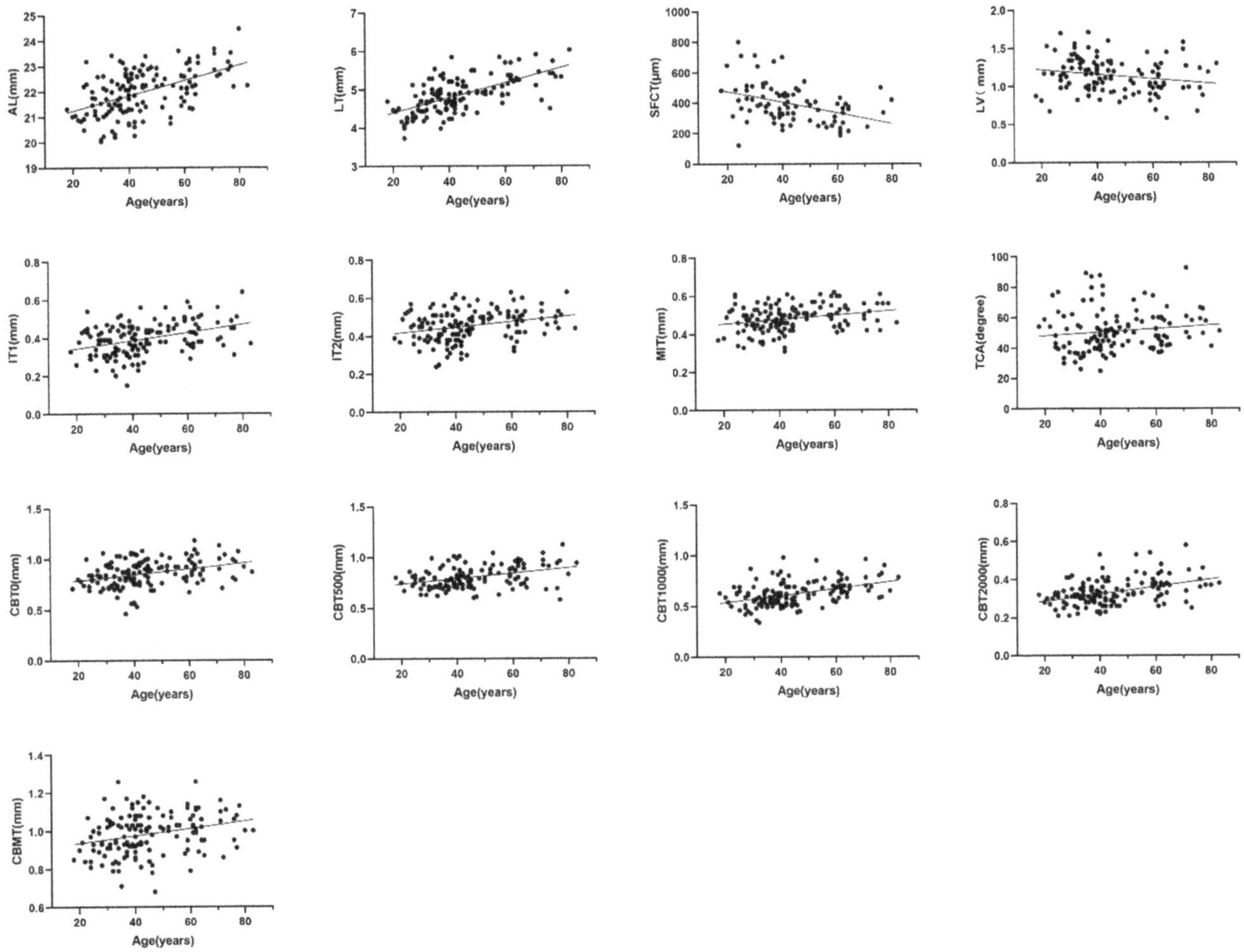

FIGURE 3 | Scatter diagram of the correlation between age and AL, LT, SFCT, LV, IT1, IT2, MIT, TCA, CBT00, CBT500, CBT1000, and CBMT (Spearman's rank correlation, $P < 0.05$).

people (0.419 ± 0.236 mm) (11). This result is in accordance with the findings of previous studies on older patients, which suggested that increased LT and LV were risk factors for angle closure (10, 11, 24). Our study indicated that larger LT and LV also played a part in the onset of PACD in younger patients.

It was interesting to note that while younger patients had shorter ALs and thinner lenses than older patients, their LV and LV/LT were larger, which suggests that the lenses of younger PACD patients significantly moved forward. This result was consistent with the studies of Ozaki et al. (10) and Nongpiur et al. (11), who found a poor correlation between LV and LT. Thus, according to the findings of Nongpiur et al. (10), the increase in LV in younger PACD patients can be related to zonular laxity. Since younger PACD patients were free of abnormal lens zonules due to trauma or other eye lesions, and the zonules of youth were less likely to degenerate (25), the strain of the lens zonules was probably related to ciliary bodies. Gohdo et al. (9) speculated that a thinner ciliary body may cause advancement and thickening of the lens. He et al. (16) believed that the reduced thickness of the ciliary body might be due to muscular atrophy, and a thinner ciliary body might cause anterior positioning of the ciliary processes and loosening of the zonules, resulting in anterior advancement of the lens. Our study found that younger patients had thinner and more anteriorly rotated ciliary bodies than older patients, suggesting that younger patients have inadequate ciliary muscle strength, which is probably the anatomical basis for anterior advancement of the lens in younger patients.

Our study also found that compared with older patients, younger patients had thinner irises and thicker choroids, which is consistent with previous studies in normal populations showing iris thickening with age, while the SFCT thinning with age (12, 26, 27). This result was also in accordance with the findings that choroid thickness and iris thickness were negatively correlated in the studies of Huang et al. (28) and Li et al. (29). Iris, ciliary body, and choroid all originate from uvea that are filled with blood vessels from the same arterial system (ophthalmic artery), so we speculated that blood flow might play an important role in this connection. Both the long posterior ciliary artery (LPCA) and the short posterior ciliary artery (SPCA) stem from the ophthalmic artery. The thinner iris and ciliary body might represent smaller

TABLE 3 | Intraclass correlation coefficient (ICC).

Parameters	ICC value	*P*
ACD (mm)	0.994	<0.001
ACW (mm)	0.9	<0.001
PD (mm)	0.911	<0.001
LV (mm)	0.996	<0.001
AOD500 (mm)	0.954	<0.001
ACA (degree)	0.956	<0.001
IT1 (mm)	0.836	<0.001
IT2 (mm)	0.794	<0.001
IT3 (mm)	0.925	<0.001
IT4 (mm)	0.932	<0.001
IC (mm)	0.904	<0.001
TCA (degree)	0.887	<0.001
CBT0 (mm)	0.918	<0.001
CBT500 (mm)	0.778	<0.001
CBT1000 (mm)	0.888	<0.001
CBT2000 (mm)	0.526	0.02
CBMT (mm)	0.916	<0.001

vascular diameters and increased blood flow resistance of the LPCA, resulting in increased blood flow of the SPCA, which was characterized by thickening of the choroid (28).

The correlation between ocular biometric parameters and the age of patients with PACD was analyzed in our study. We found that the AL, LT, IT, TCA, and CBT were positively associated with age, while the LV and SFCT were negatively correlated with age. There has been no systematic study that analyzed the relationship between ocular biometric parameters and age in PACD patients, but previous studies of normal populations have shown that the AL,TCA,CBT, and SFCT were negatively correlated with age (12, 16, 26, 27, 30–33), while the LT, LV, and IT were positively associated with age (12, 23). The correlations between age and LT, IT, and SFCT in this study were consistent with those in normal people, but the correlations between age and AL, LV, CBT, and TCA were opposite to those in the normal population. We speculate that the main reason for this inconsistency might be the different study subjects. Previous studies have analyzed the trend of ocular biometric parameters changing with age in normal populations, but in our study, the subjects were two groups of PACD patients onset at different ages, which meant that the ocular structure of older patients was not simply the state of young patients becoming older. These anatomical features of shorter AL, larger LV, and thinner and more anteriorly rotated ciliary body in younger PACD patients which are distinguished from the changing trend in normal people, might together lead to earlier onset of the disease. In addition, according to previous studies (7, 8, 21, 34), these anatomical characteristics in young patients were also risk factors for the occurrence of malignant glaucoma after filtering surgery.

A main limitation of our study was selection bias at baseline. The study was clinic-based and the sample size was not large, and thus may not be representative of the population as a whole. Besides, the different groups of angle closure (PACS, PAC, and PACG) gave a heterogenous group. So further large-scale cohort study and subgroup analyses are needed. It would also be interesting to qualitatively classify the patients into different mechanisms of angle closure and compare their frequency in different age groups.

CONCLUSION

In conclusion, the ocular biometric parameters in young patients were significantly different from those of older patients. The characteristics of anteriorly located lenses, thinner and anteriorly positioned ciliary bodies, thicker choroids, and shorter axial lengths in younger patients were probably important anatomical bases for the early onset of PACD and high risk of malignant glaucoma after filtering surgery.

ETHICS STATEMENT

The studies involving human participants were reviewed and approved by the Human Research Ethics Committee of Zhongshan Ophthalmic Center of Sun Yat-sen University in Guangzhou (Ethical No: 2021KYPJ003). Written informed consent for participation was not required for this study in accordance with the national legislation and the institutional requirements.

AUTHOR CONTRIBUTIONS

Design and conduct of the study by SL and XL. Collection of the data by SL, LF, ML, YLin, and YS. Analysis of the data by SL, HX, and LC. Preparation of the manuscript SL, CZ, YLiu, and XL. Review and final approval of the manuscript by all the authors.

REFERENCES

1. Resnikoff S, Pascolini D, Etya'ale D, Kocur I, Pararajasegaram R, Pokharel G, et al. Global data on visual impairment in the year 2002. *Bull World Health Organ.* (2004) 82:844–51. doi: 10.1076/opep.11.2.67.28158
2. Cheng JW, Cheng SW, Ma XY, Cai JP, Li Y, Wei RL. The prevalence of primary glaucoma in mainland China: a systematic review and meta-analysis. *J Glaucoma.* (2013) 22:301–6. doi: 10.1097/IJG.0b013e31824083ca
3. Tham YC, Li X, Wong TY, Quigley HA, Aung T, Cheng CY. Global prevalence of glaucoma and projections of glaucoma burden through 2040:

a systematic review and meta-analysis. *Ophthalmology.* (2014) 121:2081–90. doi: 10.1016/j.ophtha.2014.05.013

4. Badlani VK, Quinones R, Wilensky JT, Hawkins A, Edward DP. Angle-closure glaucoma in teenagers. *J Glaucoma.* (2003) 12:198–203. doi: 10.1097/00061198-200306000-00003
5. Ritch R, Chang BM, Liebmann JM. Angle closure in younger patients. *Ophthalmology.* (2003) 110:1880–9. doi: 10.1016/S0161-6420(03)00563-3
6. Wiggs J, Pasquale L. Genetics of glaucoma. *Hum Mol Genet.* (2017) 26:R21–7. doi: 10.1093/hmg/ddx184
7. Wang Z, Huang J, Lin J, Liang X, Cai X, Ge J. Quantitative measurements of the ciliary body in eyes with malignant glaucoma after trabeculectomy using ultrasound biomicroscopy. *Ophthalmology.* (2014) 121:862–9. doi: 10.1016/j.ophtha.2013.10.035
8. Chen XX, Guo XX, Xu XY, Xiao H, Liu X. Is thicker choroid a risk factor for malignant glaucoma? *Ophthalmic Res.* (2018) 60:161–8. doi: 10.1159/000490914
9. Gohdo T, Tsumura T, Iijima H, Kashiwagi K, Tsukahara S. Ultrasound biomicroscopic study of ciliary body thickness in eyes with narrow angles. *Am J Ophthalmol.* (2000) 129:342–6. doi: 10.1016/S0002-9394(99)00353-0
10. Nongpiur ME, He M, Amerasinghe N, Friedman DS, Tay WT, Baskaran M, et al. Lens vault, thickness, and position in chinese subjects with angle closure. *Ophthalmology.* (2011) 118:474–9. doi: 10.1016/j.ophtha.2010.07.025
11. Ozaki M, Nongpiur ME, Aung T, He M, Mizoguchi T. Increased lens vault as a risk factor for angle closure: confirmation in a Japanese population. *Graefes Arch Clin Exp Ophthalmol.* (2012) 250:1863–8. doi: 10.1007/s00417-012-2011-y
12. Sun JH, Sung KR, Yun SC, Cheon MH, Tchah HW, Kim MJ, et al. Factors associated with anterior chamber narrowing with age: an optical coherence tomography study. *Invest Ophthalmol Vis Sci.* (2012) 53:2607–10. doi: 10.1167/iovs.11-9359
13. Razeghinejad MR, Banifatemi M. Ocular biometry in angle closure. *J Ophthalmic Vis Res.* (2013) 8:17–24.
14. Ku JY, Nongpiur ME, Park J, Narayanaswamy AK, Perera SA, Tun TA, et al. Qualitative evaluation of the iris and ciliary body by ultrasound biomicroscopy in subjects with angle closure. *J Glaucoma.* (2014) 23:583–8. doi: 10.1097/IJG.0b013e318285fede
15. Zhou M, Wang W, Huang W, Gao X, Li Z, Li X, et al. Is increased choroidal thickness association with primary angle closure? *Acta Ophthalmol.* (2014) 92:e514–20. doi: 10.1111/aos.12403
16. He N, Wu L, Qi M, He M, Lin S, Wang X, et al. Comparison of ciliary body anatomy between American Caucasians and Ethnic Chinese using ultrasound biomicroscopy. *Curr Eye Res.* (2016) 41:485–91. doi: 10.3109/02713683.2015.1024869
17. Prum BE, Herndon LW, Moroi SE, Mansberger SL, Stein JD, Lim MC, et al. Primary angle closure preferred practice pattern® guidelines. *Ophthalmology.* (2016) 123:P1–40. doi: 10.1016/j.ophtha.2015.10.049
18. Pavlin CJ, Harasiewicz K, Sherar MD, Foster FS. Clinical use of ultrasound biomicroscopy. *Ophthalmology.* (1991) 98:287–95. doi: 10.1016/S0161-6420(91)32298-X
19. Nongpiur ME, Sakata LM, Friedman DS, He M, Chan YH, Lavanya R, et al. Novel association of smaller anterior chamber width with angle closure in Singaporeans. *Ophthalmology.* (2010) 117:1967–73. doi: 10.1016/j.ophtha.2010.02.007
20. Wang B, Sakata LM, Friedman DS, Chan YH, He M, Lavanya R, et al. Quantitative Iris parameters and association with narrow angles. *Ophthalmology.* (2010) 117:11–7. doi: 10.1016/j.ophtha.2009.06.017
21. Huang J, Wang Z, Wu Z, Li Z, Lai K, Ge J. Comparison of ocular biometry between eyes with chronic primary angle-closure glaucoma and their fellow eyes with primary angle-closure or primary angle-closure suspect. *J Glaucoma.* (2015) 24:323–7. doi: 10.1097/IJG.0b013e31829e55cd
22. Guo C, Zhao Z, Zhang D, Liu J, Li J, Zhang J, et al. Anterior segment features in nanophthalmos with secondary chronic angle closure glaucoma: an ultrasound biomicroscopy study. *Invest Ophthalmol Vis Sci.* (2019) 60:2248–56. doi: 10.1167/iovs.19-26867
23. Richdale K, Sinnott LT, Bullimore MA, Wassenaar PA, Schmalbrock P, Kao CY, et al. Quantification of age-related and per diopter accommodative changes of the lens and ciliary muscle in in the emmetropic human eye. *Invest Ophthalmol Vis Sci.* (2013) 54:1095–105. doi: 10.1167/iovs.12-10619
24. Gupta B, Angmo D, Yadav S, Dada T, Gupta V, Sihota R. Quantification of iridotrabecular contact in primary angle-closure disease. *J Glaucoma.* (2020) 29:681–8. doi: 10.1097/IJG.0000000000001572
25. Farnsworth P, Shyne S. Anterior zonular shifts with age. *J Exp Eye Res.* (1979) 28:291–7. doi: 10.1016/0014-4835(79)90091-5
26. Wei WB, Xu L, Jonas JB, Shao L, Du KF, Wang S, et al. Subfoveal choroidal thickness: the Beijing eye study. *Ophthalmology.* (2013) 120:175–80. doi: 10.1016/j.ophtha.2012.07.048
27. Aknin I, Pradat P. Choroidal thickness in healthy eyes using enhanced depth imaging optical coherence tomography and comparison with cases of retinitis pigmentosa. *J Fr Ophtalmol.* (2018) 41:933–8. doi: 10.1016/j.jfo.2018.04.013
28. Huang W, Gao X, Li X, Wang J, Chen S, Wang W, et al. Anterior and posterior ocular biometry in healthy Chinese subjects: data based on AS-OCT and SS-OCT. *PloS one.* (2015) 10:e0121740. doi: 10.1371/journal.pone.0121740
29. Li S, Wu G, Chen C, Shen L, Zhang Z, Gao F, et al. Association between choroidal thickness and anterior chamber segment in eyes with narrow or open-angle. *Int J Ophthalmol.* (2016) 9:1143–7. doi: 10.18240/ijo.2016.08.10
30. Cheon MH, Sung KR, Choi EH, Kang SY, Cho JW, Lee S, et al. Effect of age on anterior chamber angle configuration in Asians determined by anterior segment optical coherence tomography; clinic-based study. *Acta Ophthalmol.* (2010) 88:e205–10. doi: 10.1111/j.1755-3768.2010.01960.x
31. Henzan IM, Tomidokoro A, Uejo C, Sakai H, Sawaguchi S, Iwase A, et al. Ultrasound biomicroscopic configurations of the anterior ocular segment in a population-based study: the Kumejima study. *Ophthalmology.* (2010) 117:1720–8, 1728.e1. doi: 10.1016/j.ophtha.2010.01.045
32. Zong Y, Xu Q, Jiang C, Zhu H, Yu J, Sun X. Measurement of and factors associated with the anterior chamber volume in healthy Chinese adults. *J Ophthalmol.* (2017) 2017:6762047. doi: 10.1155/2017/6762047
33. Jiang Y, Wang D, Wang W, Chen F, Wang L, Scheetz J, et al. Five-year changes in anterior segment parameters in an older population in urban southern China: the Liwan eye study. *Br J Ophthalmol.* (2020) 104:582–7. doi: 10.1136/bjophthalmol-2019-313827
34. Zhang XL, Li A, Teng LL, Du SL, Zhu YY, Ge J. Primary chronic angle-closure glaucoma in younger patients. *Int J Ophthalmol.* (2007) 2007:613–7. doi: 10.1017/S0952523807080649

28

Vogt-Koyanagi-Harada Syndrome Mimicking Acute Angle-Closure Glaucoma in a Patient Infected with Human Immunodeficiency Virus

*Xue Bai and Rui Hua**

Department of Ophthalmology, First Hospital of China Medical University, Shenyang, China

***Correspondence:**
Rui Hua
woodshua@126.com

Vogt-Koyanagi-Harada disease (VKH) is a rare multisystemic inflammatory autoimmune disorder. Glaucoma secondary to VKH frequently occurs during the recurrent phase of anterior uveitis; however, acute angle-closure glaucoma (ACG) secondary to both VKH and human immunodeficiency virus (HIV) infection has rarely been reported. We describe a case of secondary acute ACG involving VKH, characterized by sudden vision loss, moderately elevated intraocular pressure (IOP), shallow anterior chamber, and fully or partially closed angle, in an HIV-infected patient. Both VKH and HIV infection contributed to the occurrence of ACG due to the leakage and forward rotation of the ciliary body, as well as choroidal effusion. The deterioration of IOP and serous macular detachment were observed after initial corticosteroid therapy. Visual acuity and IOP were improved with subretinal fluid absorption after continued corticosteroid therapy. Understanding the response of IOP and serous macular detachment after corticosteroid therapy is important for clinical practice.

Keywords: Vogt-Koyanagi-Harada, human immunodeficiency virus, secondary angle-closure glaucoma, choroidal effusion, optical coherence tomography

INTRODUCTION

Human immunodeficiency virus (HIV) is a lentivirus that infects cells of the human immune system, causing its dysfunction (1). In 2017, an estimated 36.9 million people worldwide had HIV infection, according to the World Health Organization (2). The incidence rate of HIV-related eye diseases has increased correspondingly and is considered one of the most common complications of acquired immune deficiency syndrome. Human immunodeficiency virus-related eye diseases mainly include ocular eye microangiopathy, opportunistic infections, tumors, and immune reconstitution inflammatory syndrome (3). Vogt-Koyanagi-Harada disease (VKH) is a rare multisystemic inflammatory autoimmune disorder characterized by panuveitis, accompanied by neurological and cutaneous manifestations (4). Glaucoma secondary to VKH can be observed at any time after the onset of uveitis, which frequently occurs during the recurrent phase of anterior

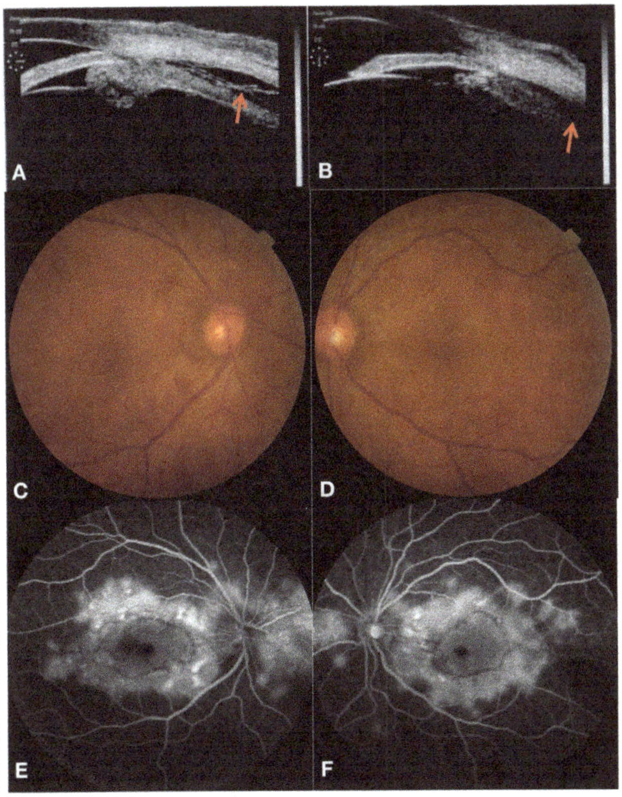

FIGURE 1 | Acute angle-closure glaucoma secondary to Vogt-Koyanagi-Harada disease at initial visit. Ultrasound biomicroscopy revealed both leakage (red arrow) and forward rotation of the ciliary body and secondary angle-closure in bilateral eyes [**(A)** right eye, **(B)** left eye]. Color fundus photograph showed multifocal serous retinal detachments with hyperaemic optic discs in both eyes [**(C)** right eye, **(D)** left eye]. Typical "multiple lake" hyperfluorescence and optic disc leakage are found in the late stage of fundus fluorescein angiography [**(E)** right eye, **(F)** left eye].

uveitis, owing to posterior iris adhesion and pupil block, anterior angle occlusion, trabecular meshwork inflammation, inflammatory cells being closed to the trabecular meshwork, and the long-term use of glucocorticoids (5).

Certain patients diagnosed with VKH can develop acute angle-closure glaucoma (ACG), with ACG as the first symptom, including a sudden or gradual increment in intraocular pressure (IOP), shallow anterior chamber, and aqueous flare often accompanied by choroiditis and optic disc oedema (6). However, acute ACG secondary to both VKH and HIV infection has rarely been reported. Herein, we present a case of VKH mimicking acute ACG in an HIV-infected patient and investigate its underlying pathogenesis.

CASE PRESENTATION

A 55-year-old man infected with HIV complained of pain in both eyes, headache, and epicranium ache for 2 days with an episode of fever (38.5°C). In addition, he did not have any systemic symptoms of HIV infection. The patient had normal best-corrected visual acuity (BCVA) for both eyes (the decimal vision for both eyes was 1.0). His symptoms mainly included bilateral conjunctival oedema and superficial scleral hyperaemia without corneal oedema. Shallow peripheral anterior chamber depth (PACD) was evaluated for both eyes on slit-lamp microscopy, which was about one-quarter of the corneal thickness at the 6 o'clock position. In addition, his IOPs were 19 and 21 mmHg in the right and left eye, respectively. Central corneal thickness was 505 mm in the right eye and 494 mm in the left eye. Moreover, ultrasound biomicroscopy (UBM) revealed shallow anterior chambers (central anterior chamber depth of 1.75 mm in the right eye and 1.85 mm in the left eye) and angle closure in both eyes (**Figure 1**). Therefore, the patient's condition was diagnosed as acute ACG in both eyes.

Unfortunately, the patient's BCVA decreased to 0.15 and 0.12 in the right and the left eye, respectively, 1 day later with keratic precipitate (dust type), which indicated acute uveitis. We realized that the previous UBM had already revealed both leakage and forward rotation of the ciliary body. Multifocal serous retinal detachments with hyperaemic optic discs were detected in both eyes through dilated pupils. Moreover, typical "multiple lake" hyperfluorescence and optic disc leakage in the late phase were also observed via fundus fluorescein angiography (**Figure 1**). In addition, optical coherence tomography (OCT) revealed multifocal serous retinal detachments with choroidal effusion in both eyes (**Figure 2**), also confirmed by ocular B ultrasonography. Finally, we revised the previous diagnosis to binocular VKH with secondary ACG, without extraocular signs of VKH. The laboratory results for uveitis included antinuclear antibody (ANA: +1:100 [granular type]) and anti-U1RNP antibody (positive). In addition, the laboratory results for HIV infection revealed that his CD4^{+} T-cell count was 296 cells/μl.

After the administration of 105 mg prednisone once a day for 1 week, the IOPs of the right and left eye increased to 23 and 26 mmHg, respectively, with the aggravation of the serous retinal detachment (**Figure 2**). After continued corticosteroid therapy for 2 weeks, the patient's BCVA in both eyes improved to 1.0. The IOPs of the right and left eye were 16 and 14 mmHg, respectively. The multifocal serous retinal detachments resolved, and subretinal fluid (SRF) was completely absorbed in the OCT. The PACD regressed from about one-quarter corneal thickness to full (normal) thickness when examined by slit-lamp microscopy. Further treatment included 95 mg prednisone for 1 week, 85 mg prednisone for 1 week, 75 mg prednisone for 2 weeks, and 60 mg prednisone for 10 days, at which point oral prednisone was reduced by 5 mg per week. Six months after the onset of VKH, normal macular structures were obtained with the complete absorption of SRF (**Figure 2**). However, at this stage, dotted hypoperfusion of choroidal capillaries can still be observed in OCT angiography (**Figure 3**).

This study was reviewed and approved by the Institutional Review Board of the First Hospital of China Medical University, and written informed consent was obtained from the participant for the publication of this case report (including all data and images).

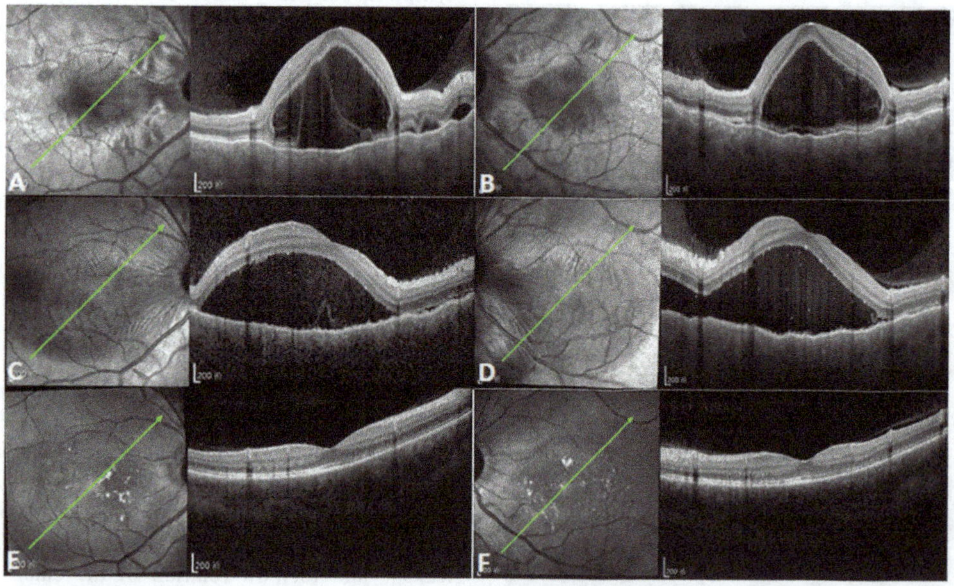

FIGURE 2 | Increased subretinal fluid after initial corticosteroid therapy. **(A,B)** Optical coherence tomography (OCT) showing multifocal serous retinal detachments with choroidal effusion in both eyes (left illustrations indicate the orientation of OCT scanning profile). **(C,D)** Subretinal fluid (SRF) increased and the coalescence of previous multifocal serous retinal detachments was observed in both eyes after initial corticosteroid therapy [left illustrations indicate the orientation of OCT scanning profile, and point-to-point follow-up mode was used for **(A,C)**, **(B,D)**]. **(E,F)** OCT showing complete absorption of SRF with normal macular structure 6 months after the onset of Vogt-Koyanagi-Harada disease [left illustrations indicate the orientation of OCT scanning profile, and point-to-point follow-up mode was used for **(A,E)**, **(B,F)**].

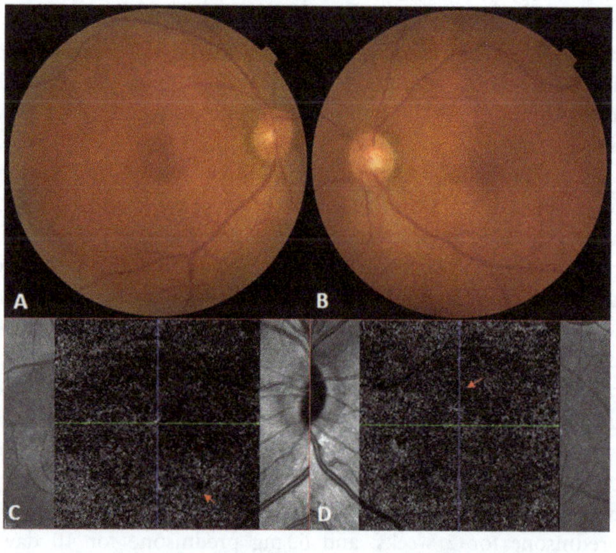

FIGURE 3 | Recovery from Vogt-Koyanagi-Harada disease. **(A,B)** The fundus appears normal in the right and left eyes, respectively, after systemic corticosteroid therapy. **(C,D)** Optical coherence tomography angiography still shows bilateral dotted hypoperfusion of the choroidal capillaries [red arrows; **(C)**: right eye; **(D)**: left eye] 6 months after the onset of Vogt-Koyanagi-Harada disease.

DISCUSSION

In this study, we present a rare case of secondary ACG involving VKH and HIV infection. Acute ACG as the first ocular manifestation of VKH is not common, and its pathogenesis may be acute inflammatory oedema, damage to the blood-aqueous humor barrier in the ciliary body, or the forward rotation of the iris and lens (7). In addition, HIV can also cause secondary glaucoma due to immune system damage and anti-optic nerve antibodies, anti-retinal antibodies, and cell lining proteins (α-fodrin) observed in the serum of HIV-infected patients (8, 9). Moreover, HIV-infected patients, who mainly have T-cell immune deficiency, can experience choroidal effusion, leading to secondary ACG with increased IOP (10). Kaushik et al. first reported a case of ACG secondary to tubercular choroidal granuloma with a mechanism similar to this case, including anterior rotation of the ciliary body at the scleral spur following the development of an inflammatory ciliochoroidal detachment (11).

To our knowledge, glucocorticoids are the first-line agents for the treatment of VKH. Glucocorticoid therapy administered during the acute phase slows down the chronic process and effectively prevents its onset in many patients. The combination of glucocorticoids and immunosuppressive drugs can help in both early vision recovery and the effective suppression of inflammation (12). In this study, unfortunately, the patient's IOP increased further after the initial systematic corticosteroid therapy, which may be partially due to the dominant hormone-sensitive genes (13). However, we did not assess the corresponding genes. In addition, glucocorticoids can inhibit phagocytosis of the trabecular cells, leading to a deposition of debris in the trabecular meshwork, blocking the outflow of aqueous humor, and increasing the IOP (14).

In this patient, the inflammation subsided after continued glucocorticoid treatment for 2 weeks, the acute inflammatory oedema of the ciliary body was reduced, the iris septum receded, and the anterior chamber angle opened (15). The serous macular detachment was aggravated after the initial corticosteroid therapy in this study. One possible explanation may be the presence of glucocorticoid and halocorticoid receptors in both retinal and choroidal vascular tissues; the combination of endogenous and exogenous glucocorticoids with the glucocorticoid receptor leads to an increase in the choroidal vascular dilation and permeability, increasing choroidal hydrostatic pressure (16). Hypoperfusion of choroidal capillaries after corticosteroid therapy also leads to the aggravation of retinal detachment (17). In this case, OCT angiography found dotted hypoperfusion of choroidal capillaries 6 months after the onset of VKH. Previously, we reported that in VKH cases, the vascular density of choriocapillaris increased significantly from 61.6 ± 2.2% at baseline to 65.1 ± 0.8, 65.7 ± 0.7, 66.1 ± 0.7, and 66.0 ± 2.0% at 1, 2, 3, and 6 months after glucocorticoid therapy, respectively (18).

Due to their anti-inflammatory and immunosuppressive effects, glucocorticoids can reduce the synthesis of inflammatory cytokines, inhibit the accumulation of inflammatory cells at inflammatory sites, reduce capillary permeability, and destroy the blood-retinal barrier, thereby reducing exudation, inhibiting tissue swelling, and reducing exudate retention, improving oedema, and promoting absorption of the SRF (19).

Increased autoimmunity and rheumatic diseases were observed in HIV-positive patients due to a disruption of the Thl/Th2 balance, stimulation of autoantibodies, chronic immune activation, immune confusion caused by HIV molecular mimicry, and increased cytotoxic T-cell response and immune dysregulation (20). The combined occurrence of VKH with HIV infection may be because they seem to act on similar cell lines (T lymphocytes) leading to immune dysfunction (21). Similarly, Graves' disease in HIV patients is associated with naive and primary thymic emigrant CD4+ T-cell recovery and inappropriate autoantibody production (22). In addition, the deterioration of Behçet's disease also has been associated with chronic HIV infection, and antiretroviral therapy for HIV will relieve the symptoms of Behçet's disease (20). Finally, posterior scleritis may develop several months after a significant rise in CD4+ T-lymphocytes, even after several years, in HIV patients (23).

This case study has some limitations; we missed information about the HIV status of the patient, including the viral load. In addition, we did not follow-up on the patient's HIV treatment to investigate its effect on the progress of VKH and secondary ACG. Finally, the UBM results from the follow-up were lost, and we had to use a slit-lamp microscope to evaluate the opening of the PACD.

In summary, this is the first report of secondary ACG in a patient with VKH and HIV infection. Both VKH and HIV infection contributed to the occurrence of ACG due to the leakage and forward rotation of the ciliary body and choroidal effusion. In clinical practice, it is important to understand the response of IOP and serous macular detachment after corticosteroid therapy.

ETHICS STATEMENT

The studies involving human participants were reviewed and approved by the Institutional Review Board of the First Hospital of China Medical University. The patients/participants provided their written informed consent to participate in this study. Written informed consent was obtained from the individual(s) for the publication of any potentially identifiable images or data included in this article.

AUTHOR CONTRIBUTIONS

RH conceived of and designed the study, acquired the data, responsible for administrative, technical, material support, and supervised the study. RH and XB developed the methodology, analyzed and interpreted the data, wrote, reviewed, and revised the manuscript. All authors contributed to the article and approved the submitted version.

REFERENCES

1. Ruiz-Cruz M, Ávila-Rios S, Ormsby CE, Ablanedo-Terrazas Y, Alvarado-de la Barrera C, Kuri-Cervantes L, et al. Cytokine profiles in aqueous humor and plasma of HIV-infected individuals with ocular syphilis or cytomegalovirus retinitis. *Ocul Immunol Inflamm.* (2018) 26:74–81. doi: 10.1080/09273948.2016.1268170
2. Zhao Y, Wu Z, McGoogan JM, Shi CX, Li A, Dou Z, et al. Immediate antiretroviral therapy decreases mortality among patients with high CD4 counts in China: a nationwide, retrospective cohort study. *Clin Infect Dis.* (2018) 66:727–34. doi: 10.1093/cid/cix878
3. Yen Y-F, Feng J-Y, Su VY-F, Chuang P-H, Ko M-C, Chen C-C, et al. Human immunodeficiency virus infection increases the risk of incident uveitis among people living with HIV/AIDS. *J Acquir Immune Defic Syndr.* (2018) 79:149-57. doi: 10.1097/QAI.0000000000001782
4. Street D, Sivaguru A, Sreekantam S, Mollan SP. Vogt-Koyanagi-Harada disease. *Pract Neurol.* (2019) 19:364–7. doi: 10.1136/practneurol-2018-002152
5. Wada S, Kohno T, Yanagihara N, Hirabayashi M, Tabuchi H, Shiraki K, et al. Ultrasound biomicroscopic study of ciliary body changes in the post-treatment phase of Vogt-Koyanagi-Harada disease. *Br J Ophthalmol.* (2002) 86:1374–9. doi: 10.1136/bjo.86.12.1374
6. Lavezzo MM, Sakata VM, Morita C, Rodriguez EEC, Abdallah SM, da Silva FTG, et al. Vogt-Koyanagi-Harada disease: review of a rare autoimmune

disease targeting antigens of melanocytes. *Orphanet J Rare Dis.* (2016) 11:29. doi: 10.1186/s13023-016-0412-4

7. Yao J, Chen Y, Shao T, Ling Z, Wang W, Qian S. Bilateral acute angle closure glaucoma as a presentation of Vogt-Koyanagi-Harada syndrome in four Chinese patients: a small case series. *Ocul Immunol Inflamm.* (2013) 21:286–91. doi: 10.3109/09273948.2013.792937
8. Trivli A, Koliarakis I, Terzidou C, Goulielmos GN, Siganos CS, Spandidos DA, et al. Normal-tension glaucoma: pathogenesis and genetics. *Exp Ther Med.* (2019) 17:563–74. doi: 10.3892/etm.2018.7011
9. Babizhayev MA. Generation of reactive oxygen species in the anterior eye segment. Synergistic codrugs of N-acetylcarnosine lubricant eye drops and mitochondria-targeted antioxidant act as a powerful therapeutic platform for the treatment of cataracts and primary open-angle glaucoma. *BBA Clin.* (2016) 6:49–68. doi: 10.1016/j.bbacli.2016.04.004
10. Ullman S, Wilson RP, Schwartz L. Bilateral angle-closure glaucoma in association with the acquired immune deficiency syndrome. *Am J Ophthalmol.* (1986) 101:419–24. doi: 10.1016/0002-9394(86)90639-2
11. Kaushik S, Singh R, Arora A, Joshi G, Sharma K, Tigari B. Acute angle closure secondary to tubercular choroidal granuloma. *J Glaucoma.* (2017) 26:e264–7. doi: 10.1097/IJG.0000000000000796
12. Du L, Kijlstra A, Yang P. Vogt-Koyanagi-Harada disease: novel insights into pathophysiology, diagnosis and treatment. *Prog Retin Eye Res.* (2016) 52:84–111. doi: 10.1016/j.preteyeres.2016.02.002
13. Becker B, Kolker AE, Roth FD. Glaucoma family study. *Am J Ophthalmol.* (1960) 50:557–67. doi: 10.1016/0002-9394(60)90233-6
14. Al Obeidan SA, Osman ES, Mousa A, Al-Muammar AM, Abu El-Asrar AM. Long-term evaluation of efficacy and safety of deep sclerectomy in uveitic glaucoma. *Ocul Immunol Inflamm.* (2015) 23:82–9. doi: 10.3109/09273948.2013.870213
15. Yang P, Liu X, Zhou H, Guo W, Zhou C, Kijlstra A. Vogt-Koyanagi-Harada disease presenting as acute angle closure glaucoma at onset. *Clin Exp Ophthalmol.* (2011) 39:639–47. doi: 10.1111/j.1442-9071.2011.02523.x
16. Behar-Cohen F, Zhao M. Corticosteroids and the retina: a role for the mineralocorticoid receptor. *Curr Opin Neurol.* (2016) 29:49–54. doi: 10.1097/WCO.0000000000000284
17. Daruich A, Matet A, Dirani A, Bousquet E, Zhao M, Farman N, et al. Central serous chorioretinopathy: recent findings and new physiopathology hypothesis. *Prog Retin Eye Res.* (2015) 48:82–118. doi: 10.1016/j.preteyeres.2015.05.003
18. Hua R, Wang N, Liu L, Ning H. Improvement of vascular density of macular capillaries in acute Vogt-Koyanagi-Harada disease after glucocorticoid therapy. *Clin Exp Ophthalmol.* (2021) 49:524–7. doi: 10.1111/ceo.13932
19. Bordaberry MF. Vogt-Koyanagi-Harada disease: diagnosis and treatments update. *Curr Opin Ophthalmol.* (2010) 21:430–5. doi: 10.1097/ICU.0b013e32833eb78c
20. Roscoe C, Kinney R, Gilles R, Blue S. Behcet's disease diagnosed after acute HIV infection: viral replication activating underlying autoimmunity? *Int J STD AIDS.* (2015) 26:432–5. doi: 10.1177/0956462414539667
21. Priya D, Sudharshan S, Biswas J. Management of a rare presentation of Vogt-Koyanagi-Harada disease in human immunodeficiency virus/acquired immunodeficiency disease syndrome patient. *Indian J Ophthalmol.* (2017) 65:413–6. doi: 10.4103/ijo.IJO_544_16
22. Sheikh V, Dersimonian R, Richterman AG, Porter BO, Natarajan V, Burbelo PD, et al. Graves' disease as immune reconstitution disease in HIV-positive patients is associated with naive and primary thymic emigrant CD4(+) T-cell recovery. *AIDS.* (2014) 28:31–9. doi: 10.1097/QAD.0000000000000006
23. Che X, Jiang J, Qian Y, Li Q, Zhang Y, Wang Z. Case report-immune recovery posterior scleritis in a HIV positive patient. *BMC Ophthalmol.* (2020) 20:262. doi: 10.1186/s12886-020-01529-3

29

A Case of Perifoveal Exudative Vascular Anomalous Complex with a Good Prognosis

Min Fu[1†], Pan Hu[1†], Gang Zhang[2], Ludonghan Huang[1], Huan Xu[1], Ju Huang[1], Meihui Wu[3] and Yanli Chen[1]*

[1] Department of Ophthalmology, Daping Hospital of Army Characteristic Medical Center, Chongqing, China, [2] Department of Medicine, 953 Hospital of People's Liberation Army (PLA), Xizang, China, [3] Nursing Teaching and Research Section, Daping Hospital of Army Characteristic Medical Center, Chongqing, China

Correspondence:
Yanli Chen
252526323@qq.com

† These authors have contributed equally to this work and share first authorship

Significance: Perifoveal exudative vascular anomalous complex (PEVAC) is a unique clinical lesion. It manifests as isolated lesions and is easily misdiagnosed. Thus far, few PEVAC case reports have been published. PEVAC is typically inconsistent with other reported macular lesions.

Purpose: To report our 24-month follow-up experience on the treatment of PEVAC with a micropulse laser (MPL).

Case Report: A 56-year-old Chinese woman with no history of other diseases complained of decreased vision in her left eye that had persisted for more than 1 year. Comprehensive ophthalmic examinations were performed, including a vision test, slit lamp fundus exam, optical coherence tomography (OCT), optical coherence tomography angiography (OCT-A), fluorescein fundus angiography (FFA) and indocyanine green angiography (ICGA). Intravitreal injection of ranibizumab was ineffective, and bleeding, exudation and visual acuity were not improved. After two rounds of micropulse laser (MPL) treatment, the patient was followed up, and the prognosis was good.

Conclusion: PEVAC is very rare, and early diagnosis is important, as the lesions readily cause irreversible damage. Our results indicate that an MPL can be used as an alternative treatment for PEVAC patients.

Keywords: perifoveal exudative vascular anomalous complex (PEVAC), micropulse laser (MPL), age-related macular degeneration (AMD), case report, good prognosis

INTRODUCTION

Perifoveal exudative vascular anomalous complex (PEVAC) is a unique clinical lesion. It manifests as isolated lesions in close proximity to the macula; thus, it is easily misdiagnosed. PEVAC is an elusive, rare lesion that has mainly been reported in case studies and is usually non-responsive to anti-vascular endothelial growth factor (VEGF) treatment. In the absence of capillary ischemia or inflammation, the pathogenesis of PEVAC may be progressive degeneration of retinal endothelial cells, which may also explain the ineffectiveness of anti-VEGF treatment (1, 2). In summary, PEVAC is an isolated perifoveal vascular lesion. The characteristics of PEVAC patients according to optical coherence tomography (OCT) are consistent in existing reports. Patients with PEVAC may have diabetes or hypertension; additionally, PEVAC can occur in healthy individuals or in

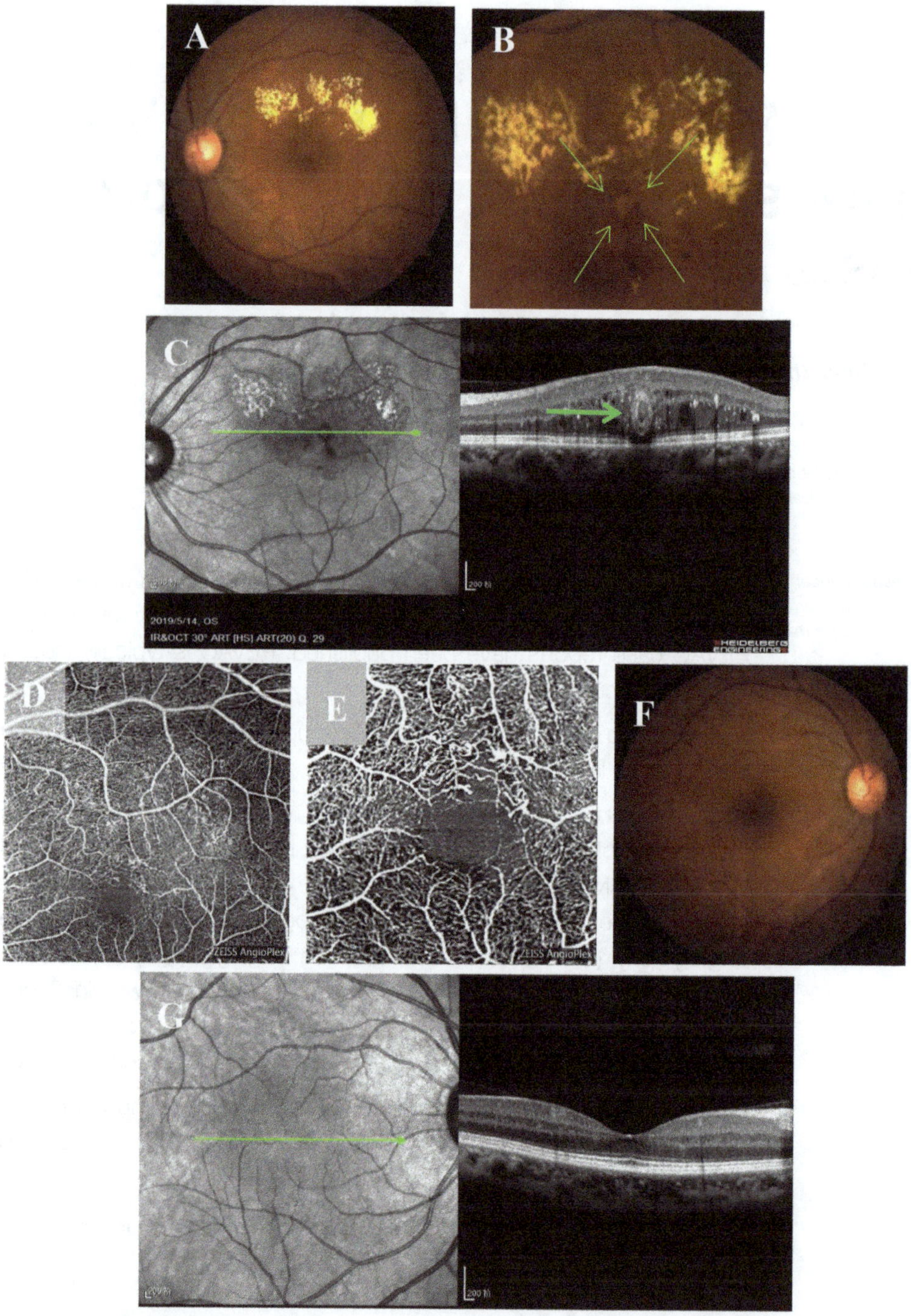

FIGURE 1 | Multimodal imaging at the initial visit. **(A)** Fundus examination of the left eye shows an isolated off-white lesion near the macular area and a large level of muddy-like exudate above the macular area. **(B)** An enlarged image of the lesion. **(C)** OCT imaging shows off-white lesions on transverse scanning; the lesions are bright on the outside and black on the inside with an oval ring reflection (bold green arrow), strong point reflection between layers, and edema between layers. **(D)** OCT-A shows sparse blood vessels, superficial vascular dilatation, and a tangled nodule beside the vessels. **(E)** Enlarged OCT-A image. **(F,G)** The fundus and OCT of the right eye are normal.

those with myopic macular degeneration and age-related macular degeneration (AMD). It may also be related to type 3 neovascularization (T3NV)/retinal angiomatous proliferation (RAP), which is inconsistent with the clinical features of macular telangiectasia type 1 (MacTel 1) and RAP. Therefore, clinicians should be aware of the possibility that patients may have this special perifoveal disease and should focus on its relatively poor prognosis and potential prolonged recovery time.

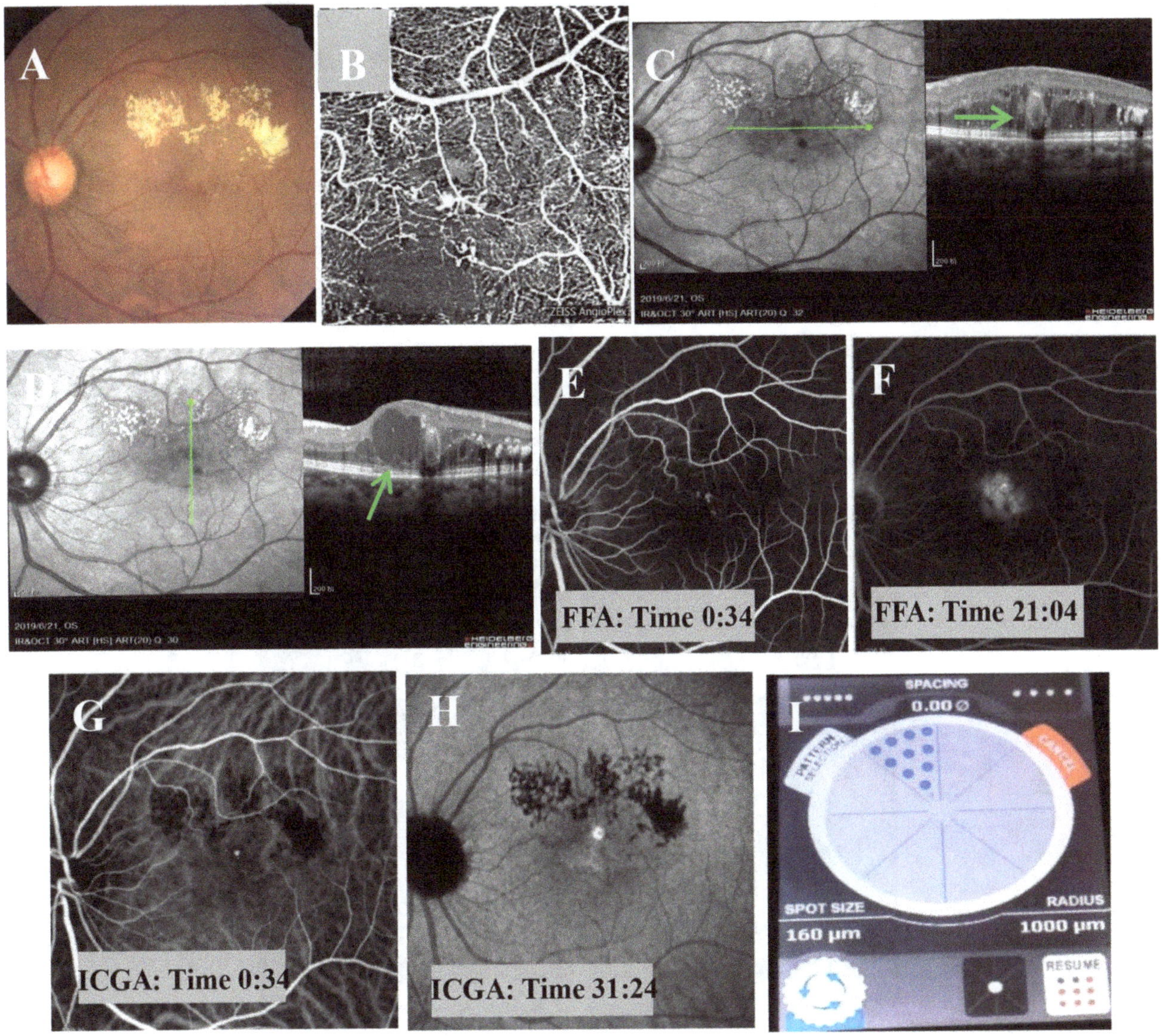

FIGURE 2 | Fundus examination one month after intravitreal injection of anti-VEGF. **(A)** Fundus examination shows muddy-like exudation above the macular area, punctate hemorrhage, and no obvious change in the off-white lesions adjacent to the macula. **(B)** OCT-A shows sparse blood vessels, dilated superficial blood vessels, and a tangled nodule beside the blood vessels. **(C,D)** OCT imaging shows macular edema, dot-like hyperreflexia between layers, light on the outside and black on the inside, with no obvious change in oval structure (bold green arrow), and cystic edema in some parts of the macular area (bold green arrow). **(E,F)** FFA shows a strong fluorescent focus with a clear boundary near the macula in the early stage and obvious leakage in the later stage. **(G,H)** ICGA shows well-defined, strong fluorescence near the macula in the early stage, but no obvious leakage in the later stage. **(I)** The MPL treatment was delivered in a fan shape, covering the focus and the upper edema area.

CASE REPORT

A 56-year-old Chinese woman without diabetes and other diseases presented with visual acuity deterioration in her left eye for over 1 year. Ophthalmic examination revealed that her right eye vision was 20/20, her left eye vision was 20/160, and the anterior segment of both eyes was normal. However, fundus examination of the left eye showed an isolated off-white lesion near the macular area and a large amount of muddy-like exudates above the macular area (**Figure 1A**). An enlarged image of the lesion (**Figure 1B**). OCT images showed off-white lesions in the cross-sectional scan that were bright around the edges and black on the inside, with an oval circular reflex, a strong point-like reflex and edema between the layers (**Figure 1C**). An OCT-A scan showed sparse blood vessels with dilated superficial blood vessels and an adjacent tangled nodule (**Figure 1D**). Enlarged OCT-A image (**Figure 1E**). The fundus and OCT of the right eye were normal (**Figures 1F,G**).

Based on these prominent clinical features, the patient was diagnosed with PEVAC. Therefore, an intravitreal injection of anti-VEGF treatment was administered. One month after the injection, the following findings were observed, as shown in

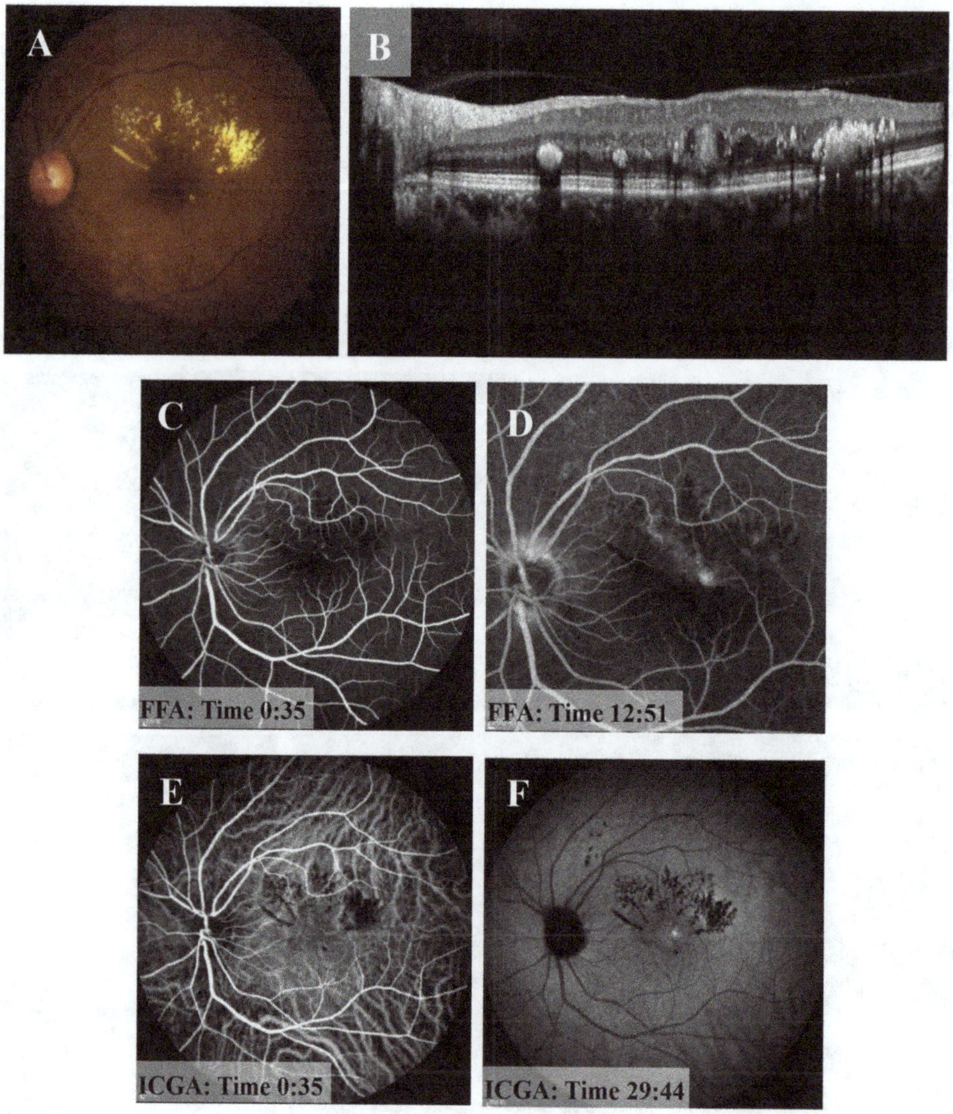

FIGURE 3 | One month after the second MPL treatment. **(A)** Fundus examination of the left eye shows muddy-like exudation above the macular area and that the off-white lesions had shrunken. **(B)** OCT shows that the oval structure in macular area had become more solid and that the cavity structure had disappeared. **(C,D)** FFA shows strong fluorescent light spots near the macular area in the early stage and slight leakage in the later stage. **(E,F)** ICGA shows a light spot near macular area in the early stage, and there was no leakage in the later stage.

Figures 2A–H. Bleeding and focal exudation were still present, and the patient's visual acuity and focality were not improved.

The suggestion of PDT treatment was refused because of the high price and lack of guaranteed efficacy. Instead, MPL treatment (QUANTEL MEDICAL) was chosen, the effect of which is uncertain, after communicating with the patient, who signed the informed consent form and subsequently received a total of 2 MPL treatments. The MPL treatment was delivered in a fan shape, covering the focus and the upper edema area. The parameters were as follows, 577 nm, 160 μm, 300 mw, 0.2 s, duty cycle 5% and spacing 0 (**Figure 2I**). The patient underwent two MPL treatments one month apart. One month after the second MPL treatment, examination of the left eye showed that the exudation and edema were significantly improved (**Figures 3A–F**). After 24 months of follow-up, the prognosis of the patient was good, and the visual acuity recovered to 20/50. Examination of the left eye showed that the exudation and edema were significantly improved and that the lesions had disappeared (**Figures 4A–D**).

DISCUSSION

In 2011, Querques et al. (1) reported PEVAC for the first time. An increasing number of researchers have begun investigating PEVAC, although its pathogenesis remains unclear (1–6). In 2017, studies across 15 centers (2) showed that PEVAC is an isolated, perifoveal, angiomatous lesion that generally occurs in healthy patients but can also be accompanied by AMD and myopic macular degeneration. PEVAC has a slight or poor response to anti-VEGF treatments. The possible

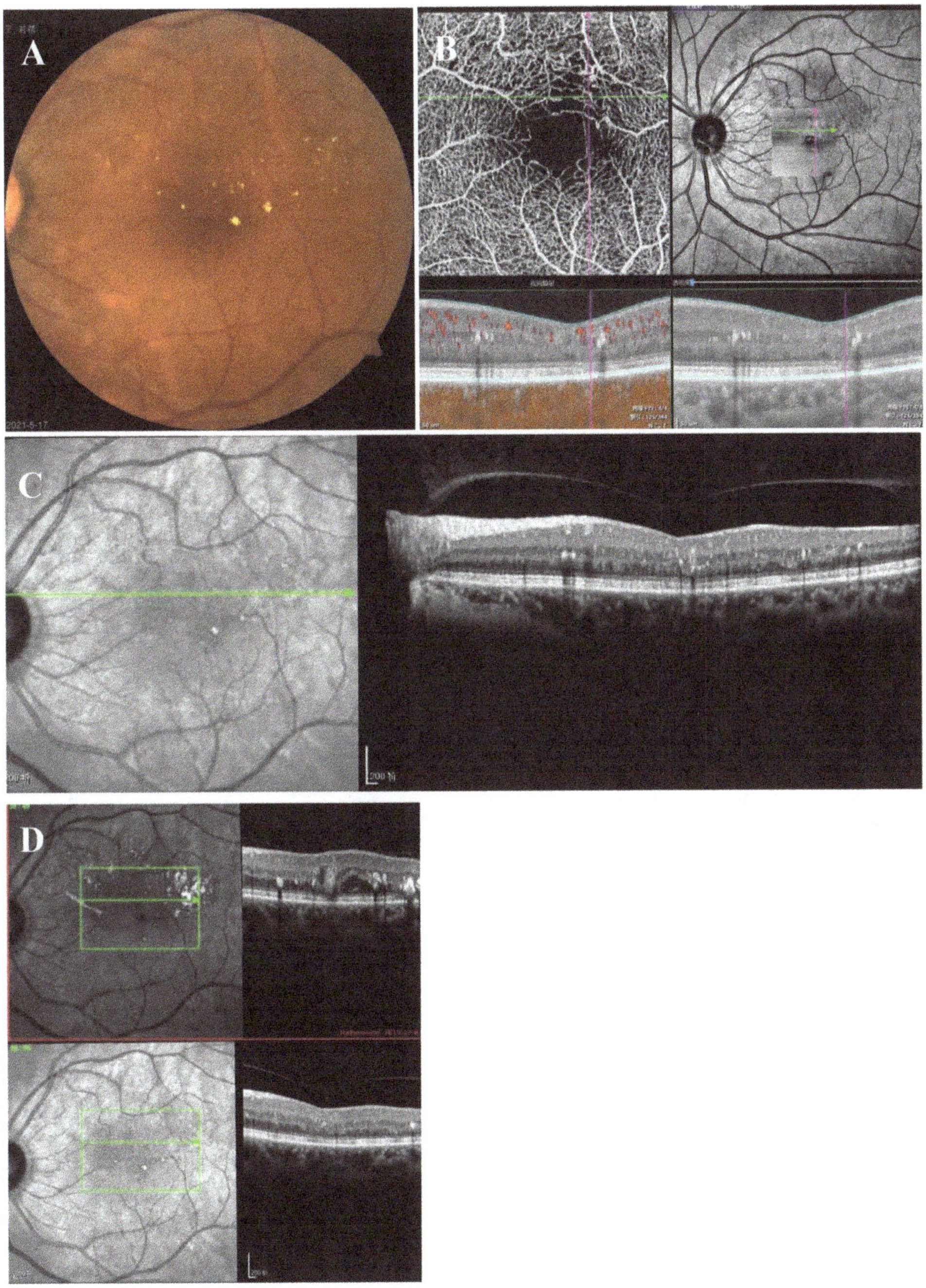

FIGURE 4 | Twenty-four months after MPL treatment. **(A)** Exudates are scattered above the macular area. **(B)** OCT-A shows sparse vessels in the upper arch ring and that the tumor-like dilatation had disappeared. **(C)** OCT shows that the tumor-like structure had disappeared, and there are a few punctate hyperreflections between the layers. **(D)** In the OCT comparison chart, the tumor-like structure had disappeared.

reasons are as follows (1): first, under an absence of capillary ischemia or inflammation, progressive retinal endothelial cell degeneration may trigger the vasogenic cellular mechanism for PEVAC; and second, the disease may be related to T3NV /RAP. In 2019, Venkatsh et al. (4) and Zhengwei Zhang et al. (6) reported the case of a patient with diabetes with PEVAC in whom anti-VEGF injection treatment was ineffective, which further indicated that PEVAC may not only occur in healthy eyes.

PEVAC should be distinguished from other periretinal vascular abnormalities. In a recent study, Mrejen-Uretsky et al. (3) reported that PEVAC may be misdiagnosed as other diseases, such as MacTel 1 and RAP. Attention should be given by clinicians to the possibility of PEVAC in the differential diagnosis. However, through multimodal imaging analysis, the characteristic imaging findings of PEVAC are obvious. For example, OCT shows that the lesion has a strong reflective ring wall and internal dark cavity, and OCT-A shows blood flow in the lesion.

RAP (T3NV) (7–10) is a special type of neovascular age-related macular degeneration (nARMD) that usually presents as isolated perifoveal vascular lesions. Stage 1 RAP is usually accompanied by small retinal edema without obvious hard exudation. PEVAC is easily confused with stage 1 RAP (11–13), but their morphologies are different on OCT. PEVAC appears as a circle-like lesion with a highly reflective signal wall and a cavity that contains a substance with uncertain reflective signals. In contrast, stage 1 RAP manifests as a hyperreflective focus without a hyperreflective wall. In addition, RAP is considered to have a poor prognosis. Anti-VEGF drugs are the first choice of therapy for nARMD; many studies have confirmed their effectiveness for the treatment of RAP (11–13), but intravitreal injection of anti-VEGF for PEVAC has no obvious effect.

Retinal arterial macroaneurysms (RAMs) are pathological dilations of the retinal artery, and most occur in elderly women over 60 years old. RAMs are associated with hypertension, diabetes, heart disease and other systemic conditions. These macroaneurys have variable clinical manifestations and are easily misdiagnosed as exudative AMD, diabetic retinopathy (DR), branch retinal vein occlusion (BRVO), telangiectasia and other hemorrhagic diseases with similar manifestations (14, 15). Unlike PEVAC, large aneurysms of the retinal artery are usually saccular or fusiform dilations of the large artery at the first three bifurcations of the central retinal artery, relatively far from the fovea (16). Most patients with retinal aneurysms have good vision after treatment (14). This is contrary to the poor vision prognosis after treatment in most patients with PEVAC (1–3).

Macular telangiectasia type 1 (MacTel 1) usually occurs in young patients and is characterized by multiple telangiectasias and microangiomas involving the temporal side of the macula. Furthermore, it is often accompanied by macular edema and hard exudation. Intravitreal injection of anti-VEGF treatment is effective (7). PEVAC exhibits perifoveal, large isolated aneurysmal changes, and two lesions have been reported in rare cases (2, 6). The common imaging feature of these PEVAC and MacTel 1 lesions is a sparse capillary network around the lesion (2, 3, 17). The relationship between PEVAC and MacTel 1 needs to be further investigated.

MPL is a repeatable, inexpensive, and minimally damaging treatment (18). The main mechanism of MPL is direct blockage of leaking microangiomas and moderate destruction of the decompensated retinal pigment epithelium (RPE) by the generation of photocoagulation. The surrounding RPE cells are then activated and proliferated, and then the function of the blood-retinal barrier is repaired and reconstructed. MPL treatment may reduce the local inflammatory response by deactivating retinal microglia. Light induces an effect on the optic nerve omentum, which causes a series of cytokine changes (19, 20).

In conclusion, according to our findings, our patient's bleeding and exudation were not alleviated by the first injection of anti-VEGF, and no improvement in vision or lesions was observed. After communication with the patient, subsequent treatment with MPL was initiated, and a beneficial treatment effect was obtained. The selective RPE injury mechanism of MPL may not be the main factor for PEVAC treatment. Instead, the photoinduced biological effect on neuroretinal tissues and cells may be responsible for improving the clinical effect of MPL in PEVAC treatment. More samples should be obtained in future in-depth research. Since PEVAC is extremely rare, retinal vein occlusion (RVO), RAP, DR and other microaneurysm-like lesions could be selected to observe the therapeutic effect and increase the applicability of MPL in further research.

CONCLUSION

PEVAC appeared as a single aneurysm with exudation in this patient, and intravitreal injection of anti-VEGF was ineffective. Subsequently, two MPL treatments were administered, and a sustained positive functional result was obtained. Therefore, the pathogenesis of PEVAC and its effective treatment with MPL are worthy of further study. Here, we presented our experience with MPL to provide valuable information about this treatment to clinicians.

ETHICS STATEMENT

The studies involving human participants were reviewed and approved by Ethics Committee, Daping Hospital of Army Characteristic Medical Center, Chongqing, China. The patients/participants provided their written informed consent to participate in this study. Written informed consent was obtained from the individual(s) for the publication of any potentially identifiable images or data included in this article.

AUTHOR CONTRIBUTIONS

The data were analyzed and the manuscript was drafted by MF and PH. The manuscript was revised by YC. The results were analyzed and conclusions were made by MF, PH, and YC. Data were collected by LH, HX, and JH. The data were analyzed and integrated by GZ and MW. The final manuscript was read and approved by all authors.

REFERENCES

1. Querques G, Kuhn D, Massamba N, Leveziel N, Querques L, Souied EH. Perifoveal exudative vascular anomalous complex. *J Fr Ophtalmol.* (2011) 34:559.e1–4. doi: 10.1016/j.jfo.2011.03.002
2. Sacconi R, Freund KB, Yannuzzi LA, Dolz-Marco R, Souied E, Capuano V, et al. The expanded spectrum of perifoveal exudative vascular anomalous complex. *Am J Ophthalmol.* (2017) 184:137–46. doi: 10.1016/j.ajo.2017.10.009
3. Mrejen S, Le HM, Nghiem-Buffet S, Tabary S, Quentel G, Cohen SY. Insights into perifoveal exudative vascular anomalous complex. *Retina.* (2020) 40:80–6. doi: 10.1097/IAE.0000000000002435
4. Venkatesh R, Yadav NK, Bavaharan B, Prabhu V, Sinha S. multimodal imaging in perifoveal exudative vascular anomalous complex with co-existent diabetic retinopathy. *Clin Exp Optom.* (2019) 102:528–32. doi: 10.1111/cxo.12868
5. Ayachit AG, Sacconi R, Ayachit GS, Joshi S, Querques G. Perifoveal exudative vascular anomalous complex-like lesion as a complication of prepapillary arterial loops. *Ophthalmic Surg Lasers Imaging Retina.* (2018) 49:974–8. doi: 10.3928/23258160-20181203-11
6. Zhang Z, Xu L, Wu Z, Zhang J. Case report: perifoveal exudative vascular anomalous complex in a Chinese patient with diabetes mellitus. *Optometry Vis Sci.* (2019) 96:531–5. doi: 10.1097/OPX.0000000000001401
7. Yannuzzi LA, Bardal AM, Freund KB, Chen KJ, Eandi CM, Blodi B. Idiopathic macular telangiectasia. *Arch Ophthalmol.* (2006) 124:450–60. doi: 10.1001/archopht.124.4.450
8. Su D, Lin S, Phasukkijwatana N, Chen X, Tan A, Freund KB, et al. An updated staging system of type 3 neovascularization using spectral domain optical coherence tomography. *Retina.* (2016) 36(Suppl. 1):S40–9. doi: 10.1097/IAE.0000000000001268
9. Yannuzzi LA, Negrão S, Iida T, Carvalho C, Rodriguez-Coleman H, Slakter J, et al. Retinal angiomatous proliferation in age-related macular degeneration. *Retina.* (2012) 32(Suppl 1.):416–34. doi: 10.1097/IAE.0b013e31823f9b3b
10. Kataoka K, Takeuchi J, Nakano Y, Fujita, A, Kaneko H, Ito Y, et al. Characteristics and classification of type 3 neovascularization with b-scan flow overlay and en face flow images of optical coherence tomography angiography. *Retina.* (2020) 40:109–20. doi: 10.1097/IAE.0000000000002357
11. Meyerle CB, Freund KB, Iturralde D, Spaide RF, Sorenson JA, Slakter JS, et al. Intravitreal bevacizumab (Avastin) for retinal angiomatous proliferation. *Retina.* (2007) 27:451–7. doi: 10.1097/IAE.0b013e318030ea80
12. Lai TY, Chan WM, Liu DT, Lam DS. Ranibizumab for retinal angiomatous proliferation in neovascular age-related macular degeneration. *Graefes Arch Clin Exp Ophthalmol.* (2007) 245:1877–80. doi: 10.1007/s00417-007-0679-1
13. Tsaousis KT, Konidaris VE, Banerjee S, Empeslidis T. Intravitreal aflibercept treatment of retinal angiomatous proliferation: a pilot study and short - term efficacy. *Graefes Arch Clin Exp Ophthalmol.* (2015) 253:663–5. doi: 10.1007/s00417-014-2835-8
14. Pitkänen L, Tommila P, Kaarniranta K, Jääskeläinen JE, Kinnunen K. Retinal arterial macroaneurysms. *Acta ophthalmol.* (2014) 92:101–4. doi: 10.1111/aos.12210
15. Abdelkader E, Yip KP, Cornish KS. Pneumatic displacement of submacular hacmorrhage. *Saudi J Ophthalmol.* (2016) 30:221–6. doi: 10.1016/j.sjopt.2016.10.002
16. Hughes EL, Dooley IJ, Kennelly KP, Doyle F, Siah WF, Connell P. Angiographic features and disease outcomes of symptomatic retinal arterial macroaneurysms. *Graefes Arch Clin Exp Ophthalmol.* (2016) 254:2203–7. doi: 10.1007/s00417-016-3388-9
17. Yannuzzi NA, Gregori NZ, Roisman L, Gupta N, Goldhagen BE, Goldhardt R. Fluorescein angiography versus optical coherence tomography angiography in macular telangiectasia type i treated with bevacizumab therapy. *Ophth Surg Lasers Imaging Retina.* (2017) 48:263–6. doi: 10.3928/23258160-20170301-12
18. Schmidt-Erfurtha U, Garcia-Arumib J, Bandello F, Berg K, Chakravarthy U, Gerendas BS, et al. Guidelines for the management of diabetic macular edema by the european society of retina specialists (EURETINA). *Ophthalmologica.* (2017) 237:185–222. doi: 10.1159/000458539
19. Midena E, Micera A, Frizziero L, Pilotto E, Esposito G, Bini S. Sub-threshold micropulse laser treatment reduces inflammatory biomarkers in aqueous humour of diabetic patients with macular edema. *Sci Rep.* (2019) 9:10034. doi: 10.1038/s41598-019-46515-y
20. Midena E, Bini S, Martini F, Enrica C, Pilotto E, Micera A, et al. Changes of aqueous humor müller cells' biomarkers in human patients affected by diabetic macular edema after subthreshold micropulse laser treatment. *Retina.* (2020) 40:126–34. doi: 10.1097/IAE.0000000000002356

Permissions

All chapters in this book were first published by Frontiers; hereby published with permission under the Creative Commons Attribution License or equivalent. Every chapter published in this book has been scrutinized by our experts. Their significance has been extensively debated. The topics covered herein carry significant findings which will fuel the growth of the discipline. They may even be implemented as practical applications or may be referred to as a beginning point for another development.

The contributors of this book come from diverse backgrounds, making this book a truly international effort. This book will bring forth new frontiers with its revolutionizing research information and detailed analysis of the nascent developments around the world.

We would like to thank all the contributing authors for lending their expertise to make the book truly unique. They have played a crucial role in the development of this book. Without their invaluable contributions this book wouldn't have been possible. They have made vital efforts to compile up to date information on the varied aspects of this subject to make this book a valuable addition to the collection of many professionals and students.

This book was conceptualized with the vision of imparting up-to-date information and advanced data in this field. To ensure the same, a matchless editorial board was set up. Every individual on the board went through rigorous rounds of assessment to prove their worth. After which they invested a large part of their time researching and compiling the most relevant data for our readers.

The editorial board has been involved in producing this book since its inception. They have spent rigorous hours researching and exploring the diverse topics which have resulted in the successful publishing of this book. They have passed on their knowledge of decades through this book. To expedite this challenging task, the publisher supported the team at every step. A small team of assistant editors was also appointed to further simplify the editing procedure and attain best results for the readers.

Apart from the editorial board, the designing team has also invested a significant amount of their time in understanding the subject and creating the most relevant covers. They scrutinized every image to scout for the most suitable representation of the subject and create an appropriate cover for the book.

The publishing team has been an ardent support to the editorial, designing and production team. Their endless efforts to recruit the best for this project, has resulted in the accomplishment of this book. They are a veteran in the field of academics and their pool of knowledge is as vast as their experience in printing. Their expertise and guidance has proved useful at every step. Their uncompromising quality standards have made this book an exceptional effort. Their encouragement from time to time has been an inspiration for everyone.

The publisher and the editorial board hope that this book will prove to be a valuable piece of knowledge for researchers, students, practitioners and scholars across the globe.

List of Contributors

Xinbo Gao, Liming Chen, Bingru Zheng, Simin Zhang, Chengguo Zuo and Mingkai Lin
State Key Laboratory of Ophthalmology, Guangdong Provincial Key Laboratory of Ophthalmology and Visual Science, Zhongshan Ophthalmic Center, Sun Yat-sen University, Guangzhou, China

Yuying Zhou, Jiawei Ren, Huishan Lin and Huanling Hu
State Key Laboratory of Ophthalmology, Zhongshan Ophthalmic Center, Sun Yat-sen University, Guangzhou, China

Haijun Gong
State Key Laboratory of Ophthalmology, Guangdong Provincial Key Laboratory of Ophthalmology and Visual Science, Zhongshan Ophthalmic Center, Sun Yat-sen University, Guangzhou, China
Guangdong Provincial Key Laboratory of Malignant Tumor Epigenetics and Gene Regulation, Department of Ophthalmology, Sun Yat-sen Memorial Hospital, Sun Yat-sen University, Guangzhou, China

Ziyi Zhu, Yongan Meng, Manyun Xie, Youling Liang, Bin Yan, Liang Zhou and Pingbo Ouyang
Department of Ophthalmology, The Second Xiangya Hospital, Central South University, Changsha, China

Igor Kozak
Hunan Clinical Research Center of Ophthalmic Disease, Changsha, China

Xiaoxi Yao
Moorfields Eye Hospital UAE, Abu Dhabi, United Arab Emirates

Jing Luo
Department of Ophthalmology, The Second Xiangya Hospital, Central South University, Changsha, China Shenzhen College of International Education, Shenzhen, China

Yingting Zhu, Yuwen Wen and Yehong Zhuo
State Key Laboratory of Ophthalmology, Zhongshan Ophthalmic Center, Sun Yat-sen University, Guangzhou, China

Lei Fang, Shufen Lin, Xiaodi Zhou and Pingping Liu
State Key Laboratory of Ophthalmology, Zhongshan Ophthalmic Center, Sun Yat-sen University, Guangzhou, China

Julius Oatts and Ying Han
Department of Ophthalmology, School of Medicine, University of California, San Francisco, San Francisco, CA, United States

Yihua Su
State Key Laboratory of Ophthalmology, Zhongshan Ophthalmic Center, Sun Yat-sen University, Guangzhou, China
The First Affiliated Hospital, Sun Yat-sen University, Guangzhou, China

Chun Yan, Fan Li, Xiaoyuan Ye, Lishi Su, Yixin Hu, Jiawen Luo and Wei Chi
State Key Laboratory of Ophthalmology, Zhongshan Ophthalmic Center, Sun Yat-sen University, Guangzhou, China

Min Hou
Department of Ophthalmology, Luoyang Central Hospital, Zhengzhou University, Luoyang, China

Xu Dong
State Key Laboratory of Ophthalmology, Guangdong Provincial Key Laboratory of Ophthalmology and Visual Science, Zhongshan Ophthalmic Center, Sun Yat-sen University, Guangzhou, China
The Fourth People's Hospital of Shenyang, Shenyang, China

Hui Xiao, Yimin Zhong, Yunlan Ling, Xiaoyu Xu and Xing Liu
State Key Laboratory of Ophthalmology, Zhongshan Ophthalmic Center, Sun Yat-sen University, Guangdong Provincial Key Laboratory of Ophthalmology and Visual Science, Guangdong Provincial Clinical Research Center for Ocular Diseases, Guangzhou, China

Pei-Yao Chang
Department of Ophthalmology, Far Eastern Memorial Hospital, New Taipei City, Taiwan
Department of Medicine, National Taiwan University Hospital, Taipei, Taiwan
Department of Healthcare Administration, Asia University, Taichung, Taiwan
Department of Electrical Engineering, Yuan Ze University, Taoyuan City, Taiwan

Jia-Kang Wang
Department of Ophthalmology, Far Eastern Memorial Hospital, New Taipei City, Taiwan
Department of Medicine, National Taiwan University Hospital, Taipei, Taiwan
Department of Electrical Engineering, Yuan Ze University, Taoyuan City, Taiwan
Department of Healthcare Administration and Department of Nursing, Oriental Institute of Technology, New Taipei City, Taiwan

Jiun-Yi Wang
Department of Ophthalmology, Far Eastern Memorial Hospital, New Taipei City, Taiwan
Department of Medicine, National Taiwan University Hospital, Taipei, Taiwan
Department of Electrical Engineering, Yuan Ze University, Taoyuan City, Taiwan
Department of Healthcare Administration and Department of Nursing, Oriental Institute of Technology, New Taipei City, Taiwan
Department of Medical Research, China Medical University Hospital, China Medical University, Taichung, Taiwan

Tzu-Lun Huang
Department of Ophthalmology, Far Eastern Memorial Hospital, New Taipei City, Taiwan
Department of Electrical Engineering, Yuan Ze University, Taoyuan City, Taiwan

Yung-Ray Hsu
Department of Ophthalmology, Far Eastern Memorial Hospital, New Taipei City, Taiwan
Department of Medicine, National Taiwan University Hospital, Taipei, Taiwan
Department of Electrical Engineering, Yuan Ze University, Taoyuan City, Taiwan

Bingjie Qiu, Xinyuan Zhang, Qiyun Wang, Yao Nie and Xiaosi Chen
Beijing Tongren Eye Center, Beijing Institute of Ophthalmology, Beijing Tongren Hospital, Capital Medical University, Beijing, China
Beijing Retinal Choroidal Vascular Diseases Study Group, China

Lin Zhao
Beijing Tongren Eye Center, Beijing Institute of Ophthalmology, Beijing Tongren Hospital, Capital Medical University, Beijing, China

Yanhong Wang
Department of Epidemiology and Biostatistics, Institute of Basic Medical Sciences Chinese Academy of Medical Sciences & School of Basic Medicine Peking Union Medical College, Beijing, China

Carol Y. L. Cheung
Department of Ophthalmology and Visual Sciences, The Chinese University of Hong Kong, Hong Kong, China

Wei Lin and Meng Feng
School of Basic Medicine, Shandong First Medical University and Shandong Academy of Medical Science, Shandong Provincial Hospital Affiliated to Shandong First Medical University, Jinan, China

Qingxu Wang
Jinan Mingshui Eye Hospital, Jinan, China

Zhongyu Ma
The First Clinical Medical College of Shandong University of Traditional Chinese Medicine, Jinan, China

Wenqi Wang and Xiao Xie
Eye Hospital of Shandong First Medical University (Shandong Eye Hospital), Jinan, China
State Key Laboratory Cultivation Base, Shandong Provincial Key Laboratory of Ophthalmology, Qingdao, China
Shandong Eye Institute, Shandong First Medical University and Shandong Academy of Medical Sciences, Qingdao, China
The First Clinical Medical College of Shandong University of Traditional Chinese Medicine, Jinan, China

Wenhao Li
Computer Department of Southwest University of Science and Technology, Mianyang, China

Tong Liu
Department of Medicine, Xizang Minzu University, Xianyang, China

Tingting Liu, Ge Tian, Jinyan Wang, Jitian Guan and Xunchang Wang
Eye Hospital of Shandong First Medical University (Shandong Eye Hospital), Jinan, China
State Key Laboratory Cultivation Base, Shandong Provincial Key Laboratory of Ophthalmology, Shandong Eye Institute, Qingdao, China
Shandong First Medical University and Shandong Academy of Medical Sciences, Qingdao, China
School of Ophthalmology, Shandong First Medical University, Jinan, China

Jingwen Jiang, Gongpeng Sun, Xiaoling Wang, Zuohuizi Yi, Mei Fu, Xueying Yang, Hongmei Zheng and Changzheng Chen
Eye Center, Renmin Hospital of Wuhan University, Wuhan, China

Qingjun Zhou
State Key Laboratory Cultivation Base, Shandong Provincial Key Laboratory of Ophthalmology, Shandong Eye Institute, Qingdao, China
Shandong First Medical University and Shandong Academy of Medical Sciences, Qingdao, China
School of Ophthalmology, Shandong First Medical University, Jinan, China
Qingdao Eye Hospital of Shandong First Medical University, Qingdao, China

Qingmei Miao and Jiajia Yuan
Eye Center, Renmin Hospital of Wuhan University, Wuhan, China

Dan Wang
Department of Ophthalmology, Tongji Hospital, Tongji Medical College, Huazhong University of Science and Technology, Wuhan, China

Bin Li
Department of Ophthalmology, Tongji Hospital, Tongji Medical College, Huazhong University of Science and Technology, Wuhan, China
Neurophth Biotechnology Co., Ltd. Wuhan, China

Hongmei Zhao, Jian Yu, Yuan Zong, Chunhui Jiang and Gezhi Xu
Department of Ophthalmology and Vision Science, Eye and Ear, Nose and Throat Hospital, Fudan University, Shanghai, China
Key Laboratory of Myopia of State Health Ministry, Shanghai, China
Key Laboratory of Visual Impairment and Restoration of Shanghai, Shanghai, China
National Health Commission (NHC) Key Laboratory of Myopia, Fudan University, Shanghai, China
Key Laboratory of Myopia, Chinese Academy of Medical Sciences, Shanghai, China

Haohao Zhu
Department of Ophthalmology, Shanghai Fifth People's Hospital, Fudan University Shanghai, China

Xin Wen, Zijing Li, Jianhui Xiao, Xuane Liu, Yichi Zhang and Yuqing Lan
Guangdong Provincial Key Laboratory of Malignant Tumor Epigenetics and Gene Regulation, Department of Ophthalmology, Sun Yat-sen Memorial Hospital, Sun Yat-sen University, Guangzhou, China

Jingyi Cheng and Xiangmei Kong
Department of Ophthalmology and Visual Science, Eye, Ear, Nose and Throat Hospital, Fudan University, Shanghai, China
Key Laboratory of Myopia, Ministry of Health, Fudan University, Shanghai, China
Shanghai Key Laboratory of Visual Impairment and Restoration, Fudan University, Shanghai, China

Xinghuai Sun
Department of Ophthalmology and Visual Science, Eye, Ear, Nose and Throat Hospital, Fudan University, Shanghai, China
Key Laboratory of Myopia, Ministry of Health, Fudan University, Shanghai, China
Shanghai Key Laboratory of Visual Impairment and Restoration, Fudan University, Shanghai, China
State Key Laboratory of Medical Neurobiology, Institutes of Brain Science, Fudan University, Shanghai, China

Ziqing Feng, Gengyuan Wang, Meng Li, Peng Xiao and Jin Yuan
State Key Laboratory of Ophthalmology, Guangdong Provincial Key Laboratory of Ophthalmology and Visual Science, Guangdong Provincial Clinical Research Center for Ocular Diseases, Zhongshan Ophthalmic Center, Sun Yat-sen University, Guangzhou, China

Honghui Xia, Guoxia Liang and Tingting Dong
Department of Ophthalmology, Zhaoqing Gaoyao People's Hospital, Zhaoqing, China

Yunru Liao
Department of Ophthalmology, Sun Yat-sen Memorial Hospital, Sun Yat-sen University, Guangzhou, China
Department of Glaucoma, Zhongshan Ophthalmic Center, Sun Yat-sen University, Guangzhou, China
State Key Laboratory of Ophthalmology, Zhongshan Ophthalmic Center, Sun Yat-sen University, Guangzhou, China

Zhenlan Yang, Rui Zeng and Jing Wang
Department of Ophthalmology, Sun Yat-sen Memorial Hospital, Sun Yat-sen University, Guangzhou, China

Zhigao Liu and Shuya Wang
First Clinical Medical College, Shandong University of Traditional Chinese Medicine, Jinan, China

Yu Wang
Department of Ophthalmology, Jinan Aier Eye Hospital, Jinan, China

Aihua Ma
Department of Pediatrics, Shandong Provincial Hospital Affiliated to Shandong First Medical University, Jinan, China

Bojun Zhao
First Clinical Medical College, Shandong University of Traditional Chinese Medicine, Jinan, China
Department of Ophthalmology, Shandong Provincial Hospital Affiliated to Shandong First Medical University, Jinan, China

Kun Wei, Jinyi Xu, Dingqiao Wang and Zhongshu Tang
State Key Laboratory of Ophthalmology, Zhongshan Ophthalmic Center, Sun Yat-sen University, Guangzhou, China

Liang Wang, Manhong Li, Hongxiang Yan, Lei Wu, Jing Fan, Yi Zhou, Kaili Gou, Zifeng Zhang and Yusheng Wang
Department of Ophthalmology, Eye Institute of Chinese PLA, Xijing Hospital, Fourth Military Medical University, Xi'an, China

Jun Zhu
State Key Laboratory of Cancer Biology, Institute of Digestive Diseases, Xijing Hospital, Fourth Military Medical University, Xi'an, China

Xinxing Guo
Wilmer Eye Institute, Johns Hopkins University, Baltimore, MD, United States

Shaoyang Zheng
State Key Laboratory of Ophthalmology, Zhongshan Ophthalmic Center, Sun Yat-sen University, Guangzhou, China

Qian Wang, Fei Yu, Weihua Li, Xinyue Du, Xuan Zhao and Saiqun Li
State Key Laboratory of Ophthalmology, Zhongshan Ophthalmic Center, Sun Yat-sen University, Guangdong Provincial Key Laboratory of Ophthalmology and Visual Science, Guangdong Provincial Clinical Research Center for Ocular Diseases, Guangzhou, China

Naiyang Li
Eye Center, Zhongshan City People's Hospital, Zhongshan, China

Yali Wu
Department of Ophthalmology, The First Affiliated Hospital of USTC, Division of Life Sciences and Medicine, University of Science and Technology of China, Hefei, China
The First Affiliated Hospital of Kunming Medical University, Kunming, China

Qing Cun, Yijin Tao, Wenyan Yang, Jia Wei, Daoqing Fan, Ying Zhang and Hua Zhong
The First Affiliated Hospital of Kunming Medical University, Kunming, China

Qin Chen
The First Affiliated Hospital of Nanjing Medical University, Nanjing, China

Shasha Yang, Zongyin Gao and Haijiang Qiu
Department of Ophthalmology, Guangzhou First People's Hospital, School of Medicine, South China University of Technology, Guangzhou, China

Lan Mi
State Key Laboratory of Ophthalmology, Zhongshan Ophthalmic Center, Sun Yat-sen University, Guangzhou, China

Kazutaka Kamiya
Visual Physiology, School of Allied Health Sciences, Kitasato University, Kanagawa, Japan

Yuji Ayatsuka and Yudai Kato
Cresco Ltd., Tokyo, Japan

Nobuyuki Shoji
Department of Ophthalmology, School of Medicine, Kitasato University, Kanagawa, Japan

Yosai Mori and Kazunori Miyata
Department of Ophthalmology, Miyata Eye Hospital, Miyazaki, Japan

Meng Chen
Zaozhuang Shizhong District People's Hospital, Zaozhuang, China

Yuan Liu and Lei Fang
State Key Laboratory of Ophthalmology, Zhongshan Ophthalmic Center, Sun Yat-sen University, Guangzhou, China

Xue Bai and Rui Hua
Department of Ophthalmology, First Hospital of China Medical University, Shenyang, China

Min Fu, Pan Hu, Ludonghan Huang, Huan Xu, Ju Huang and Yanli Chen
Department of Ophthalmology, Daping Hospital of Army Characteristic Medical Center, Chongqing, China

Gang Zhang
Department of Medicine, 953 Hospital of People's Liberation Army (PLA), Xizang, China

Meihui Wu
Nursing Teaching and Research Section, Daping Hospital of Army Characteristic Medical Center, Chongqing, China

Index

www.ingramcontent.com/pod-product-compliance
Lightning Source LLC
LaVergne TN
LVHW060515210926
848485LV00005B/1085
9781639278596